Monoclonal Antibody-Based Therapy of Cancer

BASIC AND CLINICAL ONCOLOGY

Editor

Bruce D. Cheson, M.D.

National Cancer Institute
National Institutes of Health
Bethesda, Maryland

1. Chronic Lymphocytic Leukemia: Scientific Advances and Clinical Developments, *edited by Bruce D. Cheson*
2. Therapeutic Applications of Interleukin-2, *edited by Michael B. Atkins and James W. Mier*
3. Cancer of the Prostate, *edited by Sakti Das and E. David Crawford*
4. Retinoids in Oncology, *edited by Waun Ki Hong and Reuben Lotan*
5. Filgrastim (r-metHuG-CSF) in Clinical Practice, *edited by George Morstyn and T. Michael Dexter*
6. Cancer Prevention and Control, *edited by Peter Greenwald, Barnett S. Kramer, and Douglas L. Weed*
7. Handbook of Supportive Care in Cancer, *edited by Jean Klastersky, Stephen C. Schimpff, and Hans-Jörg Senn*
8. Paclitaxel in Cancer Treatment, *edited by William P. McGuire and Eric K. Rowinsky*
9. Principles of Antineoplastic Drug Development and Pharmacology, *edited by Richard L. Schilsky, Gérard A. Milano, and Mark J. Ratain*
10. Gene Therapy in Cancer, *edited by Malcolm K. Brenner and Robert C. Moen*
11. Expert Consultations in Gynecological Cancers, *edited by Maurie Markman and Jerome L. Belinson*
12. Nucleoside Analogs in Cancer Therapy, *edited by Bruce D. Cheson, Michael J. Keating, and William Plunkett*
13. Drug Resistance in Oncology, *edited by Samuel D. Bernal*
14. Medical Management of Hematological Malignant Diseases, *edited by Emil J Freireich and Hagop M. Kantarjian*
15. Monoclonal Antibody-Based Therapy of Cancer, *edited by Michael L. Grossbard*
16. Medical Management of Chronic Myelogenous Leukemia, *edited by Moshe Talpaz and Hagop M. Kantarjian*

ADDITIONAL VOLUMES IN PREPARATION

Cancer Screening: Theory and Practice, *edited by Barnett S. Kramer, John K. Gohagan, and Philip C. Prorok*

Expert Consultations in Breast Cancer: Critical Pathways and Clinical Decision Making, *edited by William N. Hait, David A. August, and Bruce Haffty*

Monoclonal Antibody-Based Therapy of Cancer

edited by

Michael L. Grossbard

*Harvard Medical School
and Massachusetts General Hospital
Boston, Massachusetts*

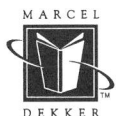

MARCEL DEKKER, INC.   NEW YORK • BASEL • HONG KONG

Library of Congress Cataloging-in-Publication Data

Monoclonal antibody-based therapy of cancer / edited by Michael L. Grossbard.
    p. cm.— (Basic and clinical oncology; 15)
  Includes index.
  ISBN 0-8247-0196-8 (alk. paper)
  1. Cancer—Immunotherapy. 2. Monoclonal antibodies—Therapeutic use. I. Grossbard, Michael L. II. Series.
  [DNLM: 1. Neoplasms—therapy. 2. Antibodies, Monoclonal—therapeutic use. QZ 266M7511 1998]
  RC271.M65M658 1998
  616.99'406—dc21
  DNLM/DLC
  for Library of Congress   98-29118
                                                                                                                                     CIP

This book is printed on acid-free paper.

Headquarters
Marcel Dekker, Inc.
270 Madison Avenue, New York, NY 10016
tel: 212-696-9000; fax: 212-685-4540

Eastern Hemisphere Distribution
Marcel Dekker AG
Hutgasse 4, Postfach 812, CH-4001 Basel, Switzerland
tel: 44-61-261-8482; fax: 44-61-261-8896

World Wide Web
http://www.dekker.com

The publisher offers discounts on this book when ordered in bulk quantities. For more information, write to Special Sales/Professional Marketing at the headquarters address above.

Copyright © 1998 by Marcel Dekker, Inc. All Rights Reserved.

Neither this book nor any part may be reproduced or transmitted in any form or by any means, electronic or mechanical, including photocopying, microfilming, and recording, or by any information storage and retrieval system, without permission in writing from the publisher.

Current printing (last digit)
10 9 8 7 6 5 4 3 2 1

PRINTED IN THE UNITED STATES OF AMERICA

Series Introduction

The current volume, *Monoclonal Antibody-Based Therapy of Cancer,* is Volume 15 in the Basic and Clinical Oncology series. Many of the advances in oncology have resulted from close interaction between the basic scientist and the clinical researcher. The current volume follows, expands on, and illustrates the success of this relationship as demonstrated by the rapidly growing field of biological approaches to cancer in general and, specifically, to monoclonal antibodies. Monoclonal antibodies are providing not only new areas of basic research, but exciting clinical results leading to the recent approval by the Food and Drug Administration of several of these agents.

As editor of the series, my goal has been to recruit volume editors who not only have established reputations based on their outstanding contributions to oncology, but also have an appreciation for the dynamic interface between the laboratory and the clinic. To date, the series has consisted of monographs on topics such as chronic lymphocytic leukemia, nucleoside analogs in cancer therapy, therapeutic applications of interleukin-2, retinoids in oncology, gene therapy of cancer, and principles of antineoplastic drug development and pharmacology. *Monoclonal Antibody-Based Therapy of Cancer* is certainly a most important addition to the series.

Volumes in progress include works on AIDS-related malignancies, secondary malignancies, chronic lymphoid leukemias, and controversies in gynecologic oncology. I anticipate that these volumes will provide a valuable contribution to the oncology literature.

Bruce D. Cheson

Preface

More than two decades have elapsed since Kohler and Milstein published their seminal article on the production of monoclonal antibodies. At that time, many scientists and clinical investigators predicted that the availability of antibody-based therapies would herald an end to traditional cancer chemotherapy and usher in an era of targeted therapies in which tumor cells could be eradicated and normal tissues spared. In retrospect, these predictions were naive and failed to account for the complexity of tumor biology and the difficulty in translating any advance from the laboratory to the bedside. Indeed, the opinion of the practicing clinician turned from optimism to skepticism after initial clinical trials of antibody-based therapies yielded few sustained clinical responses. These early clinical trials did establish several critical principles of antibody therapy and were instructive in demonstrating the obstacles to this form of therapy. Based on the lessons learned from these trials, a second generation of clinical trials began in the early 1990s in which attention was turned toward specific features of the antibody and target antigen that are critical in determining the success of antibody-based therapies.

By the middle of the 1990s, the vision of targeted therapies became a reality, with reports describing responses to antibody-based therapies appearing with increasing frequency in the medical literature. In 1997, the Anti-CD20 antibody C2B8 (Rituxan) became the first antibody approved by the FDA for the treatment of cancer (indolent B-cell NHL). Simultaneously, exciting advances were described in the development of radioimmunoconjugates, in which antibodies are used to deliver high doses of radiation therapy to malignant lymphoma cells, resulting in response rates of 70–80%. Although such dramatic advances have occurred less frequently in the treatment of solid tumors, pivotal trials currently are underway to assess the role of the 17-1A monoclonal antibody in the adjuvant therapy of colon cancer and the her-2 antibody in the therapy of breast cancer.

As the development of monoclonal antibody-based therapies begins to impact on the routine care of the cancer patient, a text describing the advances in this field becomes increasingly relevant for both the clinician and the basic scientist.

Clinicians responsible for the daily care of the cancer patient need easy access to information describing the rationale, toxicity, and benefits of antibody-based therapies. Likewise, those investigators with a laboratory-based emphasis on therapeutic antibody development can benefit from a review of the advantages and limitations of these therapies in both hematological malignancies and solid tumors as a guide toward developing the next generation of antibody-based therapeutics.

This text contains chapters describing the scientific background of antibody-based therapies along with timely and comprehensive reviews describing clinical progress in both hematological malignancies and solid tumors. It has been my privilege to work with an outstanding group of authors, many of whom have been leaders in the development of antibody-based therapies. Because many of the advances in therapy have been made initially in the hematological malignancies, several chapters are devoted to the therapy of lymphoma and leukemia. Likewise, several chapters report on exciting advances in the therapy of breast cancer, melanoma, and other solid tumors. These chapters are notable for their clinical relevance and for their description of basic principles of monoclonal antibody-based therapies that have been recognized over nearly twenty years of clinical trials. I asked the authors to focus their thoughts toward both the clinician and the scientist, since the development of further advances in this field will undoubtedly arise from a dialog between these two groups.

After extended years of preclinical studies and clinical trials, the exciting clinical advances of the past several years have led to a new enthusiasm for antibody-based therapeutics. The reader will appreciate the enthusiasm that all the authors have for the potential benefits of these therapies while understanding the obstacles that remain to be overcome in delivering these therapies to the majority of patients with cancer. Ultimately, I hope the reader will sense the renewed excitement for antibody-based therapies and their potential for both the primary and adjuvant therapy of cancer.

I am most appreciative of the assistance of Michele Sinoway of Marcel Dekker, Inc., who encouraged me to pursue this book. Likewise, Matt MacIsaac has provided superb assistance as the Production Editor. The authors all provided timely, well-written chapters with up-to-date references that will be invaluable to the reader who wishes to delve deeper into this field.

Most importantly, I dedicate this book to Sarah Jane, Lily, and my parents, who have provided incredible support and love.

Michael L. Grossbard

Contents

Series Introduction		*iii*
Preface		*v*
Contributors		*ix*
1.	Preclinical Immunotoxin Development *Walter A. Blättler and John M. Lambert*	1
2.	Delivery of Monoclonal Antibodies to the Tumor Cell *Rakesh K. Jain*	23
3.	Unconjugated Monoclonal Antibody Therapy of Lymphoma *David G. Maloney*	53
4.	Clinical Studies with Deglycosylated Ricin A-Chain Immunotoxins *Edward A. Sausville and Ellen S. Vitetta*	81
5.	Immunotoxin Therapy of Lymphoma: Studies with Anti-B4- Blocked Ricin *Pratik S. Multani and Michael L. Grossbard*	91
6.	Radioimmunoconjugate Therapy of Non-Hodgkin's Lymphoma *Thomas A. Davis and Susan J. Knox*	113
7.	Monoclonal Antibody-Based Therapy of Cutaneous T-Cell Non-Hodgkin's Lymphoma *Timothy M. Kuzel and Steven T. Rosen*	137
8.	Antibody-Based Therapies for Hodgkin's Disease *H. L. Morein and R. P. Junghans*	149

9.	Antibody-Based Therapies for the Treatment of Acute Leukemia *Pratik S. Multani and David J. Flavell*	189
10.	Immunotoxin Therapy of Graft-Versus-Host Disease *Carlos R. Bachier and Charles F. LeMaistre*	211
11.	Hematopoietic Progenitor-Cell Graft Processing and Treatment *Nadine Beauger and Denis Claude Roy*	229
12.	Monoclonal Antibody Therapy for Solid Tumors: An Overview *Panos Fidias*	281
13.	Monoclonal Antibody-Based Therapy of Breast Cancer *Francisco J. Esteva and Daniel F. Hayes*	309
14.	Monoclonal Antibody-Based Therapy of Melanoma *Marcus O. Butler and Frank G. Haluska*	339
15.	Monoclonal Antibodies in the Management of Lung Cancer *Stefan C. Grant, Ellen Early, and John Mendelsohn*	365
16.	Monoclonal Antibody-Based Immunoconjugate Therapy of Cancer: Studies with BR96-Doxorubicin *Mansoor N. Saleh, Albert F. LoBuglio, and Pamela A. Trail*	397
17.	Immunotoxin Therapy: Past Lessons and Future Directions *Ellen S. Vitetta, Maria-Ana Ghetie, and Victor Ghetie*	417
Index		*433*

Contributors

Carlos R. Bachier, M.D.   Associate Director, South Texas Cancer Institute, San Antonio, Texas

Nadine Beauger, M.Sc.   Hematopoietic Graft Engineering Laboratory, Division of Hematology-Immunology, University of Montreal and Maisonneuve-Rosemont Hospital, Montreal, Quebec, Canada

Walter A. Blättler, Dr. sc. nat.   Executive Vice President, Science and Technology, ImmunoGen, Inc., Cambridge, Massachusetts

Marcus O. Butler, M.D.   Clinical Fellow in Medicine, Harvard Medical School, and Hematology/Oncology Program, Dana-Farber/Partners CancerCare, Boston, Massachusetts

Thomas A. Davis, M.D.   Staff Physician, Division of Medical Oncology, Department of Medicine, Stanford University, Stanford, California

Ellen Early, M.D.   Fellow, Medical Oncology, Memorial Sloan-Kettering Cancer Center, New York, New York

Francisco J. Esteva, M.D.* Instructor in Medicine, Breast Cancer Program, Division of Hematology-Oncology, Vincent T. Lombardi Cancer Center, Georgetown University Medical Center, Washington, D.C.

---

* *Current affiliation:* Department of Breast Cancer Oncology, The University of Texas M. D. Anderson Cancer Center, Houston, Texas

Panos Fidias, M.D.* Hematology/Oncology Unit, Harvard Medical School and Massachusetts General Hospital, Boston, Massachusetts

David J. Flavell, B.Sc., Ph.D., M.R.C.Path. Senior Lecturer in Pathology, The Simon Flavell Leukaemia Research Unit, University of Southampton, and Southampton General Hospital, Southampton, England

Maria-Ana Ghetie, Ph.D. Assistant Professor, Cancer Immunobiology Center, The University of Texas Southwestern Medical Center at Dallas, Dallas, Texas

Victor Ghetie, Ph.D. Associate Professor, Cancer Immunobiology Center, The University of Texas Southwestern Medical Center at Dallas, Dallas, Texas

Stefan C. Grant, M.D. Assistant Professor, Department of Medicine, Cornell University Medical College, and Assistant Member, Thoracic Oncology Service, Memorial Sloan-Kettering Cancer Center, New York, New York

Michael L. Grossbard, M.D. Assistant Professor of Medicine, Harvard Medical School, and Assistant Physician, Hematology/Oncology Unit, Massachusetts General Hospital, Boston, Massachusetts

Frank G. Haluska, M.D., Ph.D. Assistant Professor of Medicine, Harvard Medical School, Division of Hematology/Oncology, Massachusetts General Hospital, and Director, Melanoma Program, Dana-Farber/Partners CancerCare, Boston, Massachusetts

Daniel F. Hayes, M.D. Associate Professor, Department of Medicine, Georgetown University Medical Center, and Clinical Director, Breast Cancer Program, Vincent T. Lombardi Cancer Center, Washington, D.C.

Rakesh K. Jain, Ph.D. Andrew Werk Cook Professor of Tumor Biology, Harvard Medical School, and Director, Edwin L. Steele Laboratory, Department of Radiation Oncology, Massachusetts General Hospital, Boston, Massachusetts

R. P. Junghans, M.D. Assistant Professor of Medicine, Biotherapeutics Development Lab, Institute of Human Genetics, Harvard Medical School, and Division of Hematology-Oncology, Beth Israel Deaconess Medical Center, Boston, Massachusetts

---

* Current affiliation: Hematology-Oncology Associates of South Texas, San Antonio, Texas.

Contributors

Susan J. Knox, M.D., Ph.D.   Associate Professor, Department of Radiation Oncology, Stanford University, Stanford, California

Timothy M. Kuzel, M.D.   Associate Professor, Division of Hematology/Oncology, Department of Medicine, Northwestern University Medical School, Chicago, Illinois

John M. Lambert, Ph.D.   Vice President, Research and Development, ImmunoGen, Inc., Cambridge, Massachusetts

Charles F. LeMaistre, M.D.   Medical Director, South Texas Cancer Institute, San Antonio, Texas

Albert F. LoBuglio, M.D.   Director, Comprehensive Cancer Center, Professor, Department of Medicine, and Associate Dean for Research, School of Medicine, University of Alabama at Birmingham, Birmingham, Alabama

David G. Maloney, M.D., Ph.D.   Assistant Professor, Division of Oncology, University of Washington, and Assistant Member, Clinical Division, Fred Hutchinson Cancer Research Center, Seattle, Washington

John Mendelsohn, M.D.   Professor, Department of Medicine, Clinical Investigation, Division of Medicine, and President, The University of Texas M. D. Anderson Cancer Center, Houston, Texas

H. L. Morein, M.D.   Research Assistant, Biotherapeutics Development Lab, Institute of Human Genetics, Harvard Medical School, and Division of Hematology-Oncology, Beth Israel Deaconess Medical Center, Boston, Massachusetts

Pratik S. Multani, M.D.   Instructor, Department of Medicine, Harvard Medical School, and Massachusetts General Hospital, Boston, Massachusetts

Steven T. Rosen, M.D.   Genevieve Teuton Professor of Medicine, Northwestern University Medical School, and Director, Robert H. Lurie Cancer Center, Chicago, Illinois

Denis Claude Roy, M.D., F.R.C.P.(C)   Associate Professor of Medicine, Division of Hematology-Immunology, and Director, Hematopoietic Graft Engineering Laboratory, University of Montreal and Maisonneuve-Rosemont Hospital, Montreal, Quebec, Canada

Mansoor N. Saleh, M.D.   Associate Professor, Department of Medicine, and

Associate Director for Clinical Research, Comprehensive Cancer Center, University of Alabama at Birmingham, Birmingham, Alabama

Edward A. Sausville, M.D., Ph.D. Associate Director, Developmental Therapeutics Program, Division of Cancer Treatment and Diagnosis, National Cancer Institute, National Institutes of Health, Rockville, Maryland

Pamela A. Trail, Ph.D. Bristol-Myers Squibb, Princeton, New Jersey

Ellen S. Vitetta, Ph.D. Director, Cancer Immunobiology Center, and Professor of Microbiology, The University of Texas Southwestern Medical Center at Dallas, Dallas, Texas

1
Preclinical Immunotoxin Development

Walter A. Blättler and John M. Lambert
ImmunoGen, Inc.,
Cambridge, Massachusetts

I. INTRODUCTION

Chemotherapeutic agents are compounds that are cytostatic or cytotoxic to tumor cells in vivo. By this definition, immunotoxins—the combination of a monoclonal antibody (MAb) and a catalytically active cytotoxic protein—are chemotherapeutic agents. The preclinical development and evaluation of immunotoxins parallels, therefore, many aspects of the development of conventional chemotherapeutic agents; i.e., cytotoxicity toward tumor cell lines in vitro and efficacy in animal tumor models have to be demonstrated, and careful safety studies have to be performed. However, immunotoxins are an attempt at improving upon the efficacy of conventional agents with novel concepts, which necessitate novel preclinical tests. It is these novel concepts and their preclinical evaluation that are the subject of this chapter.

To put the novel concepts in context it is best to summarize briefly some of the shortcomings of the current conventional chemotherapeutic agents. These agents demonstrate limited efficacy in the treatment of most tumors. Major factors contributing to this are (a) the poor ability of these agents to affect tumor cells preferentially over normal, healthy cells, (b) the intrinsic insensitivity of many tumors to most chemotherapeutic agents, and (c) the rapid induction of resistance mechanisms in tumor cells during treatment. Immunotoxins are an attempt to improve upon these three factors. By using MAbs that bind selectively to tumor cells, the cytotoxic activity should be focused onto tumors, thereby sparing healthy tissues. Toxins exert their cytotoxicity differently from any of the conventional chemotherapeutic agents, which should ensure high activity toward otherwise chemotherapy-resistant cells. In summary, the binding characteristics of the

MAb component and the unique cytotoxic mechanisms of the toxin moieties are the distinguishing features of immunotoxins. Therefore, this chapter starts with a discussion of procedures for the selection of suitable MAbs, which is followed by a summary of the work necessary to adapt several natural toxins to their role as the cytotoxic moiety of immunotoxins. The last part of the chapter will deal with efficacy and safety evaluation of the final immunotoxin.

II. SELECTION AND EVALUATION OF MONOCLONAL ANTIBODIES

A. Intact MAb vs. MAb Fragments

Immunotoxins exploit only the binding function of MAbs, which is located in the variable region of the antibody molecule. Therefore, one of the decisions one has to make is whether the whole antibody molecule should be incorporated into the immunotoxin or only fragments containing the binding function, such as the bivalent $F(ab')_2$ fragment or the monovalent Fab', Fab, sFv (single-chain variable region), or dsFv (disulfide-stabilized Fv) fragments. This decision largely affects the pharmacokinetics of the immunoconjugate, with the whole antibody conferring a much longer half-life, although the monovalent conjugates also will have some reduced binding affinity. This question was carefully analyzed by Vitetta and her colleagues with conjugates of the anti-CD22 antibody RFB4 and a deglycosylated ricin A chain. In mice, they report a $T_{1/2}$ of 37.8 h for the conjugate with the intact IgG (1) and 1.5 h for the Fab' conjugate (2). In human clinical trials, a mean $T_{1/2}$ of 7.8 h was observed for the intact IgG conjugate and of 1.5 h for the Fab' conjugate (3). However, the ultimate question is which form of the immunoconjugate is more efficacious in treating human tumors. No valid answer can be given yet, since the only data available so far for the two forms are from human Phase I clinical trials. However, as a first approximation, one might correlate efficacy directly with the total amount of immunotoxin accumulated at the tumor sites. Several studies in animal tumor models (see, for example, Ref. 4 and references cited therein), where the total accumulation of radiolabeled antibodies or different antibody fragments was measured as a percentage of the total injected dose accumulated per gram of tumor (% ID/g of tumor), demonstrated that both a long serum half-life and bivalent binding contributed to higher tumor accumulation. By this criterion, immunoconjugates should incorporate the intact IgG with its long half-life and bivalent binding. The increased immunogenicity of intact murine MAbs in comparison with fragments is likely not a relevant concern, since, in any case, the toxins used in immunotoxins are of bacterial or plant origin and rapidly elicit an immune response irrespective of the form of the antibody component.

The construction of immunotoxins by genetic engineering imposes other restrictions on the form of the antibody to be used. Since toxins have to be expressed in bacterial systems due to their toxicity to mammalian cells, and since the expression of intact immunoglobulins in bacteria has not been achieved, fusion toxins either contain sFv or dsFv fragments (5). Engineered immunotoxins suffer, therefore, from the disadvantage of having a short half-life and a low total accumulation at the tumor site, although this is counteracted somewhat by their much smaller size and better tumor penetration. Efforts are under way to generate novel antibody fragments, such as minibodies, that display longer in vivo half-lives and bivalent binding and can be produced in bacteria (4).

B. MAb Tumor Reactivity

Clearly the most important characteristic of the MAb component of an immunotoxin is its binding specificity coupled with its binding affinity or avidity. Selective binding with high avidity to tumor cells and the absence of binding to normal cells should be demonstrated to be able to fulfill the promise of tumor-specific cell killing.

Tumor reactivity has to be established at three levels: (a) at the patient population level (the percentage of patients with a given type of tumor, e.g., colon carcinoma, that have tumor cells expressing the antigen for a given MAb; (b) at the tumor biopsy level (the percentage of cells in a tumor that are expressing the antigen and, therefore, can be targeted by an immunotoxin; (c) at the cellular level (the affinity of binding and the effect of MAb binding upon the antigen).

Ideally, all tumors of a given type in all patients would express the antigen, not only for commercial reasons, but also for simplicity of treatment. No special diagnostic procedures would have to be established to demonstrate reactivity first. This goal was achieved with MAbs reactive with lymphoid tumors (6), such as anti-CD19 and anti-CD20 MAbs. These antibodies are tissue-specific rather than tumor-specific and react, therefore, with cells of all B-cell malignancies. Similarly, MAbs reactive with CD56 (NCAM), such as N901, react with all SCLC tumors because of their general reactivity with tissues of neuroendocrine origin (7,8). Very few, if any, anticarcinoma MAbs show binding to the respective tumors of all patients. Monoclonal antibodies such as C242, reactive with a carbohydrate epitope of a cell surface-associated mucin (9), or BR96 (10) and B3 (11), reactive with Le^y-associated epitopes, might be the most promising MAbs in this respect. Treatment of most carcinomas with MAbs needs, therefore, to be preceded by a diagnostic procedure that establishes the presence of the antigen.

A necessary step to the killing of cells by immunotoxins is their binding to cell surfaces. However, often an antigen is expressed heterogeneously in a tumor; i.e., only a percentage of cells express the antigen, as demonstrated by immunohistochemical staining of tissue sections or by FACS analysis with single cell suspensions. Often, fewer than 50% of cells are antigen-positive, and at first thought such tumors should not respond to immunotoxin treatment. However, it has been found in animal models that xenograft tumors having as few as 30% antigen-positive cells could be completely eradicated with a single immunoconjugate treatment (9). Analogous findings were reported from a human clinical trial with a B3-based immunotoxin where responses were seen in patients having tumors with heterogeneous expression (entry criteria was 30% positivity by immunostaining analysis) (11). Heterogeneous antigen expression should not, therefore, automatically eliminate an MAb from consideration, but should compel investigators to demonstrate preclinical efficacy against heterogeneous tumors.

At the cellular level, MAbs should bind with high avidity to be effective at low doses and should induce antigen internalization, since toxins inactivate an intracellular process. Typically, good MAbs bind with a dissociation constant (K_D) of about 10^{-10} M or lower. Also, most antigens internalize at a reasonable rate, although there are clearly exceptionally good "transport" antigens, such as the transferrin receptor, and some antigens that have an exceedingly slow internalization, such as the four-times membrane-spanning CD20 antigen (12). Some antigens cannot serve as immunotoxin targets because they are shed from the cell surface and relatively high concentrations are found in the serum of patients. Therefore, MAbs that are used diagnostically to test blood samples in order to follow the status of a disease or initially to diagnose the disease, such as anti-CEA antibodies or the anti-ovarian carcinoma antibody OC 125, are not good candidates for immunotoxins (13).

C. MAb Tumor Selectivity

Unfortunately, no cell-surface antigens have yet been identified that are expressed solely on tumor cells. Accordingly, once reactivity with tumor cells and tumor tissues has been firmly established, a great amount of preclinical effort has to be devoted to establish the degree of cross-reactivity with normal tissue and to explore the consequences of such cross-reactivity. Cross-reactivity is typically analyzed immunohistochemically using fresh frozen tissue sections. As an example from the authors' laboratories, this process is illustrated with the MAb N901, which reacts with neural cell adhesion molecules (NCAMs) and which was used for the construction of an immunotoxin to treat small-cell lung cancer (SCLC) (8). Neural cell adhesion molecules had been firmly established as markers for SCLC and other tumors of cells of neuroendocrine origin. Furthermore, it had been demonstrated that NCAMs were uniformly expressed by all cells in cell lines and in biopsies of SCLC. The immunohistochemical analysis on 27 normal tissues—specimens from three different individuals were used for most tissues—then revealed cross-reactivity with several tissues (see Table 1), the most worrisome being the strong reactivity with cardiac muscle tissue and with peripheral nerve tissue (nerve axons were negative, whereas adjacent cells, possibly

Schwann cells, were positive). This cross-reactivity finding might have dissuaded us from using MAb N901 in an immunotoxin were it not for the lack of any efficacious treatment for SCLC today and were it not that we could test the consequences of such cross-reactivity in an animal model. Immunohistochemical studies performed with tissues from cynomolgus monkeys showed the same pattern in type and degree of cross-reactivity as that for human tissues summarized in Table 1. During toxicity evaluation of the N901 immunotoxin in cynomolgus monkeys, special tests were performed to monitor for toxicity to tissues expressing NCAM. For example, possible damage to peripheral nerve tissue was monitored electrophysiologically by performing nerve conduction velocity tests. It is therefore possible to establish preclinically the safety of immunotoxins containing MAbs with cross-reactivity to normal tissue.

D. Generation of Tumor-Selective MAbs

Unfortunately, there is a paucity of MAbs useful for the treatment of cancer and in particular for the delivery of highly cytotoxic agents such as toxins. Therefore, for most tumors, and in particular for carcinomas, preclinical development of immunotoxins still must start with the generation of novel, tumor-selective monoclonal antibodies. Although the methodology to select antibodies in vitro from a large library, such as a phage display library of Fv fragments (14), allows for the rapid selection of monoclonal antibodies to cell-surface antigens, the hurdle of finding truly tumor-selective antibodies remains high and requires more knowledge about the biological and molecular differences between tumor cells and healthy cells.

III. SELECTION AND ADAPTATION OF TOXINS

A. Selection of Toxin

Of the many known natural toxins—*toxin* is used here to refer to proteinaceous, poisonous substances—only the group called *cytotoxins,* which act through a mechanism that induces cell death, is of interest for the generation of immunotoxins to treat cancer. Further, cytotoxins that are hemolytic or cytolytic upon interaction with the cell surface or cell membrane probably must be excluded, since it is difficult to imagine how to render them tumor-selective. Toxins that bind to the cell surface, get internalized, and then kill the host cell by disrupting an essential intracellular process are better candidates, because one can theoretically imagine replacing their binding function with the tumor-selective binding function of a MAb without disturbing their cytotoxic potency. Most of the known toxins with the latter characteristics, such as ricin, abrin, diphtheria toxin (DT), and *Pseudomonas* exotoxin A (PE), are of plant or bacterial origin and disrupt

Table 1 Summary of N901 and N901-Blocked Ricin (N901-bR) Reactivity on Normal Human Tissues

		N901 monoclonal antibody		N901-bR	
Organ	Tissue components	No. positive[a]/total no. tested	Reactivity[b]	No. positive[a]/total no. tested	Reactivity[b]
Adrenal gland	Cortex	3/3	2–3	3/3	2–3/a
	Medulla	2/2	3	2/2	3/a
Bladder	Urothelium	0/3	0	0/3	0
Bone marrow	Hematopoietic cells	0/1	0	0/3	0
Brain cortex	Astrocytes	3/3	3	3/3	2–3/a
	Neuropil	3/3	3	3/3	2–3/a
Breast	Acini	1/3	0–2/f	1/2	0–2/d
	Ducts	2/3	0–3	2/2	1–2/bd
Cervix	Endocervix	0/3	0	0/3	0
	Exocervix	1/2	0–1/f	0/3	0
Colon	Epithelium	2/3	0–1 (mucosa)	0/3	0
Esophagus	Epithelium	0/3	0	0/3	0
	Glands	0/3	0	0/3	0
Heart	Cardiac muscle	3/3	1–3	3/3	2–3/a
Kidney	Glomerulus	0/3	0	0/2	0
	Tubules	0/3	0	0/3	0
	Collecting tubules	0/3	0	0/3	0
Liver	Hepatocytes	0/3	0	0/3	0
	Bile ducts	2/3	0–1/f	2/3	0–3/ac
	Kupffer cells	0/3	0	0/3	0
Lung	Bronchial cells	2/3	0–1/f	0/3	0
	Alveolar cells	0/3	0	0/3	0
Lymph node	Lymphocytes	3/3	1	2/2	1–2/d
Muscle[c]	Skeletal	3/3	1–3/f[d]	0/2	0

Tissue	Subtype				
Ovary	Ovarian stroma	3/3	2-3	3/3	2-3/a
Pancreas	Endocrine cells	3/3	1-3	3/3	1-3/a
	Exocrine cells	1/3	0-1/f	1/3	0-1/d
	Ducts	1/3	0-3	0/3	0
Peripheral nerve	—	x[e]	3	3/3[f]	2/b
Prostate	Lining cells	Not done	—	2/3	0-2/d
	Glands	3/3	1-2 (single cells)	0/3	0
Skin	Epidermis	0/3	0	0/3	0
	Adnexa	0/3	0	0/3	0
Small intestine	Epithelium	3/3	1-2/f	0/3	0
Spinal cord	Neuropil	3/3	3	2/2	2-3/a
	Neurons	3/3	3	2/2	2-3/a
Spleen	Lymphocytes	3/3	1-2 (subpopulation)	3/3	1-2/d
Stomach	Epithelium	3/3	1-2/f	2/2	1-3/b
Testis	Leydig cells	3/3	3	3/3	2-3/a
	Seminiferous tubules	0/3	0	0/3	0
Thymus	Lymphocytes	2/3	0-3 (subpopulation)	3/3	1-2/d
Thyroid gland	Follicles	3/3	3	3/3	3/a
Uterus	Endometrium	0/3	0	0/2	0

[a] Positive tissues were any tissues that had observable staining.
[b] The intensity of staining was scored with the use of the following arbitrary scale: 0 = no staining, 1 = weak staining, 2 = moderate staining, and 3 = strong or maximum staining. The homogeneity/heterogeneity of staining was scored as follows: a = homogeneous staining (approximately 100% of the cells were positively stained), b = slightly heterogeneous staining (>75% of the cells were positively stained), c = moderately heterogeneous staining (approximately 50% of the cells were positively stained), d = very heterogeneous staining (<25% of the cells were positively stained), and f = focal staining (few scattered cells were positively stained).
[c] Smooth-muscle staining was variable, homogeneously positive in some cases and negative in other cases.
[d] In two additional cases, analyzed by Dr. David Dorfman, staining of skeletal muscle tissue with N901 was weak and very heterogeneous.
[e] Peripheral nerve was strongly positive (3+) in all cases where seen.
[f] Peripheral nerve axons were negative, while adjacent cells (possibly Schwann cells) were positive.

Source: Ref. 8. Reprinted with permission.

protein synthesis in the host cell in a catalytic manner. This catalytic behavior imparts one of the most important characteristics, which is the high potency of these agents. Since immunotoxins are large proteins and, therefore, have a relatively poor tumor uptake, it is essential that they be cytotoxic at very low concentrations. In addition, as mentioned earlier, MAbs should bind with K_D values smaller or equal to 10^{-10} M, and to take advantage of this binding the toxin should at least be cytotoxic to tumor cell lines in vitro at concentrations below 10^{-10} M during a relatively short exposure of the cell to the toxin.

Some of the more potent known cytotoxins, such as DT and PE, are produced by human pathogens, and humans may have a preexisting immunity against the toxin. Specifically, most humans are vaccinated against DT, which makes it a poor choice as a potential systemic therapeutic agent in the form of an immunotoxin. Apparently, only a small percentage of individuals have developed immunity against PE through exposure to *Pseudomonas* bacteria (15). Immune responses will affect the pharmacokinetic and pharmacodynamic behavior of immunotoxins and interfere with their accumulation at tumor sites.

B. Adaptation of Toxins for Incorporation into Immunotoxins

The natural toxins use an intricate process for the efficient intoxication of their target cells at low toxin concentration. They have evolved, not unlike viruses, to take advantage of some of the processes of the target cell to exert their lethal effect. First, they bind to the cell surface, which often, but not always, involves binding to chemical moieties such as complex carbohydrate ligands that are present in high numbers on cell surfaces. Binding is followed by internalization through receptor-mediated endocytosis and then transfer of the toxin or a fragment of the toxin into the cytoplasm. The final step is the inactivation of an essential cellular process, such as protein synthesis, in a catalytic fashion. Transfer to the cytoplasm involves translocation through the lipid bilayer of a cellular membrane, which is a process still poorly understood. However, when one plans to adapt natural toxins for cell-specific uses in the form of immunotoxins, it is important to realize that only the combination of all three steps—binding, translocation, and catalytic function—leads to a potent toxin and that the three functions may not act independent of each other.

In its ideal form an immunotoxin will preserve all the preceding characteristics of a natural toxin, except that it will have changed the binding specificity. The simplest notion for the preparation of an immunotoxin might, therefore, be the removal or inactivation of the portion of the toxin that is responsible for the binding and replace it with the binding portion of an antibody. This was indeed possible with PE, since in this single-chain toxin the binding function is located in a separate domain at the *N*-terminus. Removing this domain and linking the truncated toxin either by genetic engineering or by chemical linkage to an antibody or antibody fragment yielded immunotoxins with preserved potency in in vitro cytotoxicity tests (for review, see Refs. 16,17). This functional test established that the catalytic function and, in particular, the translocation function of PE are independent of the binding through the binding domain to the specific toxin receptor on human cells. These two domains become, therefore, "portable" and can be linked to diverse cell-binding agents.

Diphtheria toxin seems to be very similar at first sight. Again, binding can be located to a distinct protein domain, this time at the *C*-terminus of the toxin, and can be removed easily. However, fusion toxins between the truncated forms of DT and several cell-binding agents seemed to lack the high cytotoxicity of native DT, indicating that efficient membrane penetration depends on binding to the specific DT receptor (18). A more suitable approach may be, therefore, the use of the mutant DT CRM107, which has an 8000-fold lower binding affinity for its receptor but displayed native cytotoxicity when linked to a MAb (19).

The best-known cytotoxins from plants, ricin and abrin, are translated as single-chain proteins and then processed into the native toxin composed of an A chain and a B chain that are disulfide-linked. The lectin-type binding to galactosides could be located to the B chain and the catalytic, toxic function to the A chain, which immediately suggested that linking the A chain alone to an antibody should yield a specific immunotoxin. Unfortunately, such A chain immunotoxins displayed in vitro cytotoxicities that were much lower than that of native ricin. Not unlike DT, it was then demonstrated that binding of the B chain to galactosides is a necessary event for efficient intoxication (20). And again, the lowering of the native binding affinity by greater than 1000-fold, this time by linking affinity ligands into the two galactoside binding sites of the B chain, yielded an altered ricin, called *blocked ricin,* that displayed full ricin toxicity when linked to a MAb (21).

The development of the right form of a given toxin for incorporation into immunotoxins occurred by trial and error, largely due to the very limited knowledge of the mechanisms toxins use to reach their target in the cytoplasm. However, ways have been found to construct immunotoxins that are as cytotoxic in vitro as the native toxins and are equipped with the selectivity of their MAb components (for a review, see Ref. 22). In vivo use adds the dimensions of pharmacokinetics and pharmacodynamics. For example, plant toxins are in general glycoproteins, and their carbohydrate structures may be recognized by specific receptors in the liver and thus accelerate the elimination of such immunotoxins from circulation. Certain immunotoxins have, therefore, been constructed with deglycosylated plant toxins (23). By far the most important factor is the reaction of the immune system to the bacterial and plant toxins. Most patients promptly generate a humoral immune response that usually causes the rapid removal of the immunotoxin from circulation and prevents its targeting of tumor sites. Though it is possible to "humanize" MAbs, it remains an open question whether it is possible to "humanize" the toxin component. Alternatively, it has been proposed to replace these toxins altogether by human enzymes, such as RNases; however, it has been difficult to duplicate their potency (24).

IV. EFFICACY AND SAFETY EVALUATION OF IMMUNOTOXINS

A. Goals of Preclinical Efficacy and Safety Evaluation

The primary goal of preclinical safety evaluation of a drug candidate is to determine whether there is a chance that the drug candidate will show efficacy at tolerable doses to allow for clinical evaluation, in other words, to determine whether the drug has an acceptable risk:benefit ratio. In the case of cancer treatment, it is acceptable to take more risk for the chance of therapeutic benefit. Indeed, chemotherapeutic agents used in the treatment of cancer generally achieve efficacy only at doses that are also toxic to the patient. Since immunotoxins are chemotherapeutic agents, the preclinical safety evaluation program for an immunotoxin is, with certain notable exceptions, very similar to that for any other cytotoxic chemotherapeutic agent.

The potential for therapeutic benefit for an immunotoxin is generally demonstrated by showing that the agent can kill cancer cells in vitro. The potential risks are identified in toxicology studies in animals. The goals of toxicology evaluation are to establish a safe starting dose and dose escalation program for clinical trials in humans, to assess the target organ(s) for the toxic effects of the immunotoxin, to identify parameters to monitor in the clinic once trials in humans begin, and to determine the reversibility of any of the toxic effects. Before efficacy and safety can be evaluated properly, the immunotoxin must have all the characteristics of a well-characterized final drug product.

B. Tests and Analysis to Establish an Immunotoxin as a Well-Characterized Drug Product

The final product should be manufactured by the method intended for the preparation of material for clinical use. Indeed, it is desirable that a batch of immunotoxin be made that is of sufficient size for the entire preclinical program and a significant number of patients in the first clinical trial. The final immunotoxin product should be well characterized by biochemical methods, such as polyacrylamide gel electrophoresis and h.p.l.c. techniques, and specifications set in these assays for the appearance of the conjugate and the level of impurities, so that subsequent batches of material will have the same properties. The final product used in preclinical safety studies should also be formulated in the same vehicle as that intended for clinical use. For example, some immunotoxins, such as anti-B4-

blocked ricin (25), are formulated for clinical use at a relatively dilute concentration (100 μg/mL) that necessitates the use of a carrier protein such as human serum albumin (1 mg/mL in the case of anti-B4-blocked ricin), and the same formulation was used in all the preclinical tests. Finally, the levels of endotoxin must be below the accepted limits for the expected dosing volume, and the formulations should be sterile and particle-free.

Once an immunotoxin preparation has been made for preclinical safety evaluation and clinical use, the assays used in the research that led to the development of the immunotoxin must be adapted to provide assays for testing the identity, potency, quality, and purity of the preparation and for developing a set of specifications that each batch must satisfy in order to be released for clinical use.

Target specificity is, of course, the fundamental property of an immunotoxin. Thus, the ability of the immunotoxin to bind target cells should be assessed relative to a standard, usually unmodified antibody. Additionally, competition binding assays should be done to ensure that the immunotoxin binds to the same epitope as the original antibody. Such binding assays can be adapted for routine quality control.

Typically, it has been found that immunotoxins bind with somewhat lower affinity/avidity than the native antibodies. In the case of blocked ricin conjugates, the apparent binding avidity of the immunotoxin was about twofold less than that of native antibody (21,26). This raises an important point for immunotoxin characterization; namely, are all the molecules able to bind antigen? A twofold reduction in apparent affinity could be accounted for by complete inactivation of half the molecules. Thus, immunotoxins should be characterized by ''clearing'' experiments, using sequential incubations with excess antigen (antigen-positive cells) to see if all the immunotoxin can be absorbed (for example, Ref. 26).

Another important characterization to make is to assess whether conjugation of the antibody to a toxic effector moiety has altered in any way the specificity of the antibody. This can be evaluated by immunohistochemical studies using a panel of human tissues (three unrelated donor samples per tissue) where the staining patterns of native antibody and immunotoxin are compared (see Table 1, for example). In the cases where the target antigen and specific epitope also are found in an animal species that will be used in toxicology studies, the pattern of immunotoxin binding to the animal tissues should be assessed so that any potential toxicities due to specific tissue binding via the antibody component or the toxic effector component can be evaluated. However, one should be aware that caution is necessary when interpreting the results of immunohistochemical staining. The very nature of the technique leads to exposure of intracellular molecules, so any cross-reactivity by the antibody or the immunotoxin may be with an antigen that is not accessible in vivo and, therefore, is not relevant for potential targeted toxicities. In the authors' laboratory, in the case of one particular immunoconjugate where the toxic effector moiety was a DNA-binding drug, immunohistochemical staining could not be done since the conjugate bound to exposed DNA throughout all tissue sections. The specific binding of the conjugate only could be demonstrated in binding studies on a panel of 35 human cell lines representing all the major organs.

The mechanism of action of the toxic effector component usually is well established from prior biochemical work with the toxin. Once incorporated into an immunotoxin, the activity of the toxin moiety should be assessed to ensure that it has not become inactivated as a result of conjugation or purification. As an example, several lots of immunotoxins that incorporated blocked ricin were tested to ensure that the ability of the ricin A chain component to inactivate ribosomes, and, therefore, protein synthesis, was unaffected by conjugation (21,26).

The potency of an immunotoxin is assessed by evaluating its ability to kill antigen-positive cells, whereas the specificity of such killing is shown by using excess native antibody to block immunotoxin binding to the antigen. The selectivity of an immunotoxin for its target cells also must be demonstrated by comparison to the nonspecific toxicity of the immunotoxin for nontarget cells, in order to provide a rationale for the potential for therapeutic benefit. An example of such cytotoxicity tests for the immunotoxin N901-blocked ricin (27) is shown in Figure 1. Comparison of the cytotoxicity of an immunotoxin for an antigen-positive and an antigen-negative cell line is, of course, only valid for cell lines that are equally susceptible to being killed by the toxic effector moiety. Characterization of an immunotoxin should include both clonogenic assays (such as shown in Figure 1) to assess log kill and more rapid assays utilizing dyes such as BCECF (28). The latter assays for potency and for nonspecific toxicity (an assessment of the quality and purity of the immunotoxin to complement biochemical analysis) are more suitable for routine quality control, for which specifications can be set that must be met by all batches of immunotoxin.

C. Nonclinical Pharmacology: Evaluation of Efficacy

Once the basic parameters of specific killing of targeted antigen-positive cells and the in vitro therapeutic index have been defined, further in vitro studies to evaluate the efficacy of an immunotoxin under conditions relevant to the clinical situation fulfill an important goal of preclinical evaluation, which is to provide experimental data to guide clinical studies to allow rapid clinical development.

In vitro cytotoxicity assays can be used to assess the potency of an immunotoxin for drug-resistant cell lines. For example, anti-B4-blocked ricin was shown to be a potent killer of a B lymphoma cell line transfected with the *mdr*-1 gene in a model of multidrug resistance (Table 2), thus providing a rationale for clinical studies using the immunotoxin in patients with disease that is nonresponsive to chemotherapy. Such in vitro studies can be extended to evaluate whether an im-

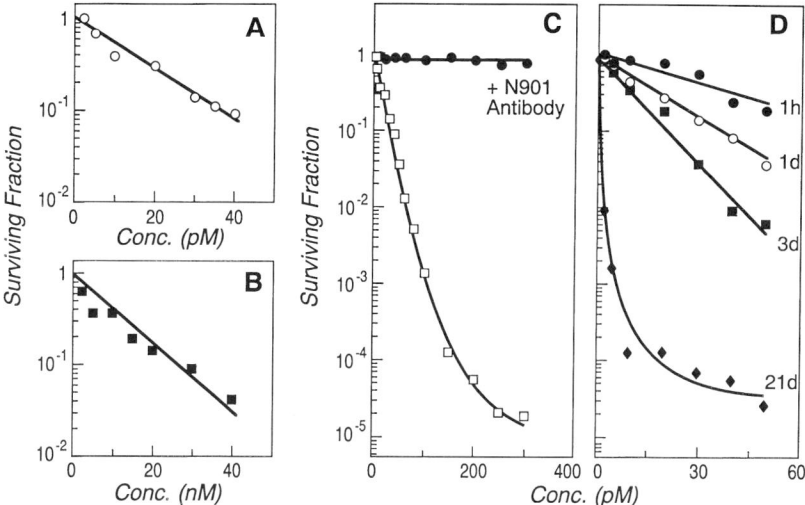

Figure 1 Cytotoxicity of the immunotoxin, N901-blocked ricin, for human cell lines. Surviving fractions of cells were determined by a direct (clonogenic) cytotoxicity assay. (A and B) Selectivity was demonstrated by exposing $CD56^+$ SW-2 cells (A) to picomolar concentrations of N901-blocked ricin for 24 hours, while $CD56^-$ Namalwa cells (B) were similarly treated with nanomolar concentrations of immunotoxin for 24 hours. (C) Specificity was demonstrated by exposing SW-2 cells for 24 hours to concentrations of immunotoxin up to 300 pM in the absence (□) or presence (●) of excess N901 antibody (0.3 µM). (D) Cytotoxicity of N901-blocked ricin for SW-2 cells after being exposed to low concentrations of immunotoxin for 1 (●), 24 (○), and 72 (□) hours, and 21 days (◆). (Reprinted, with permission, from Ref. 27.)

Table 2 Cytotoxicity of Chemotherapeutic Drugs to Namalwa and Namalwa/*mdr*-1 Cells

Drug	Namalwa IC_{37}[a]	Namalwa/*mdr*-1 IC_{37}[a]
Anti-B4-blocked ricin	8 pM	4 pM
Vincristine	0.75 nM	32 nM
Doxorubicin	5.8 nM	35 nM
Etoposide	40 nM	250 nM
Cisplatin[b]	250 nM	170 nM
4-Hydroperoxy-cyclophosphamide[b]	1 µM	1 µM

[a] IC_{37} defined as the concentration of drug that inhibits [^{3}H]-thymidine incorporation by 63% (29).
[b] Cisplatin and 4-HC are not subject to multidrug resistance.

munotoxin with a novel killing mechanism and currently used chemotherapeutic agents can act additively or synergistically. Figure 2 presents an example of experiments done to show that anti-B4-blocked ricin and doxorubicin act synergistically on the multidrug-resistance cell line Namalwa/*mdr*-1 (29,30). These assays established a rationale for combining the immunotoxin with chemotherapy in clinical trials (31).

In general, in vitro experiments to show killing of cancer cells provide a sufficient rationale for the potential therapeutic benefit of chemotherapeutic agents that in vivo studies of efficacy are not absolutely required prior to the initiation of clinical studies. Indeed, their predictive power for judging clinically active compounds from positive experimental results is not clear. Furthermore, in the case of immunotoxins, the classical models for evaluating chemotherapeutic agents cannot be used, since targeting via an antibody moiety requires the use of the specific targets, which are human tumors. Thus, in vivo efficacy evaluation can be done only in the rather artificial model systems of human tumor xenografts growing in immunodeficient mice (nude mice or severe combined immune-deficient (SCID) mice). However, with these caveats in mind, useful information can be generated in these models. One can establish that the immunotoxin has a therapeutic window in vivo, i.e., that efficacy can be demonstrated at doses that

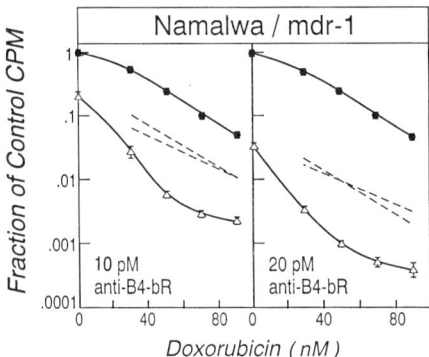

Figure 2 Isobolograms for combinations of anti-B4-blocked ricin with doxorubicin. Namalwa/*mdr*-1 cells were incubated with the indicated concentrations of the immunotoxin and doxorubicin for 72 hours and then pulsed with [^{3}H]-thymidine for 18 hours. Data are presented as the mean and standard deviation of three experiments, where the cpm incorporated into treated cells is expressed as a fraction of cpm incorporated into control cells. The solid lines with closed circles represent the killing curves for doxorubicin alone, solid lines with open triangles represent killing curves for immunotoxin combined with doxorubicin, and the broken lines represent the boundaries of the envelopes of additivity for the combination treatments. (From Ref. 29.)

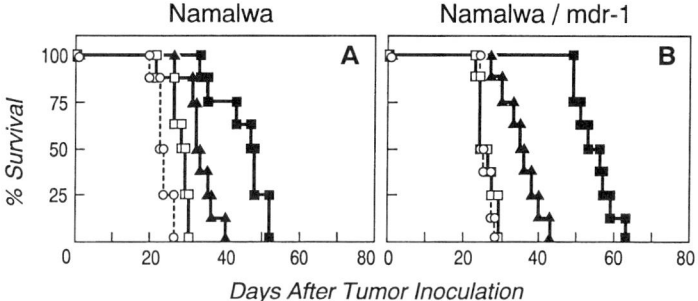

Figure 3 Survival curves for combination therapy with anti-B4-blocked ricin and doxorubicin on Namalwa and Namalwa/*mdr*-1 tumors in SCID mice. Survival as function of time after tumor inoculation (day 0) is shown for combination therapies (■) with immunotoxin (50 µg/kg/d × 5, days 7–11) and doxorubicin (3 mg/kg/d × 3q5d, beginning on day 12) on mice bearing Namalwa tumors (A) and Namalwa/*mdr*-1 tumors (B). Also shown are survival curves for tumor-bearing mice treated with (▲) immunotoxin alone (50 µg/kg/d × 5, days 7–11) or (□) doxorubicin alone (3 mg/kg/d × 3q4d, days 7–15), and survival curves for untreated mice (○). (From Ref. 29.)

cause tolerable toxicities. If this cannot be demonstrated in an ideal case (no cross-reactivity with mouse tissue, since antibodies usually originated from mice), it is unlikely that there will be a therapeutic window in the clinical situation. These models also can be used to provide further support for particular clinical studies proposed on the basis of in vitro data; clinical trials were undertaken with anti-B4-blocked ricin in combination with chemotherapy after the demonstration of synergism between anti-B4-blocked ricin, both in vitro (see, for example, Figure 2) and in vivo (Figure 3). Again, it is important to note that the immunotoxin, which kills by a mechanism not shared by current approved chemotherapeutic agents, seems to be able to reverse the multidrug-resistance phenotype (29,30).

D. Nonclinical Pharmacology: Drug Disposition

The clearance of an immunotoxin generally is assessed in the same species as used for toxicology studies. Usually, pharmacokinetic studies in mice are performed separately from toxicology studies at various dosage levels. Blood samples for pharmacokinetic studies in larger animals (for example, rabbits or monkeys) usually are taken from animals during dosing for toxicology evaluation. Ideally, pharmacokinetic analysis evaluates both the physical presence and stability of the drug, as well as the persistence of the biological activity. The important physical pharmacokinetic parameters are the peak blood levels after administration (C_{max}), the terminal half-life of clearance from the blood ($T_{1/2}$, often called the half-life of the β phase), the clearance (CL), and the total area under the concentration/time curve (AUC) (32). The pharmacokinetic data obtained in animals is used to estimate a dosing regimen for human clinical trials, and parameters calculated from bolus dosing can be used to model continuous infusion dosing (32).

Of course, extrapolation to humans assumes that a given immunotoxin will have similar pharmacokinetic parameters in humans as in an animal model. In the case of xenogeneic proteins, such as an immunotoxin made with a murine MAb and a plant or bacterial toxin, clearance rates between animals and humans do seem to be similar. However, conjugates made with human MAbs may have a longer circulation half-life in humans and, therefore, a greater AUC, and one should take account of this possibility in the design of clinical trials.

Pharmacokinetic parameters for immunotoxins should be determined using more than one assay method in order to obtain a complete picture of the behavior of the immunotoxin circulating in the blood. Each component of the immunotoxin should be measured by an ELISA specific for the antibody moiety and the toxic effector moiety. Furthermore, an assay for intact conjugate must be done; a "sandwich" ELISA can be utilized. For more precision, and to validate the ELISAs that will be adapted for measuring immunotoxin concentrations in larger animal species (e.g., monkeys) and in human serum or plasma once clinical trials have begun, the immunotoxin can be radiolabeled. Serum or plasma containing radiolabeled immunotoxins can be analyzed by biochemical techniques (e.g., polyacrylamide gels or h.p.l.c.). The aforementioned assays measure the presence of the immunotoxin protein, but it is also critical to ensure that the protein is active. Thus a bioactivity assay is necessary, using serum samples in an in vitro cytotoxicity assay. Again, such an assay can be used subsequently to test samples of human serum or plasma once clinical trials begin (see Ref. 27, for example).

Assays for each component of an immunotoxin and a bioactivity assay for intact conjugate are necessary to assess the stability of the immunotoxin in circulation. Preclinically, the immunotoxin can be incubated in human serum and human plasma and subjected to the battery of assays to assess stability and activity. Studies with radiolabeled immunotoxin can provide further support for the conclusions derived from ELISAs. If such studies demonstrate a significant rate of cleavage of the toxic effector moiety from the antibody component, it may be necessary to evaluate the toxicity, pharmacokinetics, and disposition of the free (nonconjugated) toxin effector molecule in separate (parallel) studies.

Careful pharmacokinetic analysis can be used to demonstrate product equivalency during ongoing manufacturing process development that often parallels clinical development. When changes are introduced into the manufacturing process, if it can be shown by careful studies that the immunotoxin has exactly the same pharmacokinetic parameters (as well as an identical pattern of binding, efficacy, etc.), it may be argued that clinical equivalency studies are unnecessary.

The disposition of immunotoxins generally is assessed in rodent studies using radiolabeled immunotoxin. Most often, radioiodinated (^{125}I) material is used to follow the fate of the immunotoxin as it clears from the blood. Rapid uptake by a particular organ, for example, the rapid uptake of ricin-containing immunotoxins by the liver, or concentration of Fab'-containing immunotoxins in the kidney (33), is easily determined by following a time course of biodistribution and can help identify target organs for potential toxicity and, therefore, help determine parameters to measure in the clinic.

E. Toxicology

In the evaluation of their toxicity in nonclinical animal studies, immunotoxins are treated similarly to classical chemotherapeutic agents. The goals of toxicology for cytotoxic agents are to establish the acute dose at which lethality can occur, to identify target organs for toxicity, and to determine reversibility, so that a safe starting dose and a safe dose escalation regimen can be recommended for Phase I clinical trials. The toxicology work from which a safe starting dose for clinical studies is inferred must be performed according to good laboratory practices (GLP) as described in the Code of Federal Regulations of the Food and Drug Administration (21CFR, part 58).

It is important that the dosing schedule and route be consistent with the schedule and route proposed for human clinical trials. Most cytotoxic chemotherapeutic agents are given by the intravenous route, and immunotoxins are no exception. When considering the schedule of administration, the fact that immunotoxins are xenogeneic proteins will influence both the clinical trials and the preclinical work. The value of weekly or monthly dosing, for example, is questionable due to the rapid development of an immune response to the immunotoxin, which will alter its pharmacokinetics and distribution. For example, anti-B4-blocked ricin initially was given in the clinic by daily 1-hour bolus infusions, and it was given by bolus infusions in the preclinical toxicology work prior to the first clinical trials (25). In later studies, however, the immunotoxin was given to patients by continuous infusion for periods of 1 week (34) to 1 month (35). Prior to these clinical studies, further toxicology testing was necessary to evaluate the safety of continuous infusion. A small pilot study in rats established that there was little value in dosing animals for longer than a week, since a vigorous immune response quickly removed all drug from circulation (Figure 4). Therefore, toxicology studies in monkeys were limited to 1-week infusions. In humans, however, prolonged infusions were possible (35) because the immunotoxin, since it targets an epitope found only on human B-cells, may suppress the humoral immune response (36).

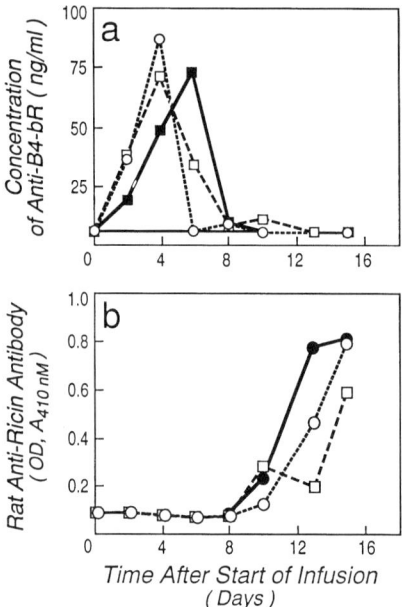

Figure 4 Evaluation of immunotoxin concentration (A) and an anti-immunotoxin humoral response (B) in Sprague-Dawley rats. Anti-B4-blocked ricin (40 µg/kg/d) was administered by continuous i.v. infusion for 14 days using a tether system. Different symbols represent data from different individual rats. Immunotoxin concentrations (A) were measured by an ELISA for the blocked ricin portion of the conjugate. Rat antiricin antibodies (B) were measured in an ELISA that takes advantage of the multivalency of antibodies: antibody was captured from serum using ricin-coated plates and detected using biotinylated ricin and a biotin-detection system.

Where immunotoxins differ from classical chemotherapeutic agents is in their targeting moiety. If the target antigen is present on normal healthy tissues, there is a chance of having antibody-directed toxicities. Thus the choice of animal species for the safety evaluation in animals must be influenced by this possibility. Generally, toxicity studies must be performed in two species, most often one rodent species (mouse or rat) and one nonrodent species. In cases where the target antigen is not expressed in any species other than human, any nonrodent species can be used, and the choice should be made based on previous toxicology experience as to how well a species predicts certain types of toxicity in humans. For example, a conjugate of anti-B4, an antibody that targets the human CD19 antigen, was recently tested in mice and rabbits for an IND application that was allowed. In cases where the target antigen is expressed in an animal species with the same distribution and expression level as in human, such species should be considered as the nonrodent animal for gathering safety data (to date, most antibodies have been of rodent origin and it is thus unlikely that rodents will share the targeted human epitope). As an example, the murine MAb N901, which targets an epitope found on the CD56 antigen (NCAM) expressed on all small-cell lung cancer cells and on normal cells of neuroendocrine origin (see Section II.C), binds to both human and nonhuman primate tissues with a similar distribution. This allowed the careful evaluation of the toxicity of the immunotoxin, N901-blocked ricin, in an animal model that would be expected to show any antibody-directed toxicities. The preclinical data obtained in these studies (7) confirmed the need for careful monitoring for potential cardiac and neurologic toxicity in Phase I studies, but did not preclude the clinical development of this agent and allowed a safe starting dose for clinical trials to be defined.

Once the appropriate animal species has been selected, toxicology studies done with each species can be divided into two types, acute bolus dosing (to establish the dose likely to cause lethality) and subacute dosing. A firm value for an LD_{50} usually is established only in acute rodent studies. Subacute dosing typically involves five successive doses of the agent or a continuous infusion for 5–7 days using at least two dose levels, a *high* toxic dose (defined as a dose that causes sublethal toxicity and that when doubled causes lethality) and a *low* toxic dose (causing minimal toxicity; doubling the dose would not result in lethality). Sometimes it may be relevant to establish a *noneffect* dose, using a third group of animals. Animals of both sexes should be used in the event of sex differences in toxic events. As just stated, although classical subacute dosing is usually for periods longer than 7 days, the nature of immunotoxins as immunogens argues for dosing for no more than 1 week.

New drug candidates usually are tested for other types of toxic events, including reproductive toxicity and genetic toxicity, and for their carcinogenicity. However, the lethal nature of cancer as a disease, and the intrinsic cytotoxic nature of anticancer drugs used in chemotherapy, mean that these types of toxicity tests often are not done, especially at the pre-IND stage. The risks from these potential toxicities are considered long-term risks that are not always relevant for the cancer patient (though they are relevant for drugs being developed for pediatric cancer patients or when treating young adults).

V. CONCLUSION

To date, hundreds of patients have been treated safely with a variety of immunotoxins. This is testimony to the fact that preclinical evaluation of these novel target-specific chemotherapeutic agents indeed does identify the important parameters for making decisions about clinical development and for the safe conduct of clinical trials.

REFERENCES

1. Ghetie V, Thorpe P, Ghetie MA, Knowles P, Uhr JW, Vitetta ES. The GLP large-scale preparation of immunotoxins containing deglycosylated ricin A chain and a hindered disulfide bond. J Immunol Methods 1991; 142:223–230.
2. Ghetie V, Ghetie MA, Uhr JW, Vitetta ES. Large-scale preparation of immunotoxins constructed with the Fab' fragment of IgG1 murine monoclonal antibodies and chemically deglycosylated ricin A chain. J Immunol Methods 1988; 112:267–277.
3. Amlot PL, Stone MJ, Cunningham D, Fay J, Newman J, Collins R, May R, McCarthy M, Richardson J, Ghetie V, Ramilo O, Thorpe PE, Uhr JW, Vitetta ES. A Phase I study of an anti-CD22-deglycosylated ricin A chain immunotoxin in the treatment of B-cell lymphomas resistant to conventional therapy. Blood 1993; 82:2624–2633.
4. Hu SZ, Shively L, Raubitschek A, Sherman M, Williams LE, Wong JYC, Shively JE, Wu AM. Minibody: a novel engineered anti-carcinoembryonic antigen antibody fragment (single-chain Fv-C_H3) which exhibits rapid, high-level targeting of xenografts. Cancer Res 1996; 56:3055–3061.
5. Reiter Y, Pastan I. Antibody engineering of recombinant Fv immunotoxins for improved targeting of cancer: disulfide-stabilized Fv immunotoxins. Clin Cancer Res 1996; 2:245–252.
6. Grossbard ML, Press OW, Appelbaum FR, Bernstein ID, Nadler LM. Monoclonal antibody-based therapies of leukemia and lymphoma. Blood 1992; 80:863–878.
7. Patel K, Moore SE, Dickson G, Rossell RJ, Beverley PC, Kemshead JT, Walsh FS. Neural cell adhesion molecule (NCAM) is the antigen recognized by monoclonal antibodies of similar specificity in small-cell lung carcinoma and neuroblastoma. Int J Cancer 1989; 44:573–578.
8. Roy DC, Ouellet S, Le Houiller C, Ariniello PD, Perreault C, Lambert JM. Elimination of neuroblastoma and small-cell lung cancer cells with an anti-neural cell adhesion molecule immunotoxin. J Natl Cancer Inst 1996; 88:1136–1145.
9. Liu C, Tadayoni BM, Bourret L, Mattocks KM, Derr SM, Widdison WC, Kedersha NL, Ariniello PD, Goldmacher VS, Lambert JM, Blättler WA, Chari RVJ. Eradication of large colon tumor xenografts by targeted delivery of maytansinoids. Proc Natl Acad Sci USA 1996; 93:8618–8623.
10. Hellström I, Garrigues HJ, Garrigues U, Hellström KE. Highly tumor-reactive, internalizing, mouse monoclonal antibodies to Le^Y-related cell surface antigens. Cancer Res 1990; 50:2183–2190.
11. Pai LH, Wittes R, Setser A, Willingham MC, Pastan I. Treatment of advanced solid tumors with immunotoxin LMB-1: an antibody linked to pseudomonas exotoxin. Nature Medicine 1996; 2:350–353.
12. Goldmacher VS, Scott CF, Lambert JM, McIntyre GD, Blättler WA, Collinson AR, Stewart JK, Chong LD, Cook S, Slayter HS, Beaumont E, Watkins S. Cytotoxicity

of gelonin and its conjugates with antibodies is determined by the extent of their endocytosis. J Cell Physiol 1989; 141:222–234.
13. Boyer CM, Lidor Y, Lottich C, Bast RC Jr. Antigenic cell surface markers in human solid tumors. Antibody Immunoconjugates Radiopharm 1988; 1:105–162.
14. Marks C, Marks JD. Phage libraries—a new route to clinically useful antibodies. N Engl J Med 1996; 335:730–733.
15. Blättler WA, Lambert JM, Goldmacher VS. Realizing the full potential of immunotoxins. Cancer Cells 1989; 1:50–55.
16. Pastan I, Fitzgerald D. Pseudomonas exotoxin: chimeric toxins. J Biol Chem 1989; 264:15,157–15,160.
17. Pastan I, Chaudhary V, Fitzgerald DJ. Recombinant toxins as novel therapeutic agents. Annu Rev Biochem 1992; 61:331–354.
18. Murphy JR, Lakkis FG, VanderSpeck JC, Anderson P. Protein engineering of diphtheria toxin. Development of receptor-specific cytotoxic agents for the treatment of human disease. In: Frankel AE, ed. Genetically Engineered Toxins. New York: Marcel Dekker, 1992:365–393.
19. Greenfield L, Johnson GV, Youle RJ. Mutations in diphtheria toxin separate binding from entry and amplify immunotoxin selectivity. Science 1987; 238:536–539.
20. Goldmacher VS, Lambert JM, Blättler WA. The specific cytotoxicity of immunoconjugates containing blocked ricin is dependent on the residual binding capacity of blocked ricin: evidence that the membrane binding and A chain translocation activities of blocked ricin cannot be separated. Biochem Biophys Res Commun 1992; 183:758–765.
21. Lambert JM, Goldmacher VS, Collinson AR, Nadler LM, Blättler WA. An immunotoxin prepared with blocked ricin: a natural plant toxin adapted for therapeutic use. Cancer Res 1991; 51:6236–6242.
22. Blättler WA, Chari RVJ, Lambert JM. In: Teicher BA, ed. Cancer Therapeutics: Experimental and Clinical Agents. Totowa, NJ: Humana Press, 1996:371–394.
23. Blackey DC, Thorpe PE. An overview of therapy with immunotoxins containing ricin or its A chain. Antibody Immunoconjugates Radiopharm 1988; 1:1–16.
24. Rybak SM, Hoogenboom HP, Meade HM, Raus JCM, Schwartz D, Youle RJ. Humanization of immunotoxins. Proc Natl Acad Sci USA 1992; 89:3165–3169.
25. Grossbard ML, Lambert JM, Goldmacher VS, Spector NL, Kinsella J, Eliseo L, Coral F, Taylor JA, Blättler WA, Epstein CL, Nadler LM. Anti-B4-blocked ricin: a Phase I trial of 7-day continuous infusion in patients with B-cell neoplasms. J Clin Oncol 1993; 11:726–737.
26. Collinson AR, Lambert JM, Liu Y, O'Dea C, Shah SA, Rasmussen RA, Goldmacher VS. Anti-CD6-blocked ricin: an anti-pan T-cell immunotoxin. Int J Immunopharmac 1994; 16:37–49.
27. Lynch TJ, Lambert JM, Coral F, Shefner J, Wen P, Blättler WA, Collinson AR, Ariniello PD, Braman G, Cook S, Esseltine D, Elias A, Skarin A, Ritz J. Immunotoxin therapy of small-cell lung cancer: a Phase I study of N901-blocked ricin. J Clin Oncol 1997; 15:723–734.
28. Sellers JR, Cook S, Goldmacher VS. A cytotoxicity assay utilizing a fluorescent dye that determines accurate surviving fractions of cells. J Immunol Methods 1994; 172: 255–264.

29. O'Connor R, Liu C, Ferris CA, Guild BC, Teicher BA, Corvi C, Liu Y, Arceci RJ, Goldmacher VS, Lambert JM, Blättler WA. Anti-B4-blocked ricin synergizes with Doxorubicin and Etoposide on multidrug-resistant and drug-sensitive tumors. Blood 1995; 86:4286–4294.
30. Liu C, Lambert JM, Teicher BA, Blättler WA, O'Connor R. Cure of multidrug-resistant human B-cell lymphoma xenografts by combinations of Anti-B4-blocked ricin and chemotherapeutic drugs. Blood 1996; 87:3892–3898.
31. Scadden DT, Doweiko J, Schenkein D, Bernstein Z, Levine AM, Besnahan J, Gere J, Esseltine D, Epstein C. A Phase I/II trial of combined immunoconjugate and chemotherapy for AIDS-related lymphoma. Blood 1993; 82 Suppl 1:386a.
32. Shah SA, Lambert JM, Goldmacher VS, Esber HJ, Levin JL, Chungi V, Zutshi A, Braman GM, Ariniello PD, Taylor JA, Blättler WA. Evaluation of the systemic toxicity and pharmacokinetics of the immunoconjugate Anti-B4-blocked ricin in non-human primates. Delivered by multiple bolus injections and by continuous infusion. Int J Immunopharmac 1993; 15:723–736.
33. Fulton RJ, Tucker TF, Vitetta ES, Uhr JW. Pharmacokinetics of tumor-reactive immunotoxins in tumor-bearing mice: effect of antibody valency and deglycosylation of the ricin A chain on clearance and tumor localization. Cancer Res 1988; 48:2618–2625.
34. Grossbard ML, Gribben JG, Freedman AS, Lambert JM, Kinsella J, Rabinowe SN, Eliseo L, Taylor JA, Blättler WA, Epstein CL, Nadler LM. Adjuvant immunotoxin therapy with Anti-B4-blocked ricin after autologous bone marrow transplantation for patients with B-cell non-Hodgkin's lymphoma. Blood 1993; 81:2263–2271.
35. McLaughlin P, Murray JL, Rosenblum M, Brewer H, LeBherz D, O'Brien S, Hagemeister FB, Epstein C, Esseltine D, Keating M. Phase I trial of Anti-B4-blocked ricin (Anti B4-bR) by 28-day continuous infusion (CI). Proc AACR 1994; 35:1501.
36. Esseltine DL, Braman GM, Park Y, Levine AM, McLaughlin P, Murray JL, Grossbard M, Lynch T, Ritz J, Nadler L, Epstein CL. Use of Anti-B4-blocked ricin as an immunosuppressant. Blood 1993; 82 Suppl 1:240a.

2
Delivery of Monoclonal Antibodies to the Tumor Cell

Rakesh K. Jain
Harvard Medical School and Massachusetts General Hospital, Boston, Massachusetts

I. INTRODUCTION

Cancer is the second leading cause of death in the United States and in many industrialized countries (1). After the primary tumor has been surgically removed and/or sterilized by radiation, the residual disease is usually managed with a variety of systemic therapies (Table 1). For these therapies to be successful, they must satisfy two requirements: (a) the relevant agent must be effective in the in vivo orthotopic microenvironment of tumors, and (b) this agent must reach the target cells in vivo in optimal quantities. The goal of our research is to examine the latter issue—the delivery of diagnostic and therapeutic agents to solid tumors and normal host tissues.

All conventional and novel therapeutic agents can be divided into three categories—molecules, particles, and cells (Table 1). A blood-borne molecule or particle that enters the tumor vasculature reaches cancer cells via distribution through the vascular compartment, transport across the microvascular wall, and transport through the interstitial compartment. For a molecule of given size, charge, and configuration, each of these transport processes may involve diffusion and convection. In addition, during the journey the molecule may bind nonspecifically to proteins or other tissue components, bind specifically to the target(s), or be metabolized (2). Although lymphokine-activated killer (LAK) cells (lymphocytes activated by the lymphokine interleukin-2) or tumor-infiltrating lymphocytes (TILs) are capable of deformation, adhesion, and migration, they encounter the same barriers that restrict their movement in tumors. Some of these

Table 1 Categorization of Agents Used in Various Conventional and Novel Therapies

Therapy	Agent		
	Molecules	Particles	Cells
Radiotherapy	✓	✓	
Chemotherapy	✓	✓	
Immunotherapy	✓	✓	✓
Gene therapy	✓	✓	✓
Hyperthermia	✓		
Phototherapy	✓	✓	

physiological parameters are also important for heat transfer in normal and tumor tissues during hyperthermic treatment of cancer (3).

The overall aim of our research is to develop a quantitative understanding of each of the aforementioned steps involved in the delivery of various agents. More specifically, our goals are to understand (a) how angiogenesis takes place and what determines blood flow heterogeneities in tumors, (b) how blood flow influences the metabolic microenvironment in tumors, and how microenvironment affects the biological properties of tumors (e.g., vascular permeability, cell adhesion), (c) how material moves across the microvascular wall, and (d) how it moves through the interstitial compartment and the lymphatics. In addition, we are examining the role of cell deformation and adhesion in the delivery of cells. Following analysis of these processes for molecules, particles, and cells, we integrate this information in a unified framework for scale-up from mice to men (Figure 1). In this chapter, I will briefly describe various experimental and theoretical approaches used in our lab, our recent findings in these six areas, and, finally, how we have taken some of these concepts from bench to bedside for potential improvement in cancer detection and treatment.

II. EXPERIMENTAL AND THEORETICAL APPROACHES

We have utilized five approaches to gain insight into the pathophysiology of solid tumors:

1. A tissue-isolated tumor that is connected to the host's circulation by a single artery and a single vein (4,5). This technique was originally developed by P. M. Gullino at the National Cancer Institute in 1961 for rats (6); we have recently adapted it to mice (7,8) and humans (9).
2. A modified Sandison rabbit ear chamber (10,11), a modified Algire

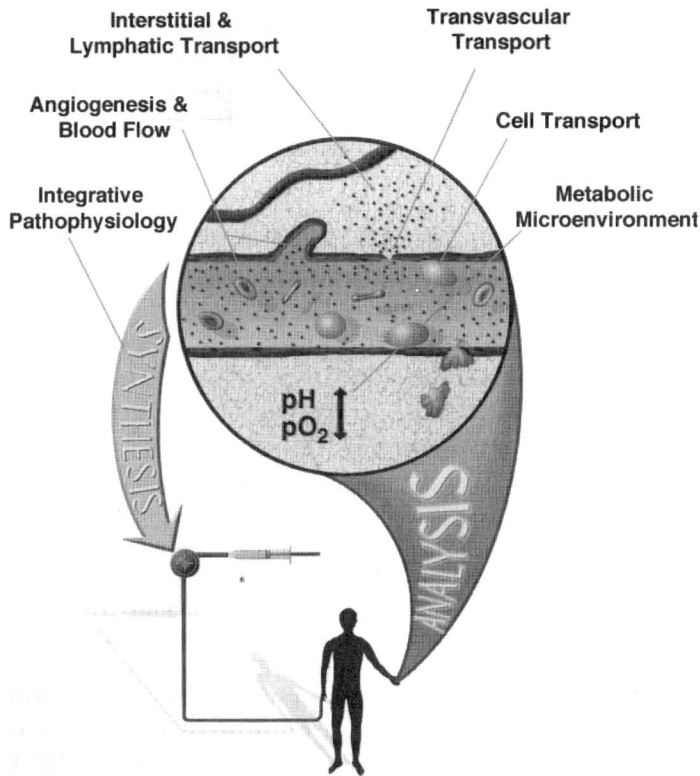

Figure 1 Quantitative understanding of various steps involved in the delivery of therapeutic agents is studied by analyzing the underlying processes and then integrating the resulting information in a unified framework. More specifically, our goal is to develop a quantitative understanding of (a) angiogenesis and blood flow, (b) metabolic microenvironment, (c) transvascular transport, (d) interstitial and lymphatic transport, (e) cell transport, and (f) systemic distribution and interspecies scale-up.

mouse dorsal chamber (12,13), and a cranial window in mice and rats (14). The ear chamber has the advantage of superior optical quality, and the mouse of working with immunodeficient and genetically engineered animals (15–17). Recently we have developed a quantitative angiogenesis assay using these windows to study the physiology of vessels induced by individual growth factors (18,19) (Figure 2). We also perfuse single vessels of tumors in these windows (20). We also utilize two acute preparations: liver and mesentery (21).

3. In vitro methods to assess the deformability, adhesion, permeability,

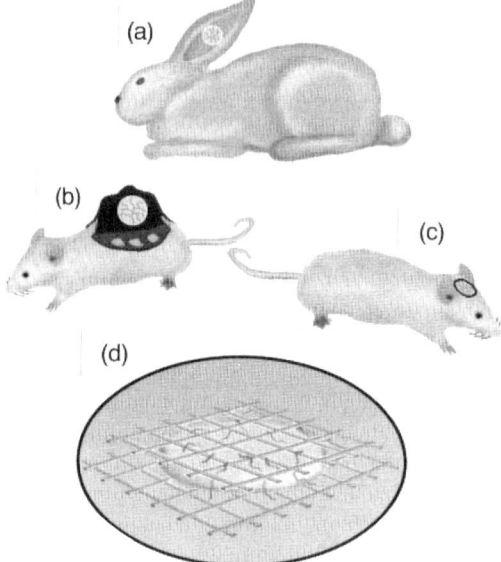

Figure 2 Various microcirculatory preparations used to study delivery of therapeutic agents in solid tumors: (a) Sandison window in the rabbit ear (11), (b) Algire window in the dorsal skin of rodents (13), (c) cranial window in rodents (14), and (d) collagen I gel, containing angiogenic factors, sandwiched between nylon mesh (3 mm $\times$ 3 mm) to permit the growth of blood vessels (18). These preparations allow noninvasive, continuous measurement of angiogenesis and blood flow; metabolites, such as pH, pO_2; transport of molecules and particles; and cell–cell interactions in vivo.

and growth stress of normal and neoplastic cells (22–26), as well as measurements of adhesion molecules' expression in intact monolayers (27,28) (Figure 3).
4. Routine molecular biology techniques (e.g., in situ hybridization, Southern, Northern, and Western blotting).
5. Mathematical models to describe and integrate the data obtained from the preceding four approaches, to scale up biodistribution data from mice to men, and to design future experiments (29–43).

Although each of these approaches has its limitations, it is their combination that has permitted us to develop the framework for tumor microcirculation and drug delivery described in this chapter.

III. DISTRIBUTION THROUGH VASCULAR SPACE

The tumor vasculature consists of both vessels recruited from the preexisting network of the host vasculature and vessels resulting from the angiogenic re-

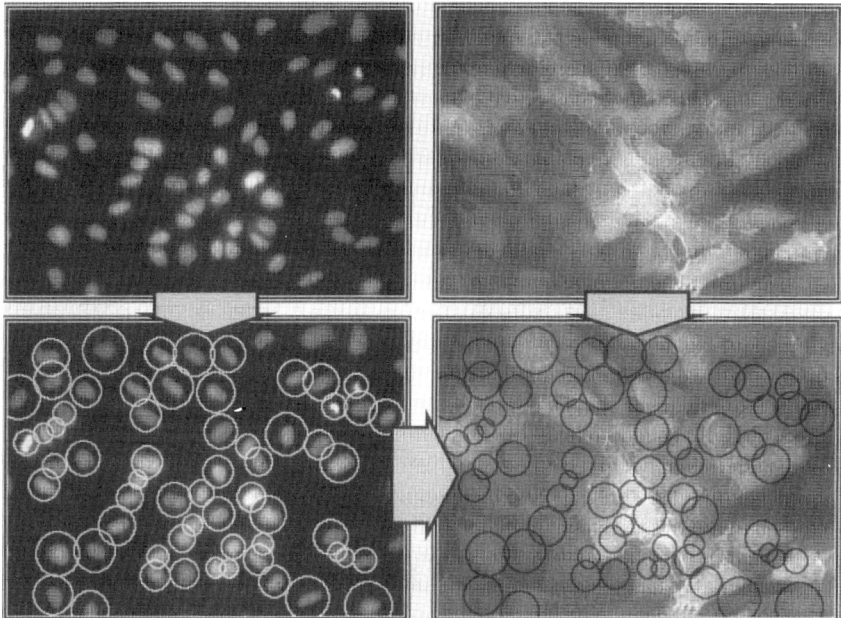

Figure 3 Targeted sampling fluorometry (TSF) allows the quantification of adhesion molecule expression over an intact cell monolayer on a cell-by-cell basis. At top are the two images acquired for analysis: the nuclei are stained with propidium iodide and the adhesion molecule is labeled with fluorescein using double immunostaining. The nuclei are first located in the propidium iodide channel, and regions of interest (ROIs) are formed around each nucleus (bottom left); these ROIs are then applied to the immunostained image to find the fluorescence intensity in each region, corresponding to one cell. The procedure yields a histogram of intensities for the monolayer. (Adapted from Ref. 27.)

sponse of host vessels to cancer cells (44,45). Movement of molecules through the vasculature is governed by the vascular morphology (i.e., the number, length, diameter, and geometric arrangement of various blood vessels) and the blood flow rate (30,46–48).

Although the tumor vasculature originates from the host vasculature and the mechanisms of angiogenesis are similar (44,49), its organization may be completely different, depending on the tumor type, its growth rate, and its location (48). The fractal dimensions and minimum path lengths of tumor vasculature are different from those of the normal host vessels (46,47,50). The architecture and blood flow are different not only among various tumor types but also between a spontaneous tumor and its transplants (45,51). For example, unlike normal tissue, where RBC velocity is dependent on vessel diameter, there is no such dependence in tumors (13,14,21). Furthermore, the RBC velocity may be an order of magnitude lower in some tumors compared to the host vessels (Figure 4). The temporal and spatial heterogeneity in tumor blood flow may, in part, be a result of elevated geometric and viscous resistance in tumor vessels (5,9,52,53), coupling between high vascular permeability and elevated interstitial fluid pressure (39), and vascular remodeling by intussusception (49) and solid stress generated by proliferating cancer cells (26).

Based on perfusion rates, four regions can be recognized in a tumor: an avascular, necrotic region, a seminecrotic region, a stabilized microcirculation region, and an advancing front (54) (Figure 5a). Intratumor blood flow distributions in spontaneous animal and human tumors are now being investigated using nuclear magnetic resonance, positron emission tomography, and functional computed tomography (35,55,56). Though limited, these results are in concert with the transplanted tumor studies: blood flow rates in necrotic and seminecrotic regions of tumors are low, whereas those in non-necrotic regions are variable and can be substantially higher than in surrounding (contralateral) host normal tissues (57). Considering these spatial and temporal heterogeneities in blood supply coupled with variations in the vascular morphology at both microscopic and macroscopic levels, it is not surprising that the spatial distribution of therapeutic agents in tumors is heterogeneous and that the average uptake decreases, in general, with an increase in tumor weight. This perfusion heterogeneity also makes it difficult to heat the tumor periphery during hyperthermia (3).

IV. METABOLIC MICROENVIRONMENT

The temporal and spatial heterogeneities in blood flow are expected to lead to a compromised metabolic microenvironment in tumors. To quantify the spatial gradients of key metabolites, we have recently adapted two optical techniques: fluorescence ratio-imaging microscopy (FRIM) and phosphorescence quenching microscopy (PQM) (58–62). As shown in Figure 6, both pH and pO_2 decrease as one moves away from tumor vessels leading to acidic and hypoxic regions in tumors. Coupled with the use of cells selected for impaired glycolytic and oxidative pathways, these methods have provided novel insight into pH regulation in tumors (63). Though low pO_2 and pH are detrimental to some therapies (e.g., radiation), they might enhance the effect of certain drugs, if the drug could be delivered in adequate quantities in those regions (64–66).

To gain further insight into tumor metabolism, we have combined two powerful approaches: magnetic resonance spectroscopy and tissue-isolated tumors. The former allows us to measure the energy level in tumors; the latter allows us to control the supply of individual substrates (e.g., glucose, oxygen) to the tumor.

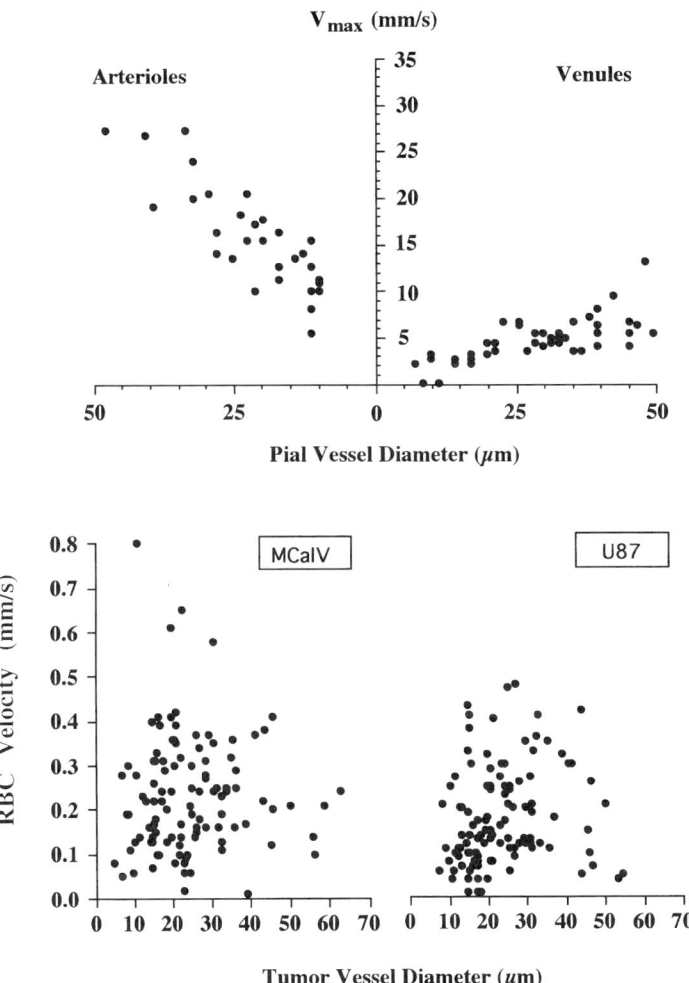

Figure 4 Blood velocity as a function of vessel diameter in (a) normal pial vessels, and (b) a human glioma (U87) xenograft on the pial surface. Note that in normal microcirculation, blood velocity is dependent on vessel diameter, whereas in tumors there is no such dependence. Furthermore, the blood velocity in tumor vessels is about an order of magnitude lower than in host vessels. (Adapted from Ref. 14.)

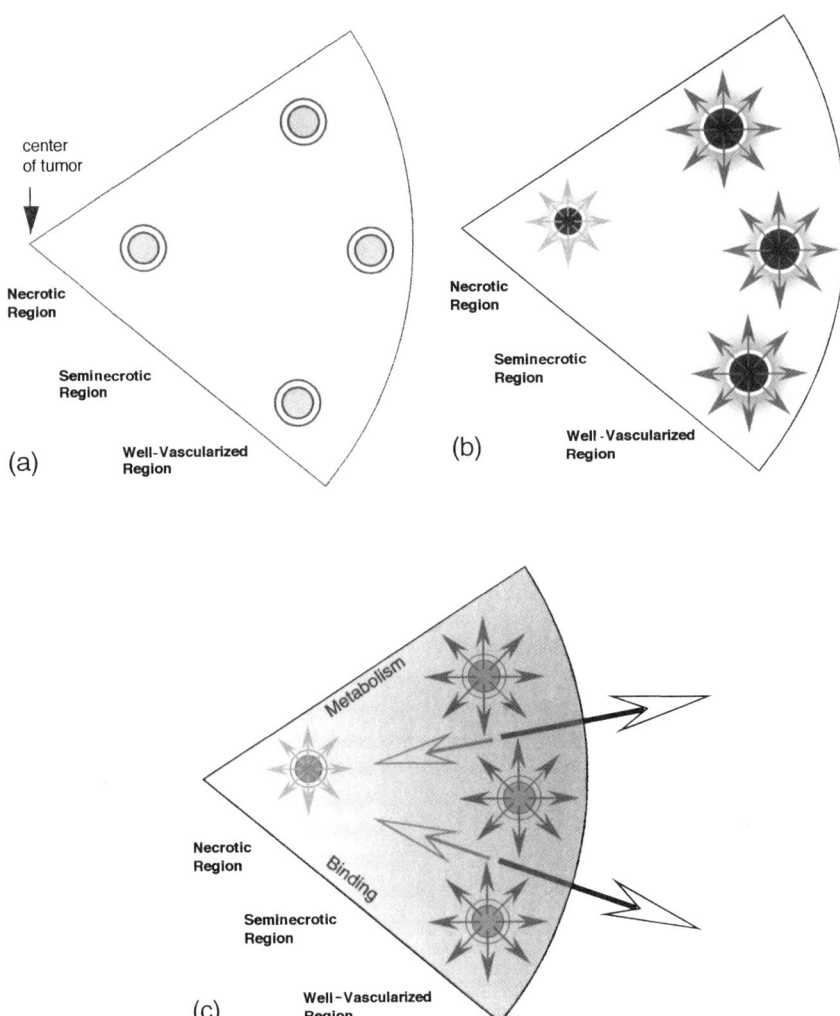

Figure 5 Physiological barriers that a blood-borne molecule encounters before it reaches a cancer cell in a solid tumor. (a) Schematic of a heterogeneously perfused tumor showing well-vascularized periphery, a seminecrotic, intermediate zone, and an avascular, necrotic central region. Note that immediately after i.v. injection, the molecules are delivered to perfused regions only. (b) Low interstitial pressure in the periphery permits adequate extravasation of fluid and macromolecules. (c) These macromolecules move toward the center by the slow process of diffusion. In addition, interstitial fluid oozing from tumor carries macromolecules with it by convection into the normal tissue. Note that the interstitial movement may be further retarded by binding. Products of metabolism may be cleared rapidly by blood. (Reproduced from Ref. 112.)

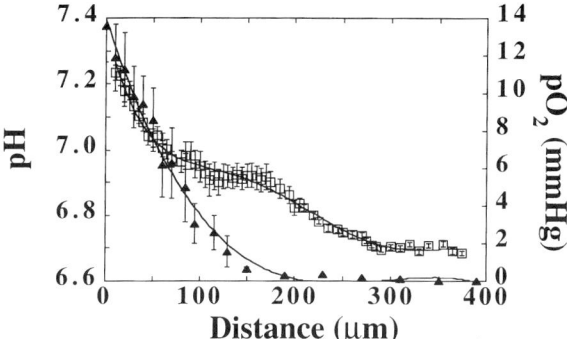

Figure 6 Spatial gradients of metabolites in tumors. pH (□) gradients measured using fluorescence ratio imaging microscopy. pO$_2$ (▲) gradients measured using phosphorescence quenching. Distance from the vessel wall, in microns, is shown on the x-axis, with zero being the vessel wall. (Adapted from Ref. 59.)

Using this combination approach, we have recently shown that solid tumors depend more on glucose than on oxygen to maintain their ATP level (67). Using a sandwich culture system, we are currently examining the relationship between the gradients of metabolites and gene expression (68).

V. TRANSPORT ACROSS THE MICROVASCULAR WALL

Once a blood-borne molecule has reached an exchange vessel, its extravasation, J_s (g/s), occurs by diffusion and convection and, to some extent, presumably by transcytosis (69). Diffusive flux is proportional to the exchange vessel's surface area, S (cm^2), and the difference between the plasma and interstitial concentrations, $C_p - C_i$ (g/m). Convection is proportional to the rate of fluid leakage, J_f (m/s), from the vessel. In turn, J_f is proportional to S and the difference between the vascular and interstitial hydrostatic pressures, $p_v - p_i$ (mm Hg), minus the osmotic reflection coefficient (σ) times the difference between the vascular and interstitial osmotic pressures, $\pi_v - \pi_i$ (mm Hg). The proportionality constant that relates transluminal diffusion flux to concentration gradients, $(C_p - C_i)$, is referred to as the vascular permeability coefficient, P (cm/s), and the constant that relates fluid leakage to pressure gradients is referred to as the hydraulic conductivity, L_p (cm/mm Hg·s). The effectiveness of the transluminal osmotic pressure difference in producing fluid movement across a vessel wall is characterized by σ, which is close to 1 for a macromolecule and close to 0 for a small molecule. Thus, the transport of a molecule across normal or tumor vessels is governed by three transport parameters (P, L_p, and σ), the surface area for exchange, and the transvascular concentration and pressure gradients.

Vascular permeability and hydraulic conductivity of tumors in general is significantly higher than that of various normal tissues (14,20,69–74), and, hence, these vessels may lack permselectivity (75) (Figure 7a,b). Positively changed molecules have a higher permeability (76). Despite increased overall permeability, not all blood vessels of a tumor are leaky (Figure 7b). Even the leaky vessels have a finite pore size, which we have been able to measure in a variety of human and rodent tumors (77), including a human colon carcinoma (LS174T) xenografted in the dorsal window (Figure 7c,d). Our hypothesis is that the large pore size in tumors represents wide interendothelial junctions (77,78). Not only does the vascular permeability vary from one tumor to the next, but within the same tumor it varies both spatially and temporally (69). The local microenvironment plays an important role in controlling vascular permeability. For example, a human glioma (HGL21) is fairly leaky when grown subcutaneously in immunodeficient mice, but it exhibits blood-brain barrier properties in the cranial window (Figure 7e,f). We have seen such site-dependent differences for other tumors in other orthotopic sites (21). Our working hypothesis is that the host–tumor interactions control the production and secretion of cytokines associated with permeability changes (e.g., vascular permeability factor (VPF)/vascular endothelium growth factor (VEGF) and its inhibitors). A better understanding of the molecular mechanisms of permeability regulation in tumors is likely to yield strategies for improved drug delivery (79).

If tumor vessels are indeed "leaky" to fluid and macromolecules, then what leads to the poor extravasation of these agents in various regions of tumors? As shown by us and others (80–93), experimental and human tumors exhibit high interstitial fluid pressure. Furthermore, the uniformly high pressure drops precipitously to normal values in the tumor's periphery or in the peritumor region (29,36,81). This may lower fluid extravasation in the high-pressure regions, especially because the oncotic and hydrostatic pressures are also equal between the intravascular and extravascular space (82,94,95). Because the transvascular transport of macromolecules in normal tissues occurs primarily by convection (69,96), convective transport of macromolecules in the center of tumors may be less than in the tumor periphery (20,29,36). Additionally, the average vascular surface area per unit tissue weight decreases with tumor growth; hence, reduced transvascular exchange would be expected in large tumors compared with small tumors (29,30).

VI. TRANSPORT THROUGH INTERSTITIAL SPACE AND LYMPHATICS

Once a molecule has extravasated, its movement through the interstitial space occurs by diffusion and convection (88). Diffusion is proportional to the con-

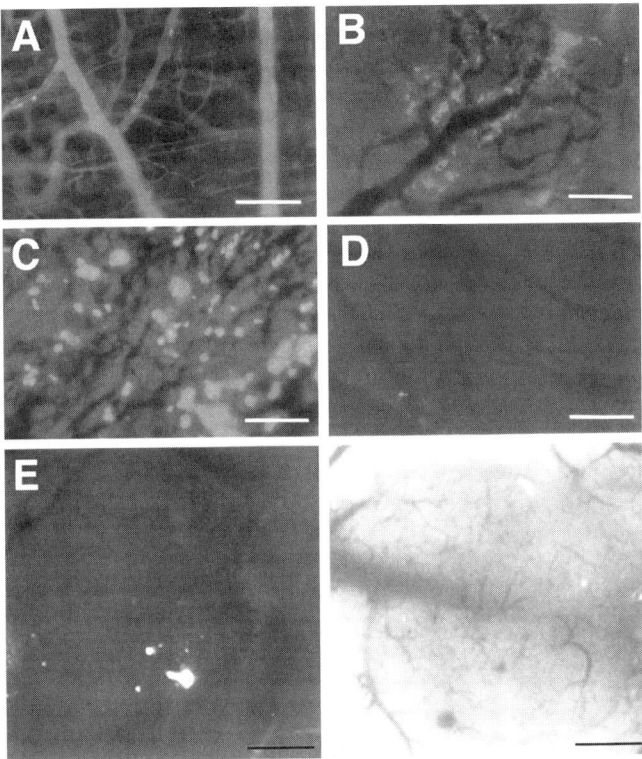

Figure 7 Transvascular transport in dorsal skin and tumors. (A) There is hardly any extravasation of 90-nm-diameter liposomes from normal vessels; (B) heterogeneous extravasation of 90-nm-diameter liposomes from LS174T tumor vessels, 48 h after injection. Note that some vessels are leaky, as indicated by the fluorescence for Rhodamine, whereas others are not. Extravasated liposomes do not diffuse far from blood vessels. (Adapted from Ref. 14.) (C) Liposomes of 400-nm-diameter (fluorescent spots) extravasate adequately from LS174T tumor. (D) Liposomes of 600-nm-diameter do not extravasate, suggesting that LS174T vessels have pore-size cutoff of about 500 nm. (Adapted from Ref. 75.) (E) The human glioma (HGL21) xenograft is permeable to Lissamin green (i.e., tumor tissue becomes green) when grown subcutaneously (Yuan and Jain, unpublished results). (F) The same glioma develops blood–brain barrier properties (i.e., impermeable to Lissamin green) when grown in the cranial window. (Adapted from Ref. 14.)

centration gradient in the interstitium, and convection is proportional to the interstitial fluid velocity, u_i (cm/s). The latter, in turn, is proportional to the pressure gradient in the interstitium. Just as the interstitial diffusion coefficient, D (cm^2/s), relates the diffusive flux to the concentration gradient, the interstitial hydraulic conductivity, K (cm^2/mm Hg·s), relates the interstitial velocity to the pressure gradient (88). Values of these transport coefficients are determined by the structure and composition of the interstitial compartment as well as the physicochemical properties of the solute molecule (97–103).

Using fluorescence recovery after photobleaching (FRAP) we have found D of various molecules to be about one-third that in water (104) and similar to that in the host tissue (98). Similarly, the value of K for a human colon carcinoma xenograft (LS174T) measured using two different methods (105,106) was found to be higher than that of a hepatoma (103), which in turn was higher than that of the liver. Given these relatively high values of D and K, why do exogenously injected macromolecules not distribute uniformly in tumors? As discussed next, there are two reasons for this apparent paradox.

The time constant for a molecule with diffusion coefficient D to diffuse across distance L is approximately $L^2/4D$. For diffusion of IgG in tumors, this time constant is on the order of 1 hour for a 100-μm distance, days for a 1-mm distance, and months for a 1-cm distance. So for a 1-mm tumor, diffusional transport would take days; and for a 1-cm tumor, it would take months. If the central vessels have collapsed completely due to cellular proliferation (26) and interstitial matrix rearrangement, there would be no delivery of macromolecules by blood flow to this necrotic center. Binding may further retard the transport in tumors (31,32,104,107–111). The role of binding is clearly illustrated in Figure 8, which compares the rate of fluorescence recovery of a photobleached spot in tumor tissue injected with a nonspecific vs. specific IgG. In addition to the heterogeneity in D in tumors, the most unexpected result of these photobleaching studies was the large extent (30–40%) of nonspecific binding (104).

As mentioned earlier, interstitial fluid pressure is high in the center of tumors and low in the periphery and surrounding tissue (29,36,81). Therefore, one would expect interstitial fluid motion from the tumor's periphery into the surrounding normal tissue (Figure 5b,c). In various animal and human (xenograft) tumors studied to date, 6–14% of plasma entering the tumor has been found to leave from the tumor's periphery (69,112). This fluid leakage leads to a radially outward interstitial fluid velocity of 0.1–0.2 μm/s at the periphery of a 1-cm "tissue-isolated" tumor (69). [The radially outward velocity is likely to be an order of magnitude lower in a tumor grown in the subcutaneous tissue or muscle (29)]. A macromolecule at the tumor periphery has to overcome this outward convection to diffuse into the tumor. The relative contribution of this mechanism of heterogeneous distribution of antibodies in tumors may be smaller than the contribution of heterogeneous extravasation due to elevated pressure and necrosis (29).

Delivery of MAbs to the Tumor Cell 35

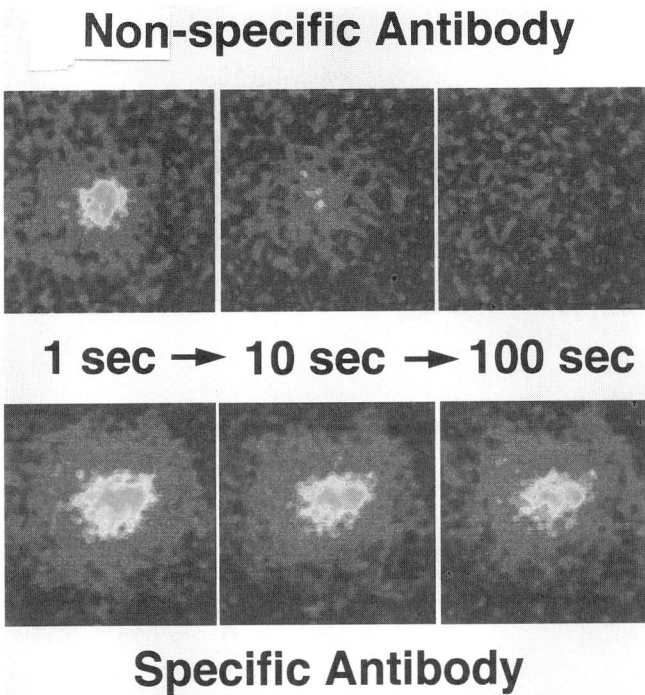

Figure 8 Role of binding in the interstitial transport in tumors, measured using fluorescence recovery after photobleaching. (a) Recovery of a photobleached spot is complete in about 100 s for a nonspecific monoclonal antibody. (b) Recovery is incomplete for an antibody against carcino-embryonic antigen, present on the surface of many carcinoma cells. (Adapted from Ref. 104.)

In most normal tissues, extravasated macromolecules are taken up by the lymphatics and brought back to the central circulation. Because of the lack of functional lymphatics within the tumor, the fluid and macromolecules oozing from the tumor surface must be picked by the peritumor host lymphatics (30). To characterize the transport into and within the lymphatic capillaries, we have recently developed a mouse tail model (113). We have measured uptake and transport in this model using a macroscopic approach (RTD analysis) and a microscopic approach (FRAP) (114,115). Our current efforts are directed toward uncovering mechanisms of lymphangiogenesis (116) and understanding changes in lymphatic transport in the presence of a tumor (117).

VII. TRANSPORT OF CELLS

So far we have discussed the parameters that govern the transport of molecules and particles (e.g., liposomes) in tumors. When a leukocyte enters a blood vessel, it may continue to move with flowing blood, collide with the vessel wall, adhere transiently or stably, and finally extravasate. These interactions are governed by both local hydrodynamic forces and adhesive forces. The former are determined by the vessel diameter and fluid velocity, and the latter by the expression, strength, and kinetics of bond formation between adhesion molecules and by the surface area of contact (118,119). Deformability of cells affects both types of forces. Despite their importance in immunotherapy and gene therapy, the determinants of cell transport in tumors have not been examined.

Using intravital microscopy, we have recently shown that rolling of endogenous leukocytes is generally low in tumor vessels, whereas stable adhesion (≥ 30 s) is comparable between normal and tumor vessels (Figure 9a,b) (120). On the other hand, both rolling and stable adhesion are nearly zero in angiogenic vessels induced in collagen gels by bFGF or VEGF/VPF, two of the most potent angiogenic factors (18). Whether the latter is due to a low flux of leukocytes into angiogenic vessels and/or to downregulation of adhesion molecules in these immature vessels is currently under investigation. The age of the animal also plays an important role in leukocyte–endothelial interactions (121).

To gain further insight into the type of cells that adhere to tumor vessels, we examined the localization of IL-2 activated natural killer (A-NK) cells in normal and tumor tissues in mice using positron emission tomography (22,122). Following systemic injection, we found that these cells localized primarily in the lungs immediately after injection and a nondetectable number of cells arrived in the tumor (22). These findings were consistent with our previous work on the deformability of these cells using micropipet aspiration technique, in which we showed that IL-2 activation makes these cells rigid and predicted their mechanical entrapment in the lung microcirculation (24,123). Constitutive expression of certain adhesion molecules in the lung vasculature also facilitates their localization in the lungs (124).

One approach to reduce lung entrapment is to reduce the rigidity of these cells (125). Instead, to circumvent the lung, we decided to inject A-NK cells into the blood supply of tumors, and we found that A-NK cells, both xenogenic and syngeneic, adhered to blood vessels in three different tumor models (122, 126,127). These results also supported the hypothesis that the endogenous cells that adhere to tumor vessels after systemic IL-2 injection are mostly activated lymphocytes (128).

To find out the adhesion molecules involved in the A-NK cell adhesion to tumor vessels, we utilized two in vitro approaches. In the first approach, we simulated the tumor vasculature in vitro by incubating the human umbilical vein

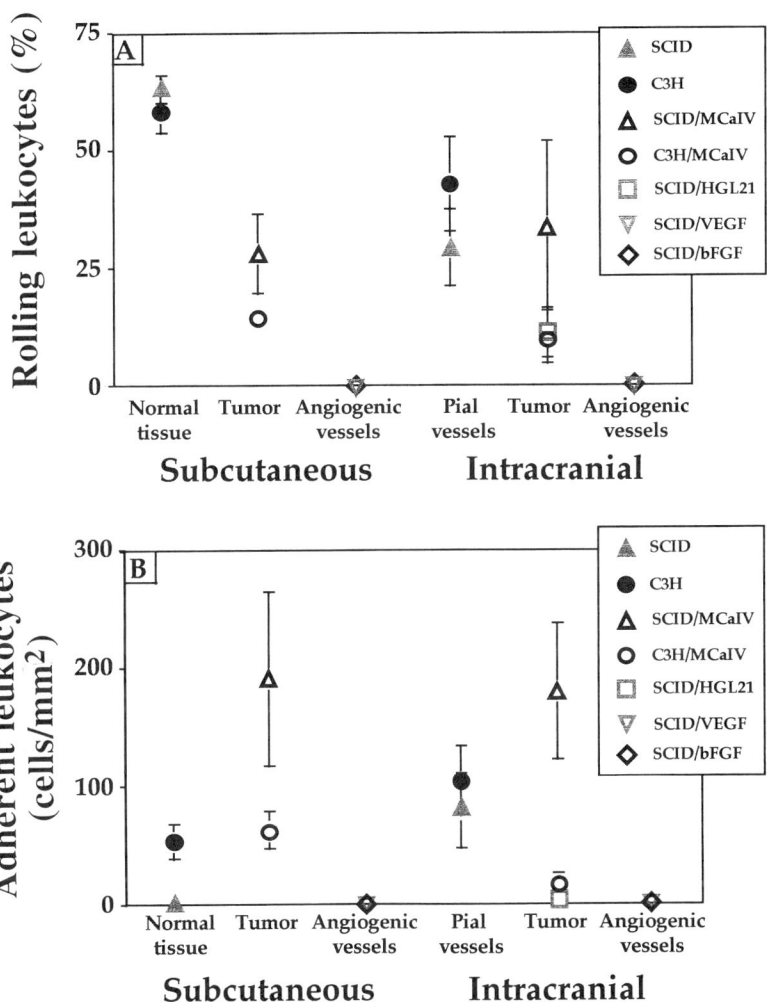

Figure 9 Leukocyte–endothelial interactions in normal and tumor (120) and angiogenic (18) vessels in the dorsal skin window and the cranial window: (A) rolling, and (B) adhesion. Note that rolling is significantly reduced in tumor vessels compared to host vessels, whereas stable adhesion is similar in both vessel types. Both rolling and adhesion are negligible in angiogenic vessels.

endothelial cells (HUVECs) in the tumor interstitial fluid collected using a micropore chamber (6,38,64,129). Using targeted sampling fluorometry (Figure 3), we were able to quantify the expression of relevant adhesion molecules on the HUVEC monolayers (27). To determine the relative contributions of these molecules in adhesion under physiological flow conditions, we utilized the flow chamber (23). Using appropriate antibodies, we found that molecules upregulated on the HUVECs include ICAM-1 and VCAM-1, which bind to CD18 and VLA-4 on the A-NK cells. We also observed sporadic upregulation of E-selectin. We were able to confirm the role of these molecules in vivo by treating A-NK cells with antibodies against CD18 and VLA-4 prior to injecting them into the arterial supply of tumors. As in our in vitro studies, blocking these adhesion molecules nearly eliminated the adhesion of A-NK cells to tumor vessels (129).

What leads to the upregulation of these molecules in the tumor vasculature? We already knew that these molecules can be upregulated by TNF-α and a protein of 90-kD molecular weight (p90) secreted by some neoplastic cells (118,130,131) and downregulated by TGF-β (132–134). We wanted to find out if there are other molecules present in the tumor milieu that are also inducing this upregulation. Since tumor growth and metastasis are angiogenesis dependent, we decided to focus on the two most potent angiogenic molecules, bFGF and VEGF/VPF (44,124,135). We found that VEGF can mimic tumor interstitial fluid and upregulate these molecules (17). On the other hand, bFGF exhibited no effect when used alone, but abrogated the upregulation induced by VEGF or TNF-α (129). These findings were in concert with earlier reports that bFGF retards the transmigration of lymphocytes across endothelial monolayer (136) and reduces adhesion of endothelial cells to collagen (137). They also offer a possible explanation for lower leukocyte–endothelial interactions in tumors; bFGF might have downregulated adhesion molecules in these tumors. Our current efforts are directed toward defining interactions between angiogenic and adhesion molecules using various in vitro and in vivo approaches, including genetically engineered mice (15,17,124).

VIII. PHARMACOKINETIC MODELING: SCALE-UP FROM MOUSE TO HUMAN

So far we have analyzed each of the steps in the delivery of molecules and cells to and within solid tumors. Can we take this information and integrate it in a unified framework? We have been successful to some extent in this endeavor, using physiologically based pharmacokinetic modeling. This approach, pioneered in the 1960s by two chemical engineers, K. Bischoff and R. L. Dedrick, has been applied successfully to describe and scale up the biodistribution of low-molecular-weight agents (for a review, see Refs. 3,138,139). We have extended this approach to macromolecules and cells (33,34,140–142).

In this approach, a mammalian body is represented by a number of physiological compartments interconnected anatomically (Figure 10). The volume and blood flow rate to each of these compartments/organs are known or can be measured. The parameters that characterize transport across the subcompartments (i.e., vascular, interstitial, and cellular) and the metabolism of various agents are not generally known and cannot easily be measured. Our philosophy has been to use as many measured parameters as possible and to estimate the remaining parameters by fitting the model to the murine biodistribution data. By scaling up the parameters using well-defined scale-up laws (138), we then predict the biodistribution in human patients and compare with clinical data. Discrepancies between predictions and actual data help us in identifying interspecies differences and force us to question our model assumptions. This is an evolutionary process; as our understanding of underlying physiology and biochemistry improves, the relevant parameters are modified and the model is refined further. The model is useful not only for designing murine experiments and/or clinical trials, but also in identifying the sensitive parameters that need careful measurement and analysis. If we need detailed spatial information about a tissue/organ, then we develop a distributed parameter model for that organ, e.g., tumor (29–34,37,143,144). Although simple in principle, this cyclic approach of analysis and synthesis has

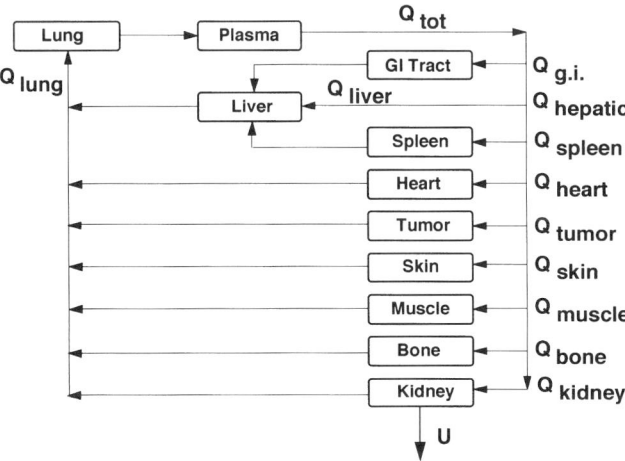

Figure 10 Schematic of physiologically based kinetic model to describe the biodistribution of molecules and cells in a mammalian system. Such an approach permits interspecies scale-up of biodistribution. (Adapted from Ref. 33.)

served as a useful paradigm for developing a deeper understanding of drug and cell distribution in normal and malignant tissues. The level of sophistication of these models is likely to improve with our understanding of underlying principles (46).

IX. BENCH TO BEDSIDE

The physiologic factors that contribute to the poor delivery of therapeutic agents to tumors include heterogeneous blood supply, interstitial hypertension, relatively long transport distances in the interstitium, and cellular heterogeneities (Figure 5). How can these physiologic barriers be exploited or overcome? Can we take our findings about these barriers from the bench to the bedside? Two recently developed strategies that have the potential to improve the detection and treatment of solid tumors in patients are described here.

As stated earlier, all solid tumors in patients exhibit interstitial hypertension (Table 2), provided the patient has not received any antiedema treatment (85). We have also shown theoretically and confirmed experimentally that IFP rises quite steeply in the tumor boundary (36,81). We have used this knowledge in improving the design of the needle used by radiologists to localize the tumor for surgical excision (145). We can facilitate the needle placement in a tumor by placing a pressure sensor in the needle. Since tumors begin to exhibit interstitial

Table 2 Interstitial Pressure in Normal and Neoplastic Human Tissues (mmHg)

Tissue type	Number	Median	Range
Normal skin	5	0.4	−1.0– 3.0
Normal breast	8	0.0	−0.5– 3.0
Head/neck carcinomas	27	19.0	1.5–79.0
Cervical carcinomas	26	23.0	6.0–94.0
Lung carcinomas	26	10.0	1.0–27.0
Metastatic melanomas	14	21.0	0.0–60.0
Metastatic melanomas	12	14.5	2.0–41.0
Breast carcinomas	13	29.0	5.0–53.0
Breast carcinomas	8	15.0	4.0–33.0
Brain tumors	17	7.0	2.0–15.0
Brain tumors	11	1.0	−0.5– 8.0
Colorectal liver mets	8	21.0	6.0–45.0
Lymphomas	7	4.5	1.0–12.5
Renal cell carcinoma	1	38.0	—

hypertension almost from the onset of angiogenesis (95), this needle may be able to help in localizing early disease. The same concept may be useful in optimizing location and infusion pressure of needles employed in intratumor infusion of therapeutic agents (105) and for monitoring response to therapy (92).

Several physical agents (e.g., radiation, heat) and chemical agents (e.g., vasoactive drugs) may lead to an increase in tumor blood flow or vascular permeability (51,69,146–151) or to lower pH (64,66). Another approach may be based on increasing the interstitial transport rate of molecules by increasing K or D enzymatically (103,105,112) or by using multistep approaches (34,42,152,153). We have used several physical and chemical agents to lower IFP in tumors (13,106,154–159). Since microvascular and interstitial pressures in tumors are approximately equal, any change in one is followed rapidly by a similar change in the other, and thus the convective enhancement disappears rapidly (40,82,160,161). By adapting a poroelastic model to solid tumors, we have calculated theoretically and confirmed experimentally that the time constant of pressure transmission across the tumor vasculature is on the order of 10 s (40). During such a short time, the convective enhancement is calculated to be very small ($\sim$1%). However, if the vascular pressure is increased repeatedly and if the transvascular transport is unidirectional or if the molecule binds avidly in the extravascular region, then we can, in principle, increase drug delivery to solid tumors significantly (Figure 11).

In contrast, the physiologic barriers discussed here may be less of a problem for (a) radioimmunodetection, (b) treating leukemias, lymphomas, and small tumors (e.g., micrometastases) in which the physiological barriers are not yet fully established, (c) treatment of adequately perfused, low-pressure regions of large tumors for debulking, and (d) treatment with antibodies or other agents directed against the host cells (e.g., tumor endothelial cells, fibroblasts) or the subendothelial matrix. These physiologic barriers also may pose fewer problems for treatment with a molecule or cell that has nearly 100% specificity for cells in the tumor. Until such selective molecules or cells are developed, methods are urgently needed to overcome or exploit these physiologic barriers in tumors. It is hoped that an improved understanding of transport in tumors will help in developing these strategies (162).

ACKNOWLEDGMENTS

I am grateful to my former and current collaborators who have made working on this difficult and often frustrating problem a real joy. They and others working independently on this problem have contributed significantly to the accomplishments summarized in this chapter. I wish to thank Pietro M. Gullino, Marcos Intaglietta, and Herman D. Suit for their encouragement, wise counsel, and un-

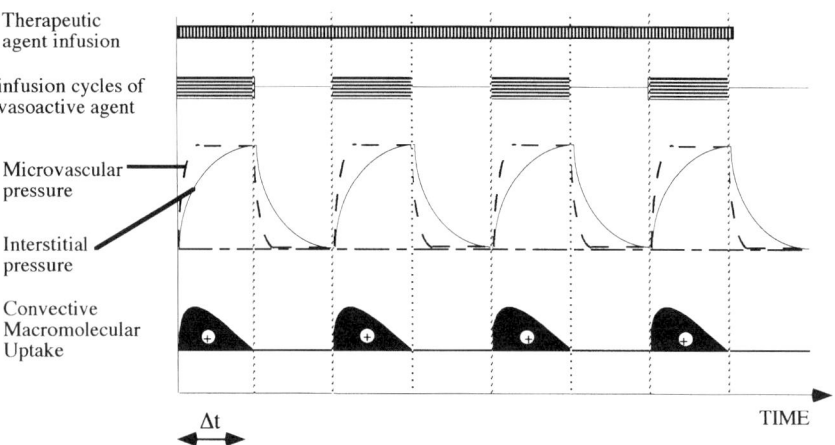

Figure 11 A novel approach to increase convective transport of molecules across tumor vessels based on the finding that there is a ~10-s delay in the transmission of intravascular pressure to the interstitial compartment. For this approach to work, the transvascular transport has to be unidirectional, *or* the extravasated molecule must bind avidly so that it does not intravasate when the intravascular pressure is lower than interstitial pressure. (Adapted from Ref. 40.)

conditional support. I also thank Carol Lyons for typing this manuscript, Stuart Friedrich for his help with the references, Lance Munn for his help with Figures 1–3, Fan Yuan with Figures 4 and 7, Gabriel Helmlinger with Figure 6, David Berk with Figure 8, Dai Fukumura with Figure 9, Larry Baxter with Figure 10, Paolo Netti with Figure 11, and Yves Boucher with Table 2. Research described here was supported primarily by grants from the National Cancer Institute, the National Science Foundation, and the American Cancer Society.

An earlier version of this chapter was published as ''1995 Whitaker Lecture: Delivery of Molecules, Particles and Cells to Solid Tumors,'' in the *Annals of Biomedical Engineering*, 24:457–473 (1996). The author thanks the Biomedical Engineering Society for allowing him to reproduce that article.

REFERENCES

1. Beardsley T. Trends in cancer epidemiology: a war not won. Scientific American 1994; 270:118–126.
2. Jain RK. Barriers to drug delivery in solid tumors. Scientific American 1994; 271: 58–65.

3. Jain RK. Transport phenomena in tumors. Advances Chemical Engineering 1994; 20:129–200.
4. Sevick EM, Jain RK. Blood flow and venous pH of tissue-isolated Walker 256 carcinoma during hyperglycemia. Cancer Res 1988; 48:1201–1207.
5. Sevick EM, Jain RK. Geometric resistance to blood flow in solid tumors perfused ex vivo: effects of tumor size and perfusion pressure. Cancer Res 1989; 49:3506–3512.
6. Gullino PM. Techniques in tumor pathophysiology. In: Busch H, ed. Methods in Cancer Research. New York: Academic Press, 1970:45–92.
7. Kristjansen PE, Roberge S, Lee I, Jain RK. Tissue-isolated human tumor xenografts in athymic nude mice. Microvasc Res 1994; 48:389–402.
8. Kristjansen PEG, Brown TJ, Shipley LA, Jain RK. Intratumor pharmacokinetics, flow resistance, and metabolism during gemcitabine infusion in ex vivo perfused human small cell lung cancer. Clin Cancer Res 1996; 2:359–367.
9. Less JR, Posner MC, Skalak T, Wolmark N, Jain RK. Geometric resistance to blood flow and vascular network architecture in human colorectal carcinoma. Microcirculation 1997; 4:25–33.
10. Dudar TE, Jain RK. Microcirculatory flow changes during tissue growth. Microvasc Res 1983; 25:1–21.
11. Zawicki DF, Jain RK, Schmid-Schoenbein GW, Chien S. Dynamics of neovascularization in normal tissue. Microvasc Res 1981; 21:27–47.
12. Leunig M, Yuan F, Berk DA, Gerweck LE, Jain RK. Angiogenesis and growth of isografted bone: quantitative in vivo assay in nude mice. Lab Investigation 1994; 71:300–307.
13. Leunig M, Yuan F, Menger MD, et al. Angiogenesis, microvascular architecture, microhemodynamics, and interstitial fluid pressure during early growth of human adenocarcinoma LS174T in SCID mice. Cancer Res 1992; 52:6553–6560.
14. Yuan F, Salehi HA, Boucher Y, Vasthare US, Tuma RF, Jain RK. Vascular permeability and microcirculation of gliomas and mammary carcinomas transplanted in rat and mouse cranial windows. Cancer Res 1994; 54:4564–4568.
15. Yamada S, Mayadas T, Yuan F, et al. Rolling in P-selectin deficient mice is reduced but not eliminated in the dorsal skin. Blood 1995; 86:3487–3492.
16. Milstone DS, Fukumura D, Padget RC, et al. Mice lacking E-selectin show normal rolling but reduced arrest of leukocytes on cytokine-activated microvascular endothelium. Microcirculation 1998. In press.
17. Detmar M, Brown LF, Schön MP, et al. Tortuous blood vessels and enhanced leukocyte adhesion in VEGF transgenic mice. J Invest Derm 1998. In press.
18. Dellian M, Witwer BP, Salehi HA, Yuan F, Jain RK. Quantitation and physiological characterization of bFGF and VEGF/VPF induced vessels in mice: effect of microenvironment on angiogenesis. Am J Pathol 1996; 149:59–72.
19. Jain RK, Schlenger K, Höckel M, Yuan F. Quantitative angiogenesis assays: Progress and problems. Nature Medicine 1997; 3:1203–1208.
20. Lichtenbeld HC, Yuan F, Michel CC, Jain RK. Perfusion of single tumor microvessels: application to vascular permeability measurement. Microcirculation 1996; 3:349–357.
21. Fukumura D, Yuan F, Monsky WL, Chen Y, Jain RK. Effect of host microenviron-

ment on the microcirculation of human colon adenocarcinoma. Am J Pathol 1997; 150:713–725.
22. Melder RJ, Brownell AL, Shoup TM, Brownell GL, Jain RK. Imaging of activated natural killer cells in mice by positron emission tomography: preferential uptake in tumors. Cancer Res 1993; 53:5867–5871.
23. Munn LL, Melder RJ, Jain RK. Analysis of cell flux in the parallel plate flow chamber: implications for cell capture studies. Biophys J 1994; 67:889–895.
24. Sasaki A, Jain RK, Maghazachi AA, Goldfarb RH, Herberman RB. Low deformability of lymphokine-activated killer cells as a possible determinant of in vivo distribution. Cancer Res 1989; 49:3742–3746.
25. Traykov TT, Jain RK. Effect of glucose and galactose on red blood cell membrane deformability. Int J Microcirculation: Clinical Experimental 1987; 6:35–44.
26. Helmlinger G, Netti PA, Lichtenbeld HC, Melder RJ, Jain RK. Solid stress inhibits the growth of multicellular tumor spheroids. Nature Biotechnol 1997; 15:778–783.
27. Munn L, Koenig GC, Jain RK, Melder R. Kinetics of adhesion molecule expression and spatial organization using targeted sampling fluorometry. BioTechniques 1995; 19:622–631.
28. Jain RK, Munn LL, Fukumura D, Melder RJ. Methods for the in vitro and in vivo quantification of adhesion between leukocytes and vascular endothelium. In: Morgan JR, Yarmush ML, eds. Methods in Molecular Medicine—Methods in Tissue Engineering. Totowa, NJ: Humana Press, 1998:Chapter 41.
29. Baxter LT, Jain RK. Transport of fluid and macromolecules in tumors. I. role of interstitial pressure and convection. Microvasc Res 1989; 37:77–104.
30. Baxter LT, Jain RK. Transport of fluid and macromolecules in tumors. II. role of heterogeneous perfusion and lymphatics. Microvasc Res 1990; 40:246–263.
31. Baxter LT, Jain RK. Transport of fluid and macromolecules in tumors. III. role of binding and metabolism. Microvasc Res 1991; 41:5–23.
32. Baxter LT, Jain RK. Transport of fluid and macromolecules in tumors. IV. a microscopic model of the perivascular distribution. Microvasc Res 1991; 41:252–272.
33. Baxter LT, Zhu H, Mackensen DG, Butler WF, Jain RK. Biodistribution of monoclonal antibodies: scale-up from mouse to man using a physiologically based pharmacokinetic model. Cancer Res 1995; 55:4611–4622.
34. Baxter LT, Zhu H, Mackensen DG, Jain RK. Physiologically based pharmacokinetic model for specific and nonspecific monoclonal antibodies and fragments in normal tissues and human tumor xenografts in nude mice. Cancer Res 1994; 54: 1517–1528.
35. Eskey CJ, Wolmark N, McDowell CL, Domach MM, Jain RK. Residence time distributions of various tracers in tumors: implications for drug delivery and blood flow measurement. J Nat Cancer Inst 1994; 86:293–299.
36. Jain RK, Baxter LT. Mechanisms of heterogeneous distribution of monoclonal antibodies and other macromolecules in tumors: significance of elevated interstitial pressure. Cancer Res 1988; 48:7022–7032.
37. Jain RK, Wei J. Dynamics of drug transport in solid tumors: Distributed parameter model. J Bioengineering 1977; 1:313–329.
38. Jain RK, Wei J, Gullino PM. Pharmacokinetics of methotrexate in solid tumors. J Pharmacokin Biopharmaceutics 1979; 7:181–194.

39. Netti PA, Roberge S, Boucher Y, Baxter LT, Jain RK. Effect of transvascular fluid exchange on arterio-venous pressure relationship: Implication for temporal and spatial heterogeneities in tumor blood flow. Microvasc Res 1996; 52:27–46.
40. Netti PA, Baxter LT, Boucher Y, Skalak R, Jain RK. Time-dependent behavior of interstitial pressure in solid tumors: Implications for drug delivery. Cancer Res 1995; 55:5451–5458.
41. Pierson RN, Price DC, Wang J, Jain RK. Extracellular water measurements: Organ tracer kinetics of bromide and sucrose in rats and man. Am J Physiol 1978; 235: 254–264.
42. Yuan F, Baxter LT, Jain RK. Pharmacokinetic analysis of two-step approaches using bifunctional and enzyme-conjugated antibodies. Cancer Res 1991; 51:3119–3130.
43. Netti P, Baxter LT, Boucher Y, Skalak R, Jain RK. Analysis of macro and microscopic fluid transport mechanisms in living tissues. AIChE J 1997; 43:818–834.
44. Folkman J. Tumor angiogenesis. In: Mendelsohn PM, Howley MAP, Liotta LA, eds. The Molecular Basis of Cancer. Philadelphia: W.B. Saunders, 1995:206–232.
45. Jain RK. Determinants of tumor blood flow: a review. Cancer Res 1988; 48:2641–2658.
46. Baish JW, Gazit Y, Berk DA, Nozue M, Baxter LT, Jain RK. A novel approach to examine the role of vascular heterogeneity in nutrient and drug delivery for tumors: an invasion percolation model. Microvasc Res 1996; 51:327–346.
47. Gazit Y, Berk DA, Leunig M, Baxter LT, Jain RK. Scale-invariant behavior and vascular network formation in normal and tumor tissue. Phys Rev Lett 1995; 75: 2428–2431.
48. Less JR, Skalak TC, Sevick EM, Jain RK. Microvascular architecture in a mammary carcinoma: branching patterns and vessel dimensions. Cancer Res 1991; 51: 265–273.
49. Patan S, Munn L, Jain RK. Intussusceptive microvascular growth in solid tumors: a novel mechanism of tumor angiogenesis. Microvasc Res 1996; 51:260–272.
50. Gazit Y, Baish JW, Safabakhsh N, Leunig M, Baxter LT, Jain RK. Fractal characteristics of tumor vascular architecture: significance and implications. Microcirculation 1997; 4:395–402.
51. Jain RK, Ward-Hartley KA. Tumor blood flow: characterization, modifications and role in hyperthermia. IEEE Transactions in Sonics and Ultrasonics 1984; 31:504–526.
52. Sevick EM, Jain RK. Viscous resistance to blood flow in solid tumors: effect of hematocrit on intratumor blood viscosity. Cancer Res 1989; 49:3513–3519.
53. Sevick EM, Jain RK. Effect of red blood cell rigidity on tumor blood flow: increase in viscous resistance during hyperglycemia. Cancer Res 1991; 51:2727–2730.
54. Endrich B, Reinhold HS, Gross JF, Intaglietta M. Tissue perfusion inhomogeneity during early tumor growth in rats. J Natl Cancer Inst 1979; 62:387–395.
55. Eskey CJ, Koretsky AP, Domach MM, Jain RK. 2H-Nuclear magnetic resonance imaging of tumor blood flow: spatial and temporal heterogeneity in a tissue-isolated mammary adenocarcinoma. Cancer Res 1992; 52:6010–6019.
56. Hamberg LM, Kristjansen PE, Hunter GJ, Wolf GL, Jain RK. Spatial heterogeneity

in tumor perfusion measured with functional computed tomography at 0.05 microliter resolution. Cancer Res 1994; 54:6032–6036.
57. Vaupel P, Jain RK. Tumor Blood Supply and Metabolic Microenvironment: Characterization and Therapeutic Implications. Stuttgart: Gustav Fischer Publications, 1991.
58. Dellian M, Helmlinger G, Yuan F, Jain RK. Fluorescence ratio imaging and optical sectioning: effect of glucose on spatial and temporal gradients. Brit J Cancer 1996; 74:1206–1215.
59. Helmlinger G, Yuan F, Dellian M, Jain RK. Interstitial pH and pO_2 gradients in solid tumors in vivo: simultaneous high-resolution measurements reveal a lack of correlation. Nature Medicine 1997; 3:177–182.
60. Martin GR, Jain RK. Fluorescence ratio imaging measurement of pH gradients: calibration and application in normal and tumor tissues. Microvasc Res 1993; 46:216–230.
61. Martin GR, Jain RK. Noninvasive measurement of interstitial pH profiles in normal and neoplastic tissue using fluorescence ratio imaging microscopy. Cancer Res 1994; 54:5670–5674.
62. Torres-Filho IP, Leunig M, Yuan F, Intaglietta M, Jain RK. Noninvasive measurement of microvascular and interstitial oxygen profiles in a human tumor in SCID mice. Proc Nat Acad Sci USA 1994; 91:2081–2085.
63. Helmlinger G, Sckell A, Dellian M, Jain RK. Acid production in variant, glycolysis-deficient and parental tumors in vivo: evidence for a role of the pentose cycle. Submitted 1998.
64. Jain RK, Shah SA, Finney PL. Continuous noninvasive monitoring of pH and temperature in rat Walker 256 carcinoma during normoglycemia and hyperglycemia. J Natl Cancer Inst 1984; 73:429–436.
65. Nozue M, Lee I, Manning JM, Manning LR, Jain RK. Oxygenation in tumors by modified hemoglobins. J Surg Oncol 1996; 62:109–114.
66. Ward KA, Jain RK. Response of tumours to hyperglycaemia: characterization, significance and role in hyperthermia. Int J Hyperthermia 1988; 4:223–250.
67. Eskey CJ, Koretsky AP, Domach MM, Jain RK. Role of oxygen vs. glucose in energy metabolism in a mammary carcinoma perfused ex vivo: direct measurement by 31P NMR. Proc Natl Acad Sci USA 1993; 90:2646–2650.
68. Helmlinger G, Endo M, Hlatky L, Ferrara N, Friedrich S, Jain RK. Dynamics of oxygen gradient-induced angiogenesis via endothelial VEGF. Submitted 1997.
69. Jain RK. Transport of molecules across tumor vasculature. Cancer Metastasis Reviews 1987; 6:559–593.
70. Dvorak HF, Brown LF, Detmar M, Dvorak AM. Vascular permeability factor/vascular endothelial growth factor, microvascular hyperpermeability, and angiogenesis. Am J Pathol 1995; 146:1029–1039.
71. Gerlowski LE, Jain RK. Microvascular permeability of normal and neoplastic tissues. Microvasc Res 1986; 31:288–305.
72. Sevick EM, Jain RK. Measurement of capillary filtration coefficient in a solid tumor. Cancer Res 1991; 51:1352–1355.
73. Yuan F, Leunig M, Berk DA, Jain RK. Microvascular permeability of albumin, vascular surface area, and vascular volume measured in human adenocarcinoma

LS174T using dorsal chamber in SCID mice. Microvasc Res 1993; 45:269–289.
74. Yuan F, Leunig M, Huang SK, Berk DA, Papahadjopoulos D, Jain RK. Microvascular permeability and interstitial penetration of sterically stabilized (stealth) liposomes in a human tumor xenograft. Cancer Res 1994; 54:3352–3356.
75. Yuan F, Dellian M, Fukumura D, et al. Vascular permeability in a human tumor xenograft: molecular size-dependence and cutoff size. Cancer Res 1995; 55:3752–3756.
76. Dellian M, Yuan F, Trubetskoy V, Torchilin V, Jain RK. Vascular permeability in a human tumor xenograft: molecular charge dependence. Submitted 1998.
77. Hobbs S, Monsky W, Yuan F, et al. Regulation of transport pathways in tumor vessels: role of tumor type and host microenvironment. Proc Natl Acad Sci USA 1998. In press.
78. Roberts WG, Palade G. Neovasculature induced by vascular endothelial growth factor is fenestrated. Cancer Res 1997; 57:1207–1211.
79. Yuan F, Chen Y, Dellian M, Safabakhsh N, Ferrara N, Jain RK. Time-dependent changes in vascular permeability and morphology in established human tumor xenografts induced by an anti-VEGF/VPF antibody. Proc Natl Acad Sci USA 1996; 93:14,765–14,770.
80. Arbit E, Lee J, DiResta G. Interstitial hypertension in human brain tumors: possible role in peritumoral edema formulation. In: Nagai H, Kamiya K, Ishi S, eds. Intracranial Pressure. Vol. IX. Tokyo: Springer-Verlag, 1994:609–614.
81. Boucher Y, Baxter LT, Jain RK. Interstitial pressure gradients in tissue-isolated and subcutaneous tumors: implications for therapy. Cancer Res 1990; 50:4478–4484.
82. Boucher Y, Jain RK. Microvascular pressure is the principal driving force for interstitial hypertension in solid tumors: implications for vascular collapse. Cancer Res 1992; 52:5110–5114.
83. Boucher Y, Lee I, Jain RK. Lack of general correlation between interstitial fluid pressure and pO_2 in tumors. Microvasc Res 1995; 50:175–182.
84. Boucher Y, Kirkwood JM, Opacic D, Desantis M, Jain RK. Interstitial hypertension in superficial metastatic melanomas in humans. Cancer Res 1991; 51:6691–6694.
85. Boucher Y, Salehi H, Witwer B, Harsh GR, Jain RK. Interstitial fluid pressure in intracranial tumors in patients and in rodents: effect of anti-edema therapy. Brit J Cancer 1997; 75:829–836.
86. Curti BD, Urba WJ, Alvord WG, et al. Interstitial pressure of subcutaneous nodules in melanoma and lymphoma patients: changes during treatment. Cancer Res 1993; 53:2204–2207s.
87. Gutmann R, Leunig M, Feyh J, et al. Interstitial hypertension in head and neck tumors in patients: correlation with tumor size. Cancer Res 1992; 52:1993–1995.
88. Jain RK. Transport of molecules in the tumor interstitium: a review. Cancer Res 1987; 47:3039–3051.
89. Less JR, Posner MC, Boucher Y, Borochovitz D, Wolmark N, Jain RK. Interstitial hypertension in human breast and colorectal tumors. Cancer Res 1992; 52:6371–6374.
90. Nathanson SD, Nelson L. Interstitial fluid pressure in breast cancer, benign breast conditions, and breast parenchyma. Ann Surg Oncol 1994; 1:333–338.

91. Roh HD, Boucher Y, Kalnicki S, Buchsbaum R, Bloomer WD, Jain RK. Interstitial hypertension in carcinoma of uterine cervix in patients: possible correlation with tumor oxygenation and radiation response. Cancer Res 1991; 51:6695–6698.
92. Znati CA, Karasek K, Faul C, et al. Interstitial fluid pressure changes in cervical carcinomas in patients undergoing radiation therapy: a potential prognostic factor. Submitted 1998.
93. Znati CA, Rosenstein M, Boucher Y, Epperly MW, Bloomer WD, Jain RK. Effect of radiation on interstitial fluid pressure and oxygenation in a human colon carcinoma xenograft. Cancer Res 1996; 56:964–968.
94. Stohrer M, Boucher Y, Stangassinger M, Jain RK. Oncotic pressure in human tumor xenografts. Proc AACR 1995.
95. Boucher Y, Leunig M, Jain RK. Tumor angiogenesis and interstitial hypertension. Cancer Res 1996; 56:4264–4266.
96. Rippe B, Haraldsson B. Fluid and protein fluxes across small and large pores in the microvasculature. Application of two-pore equations. *Acta Physiol Scand* 1987; 131:411–428.
97. Berk DA, Yuan F, Leunig M, Jain RK. Fluorescence photobleaching with spatial Fourier analysis: measurement of diffusion in light-scattering media. Biophys J 1993; 65:2428–2436.
98. Chary SR, Jain RK. Direct measurement of interstitial convection and diffusion of albumin in normal and neoplastic tissues by fluorescence photobleaching. Proc Natl Acad Sci USA 1989; 86:5385–5389.
99. Johnson EM, Berk DA, Jain RK, Deen WM. Diffusion and partitioning of proteins in charged agarose gels. Biophys J 1995; 68:1561–1568.
100. Johnson EM, Berk DA, Jain RK, Deen WM. Hindered diffusion in agarose gels: test of effective medium model. Biophys J 1996; 70:1017–1026.
101. Johnson M, Berk DA, Blankschtein D, Golan DE, Jain RK, Langer R. Lateral diffusion of small compounds in human stratum corneum and model lipid bilayer systems. Biophys J 1996; 71:2656–2668.
102. Nugent LJ, Jain RK. Extravascular diffusion in normal and neoplastic tissues. Cancer Res 1984; 44:238–244.
103. Swabb EA, Wei J, Gullino PM. Diffusion and convection in normal and neoplastic tissues. Cancer Res 1974; 34:2814.
104. Berk DA, Yuan F, Leunig M, Jain RK. Direct in vivo measurement of targeted binding in a human tumor xenograft. Proc Natl Acad Sci USA 1997; 94:1785–1790.
105. Boucher Y, Brekken C, Netti PA, Baxter LT, Jain RK. Intratumoral infusion of fluid: estimation of hydraulic conductivity and compliance and implications for the delivery of therapeutic agents. Brit J Cancer 1998. In press.
106. Znati CA, Boucher Y, Rosenstein M, Turner D, Watkins S, Jain RK. Effect of radiation on the interstitial matrix and hydraulic conductivity of tumors. Submitted 1998.
107. Juweid M, Neumann R, Paik C, et al. Micropharmacology of monoclonal antibodies in solid tumor: direct experimental evidence for a binding site barrier. Cancer Res 1992; 52:5144.
108. Kaufman EN, Jain RK. Quantification of transport and binding parameters using

fluorescence recovery after photobleaching. Potential for in vivo applications. Biophys J 1990; 58:873–885.
109. Kaufman EN, Jain RK. Measurement of mass transport and reaction parameters in bulk solution using photobleaching. Reaction limited binding regime. Biophys J 1991; 60:596–610.
110. Kaufman EN, Jain RK. Effect of bivalent interaction upon apparent antibody affinity: experimental confirmation of theory using fluorescence photobleaching and implications for antibody binding assays. Cancer Res 1992; 52:4157–4167.
111. Kaufman EN, Jain RK. In vitro measurement and screening of monoclonal antibody affinity using fluorescence photobleaching. J Immunological Methods 1992; 155:1–17.
112. Jain RK. Delivery of novel therapeutic agents in tumors: physiological barriers and strategies. J Natl Cancer Inst 1989; 81:570–576.
113. Leu AJ, Berk DA, Yuan F, Jain RK. Flow velocity in the superficial lymphatic network of the mouse tail. Am J Physiol 1994; 267:H1507–H1513.
114. Berk DA, Swartz MA, Leu AJ, Jain RK. Transport in lymphatic capillaries: II. Microscopic velocity measurement with fluorescence recovery after photobleaching. Am J Physiol 1996; 270:H330–H337.
115. Swartz MA, Berk DA, Jain RK. Transport in lymphatic capillaries: I. Macroscopic measurements using residence time distribution theory. Am J Physiol 1996; 270:H324–H329.
116. Jeltsch M, Kaipainen A, Joukov V, et al. Hyperplasia of lymphatic vessels in VEGF-C transgenic mice. Science 1997; 276:1423–1425.
117. Leu A, Berk DA, Alitalo K, Jain RK. Molecular and functional evaluation of initial lymphatics in a murine sarcoma. Submitted 1998.
118. Melder RJ, Munn LL, Yamada S, Ohkubo C, Jain RK. Selectin and integrin mediated T lymphocyte rolling and arrest on TNF-α-activated endothelium is augmented by erythrocytes. Biophys J 1995; 69:2131–2138.
119. Munn LL, Melder RJ, Jain RK. Role of erythrocytes in leukocyte-endothelial interactions: mathematical model and experimental validation. Biophys J 1996; 71:466–478.
120. Fukumura D, Salehi H, Witwer B, Tuma RF, Melder RJ, Jain RK. TNF-alpha-induced leukocyte-adhesion in normal and tumor vessels: effect of tumor type, transplantation site and host. Cancer Res 1995; 55:4824–4829.
121. Yamada S, Melder RJ, Leunig M, Ohkubo C, Jain RK. Leukocyte-rolling increases with age. Blood 1995; 86:4707–4708.
122. Melder RJ, Elmaleh D, Brownell AL, Brownell GL, Jain RK. A method for labeling cells for positron emission tomography (PET) studies. J Immunological Methods 1994; 175:79–87.
123. Melder RJ, Jain RK. Kinetics of interleukin-2 induced changes in rigidity of human natural killer cells. Cell Biophysics 1992; 20:161–176.
124. Jain RK, Koenig G, Dellian M, Fukumura D, Munn LL, Melder RJ. Leukocyte-endothelial adhesion and angiogenesis in tumors. Cancer Metastasis Rev 1996; 15:195–204.
125. Melder RJ, Jain RK. Reduction of rigidity in human activated natural killer cells by thioglycollate treatment. J Immunological Methods 1994; 175:69–77.

126. Melder RJ, Salehi HA, Jain RK. Localization of activated natural killer cells in MCaIV mammary carcinoma grown in cranial windows in C3H mice. Microvasc Res 1995; 50:35–44.
127. Sasaki A, Melder RJ, Whiteside TL, Herberman RB, Jain RK. Preferential localization of human adherent lymphokine-activated killer cells in tumor microcirculation. J Natl Cancer Inst 1991; 83:433–437.
128. Ohkubo C, Bigos D, Jain RK. Interleukin-2 induced leukocyte adhesion to the normal and tumor microvascular endothelium in vivo and its inhibition by dextran sulfate: implications for vascular leak syndrome. Cancer Res 1991; 51:1561–1563.
129. Melder RJ, Koenig G, Witwer BP, Safabakhsh N, Munn LL, Jain RK. During angiogenesis, vascular endothelial growth factor and basic fibroblast growth factor regulate natural killer cell adhesion to tumor endothelium. Nature Medicine 1996; 2:992–997.
130. Jallal B, Powell F, Zachwieja J, et al. Suppression of tumor growth in vivo by local and systemic 90K level increase. Cancer Res 1995; 55:3223–3227.
131. Melder RJ, Koenig G, Munn LL, Jain RK. Adhesion of activated natural killer cells to TNF-alpha treated endothelium under physiological flow conditions. Natural Immunity 1997; 15:154–163.
132. Gamble JR, Vadas MA. Endothelial adhesiveness for blood neutrophils is inhibited by transforming growth factor-beta. Science 1988; 242:97–99.
133. Gamble JR, Vadas MA. Endothelial cell adhesiveness for human T lymphocytes is inhibited by transforming growth factor-beta. J Immunology 1991; 146:1149–1154.
134. Gamble JR, Khew-Goodall Y. Transforming growth factor-beta inhibits E-selectin expression on human endothelial cells. J Immunology 1993; 150:4494–4503.
135. Fidler IJ. Modulation of the organ microenvironment for treatment of cancer metastasis. J Natl Cancer Inst 1995; 87:1588–1592.
136. Kitayama J, Nagawa J, Yasuhara H, et al. Suppressive effect of basic fibroblast growth factor on transendothelial emigration of CD4(+) T-lymphocyte. Cancer Res 1994; 54:4729–4733.
137. Haying JB, Williams SK. Reduced adhesion of human microvascular endothelial cells to collagen in response to basic FGF is mediated by $\beta 1$ integrin. FASEB J 1994; 8:Abstr. 263.
138. Dedrick RL. Animal scale-up. J Pharmacokinetics Biopharmaceutics 1973; 1:435–461.
139. Gerlowski LE, Jain RK. Physiologically based pharmacokinetic modeling: principles and applications. J Pharmaceut Sci 1983; 72:1103–1127.
140. Zhu H, Melder R, Baxter L, Jain RK. Physiologically based kinetic model of effector cell biodistribution in mammals: implications for adoptive immunotherapy. Cancer Res 1996; 56:3771–3781.
141. Zhu H, Baxter L, Jain RK. Potential and limitations of radioimmunodetection and radioimmunotherapy with monoclonal antibodies: evaluation using a physiologically-based pharmacokinetic model. J Nucl Med 1997; 38:731–741.
142. Zhu H, Jain RK, Baxter LT. Tumor pretargeting for radioimmunodetection and radioimmunotherapy: evaluation using a physiologically based pharmacokinetic model. J Nucl Med 1998; 39:65–76.

143. Jain RK. Effect of inhomogeneities and finite boundaries on temperature distribution in a perfused medium with application to tumors. Trans. ASME J Biomechanical Engineering 1978; 100:235–241.
144. Jain RK. Transient temperature distributions in an infinite perfused medium due to a time-dependent, spherical heat source. Trans ASME J Biomechanical Engineering 1979; 101:82–86.
145. Jain RK, Boucher Y, Stacey-Clear A, Moore R, Kopans D. Method for locating tumors prior to needle biopsy, U.S. Patent Number 5,396,897, March 14, 1995.
146. Dudar TE, Jain RK. Differential response of normal and tumor microcirculation to hyperthermia. Cancer Res 1984; 44:605–612.
147. Fukumura D, Yuan F, Endo M, Jain RK. Role of nitric oxide in tumor microcirculation: blood flow, vascular permeability, and leukocyte-endothelial interactions. Am J Pathol 1997; 150:713–725.
148. Gerlowski LE, Jain RK. Effect of hyperthermia on microvascular permeability to macromolecules in normal and tumor tissues. Int J Microcirculation: Clinical Experimental 1985; 4:363–372.
149. Kristensen CA, Nozue M, Boucher Y, Jain RK. Reduction of interstitial fluid pressure after TNF-alpha treatment of human melanoma xenografts. Brit J Cancer 1996; 74:533–536.
150. Kristensen CA, Roberge S, Jain RK. Effect of tumor necrosis factor-alpha on vascular resistance, nitric oxide production, glucose and oxygen consumption in perfused, tissue-isolated human melanoma xenografts. Clin Cancer Res 1997; 3:319–324.
151. Fukumura D, Jain RK. Role of nitric oxide in angiogenesis and microcirculation in tumors. Cancer Metastasis Rev 1998. In press.
152. Baxter LT, Jain RK. Pharmacokinetic analysis of the microscopic distribution of enzyme-conjugated antibodies and prodrugs: comparison with experimental data. Brit J Cancer 1996; 73:447–456.
153. Baxter LT, Yuan F, Jain RK. Pharmacokinetic analysis of the perivascular distribution of bifunctional antibodies and haptens: comparison with experimental data. Cancer Res 1992; 52:5838–5844.
154. Kristjansen PE, Boucher Y, Jain RK. Dexamethasone reduces the interstitial fluid pressure in a human colon adenocarcinoma xenograft. Cancer Res 1993; 53:4764–4766.
155. Lee I, Boucher Y, Jain RK. Nicotinamide can lower tumor interstitial fluid pressure: mechanistic and therapeutic implications. Cancer Res 1992; 52:3237–3240.
156. Lee I, Boucher Y, Demhartner TJ, Jain RK. Changes in tumor blood flow, oxygenation and interstitial fluid pressure induced by pentoxifylline. Brit J Cancer 1994; 69:492–496.
157. Lee I, Demhartner TJ, Boucher Y, Jain RK, Intaglietta M. Effect of hemodilution and resuscitation on tumor interstitial fluid pressure, blood flow, and oxygenation. Microvas Res 1994; 48:1–12.
158. Leunig M, Goetz AE, Dellian M, et al. Interstitial fluid pressure in solid tumors following hyperthermia: possible correlation with therapeutic response. Cancer Res 1992; 52:487–490.
159. Leunig M, Goetz AE, Gamarra F, Zetterer G, Messmer K, Jain RK. Photodynamic

therapy-induced alterations in interstitial fluid pressure, volume and water content of an amelanotic melanoma in the hamster. Brit J Cancer 1994; 69:101–103.
160. Zlotecki RA, Baxter LT, Boucher Y, Jain RK. Pharmacologic modification of tumor blood flow and interstitial fluid pressure in a human tumor xenograft: network analysis and mechanistic interpretation. Microvasc Res 1995; 50:429–443.
161. Zlotecki RA, Boucher Y, Lee I, Baxter LT, Jain RK. Effect of angiotensin II induced hypertension on tumor blood flow and interstitial fluid pressure. Cancer Res 1993; 53:2466–2468.
162. Jain RK. Delivery of molecular medicine to solid tumors. Science 1996; 271:1079–1080.

3
Unconjugated Monoclonal Antibody Therapy of Lymphoma

David G. Maloney
University of Washington and Fred Hutchinson Cancer Research Center, Seattle, Washington

I. INTRODUCTION

Despite initial sensitivity to chemotherapy, and even the induction of complete remissions, patients with advanced-stage low-grade B-cell malignancies are not cured by conventional chemotherapy. The disease usually follows a continuously relapsing course characterized by increased chemoresistance and decreasing host tolerance to the side effects of therapy. While some patients with the aggressive non-Hodgkin's lymphomas (NHLs) are cured by combination chemotherapy, many patients relapse and subsequently are not candidates for, or fail, salvage therapy with high-dose therapy and stem-cell transplantation. Additional agents with greater tumor specificity are needed, and the use of antibodies against tumors has generated a great deal of interest.

Directing the immune system to attack cancer has been tried using a variety of methods for many years. Nearly 100 years ago Ehrlich proposed what has been termed the ''magic bullet'' idea of using antibodies to target cancer (1). However, it was not until the development of monoclonal antibody technology by Kohler and Milstein that antibodies with defined specificity for a target antigen could be produced (2). This made antibody therapy a possibility. Subsequent advances in molecular biology have made it possible to produce altered antibodies or antibody fragments, resulting in the many new agents that are entering the clinical arena for cancer therapy. Among the areas of antibody therapy that has demonstrated the most promise is the treatment of hematologic malignancies, specifically the B- and T-cell non-Hodgkin's lymphomas. Approaches utilizing unconjugated, toxin-conjugated, and radiolabeled antibodies have demonstrated promising antitumor activity. This review will focus on the use of unconjugated monoclonal antibodies directed against lymphoid cell-surface antigens for the treatment of B- and T-cell lymphomas.

The recent FDA approval for marketing of the chimeric Anti-CD20 antibody IDEC-C2B8 (Rituxan) for the treatment of relapsed low-grade B-cell lymphoma represents the first monoclonal antibody approved for cancer therapy. This chimeric unconjugated antibody and its target, the CD20 antigen, both have characteristics that are responsible for the clinical activity observed. This new treatment will provide additional options for the management of patients with CD20-expressing lymphomas and ushers into the clinic the reality of immunotherapy from experimental and clinical laboratory studies. Hopefully, this is the first of many new treatments that will provide greater tumor specificity with less host toxicity that will ultimately, either alone or in combination with standard chemotherapy, alter the natural history of low-grade or relapsed NHL patients.

The success of these antibody-based approaches for the treatment of lymphoma can be traced to careful consideration of the characteristics of the target antigen, the tumor, and the antibody. These will be reviewed here.

II. LYMPHOID ANTIGENS

The lymphoid malignancies are composed of clonal expansions of B- or T-lymphocytes. Both the B-cell and T-cell phenotypes express tumor-specific antigens as well as lineage-specific antigens. The B-cell surface immunoglobulin (idiotype) and the T-cell antigen receptor are proteins formed by recombination of multiple gene segments, and the sequence and structure of the antigen receptor are unique to each patient's malignant clone. These proteins can be targeted as tumor-specific antigens using anti-idiotypic or anticlonotypic monoclonal antibodies. Treatment with patient-specific anti-idiotype antibodies was one of the first approaches to demonstrate clinical antitumor activity in patients with relapsed B-cell non-Hodgkin's lymphoma (3). Despite significant activity, the implementation of this therapy is difficult, because each antibody has to be custom made for each patient.

In addition to the antigen receptors, B- and T-cell lymphomas express a large number of antigens, some of which are more or less restricted to the B-cell or T-cell lineages. These antigens can be used as targets for immunotherapy, with the advantage that a single antibody would be expected to react with tumor cells from all patients with the tumor type that expresses the target antigen. The downside of this approach is that these lineage-specific antigens are also expressed on some normal B- or T-cells of the patient, thus decreasing the "tumor specificity" of the treatment. The degree that this presents a problem is determined by the number and type of normal cells that express the target antigen.

Table 1 Characteristics of Selected Lymphoma Tumor Antigens

Antigen	Distribution	Modulation	Mutation	Function
CD20	B-cells	No	No	Ca^{2+} channel
CD19	B-cells	Yes	No	Signal transduction complex
Ig idiotype	B-cells	Yes	Yes	Antigen receptor
CD40	B-cells	Yes	No	Costimulatory molecule receptor
CD22	B-cells	Yes	No	Adhesion receptor
CD25	T-cells	Yes	No	IL-2 receptor alpha
HLA-DR	B-cells T-cells	No	Yes	Antigen presentation
CD5	T-cells B-cell CLL	Yes	No	Ligand for CD72
CD52	T-cells B-cells Monocytes platelets/other	No	Yes	Unknown
CD10	Pre-B-cells Some B-cells Some T-cells	Yes	No	Zinc metalloprotease
CD4	T-cells	Yes	No	T-cell antigen recognition
CD21	B-cells	?	No	EBV/C3d receptor on B-cells

The most well-characterized and -utilized targets for immunotherapy have included CD20, immunoglobulin idiotype, CD52, CD19, CD22, CD5, HLA-DR, CD40, and CD25. While each antigen is different, a number of factors must be considered when applying an antibody-based treatment directed against an antigen on the tumor cell. A sampling of the most promising of these antigens and their characteristics is shown in Table 1.

III. ANTIGEN CHARACTERISTICS TO CONSIDER FOR ANTIBODY THERAPY

A. Tissue Distribution

Foremost is the tissue distribution of the target antigen. Ideally, the antigen is expressed only on the tumor cells and not on host cells, and especially not on any critical host tissue types. As an example, the antigen CD52 is widely expressed on both B- and T-cells, and treatment with the CAMPATH-1H antibody can cause profound immunosuppression in addition to antitumor effects (4). In contrast, as just discussed, the antigen receptor (immunoglobulin idiotype) is nearly tumor specific, and treatment with anti-idiotype antibodies causes minimal toxicity. Many of the other B- and T-cell antigens are lineage specific and do not appear to be expressed on other critical host tissues. Thus, if the treatment is successful in eliminating all of the cells expressing the target antigen, there would also be depletion of the normal cells expressing the antigen. In cases where the antigen is not expressed on early lymphoid cells or on stem cells, the normal cells would be expected to repopulate following antibody treatment. Very careful consideration of antigen expression is required to minimize toxicity, especially when using a toxin or radiolabeled antibody.

A second consideration is the antigen density on the cell surface. In nearly all cases a higher density of antigen results in greater antitumor effect. An additional important factor includes the disposition of the target antigen. This includes whether the antigen is stable in the cell membrane or whether it modulates off of the cell surface and internalizes rapidly following antibody binding. Secretion of the antigen into the circulation by the tumor cell or by normal cells may result in high levels of free antigen that block the antibody from reaching the tumor cells.

The answers to these questions determine the type of antibody therapy that may be applied. For example, CD20 is expressed in high copy number on the cell surface of most B-cell lymphomas (5). It is tightly integrated into the cell-surface membrane and does not modulate or internalize upon antibody binding. It is not secreted or shed into the circulation and is not present on early pre-B-cells, stem cells, or other critical host tissues. Preclinical studies demonstrated safety and B-cell depletion (6). CD20 has proven to be an excellent target for therapy with unconjugated antibodies (IDEC-C2B8) (7,8) or radiolabeled antibodies (^{131}-B1 (9,10), ^{90}Y-IDEC-2B8 (11)), but it is not a good target for immunotoxin-based therapy that requires internalization into the cell of the antibody-toxin-antigen complex. In contrast, CD19 or CD22, which has a similar level of density on the cell surface and is restricted to the B-cell subset, rapidly internalizes upon antibody binding. This antigen has been utilized as a target for delivery of a variety of ricin-based immunotoxins (12,13), whereas unmodified antibodies have shown limited activity (14).

Thus, the characteristics and the expression of the target antigens are critical in determining the outcome of antibody-based therapies.

B. Antigen Mutation Frequency

Ideally, the target antigen would have a biologic function critical to the tumor cell's existence and there would be no possibility of antigen mutation or loss.

Listed in Table 1 are the known functions and mutations of selected lymphoma antigens that have been used as targets for antibody-directed therapy. In most cases, current antibody therapies have been unable to exert a selective pressure powerful enough against the antigen-expressing cells to result in antigen-negative escape. However, several examples have been very illustrative. Early work with custom anti-idiotype MAb against the B-cell surface immunoglobulin demonstrated that idiotype variants existed in the tumor cells prior to antibody treatment (15). These were identified by isolation and sequencing of the cell-surface immunoglobulin genes that produced the idiotype structures. Variants containing a single amino acid substitution could result in loss of anti-idiotype antibody binding. Following therapy with monoclonal anti-idiotype antibodies, many patients relapsed with tumors that expressed variant immunoglobulins that no longer bound to the treatment antibody. Interestingly, complete immunoglobulin loss variants were rare, suggesting that the surface immunoglobulin may be critical to the survival of the B-cell lymphoma. The mechanism of variant generation is the result of continued activity of the recombinase activity that is important in the generation of antibody diversity and in the generation of antibody affinity maturation. Follicular lymphoma cells continue to express this activity. Thus, treatment with a single monoclonal antibody frequently resulted in the outgrowth of idiotype negative variants that in some cases could still be treated with a second or third monoclonal anti-idiotype antibody directed against other idiotopes of the tumor immunoglobulin (16). This activity is absent in chronic lymphocytic leukemias and myeloma, which may present the idiotype as a more stable antigen for immunologic attack. This demonstrates that the target itself may have different characteristics, depending on the stage and differentiation of the tumor cell. Evidence for idiotype selection demonstrates the power of anti-idiotype antibody therapy, while it also demonstrates a major limitation. Efforts to overcome this problem include treatment with multiple anti-idiotype antibodies and the use of an idiotype vaccine in the patient to generate a polyclonal anti-idiotype immune response (17). However, in animal models, anti-idiotype antibody therapy or the generation of an immune response to the immunoglobulin idiotype results in the expression of cell-surface Ig loss variants (18). It remains to be seen if this will be a problem of idiotype vaccination clinical trials.

Little is known about the mutation frequency of the lineage-specific antigens. In most cases antigen variants due to mutation have not been observed. In the case of the CD20 antigen, patients with an antitumor response to IDEC-C2B8 who subsequently relapse have continued to express CD20 reactive with the treatment antibody. More data will be available on this as this treatment becomes more widely used.

Antigen-negative variants present a problem for antibody- or immunotoxin-based treatments, where the antibody would not have an effect on antigen-negative cells. With targeted radioisotopes, however, there is the possibility that antigen-negative cells in the vicinity of antigen-positive cells would be killed due to the cross-fire effect (19). This is obviously a double-edged sword, because radiolabeled antibodies also have dose-limiting toxicities due to radiation exposure to the nearby normal cells (9,10).

C. The Biological Function of the Target Antigen

Over the past few years there has been an increasing realization of the importance of the biologic function of the target antigen. Early experience with nonlabeled anti-idiotype antibodies and recent experience with CD20 (20), CD19 (21), and CD40 (22) suggest that interaction of the antibody with the target antigen may cause direct tumor effects. This may occur through several mechanisms, including: (a) blocking of a natural ligand (for example, Anti-CD25–blocking IL-2), (b) mimicking a natural ligand (for example, anti-idiotype–simulating antigen), and (c) interfering with the functioning of the surface molecule (CD20, CD19). Each of these may cause direct effects on the tumor cell by causing or preventing cell signaling outside of the context of the normal cell cycle or without required cofactor stimulation from accessory cells. Some lymphoma cells respond to this by the induction of apoptosis.

As an example, during clinical trials with monoclonal anti-idiotype antibodies there was a poor correlation between the isotype of the murine antibody and the clinical outcome. This suggested that more may be involved in the antitumor effect than the immune-mediated mechanisms of tumor cell killing involving complement or ADCC, which are in large part dependent on the isotype of the antibody. Subsequent work found that the ability of the treatment anti-idiotype antibody to induce tyrosine phosphorylation in the patients tumor cells in vitro correlated with the effectiveness of the antitumor effect in vivo (23). This suggests that the tumor cell is triggered by the anti-idiotype antibody (?simulating antigen) in the absence of the normal cofactors required for cell proliferation (possibly CD40 ligand), which may result in programmed cell death.

In a similar fashion, in vitro effects have been reported using monoclonal antibodies against CD20 (20), CD19 (21), CD25 (24), and CD40 (22). In some cases (CD25 and anti-tac antibody) this is clearly due to the blocking of a natural ligand (IL-2); in other cases the mechanism of growth inhibition is still unknown. As an example, the Anti-CD20 antibody IDEC-C2B8 has direct antiproliferative activity against some but not all CD20-positive B-cell lines in vitro (25). DHL-4 cells are derived from a transformed follicular lymphoma patient and carry the characteristic t(14:18) translocation resulting in the overexpression of bcl-2. These cells are growth arrested by incubation with IDEC-C2B8 but not by other Anti-CD20 antibodies. Following growth arrest, the cells rapidly undergo apoptosis. The degree that this effect is responsible for the antitumor activity observed in clinical trials is not known. While this area is largely still unexplored, the antitumor effect of antibody-based therapy (especially that of unconjugated monoclonal antibodies) is likely in part dependent on such effect. Trials of immunotoxins or radiolabeled antibodies may also have some part of their antitumor activity due directly to the antibody binding to the target antigen.

IV. ANTIBODY ADMINISTRATION AND TISSUE DISTRIBUTION

In the earliest clinical trials of monoclonal antibody–based treatments, it became clear that, following intravenous administration of antibody, the antibody could rapidly be detected binding to tumor cells in the blood, bone marrow, spleen, and lymph node tissues. In most cases, when enough antibody can be administered to achieve persistent saturating antibody levels in the peripheral blood circulation, tumor cells are accessible to the antibody. In clinical trials with anti-idiotype, Anti-CD20, and other antibodies, biopsy of tumor sites following antibody administration has observed tumor cells coated with the treatment antibody. This may be due to the fact that most lymphoma masses are in vascular-rich tissues, such as lymph nodes, spleen, or bone marrow. However, a number of factors may still block antibody–tumor cell binding. These include the secretion of blocking antigen (such as anti-idiotype antibody therapy in patients with immunoglobulin- (idiotype-)-secreting lymphomas) or due to the development of an immune response against the treatment antibody (HAMA or HACA). In general, unlike the poorly perfused solid tumors, the lymphomas and leukemias are usually saturable. In most cases this has been accomplished by delivery of the antibody directly into the blood stream using intravenous administration. Recently, however, subcutaneous injection of CAMPATH-1H has been reported to be a successful method that decreases some of the infusional toxicity associated with intravenous administration of this antibody (26). It remains to be determined if this approach will have advantages in the treatment with other antibodies.

V. ANTIBODY CHARACTERISTICS

In addition to consideration of the antigen characteristics, the characteristics of the antibody used for lymphoma treatment is critical. Factors such as the type of the antibody (murine, chimeric, human), its affinity and avidity for the target antigen, and its ability to interact with the human immune effector mechanisms such as complement or immune effector cells are important. Each antibody has a pattern of recognition for its antigen and cross-reactivity with other similar structures. Some antibodies recognize different epitopes on the same target antigen and can cause different effects. For example, some Anti-CD3 antibodies are activating, whereas others block T-cell signaling. In addition, the affinity for the target antigen may also vary and may also determine whether the antibody induces target antigen modulation.

The effect of unconjugated monoclonal antibodies depends on the antibody interacting with either the human complement cascade or human ADCC effector cells or by direct effects caused by the antibody binding to the target cells. Murine immunoglobulin isotypes vary in their ability to mediate cell killing in vitro using human immune mechanisms. In general the IgG2a isotype is the most active, while murine IgG1, and IgG2b are minimally active. In contrast, the human IgG1 constant region confers the greatest ability to interact with human complement or ADCC effector cells. Currently there are few totally human Ig monoclonal antibodies in clinical trials. However, genetic engineering has made it possible to produce chimeric and humanized antibodies. Chimeric antibodies generally contain human IgG1 and human kappa constant regions with intact murine variable regions, while "humanized" antibodies are further altered by grafting only the complementarity-determining regions (CDRs) of the murine variable regions onto a human variable region framework. Chimerized or humanized antibodies have a greater ability to mediate CDC and ADCC in vitro (6), and this may in part explain the greater clinical activity of IDEC-C2B8 over prior clinical trials of the murine Anti-CD20 antibody 1F5 (27). However, direct comparison of the chimeric antibody IDEC-C2B8 with the parent murine IgG1 antibody IDEC-2B8 has not been done. Interestingly, the murine and chimeric antibodies both directly cause apoptosis in a similar rate and intensity against sensitive cell lines in vitro (25). These direct antiproliferative effects of monoclonal antibodies may also play a critical role in the activity of unconjugated antibodies in vivo. Not all antibodies are identical in this activity, thus consideration of direct effects should be undertaken. Unfortunately, we do not yet know the contribution of these direct effects to the observed antitumor clinical activity of most monoclonal antibodies.

Early studies utilized unmodified murine antibodies, and, in some patients, rapid rejection of the treatment antibody occurred through the generation of a HAMA response. In practice, treatment of patients with B-cell non-Hodgkin's lymphoma using unconjugated murine antibodies seldom results in HAMA formation, due to underlying immune dysfunction caused by the disease and possibly by prior chemotherapy. In contrast, treatment of patients with T-cell lymphomas or patients with solid cancers such as breast or colon cancer with unmodified murine antibodies rapidly induces HAMA response in nearly all patients, even if they have undergone extensive prior chemotherapy. Attachment of a radiolabel appears to increase the risk of HAMA, while attachment of a toxin (such as ricin) makes the development of HAMA and immune responses to the toxin occur in the majority of patients. The production of chimeric or humanized antibodies that contain mostly human immunoglobulin structures has markedly decreased the immune responses against the antibody in most patients.

VI. UNCONJUGATED MONOCLONAL ANTIBODY THERAPY—GENERAL PRINCIPLES

A number of important conclusions can be drawn from the early clinical trials of unconjugated monoclonal antibody therapy for lymphoma. As discussed in the previous sections, the characteristics of the target antigen are largely responsible for the success and for the failure of antibody therapy. Shown in Table 2 are the characteristics of an "ideal" tumor antigen for unconjugated monoclonal antibody therapy. Thus far, all described cell-surface antigens have fallen short of the ideal goal, but some have the majority of these factors. While each characteristic may not be absolutely essential for antitumor activity, the absence of these features will generally lead to less tumor specificity and greater host toxicity and/or increase the chance for tumor cell escape. Critical considerations for treatment with unconjugated antibodies include the following. The antigen must be present on every tumor cell, and the antigen must not be expressed on critical host tissues. Mutations in the antigen or antigen loss variants should not exist. The antigen should not modulate, be secreted, or exist in high levels in the circulation. The effector mechanisms of tumor cell kill depend on either immune-mediated effects (ADCC or complement) or direct antiproliferative effects of the antibody. The antibody characteristics are also critical in determining many of these functions. The most important concept to remember is that with unconjugated antibody therapy, the antigen must be expressed on all of the clonogenic tumor cells, and

TABLE 2 Characteristics of an Ideal Target Antigen for Unconjugated Monoclonal Antibody Therapy

---
Expressed *only* on the tumor cells
   Not expressed on critical host cells
   No significant toxicity if all of the positive cells are eliminated
Expressed on *all* of the tumor cells
Expressed in high copy number
No mutation or variant antigen expression
Antigen has a critical biological function
Antigen is necessary for tumor cell survival
Not shed or secreted
No modulation
---

there should be little chance of variant antigen or antigen loss variants that would lead to tumor escape. Those antigens that are critical to the survival of the cell are most likely those that have an important biologic function. Unconjugated antibodies that can bind to that antigen and either mimic or induce function or those that may block function may have biologic effects that result in growth inhibition or cell death.

VII. MECHANISM OF ANTITUMOR ACTIVITY BY UNCONJUGATED ANTIBODIES

The general mechanisms of tumor cell kill by unconjugated monoclonal antibodies are shown in Table 3. A major mechanism of monoclonal antibody cell kill is thought to be due to immune-mediated effects by interaction with the complement cascade or with Fc receptors on antibody-dependent cell-mediated cytotoxicity (ADCC) effector cells. These functions are generally attributes of the monoclonal antibody isotype and species. A list of the immune functions of murine and human immunoglobulin isotypes is shown in Table 4. Despite these obvious interactions with the immune system, it has been difficult to prove that immune-mediated lysis is the most important factor in eliminating tumor cells. For example, in most antibody trials, little change in total complement or in the fragments of complement fixation has been detected following antibody therapy. In a similar fashion, efforts to augment ADCC effector cells using cytokines such as IFN, G-CSF, or GM-CSF have generally not demonstrated significant increases in antitumor effect, although studies using anti-idiotype antibodies have suggested this possibility.

Over the past 15 years a number of observations have been made that indicate that direct effects of the monoclonal antibody binding to the cell-surface antigen may be important in tumor cell kill. This can be thought of in several

Table 3 Mechanisms of Antitumor Effect Using Unconjugated Monoclonal Antibodies

---

Immune-mediated effects:
   Complement-dependent lysis (CDC)
   ADCC (antibody-dependent cell-mediated cytotoxicity)
Direct antiproliferative or apoptosis-inducing effects:
   Mimic a ligand
   Block a ligand
   Interfere with function
Interact or sensitize with other modalities

Table 4 Immune Effector Functions of Human and Murine Immunoglobulin Isotypes

Species	Isotype	Interactions	
		Human ADCC	Human complement
Murine Fc	IgG1	−	±
	IgG2a	++	±
	IgG2b	−	±
	IgG3	++	±
	IgM	−	++
Human Fc	IgG1	+++	+++
	IgG2	+	++
	IgG3	+++	+++
	IgG4	+	+
	IgM	±	++++

ways. For example, CD25, a component of the IL-2 receptor, is expressed on a variety of T-cell and some B-cell malignancies. In some cases (adult T-cell leukemia/lymphoma) these cells appear to be driven by IL-2. Treatment with Anti-CD25 antibodies in vitro and in vivo can bind to the CD25 antigen without activating the receptor and can block IL-2 from signaling the receptor. This results in the inhibition of cell proliferation and even cell death by apoptosis in some cases (24). This is an example of the antibody blocking a natural ligand. In a similar fashion, the antibody may bind to and stimulate or signal the cell-surface antigen. In the case of immunoglobulin idiotype and anti-idiotype antibodies, we found that patients with the greatest response to the antibody therapy were those in whom the treatment antibody was able to induce a strong tyrosine phosphorylation signal in the pretreatment tumor cells (23). Although not proof, a possible explanation of this observation is that the antibody mimics antigen, in the absence of other essential cofactors (such as CD40L), which results in the induction of apoptosis. A third direct effect is by the inhibition of a normal biologic function of the cell-surface antigen directly by the binding of the antibody. This may be the case with treatment with anti-CD20 antibodies such as IDEC-C2B8. In this case, the CD20 molecule appears to function as a calcium channel, and antibody binding to CD20 may interfere with the control of this channel, resulting in the inhibition of the cell cycle and, in some cell lines, in the induction of apoptosis (20,25,28,29). Additional mechanisms of antitumor effect include the ability of the antibody to alter the sensitivity of the cells to standard treatments with radiation or chemotherapy. This is very poorly understood, but may be true in some cases (29).

VIII. CLINICAL TRIALS OF UNCONJUGATED MONOCLONAL ANTIBODIES FOR HEMATOLOGIC MALIGNANCIES

A brief overview of the target antigens that have been targeted with monoclonal antibody therapy is shown in Table 5. A large number of exploratory clinical trials were performed in the 1980s and early 1990s that evaluated a number of cell-surface antigens and their respective antibodies. In most cases, these clinical trials demonstrated some antitumor activity, but the tumor responses were often incomplete and of short duration. However, these trials have pointed out the importance of the characteristics of the tumor, the antigen, and the antibody in determining the effectiveness of the antibody therapy. Subsequent trials of anti-idiotype, Anti-CD20, and Anti-CD52 have demonstrated significant activity in patients with relapsed NHL or CLL, and selected clinical trials will be reviewed.

A. Immunoglobulin Idiotype

The immunoglobulin idiotype is comprised of the combinations of the variable-region gene segments and is highly mutated in most lymphomas by the process of somatic mutation and antigen selection. However, this Ig sequence is unique to the tumor cell clone. Anti-idiotype antibodies can be raised against the tumor cell-surface Ig idiotype, but this process is somewhat labor intensive and requires a custom antibody to be made for each patient with lymphoma. However, these antibodies are nearly tumor-specific probes and can be used to detect tumor cells using immunoassays and have demonstrated antitumor activity (30). In a series of trials at Stanford University, 34 patients were treated with custom-made murine anti-idiotype antibodies alone or in combination with IFN or a short course of chlorambucil (3,16,31,32). A number of observations can be made concerning these trials. First, major tumor responses were observed in patients who had failed prior chemotherapy and had large tumor burdens. Tumor responses were observed in the blood, bone marrow, lymph nodes, spleen, and liver and in extra nodal masses. In most cases, the antibody could be given with minimal infusional related toxicity, although chills, fever, and rigor were observed more frequently during the initial antibody infusions. Responses occurred in approximately 68% of patients and were complete in 18%. Interestingly, while the duration of partial remission was generally less than 1 year, six patients had complete remissions, and five of six persisted more than 5 years.

The major factor responsible for relapse was the selection of immunoglobulin idiotype variant cells that expressed surface immunoglobulin that had somatic mutations that rendered it unreactive with the treatment antibody (15). This was shown to be due to the presence at low levels of variant cells in the tumor cell population, likely as a result of somatic mutation of the hypervariable regions.

In some cases, this could be treated by utilizing second or third anti-idiotype antibodies reactive with separate idiotopes on the Ig molecule (16).

In addition, difficulty with therapy occurred because some patients' tumor cells secreted high levels of Ig idiotype into the serum that could not be overcome by administration of anti-idiotype antibody (31). Interestingly, despite the fact that murine antibodies were used in these trials, the development of HAMA immune responses was rare (10–20% in later trials), consistent with what has been observed with patients with B-cell NHL.

As noted earlier, there was a poor correlation between the isotype of the treatment antibody and outcome, and no significant changes in the serum complement levels with therapy. The antitumor activity did correlate with the ability of the treatment antibody to induce cell signaling in the pretreatment tumor cells (23), suggesting that direct effects of the interaction of the antibody with the cell surface Ig (the B-cell antigen receptor) are important.

B. Special Case of Idiotype Vaccination

Due to the difficulty of producing a custom monoclonal anti-idiotype antibody for the treatment of patients with B-cell lymphoma, several groups have now turned to isolating the cell-surface Ig from the tumor cells and formulating a tumor-specific vaccine that is used to induce an anti-idiotype antibody immune response in the patient directly. This is quicker and easier to produce, and results in a polyclonal anti-idiotype response that is directed against multiple idiotopes on the cell-surface Ig that may prevent the escape of idiotype variant cells (33). This has been shown to be true in murine models. The murine studies also indicate that the idiotype needed to be conjugated to a carrier protein and administered in an immunological adjuvant to elicit an immune response (34).

In a recently published follow-up of 41 patients treated at Stanford University with idiotype vaccination, the authors noted immune responses to the idiotype in approximately 49% of patients (17). Patients in remission following chemotherapy were more likely to develop an immune response when compared to patients with persistent tumor following chemotherapy. Of 32 patients in first CR following chemotherapy and vaccinated with idiotype conjugated to KLH with the adjuvant SAF-1, significant prolongation to tumor progression was observed for those patients with an anti-idiotype immune response (median 7.9 years) compared to those who did not (medium 1.3 years). These and other ongoing studies at the NCI suggest that the development of an immune response to the Ig idiotype may delay or prevent tumor relapse. It is still unclear if this is due only to a polyclonal anti-idiotype antibody effect or if idiotype-specific T-cell responses are also involved. It is clear that anti-idiotype antibodies can induce antitumor effects, and the proof that T-cells can do so as well is still circumstantial. In a few patients with tumor present at the time of vaccination, objective antitumor

Table 5 Selected Clinical Trials of Unconjugated Monoclonal Antibodies

Antigen	MAb	Disease	No. pts.	Dose	Response	Problems/observations	Refs.
Ig idiotype Stanford	Custom anti-idiotype (murine)	Relapsed B-cell NHL	34	400–11,500 mg qod × 2–3 wks alone, with Chl or IFN	PR—50% CR—18%	Minor infusional toxicity Serum idiotype Modulation Id negative escape Custom MAb each pt	3, 16, 31, 32
Ig idiotype	Custom anti-idiotype MAb or antisera	Relapsed B-cell NHL or CLL	2 NHL 9 CLL/PLL	Multiple regimens	1 PR others transient decrease in WBC	Minor infusional toxicity Modulation	80–88
CD20	IDEC-C2B8 Rituxan (chimeric)	Relapsed low-grade B-Cell NHL	204	375 mg/m^2 1 × each wk × 4	PR + CR 50%	Minor infusional toxicity	7, 8, 38, 39
CD52	CAMPATH1H (humanized)	CLL no prior chemo	9	30 mg, tiw × 18 wk	5 PR, 3 CR	Severe infusional tox Immunosuppression	46
CD52	CAMPATH1H (humanized)	CLL prior chemo	29	30 mg, tiw × 12 wk	11 PR, 1 CR	Severe infusional tox Immunosuppression	4

Antigen	MAb	Disease	N	Dose	Response	Toxicity	Refs
CD52	CAMPATH1H (humanized)	T-PLL	15	30 mg, tiw × 12 wk	2 PR, 9 CR	Severe infusional tox Immunosuppression	44
CD4	CMT412 (chimeric)	CTCL	15	50–200 mg single or 10–80 mg × biw × 6	14 improved transiently	Minimal tox	73, 74
CD25	Anti-Tac (murine)	HTLV-1 induced adult T cell leukemia	19	100–220 mg over 5–16 days	4 PR, 2 CR	Minimal tox	24, 71
CD5	L17F12 T-101 (murine)	CTCL B-CLL	35 25	1–500 mg Multiple schedules	Transient responses CTCL > CLL	Mild infusional tox Modulation HAMA	55–62
CD19	CLB-CD19 (murine) ± IL-2	B-cell NHL	6 7	15–250 mg × 4 days Various twice weekly	1 PR 1 PR	Minimal tox Modulation IL-2 toxicity	14, 63
CD21 and CD24	BL13 ALB9 (murine)	PTLD following organ Tx	27	0.2 mg/kg/d × 10	16/26/CR	Minimal tox	64–66
HLA-DR	Lym-1 (murine)	NHL	10	58–465 mg × 4	3 minor	Minor infusional tox	69
CR2	OKB-7	NHL	18	0.1–40 mg	None	Imaged when trace labeled	70

effects have been observed. Although still a custom process for each patient, the development of alternative methods to obtain the cell-surface immunoglobulin for vaccine formulation (molecular cloning) or the administration of DNA sequences containing the variable regions with or without cytokine sequences to stimulate an immune response directly appears feasible (33).

C. Anti-CD20 Antibody Therapy

As noted earlier, the chimeric Anti-CD20 MAb IDEC-C2B8 (Rituxan) has become the first MAb approved by the U.S. FDA for the treatment of cancer. The structure of the antibody contains variable regions from the murine IgG1 antibody IDEC-2B8 and human IgG1, kappa constant regions (6). The antibody binds with high affinity to the CD20 antigen, a B-cell-restricted antigen that is not present on precursor B-cells, stem cells, or plasma cells. It is expressed in high copy number on the surface of nearly all normal and malignant mature B-cells (35,36). It is expressed at lower levels on chronic lymphocytic leukemia cells and on only 10–20% of plasma cell or early B-cell malignancies. The antigen is held tightly in the cell membrane, and it is not shed or secreted and it does not modulate upon antigen binding. Only a small portion of the molecule is external to the cell surface, and all Anti-CD20 antibodies appear to bind to this section of the molecule, except for L26, an antibody that binds to an internal epitope of CD20 and is useful for immunophenotyping tumor sections. The antigen appears to function as a calcium channel (37), and antibodies binding to the antigen may induce growth arrest or apoptosis of some sensitive cell lines (25,28,29).

Clinical trials with Rituxan have been reported using single doses from 10 to 500 mg/m^2 (7) and multiple doses of up to four times of 375 mg/m^2 weekly (8,38,39). Two clinical trials have been presented that have treated 203 patients (a smaller trial with 37 patients and a larger trial with 166 patients), most with relapsed low-grade or follicular B-cell NHL. All patients were treated with 375 mg/m^2 weekly $\times$ 4 weeks. Overall there was an objective antitumor effect observed in approximately 50% of patients, with a time to progression of 11–13 months. Complete remissions have been observed in 10–20% of patients, and nearly identical results were observed in the two trials. Of note, however, is that a complete remission required all tumor masses to resolve to less than 1×1 cm, to be confirmed on follow-up CT evaluation and to be independently audited blind by a third party. Tumor responses were more frequent in patients with follicular lymphoma (working formulation B, C, or D) compared with those with small lymphocytic lymphoma (working formulation group A), possibly due to the lower expression of CD20 density observed in this group. Tumor responses were observed during treatment in some patients, but not until 1–3 months later in others, and some patients continued to regress for several months. Tumor responses were observed in elderly patients, those with extranodal disease, and those with peripheral blood, spleen, or bone marrow involvement. Patients refractory to chemotherapy had a decreased response rate to the antibody, but significant remissions were still observed in 25–35%. Interestingly, the response rate was more than 70% in patients who had relapsed following high-dose therapy and autologous stem-cell support (39). To date, there has been minimal experience in other B-cell histologies, such as the intermediate or high-grade NHL, mantle cell NHL, or chronic lymphocytic leukemias, although there are several ongoing studies.

In general this antibody therapy has been well tolerated, with no dose-limiting or cumulative toxicity. Infusional-related symptoms have been observed, most frequently during the initial antibody treatment. The treatment is given by a slow, escalating-rate intravenous infusion in an outpatient setting. Symptoms frequent to the initial antibody infusion include fever, chills with occasional rigors, and, more rarely, bronchospasm, cough, or mild-to-moderate hypotension. In nearly all cases these symptoms can be managed by temporarily stopping the antibody infusion and treating with acetaminophen or diphenhydramine and occasionally meperidine for severe rigors. Usually, the antibody infusion can be restarted following abatement of the symptoms and adverse reactions will not recur with the rest of the infusion or on subsequent infusions.

Because the CD20 antigen is expressed on normal B-cells as well as on most lymphoma cells, a consequence of Rituxan antibody therapy is the rapid and specific depletion of normal, circulating B-cells and tumor cells in the peripheral blood. This depletion persists for 3–9 months but does not appear to increase the risk for infection with bacterial, viral, or other pathogens. Immunoglobulin levels are largely unchanged, although IgM levels appear to be transiently depressed (8,39). Immune responses to the chimeric antibody have occurred in less than 1% of patients, and retreatment appears feasible.

Pharmacokinetics of the antibody are complex and in part dependent on the tumor burden and on the burden of normal B-cells. However, once sites are saturated, the majority of patients treated at the 375-mg/m^2 dose achieved persistent, increasing levels of antibody in the serum that persisted for 3–6 months following the fourth dose. At this time, antigen-negative escape and antigen-negative variants have not been described for CD20. However, previous experience using antibodies that can exert powerful antitumor effects suggests that this is possible.

There is minimal experience with other Anti-CD20 antibodies administered as unconjugated antibody therapy. Press et al. described four patients treated with the murine anti-CD20 antibody 1F5 and noted short-lived responses in one of these patients (27). There is anecdotal information that suggests that some antitumor activity has been observed in clinical trials of the murine Anti-CD20 antibody B1 when given as a trace-labeled imaging dose (9,10). This suggests that there may be some antitumor activity of murine Anti-CD20 antibodies, but formal comparison of trials evaluating unconjugated B1 with nonmyeloablative doses of ^{131}I-B1 have not yet been reported.

Because this antibody has been the first one introduced to the marketplace, there will likely be a time of adjustment as physicians develop the knowledge and comfort to use this new type of therapy routinely. Several new trials are under way in multiple institutions and in multiple cooperative groups that are evaluating the use of the antibody combined with or following multiple combinations of chemotherapy. Early clinical experience suggests that this will be possible. In a recent clinical trial, six infusions of Rituxan were given with six cycles of standard-dose CHOP chemotherapy. All evaluable patients responded to the combination therapy, and the majority of patients tested became PCR negative for the t(14:18) translocation (40). Toxicity was attributable largely to the chemotherapy, with minor infusional symptoms occurring during antibody administration. Longer follow-up is needed to evaluate the clinical efficacy of this combination, but hopefully this new treatment, in addition to having substantial single-agent activity, when integrated with standard therapy will be able to alter the natural history of relapsed or low-grade B-cell NHL.

D. Anti-CD52 (CAMPATH-1H)

The CD52 antigen is a 12-amino acid, 21–28-kDa glycosylphosphatidyl-inositol (GPI)-linked glycoprotein that is expressed in high levels on both T- and B-lymphocytes and at lower levels on monocytes (absent on granulocytes and stem-cell precursors). The CAMPATH-1H antibody is a human IgG1, kappa, with rat hypervariable regions directed against the CD52 antigen. The antigen does not modulate from the cell surface.

Treatment with the rat or the humanized antibodies has demonstrated antitumor activity against some lymphoid leukemias and lymphomas. Early studies demonstrated antitumor activity in a minority of patients with lymph-node-based lymphoma, but was associated with rapid clearing of tumor cells in the blood and bone marrow and to a lesser extent the spleen (41,42). Additional studies demonstrated minimal effects on the lymph nodes in patients with lymphoma and were complicated by severe immunosuppression (43). Later studies have taken advantage of the ability to clear the peripheral blood and bone marrow and have focused on the use of CAMPATH-1H to treat patients with B-cell chronic lymphocytic leukemia (CLL) and both B- and T-cell pro-lymphocytic leukemia (PLL). Significant antitumor activity has been reported in patients with T-cell PLL with 11 of 15 patients having a major remission, including nine patients with CR (44). Significant toxicity was observed, including the development of severe bone marrow failure in two patients.

In patients with CLL, significant activity has also been observed. In a recent report, 29 patients with previously treated CLL (eight with a prior response and

21 refractory) were treated with doses escalating to 30 mg 3× each week for 12 weeks. Overall there was a 42% response rate (1 CR). As seen previously, 28 of 29 patients cleared their blood, 36% cleared the bone marrow, 32% resolved splenomegaly, but only 7% cleared lymph nodes (4). In some patients, CAMPATH-1H therapy has been used in vivo to purge bone marrow prior to ABMT (45). In at least two cases, successful autografts have been performed in patients previously ineligible due to persistent bone marrow disease. In untreated CLL patients treated with intravenous or subcutaneous CAMPATH-1H at doses up to 30 mg 3× each week for 18 weeks, 8 of 9 patients had a PR ($n = 5$) or CR ($n = 3$) (46). All patients cleared the peripheral blood, and 7 of 9 cleared their bone marrow. Responses ranged from 8 to 24 months plus. Serious infection (with CMV) was reported in only one patient.

A major difficulty with the administration of this antibody has been the occurrence of severe infusional-related reactions. These are characterized by fever, chills, rigors, and hypotension and appear to be dependent on the release of cytokines TNF-alpha, IFN-gamma, and IL-6 through crosslinking of CD16 (low-affinity Fc-receptor to IgG) on NK cells (47). These symptoms are often severe and have limited the amount of antibody that can be given in a single setting. A tachyphylaxis to the infusional syndrome allows the dose to be started at a low level and then escalated to the full 30-mg dose. However, because of the wide distribution of the CD52 antigen, treatment with the CAMPATH-1H antibody also causes marked lymphocyte depletion that has resulted in profound immunosuppression associated with increased incidence of opportunistic infections (43). Prophylactic use of antibiotics has decreased this complication somewhat, but prolonged lymphopenia is often present.

Therapy with CAMPATH-1H appears to lyse tumor cells rapidly due to complement fixation. While the antigen does not modulate from the cell surface, antigen-negative variant normal T-cells have been observed to emerge in rheumatoid arthritis patients treated with low levels of the antibody (48,49). However, there have not been any reports of CD52-negative tumor cells arising posttherapy. In addition, neutralizing immune responses to CAMPATH-1H have been observed in patients with rheumatoid arthritis treated with low-dose subcutaneous injections (50). Additional ongoing studies are exploring further uses of the lymphocyte-depleting ability of the antibody for bone marrow purging (51), in the treatment of graft-vs-host disease (52), and in the treatment of patients with autoimmune diseases (53,54).

E. Other Antigens

As shown in Table 5, a large number of additional cell-surface antigens have been targeted with unconjugated monoclonal antibodies over the past 15 years.

CD5 is a T-cell antigen that is expressed on cutaneous T-cell lymphoma

(CTCL) and on a subset of B-cells (CLL). Multiple clinical trials in the 1980s demonstrated some transient clinical activity in the treatment of patents with CLL or CTCL (55–62). However, due to severe modulation of the cell-surface antigen, these responses were generally transient and incomplete. Further clinical trials have attempted to take advantage of the modulation and internalization by utilizing immunotoxins.

CD19 is a B-cell-restricted antigen, arising earlier in B-cell differentiation than CD20. Unconjugated monoclonal antibody therapy alone (63) or in combination with IL-2 (14) produced two responses in 13 patients. However, again due to significant cell-surface modulation, subsequent clinical trials have favored immunotoxin-directed approaches.

Patients with post-organ-transplant lymphoproliferative disorders that are caused by the polyclonal expansion of B-cells, generally due to EBV, appear to be sensitive to antibody therapy. Earlier clinical trials using murine antibodies have demonstrated CRs in the majority of patients (64–66). Subsequent trials have reported antidotal activity using a chimeric antibody (67,68). Trials evaluating additional antibodies in this subgroup of patients are ongoing.

Other antigens on the cell surface, such as HLA-DR, and the CR2 EBV receptor have been targeted with the Lym-1 and OKB7 MAbs, respectively (69,70). Minimal responses were observed using the murine antibodies alone, and further clinical trials have used the antibodies to target radioisotopes.

As mentioned earlier, Anti-CD25 antibody has been use in the treatment of patients with adult T-cell leukemia (ATL). In early cases, the cells appear to be driven by IL-2, and blocking of the CD25 IL-2 receptor by the Anti-TAC antibody results in the inhibition of cell growth and cell death in some cases. In early clinical trials, a murine antibody was utilized, and 6 of 19 cases had a PR ($n = 4$) or CR ($n = 2$), with the complete remissions lasting 9 months to more than 3 years. The antibody has been chimerized, and subsequent studies have focused on the use of radiolabeled antibody in this disease (24,71,72).

The CD4 antigen is expressed on T-cells of the helper subtype (Th2) and is brightly expressed on CTCL. Clinical trials targeting the CD4 antigen with a chimeric antibody, cMT412, have demonstrated antitumor activity in both skin lesions and nodules (73,74). There was some depression of the CD4 count at the higher doses. Most patients had significant improvement in their skin symptoms and signs of disease, but the improvement was transient, lasting 6–52 weeks.

Lastly, several clinical trials have attempted to decrease high-serum levels of IL-6 by treatment with an Anti-IL-6 antibody in diseases thought to be driven in part by IL-6. A clinical trial in HIV-positive patients with aggressive B-cell NHL showed that the antibody cleared the IL-6 in some cases and alleviated the symptoms of severe cachexia and fever. One of 11 patients had a PR of short duration (75). In a similar fashion, Anti-IL6 has been used to treat the symptoms due to Castlemann's disease (76). Multiple myeloma may also be driven by

IL-6, and treatment with an Anti-IL-6 demonstrated a decrease in tumor-cell proliferation in some cases as well as a decrease in symptoms (77), but showed limited antitumor activity.

IX. FUTURE DIRECTIONS

Over nearly the past 20 years, much has been learned concerning the use of monoclonal antibodies to treat cancer. Unfortunately, there has been much more hype than reality. Future trials should seek to learn from the past, to select cell-surface antigens that could be targeted using unconjugated monoclonal antibodies with the expectation of observing an antitumor effect. Careful consideration of the properties of the cell-surface molecule is required. Several new, promising agents are on the horizon. Anti-CD30 has demonstrated in vitro activity and activity in murine xenograft models for the treatment of CD30-positive anaplastic large-cell lymphoma (78). Similarly, CD40 is a key molecule controlling much of the normal communication between cells. Anti-CD40 antibodies have shown variable effects on many CD40-positive cells and activity in murine models (22,79). Clinical trials using these unconjugated antibodies have not yet been reported. Hopefully, these agents and many others will continue to be discovered and pilot trials of immunotherapy pursued with the rapid development of antibodies from the laboratory into the clinic.

X. CONCLUSION

The successful application of antibody therapy to the treatment of lymphoma can be traced to consideration of the characteristics of the antigen, the tumor cell, and the antibody. As new antigens are identified and old antigens further characterized, additional approaches will emerge. The ultimate role for unconjugated, toxin-labeled, or radiolabeled antibodies in the treatment of lymphoma remains to be defined. The approval of Rituxan (IDEC-C2B8 chimeric Anti-CD20 antibody) represents a significant advancement for the treatment of patients with B-cell lymphoma. This new agent has significant single-agent activity and a novel mechanism of action, with increased tumor specificity and decreased toxicity. The CD20 antigen is nearly an ideal target for unconjugated antibody therapy. This efficacy combined with minimal toxicity should also allow this antibody to be combined with chemotherapy or to be given as an adjuvant following standard treatments. Hopefully, these approaches will be able to reduce the minimal residual disease that remains and causes relapse in patients with the B-cell lymphomas.

REFERENCES

1. Ehrlich P. On immunity with specific reference to cell life. Proc Royal Soc London 1900; 66:424.
2. Kohler G, Milstein C. Continuous culture of fused cells secreting antibody of predefined specificity. Nature 1975; 236:495.
3. Miller RA, Maloney DG, Warnke R, Levy R. Treatment of B cell lymphoma with monoclonal anti-idiotype antibody. N Eng J Med 1982; 306:517.
4. Osterborg A, Dyer MJ, Bunjes D, et al. Phase II multicenter study of human CD52 antibody in previously treated chronic lymphocytic leukemia. European Study Group of CAMPATH-1H Treatment in Chronic Lymphocytic Leukemia. J Clin Oncol 1997; 15:1567–1574.
5. Nadler LM, Ritz, J, Hardy R, Pesando JM, Schlossman SF, Stashenko P. A unique cell surface antigen identifying lymphoid malignancies of B cell origin. J Clin Invest 1981; 67:134–40.
6. Reff ME, Carner K, Chambers KS, et al. Depletion of B cells in vivo by a chimeric mouse numan monoclonal antibody to CD20. Blood 1994; 83:435–445.
7. Maloney DG, Liles TM, Czerwinski DK, et al. Phase I clinical trial using escalating single-dose infusion of chimeric anti-CD20 monoclonal antibody (IDEC-C2B8) in patients with recurrent B-cell lymphoma. Blood 1994; 84:2457–2466.
8. Maloney DG, Grillo-Lopez AJ, White CA, et al. IDEC-C2B8 (Rituximab) anti-CD20 monoclonal antibody therapy in patients with relapsed low-grade non-Hodgkin's lymphoma. Blood 1997; 90:2188–2195.
9. Kaminski MS, Zasadny KR, Francis IR, et al. Iodine-131-anti-B1 radioimmunotherapy for B-cell lymphoma. J Clin Oncol 1996; 14:1974–1981.
10. Press OW, Eary JF, Appelbaum FR, et al. Phase II trial of 131I-B1 (anti-CD20) antibody therapy with autologous stem cell transplantation for relapsed B cell lymphomas. Lancet 1995; 346:336–340.
11. Knox SJ, Goris ML, Trisler K, et al. Yttrium-90-labeled anti-CD20 monoclonal antibody therapy of recurrent B-cell lymphoma. Clin Cancer Res 1996; 2:457–470.
12. Grossbard ML, Freedman AS, Ritz J, et al. Serotherapy of B-cell neoplasms with anti-B4-blocked ricin: a Phase I trial of daily bolus infusion. Blood 1992; 79:576–585.
13. Stone MJ, Sausville EA, Fay JW, et al. A Phase I study of bolus versus continuous infusion of the anti-CD19 immunotoxin, IgG-HD37-dgA, in patients with B-cell lymphoma. Blood 1996; 88:1188–1197.
14. Vlasveld LT, Hekman A, Vyth-Dreese FA, et al. Treatment of low-grade non-Hodgkin's lymphoma with continuous infusion of low-dose recombinant interleukin-2 in combination with the B-cell-specific monoclonal antibody CLB-CD19. Cancer Immunol Immunother 1995; 40:37–47.
15. Meeker T, Lowder J, Cleary ML, et al. Emergence of idiotype variants during treatment of B-cell lymphoma with anti-idiotype antibodies. N Eng J Med 1985; 312:1658–65.
16. Brown SL, Miller RA, Horning SJ, et al. Treatment of B-cell lymphomas with anti-

idiotype antibodies alone and in combination with alpha interferon. Blood 1989; 73: 651–661.
17. Hsu FJ, Caspar CB, Czerwinski D, et al. Tumor-specific idiotype vaccines in the treatment of patients with B-cell lymphoma—long term results of a clinical trial. Blood 1997; 89:3129–3135.
18. Weiner GJ, Kaminski MS. Idiotype variants emerging after anti-idiotype monoclonal antibody therapy of a murine B cell lymphoma. J Immunol 1989; 142:343–351.
19. Corcoran MC, Eary J, Bernstein I, Press OW. Radioimmunotherapy strategies for non-Hodgkin's lymphomas. Ann Oncol 1997; 8:133–138.
20. Tedder TF, Engel P. CD20: a regulator of cell-cycle progression of B lymphocytes. Immunol Today 1994; 15:450–454.
21. Ghetie MA, Podar EM, Ilgen A, Gordon BE, Uhr JW, Vitetta ES. Homodimerization of tumor-reactive monoclonal antibodies markedly increases their ability to induce growth arrest or apoptosis of tumor cells. Proc Natl Acad Sci USA 1997; 94:7509–7514.
22. Funakoshi S, Taub DD, Asai O, et al. Effects of CD40 stimulation in the prevention of human EBV-lymphomagenesis. Leuk Lymphoma 1997; 24:187–199.
23. Vuist WM, Levy R, Maloney DG. Lymphoma regression induced by monoclonal anti-idiotypic antibodies correlates with their ability to induce Ig signal transduction and is not prevented by tumor expression of high levels of bcl-2 protein. Blood 1994; 83:899–906.
24. Waldmann TA, Goldman CK, Bongiovanni KF, et al. Therapy of patients with human T-cell lymphotrophic virus I-induced adult T-cell leukemia with anti-Tac, a monoclonal antibody to the receptor for interleukin-2. Blood 1988; 72:1805–1816.
25. Maloney DG, Smith B, Appelbaum FR. The anti-tumor effect of monoclonal anti-CD20 antibody (mAb) therapy includes direct anti-proliferative activity and induction of apoptosis in CD positive non-Hodgkin's lymphoma (NHL) cell lines (abstr). Blood 1996; 88(10) Suppl 1:63a.
26. Bowen AL, Zomas A, Emmett E, Matutes E, Dyer MJ, Catovsky D. Subcutaneous CAMPATH-1H in fludarabine-resistant/relapsed chronic lymphocytic and B-prolymphocytic leukaemia. Br J Haematol 1997; 96:617–619.
27. Press OW, Appelbaum F, Ledbetter JA, et al. Monoclonal antibody 1F5 (anti-CD20) serotherapy of human B cell lymphomas. Blood 1987; 69:584–591.
28. Tedder TF, Forsgren A, Boyd AW, Nadler LM, Schlossman SF. Antibodies reactive with the B1 molecule inhibit cell cycle progression but not activation of human B lymphocytes. Eur J Immunol 1986; 16:881–887.
29. Demidem A, Lam T, Alas S, Hariharan K, Hanna N, Bonavida B. Chimeric anti-Cd20 (Idec-C2b8) monoclonal antibody sensitizes a B cell lymphoma cell line to cell killing by cytotoxic drugs. Cancer Biother Radiopharmaceuticals 1997; 12:177–186.
30. Hatzubai A, Maloney DG, Levy R. The use of a monoclonal anti-idiotype antibody to study the biology of a human B cell lymphoma. J Immunol 1981; 126:2397.
31. Meeker TC, Lowder J, Maloney DG, et al. A clinical trial of anti-idiotype therapy for B cell malignancy. Blood 1985; 65:1349.
32. Maloney DG, Brown S, Czerwinski DK, et al. Monoclonal anti-idiotype antibody

therapy of B cell lymphoma: the addition of a short course of chemotherapy does not prevent the emergence of idiotype negative variant cells. Blood 1992; 80:1502–1510.
33. Caspar CB, Levy S, Levy R. Idiotype vaccines for non-Hodgkins lymphoma induce polyclonal immune responses that cover mutated tumor idiotypes—comparison of different vaccine formulations. Blood 1997; 90:3699–3706.
34. Maloney DG, Kaminski MS, Burowski D, Haimovich J, Levy R. Monoclonal anti-idiotype antibodies against the murine B cell lymphoma 38C13: characterization and use as probes for the biology of the tumor in vivo and in vitro. Hybridoma 1985; 4:191.
35. Stashenko P, Nadler LM, Hardy R, Schlossman SF. Characterization of a human B lymphocyte-specific antigen. J Immunol 1980; 125:1678–1685.
36. Anderson KC, Bates MP, Slaughenhoupt BL, Pinkus GS, Schlossman SF, Nadler LM. Expression of human B cell–associated antigens on leukemias and lymphomas: a model of human B cell differentiation. Blood 1984; 63:1424–1433.
37. Bubien JK, Zhou LJ, Bell PD, Frizzell RA, Tedder TF. Transfection of the CD20 cell surface molecule into ectopic cell types generates a Ca^{2+} conductance found constitutively in B lymphocytes. J Cell Biol 1993; 121:1121–1132.
38. Maloney DG, Grillolopez AJ, Bodkin DJ, et al. Idec-C2b8—results of a Phase I multiple-dose trial in patients with relapsed non-Hodgkin's lymphoma. J Clin Oncol 1997; 15:3266–3274.
39. McLaughlin P, Cabanillas F, Grillo-Lopez AJ, et al. IDEC-C2B8 anti CD20 antibody: final report on a phase III pivotal trial in patients with relapsed low-grade or follicular lymphoma. Blood 1996; 88(10) Suppl 1:90a.
40. Czuzman MS, Grillo-Lopez AJ, Saleh M, et al. IDEC-C2B8/CHOP chemoimmunotherapy in patients with low-grade lymphoma: interim clinical and bcl-2 (PCR) results. Ann Oncol 1996; 7(suppl 1):56.
41. Hale G, Dyer MJ, Clark MR, et al. Remission induction in non-Hodgkin's lymphoma with reshaped human monoclonal antibody CAMPATH-1H. Lancet 1988; 2:1394–1399.
42. Dyer MJ, Hale G, Hayhoe FG, Waldmann H. Effects of CAMPATH-1 antibodies in vivo in patients with lymphoid malignancies: influence of antibody isotype. Blood 1989; 73:1431–1439.
43. Tang SC, Hewitt K, Reis MD, Berinstein NL. Immunosuppressive toxicity of Campath(R)-1H monoclonal antibody in the treatment of patients with recurrent low-grade lymphoma. Leuk Lymphoma 1996; 24:93–101.
44. Pawson R, Dyer MJ, Barge R, et al. Treatment of T-cell prolymphocytic leukemia with human CD52 antibody. J Clin Oncol 1997; 15:2667–2672.
45. Dyer MJ, Kelsey SM, Mackay HJ, et al. In vivo "purging" of residual disease in CLL with Campath-1H. Br J Haematol 1997; 97:669–672.
46. Osterborg A, Fassas AS, Anagnostopoulos A, Dyer MJ, Catovsky D, Mellstedt H. Humanized CD52 monoclonal antibody Campath-1H as first-line treatment in chronic lymphocytic leukaemia. Br J Haematol 1996; 93:151–153.
47. Wing MG, Moreau T, Greenwood J, et al. Mechanism of first-dose cytokine-release syndrome by CAMPATH 1-H: involvement of CD16 (FcgammaRIII) and CD11a/CD18 (LFA-1) on NK cells. J Clin Invest 1996; 98:2819–2826.

48. Brett SJ, Baxter G, Cooper H, et al. Emergence of CD52−, glycosylphosphatidylinositol-anchor-deficient lymphocytes in rheumatoid arthritis patients following Campath-1H treatment. Int Immunol 1996; 8:325–334.
49. Osterborg A, Werner A, Halapi E, et al. Clonal CD8+ and CD52− T-cells are induced in responding B-cell lymphoma patients treated with Campath-1H (anti-CD52). Eur J Haematol 1997; 58:5–13.
50. Schnitzer TJ, Yocum DE, Michalska M, et al. Subcutaneous administration of CAMPATH-1H: clinical and biological outcomes. J Rheumatol 1997; 24:1031–1036.
51. Mehta J, Powles R, Treleaven J, et al. Autologous transplantation with CD52 monoclonal antibody-purged marrow for acute lymphoblastic leukemia: long-term follow-up. Leuk Lymphoma 1997; 25:479–486.
52. Hamblin M, Marsh JC, Lawler M, et al. Campath-1G in vivo confers a low incidence of graft-versus-host disease associated with a high incidence of mixed chimaerism after bone marrow transplantation for severe aplastic anaemia using HLA-identical sibling donors. Bone Marrow Transplant 1996; 17:819–824.
53. Isaacs JD, Manna VK, Rapson N, et al. CAMPATH-1H in rheumatoid arthritis—an intravenous dose-ranging study. Br J Rheumatol 1996; 35:231–240.
54. Isaacs JD, Hazleman BL, Chakravarty K, Grant JW, Hale G, Waldmann H. Monoclonal antibody therapy of diffuse cutaneous scleroderma with CAMPATH-1H. J Rheumatol 1996; 23:1103–1106.
55. Miller RA, Maloney DG, McKillop J, Levy R. In vivo effects of murine hybridoma monoclonal antibody in a patient with T-cell leukemia. Blood 1981; 58:78.
56. Miller RA, Levy R. Response of cutaneous T cell lymphoma to therapy with hybridoma monoclonal antibody. Lancet 1981; 2:226.
57. Miller RA, Oseroff AR, Stratte PT, Levy R. Monoclonal antibody therapeutic trials in seven patients with T-cell lymphoma. Blood 1983; 62:988–995.
58. Bertram JH, Gill PS, Levine AM, et al. Monoclonal antibody T101 in T cell malignancies: a clinical, pharmacokinetic, and immunologic correlation. Blood 1986; 68:752–761.
59. Dillman RO, Shawler DL, Sobol RE, et al. Murine monoclonal antibody therapy in two patients with chronic lymphocytic leukemia. Blood 1982; 59:1026.
60. Dillman RO, Shawler DL, Dillman JB, Royston I. Therapy of chronic lymphocytic leukemia and cutaneous T-cell lymphoma with T101 monoclonal antibody. J Clin Oncol 1984; 2:881.
61. Dillman RO, Beauregard J, Shawler DL, et al. Continuous infusion of T101 monoclonal antibody in chronic lymphocytic leukemia and cutaneous T-cell lymphoma. J Biol Resp Mod 1986; 5:394–410.
62. Foon KA, Schroff RW, Bunn PA, et al. Effects of monoclonal antibody therapy in patients with chronic lymphocytic leukemia. Blood 1984; 64:1085–1093.
63. Hekman A, Honselaar A, Vuist WM, et al. Initial experience with treatment of human B cell lymphoma with anti-CD19 monoclonal antibody. Cancer Immunol Immunother 1991; 32:364–372.
64. Fischer A, Blanche S, Le BJ, et al. Anti-B-cell monoclonal antibodies in the treatment of severe B-cell lymphoproliferative syndrome following bone marrow and organ transplantation. N Engl J Med 1991; 324:1451–1456.

65. Blanche S, Le DF, Veber F, et al. Treatment of severe Epstein-Barr virus-induced polyclonal B-lymphocyte proliferation by anti-B-cell monoclonal antibodies. Two cases after HLA-mismatched bone marrow transplantation. Ann Intern Med 1988; 108:199–203.
66. Stephan JL, Le DF, Blanche S, et al. Treatment of central nervous system B lymphoproliferative syndrome by local infusion of a B cell-specific monoclonal antibody. Transplantation 1992; 54:246–249.
67. Garnier JL, Berger F, Martin X, et al. Post-transplant B-cell lymphomas—correlation of late stage B-cell differentiation and progression of disease; treatment with chimeric monoclonal antibody. Transplant Proc 1995; 27:1777.
68. Antoine C, Garnier JL, Duboust A, Bariety J, Stevenson G, Glotz D. Successful treatment of posttransplant lymphoproliferative disorder with renal graft preservation by monoclonal antibody therapy. Transplant Proc 1996; 28:2825–2826.
69. Hu E, Epstein AL, Naeve GS, et al. A phase 1a clinical trial of LYM-1 monoclonal antibody serotherapy in patients with refractory B cell malignancies. Hematol Oncol 1989; 7:155–166.
70. Scheinberg DA, Straus DJ, Yeh SD, et al. A Phase I toxicity, pharmacology, and dosimetry trial of monoclonal antibody OKB7 in patients with non-Hodgkin's lymphoma: effects of tumor burden and antigen expression. J Clin Oncol 1990; 8:792–803.
71. Waldmann TA, White JD, Goldman CK, et al. The interleukin-2 receptor: a target for monoclonal antibody treatment of human T-cell lymphotrophic virus I-induced adult T-cell leukemia. Blood 1993; 82:1701–1712.
72. Waldmann TA, White JD, Carrasquillo JA, et al. Radioimmunotherapy of interleukin-2R alpha-expressing adult T-cell leukemia with yttrium-90-labeled anti-Tac. Blood 1995; 86:4063–4075.
73. Knox SJ, Levy R, Hodgkinson S, et al. Observations on the effect of chimeric anti-CD4 monoclonal antibody in patients with mycosis fungoides. Blood 1991; 77:20–30.
74. Knox S, Hoppe RT, Maloney D, et al. Treatment of cutaneous T-cell lymphoma with chimeric anti-CD4 monoclonal antibody. Blood 1996; 87:893–899.
75. Emilie D, Wijdenes J, Gisselbrecht C, et al. Administration of an anti-interleukin-6 monoclonal antibody to patients with acquired immunodeficiency syndrome and lymphoma: effect on lymphoma growth and on B clinical symptoms. Blood 1994; 84:2472–2479.
76. Beck JT, Hsu SM, Wijdenes J, et al. Brief report: alleviation of systemic manifestations of Castleman's disease by monoclonal anti-interleukin-6 antibody. N Engl J Med 1994; 330:602–605.
77. Bataille R, Barlogie B, Lu ZY, et al. Biologic effects of anti-interleukin-6 murine monoclonal antibody in advanced multiple myeloma. Blood 1995; 86:685–691.
78. Tian ZG, Longo DL, Funakoshi S, et al. In vivo antitumor effects of unconjugated CD30 monoclonal antibodies on human anaplastic large-cell lymphoma xenografts. Cancer Res 1995; 55:5335–5341.
79. Funakoshi S, Longo DL, Beckwith M, et al. Inhibition of human B-cell lymphoma growth by CD40 stimulation. Blood 1994; 83:2787–2794.
80. Rankin EM, Hekman A, Somers R, Bokkel TCN, Huinink W. Treatment of two

patients with B cell lymphoma with monoclonal anti-idiotypic antibodies. Blood 1985; 65:1373.

81. Capel PJA, Preijers WMB, Allebes WA, Haanen C. Treatment of chronic lymphocytic leukemia with monoclonal anti-idiotypic antibody. Nether J Med 1985; 28: 112.

82. Caulfield MJ, Murthy S, Tubbs RR, Sergi J, Bukowksi RM. Treatment of chronic lymphocytic leukemia with an anti-idiotypic monoclonal antibody. Cleve Clin J Med 1989; 56:182–188.

83. Allebes WA, Preijers FW, Haanen C, Capel PJ. The development of nonresponsiveness to immunotherapy with monoclonal anti-idiotypic antibodies in a patient with B-CLL. Br J Haematol 1988; 70:295–300.

84. Allebes WA, Knops R, Bontrop RE, et al. Phenotypic and functional changes of tumour cells from patients treated with monoclonal anti-idiotypic antibodies. Scand J Immunol 1990; 32:441–449.

85. Allebes W, Knops R, Herold M, Huber C, Haanen C, Capel P. Immunotherapy with monoclonal anti-idiotypic antibodies: tumour reduction and lymphokine production. Leuk Res 1991; 15:215–222.

86. Hamblin TJ, Stevenson FK, Abdul-Ahad AK, Gordon J, Stevenson FK, Stevenson GT. Preliminary experience in treating lymphocytic leukaemia with antibody to immunoglobulin idiotypes on the cell surface. Br J Cancer 1980; 42:495.

87. Hamblin TJ, Cattan AR, Glennie MJ. Initial experience in treating human lymphoma with a chimeric univalent derivative of monoclonal anti-idiotype antibody. Blood 1987; 69:790.

88. Gordon J, Abdul-Ahad AK, Hamblin TJ, Stevenson FK, Stevenson GT. Mechanisms of tumor cell escape encountered in treating lymphocytic leukaemia with anti-idiotype antibody. Br J Cancer 1984; 49:547.

4
Clinical Studies with Deglycosylated Ricin A-Chain Immunotoxins

Edward A. Sausville
National Cancer Institute, National Institutes of Health, Rockville, Maryland

Ellen S. Vitetta
The University of Texas Southwestern Medical Center at Dallas, Dallas, Texas

I. INTRODUCTION

Deglycosylated ricin A (dgA)-chain immunotoxins (ITs) have emerged from successive efforts to improve upon undesirable features of native ricin conjugates so that therapeutic efficacy and therapeutic index would be improved. As outlined in detail elsewhere (1,2), dgA is prepared from the heterodimeric chemically oxidized ricin holotoxin by reduction and separation of the dgA and dgB chains. dgA does not bind to or damage liver cells and retains its potency when chemically conjugated to some, although not all, immunoglobulins (Igs) to form an IT.

Initial clinical studies of dgA-ITs have been conducted in non-Hodgkin's lymphoma (NHL) and Hodgkin's disease (HD). This choice of disease targets reflects a number of features of these diseases that render them especially suitable for IT therapy. These include (3): availability of highly specific monoclonal antibodies (Mabs) directed against uniquely expressed cell-surface molecules; accessibility of the tumor cells to large molecules; lack of long-term dire consequences when normal B-cells are transiently eliminated; and concomitant disease-related immunosuppression, which increases the likelihood that more than one treatment with these potentially immunogenic molecules will be possible. This chapter will focus on the initial Phase I clinical experiences with dgA-ITs.

II. ANTI-CD22-dgA IN NHL

The CD22 molecule has been used as a target for dgA via the murine Mab RFB4 (4). Vitetta et al. (3) conducted a Phase I study of the Fab'-RFB4-dgA construct in 15 patients with B-cell NHL. Patients received two to six infusions over 4 h, administered every 48 h. Cumulative dose administered was the basis for determining a maximal tolerated dose (MTD). Doses were withheld after any infusion if Grade II toxicity was encountered (moderately symptomatic, requiring treatment but not severe or life-threatening). Treatment was not resumed until improvement in toxicity was noted. Peak serum concentrations of the IT achieved in this study did not correlate with the dose administered, with peak concentrations ranging from 300 to 1500 ng/mL. The $T_{1/2}$ ranged from 48 to 121 min. Four of 14 evaluable patients made anti-IT antibodies by 28 days after initial treatment. Dose-limiting toxicity (DLT) in this trial was vascular leak syndrome (VLS), with all patients manifesting a decrease in serum albumin and an increase in body weight. Cumulative doses ranged from 12.5 to 120 mg/M^2. At cumulative doses of 75 or more mg/M^2, additional toxic manifestations included myalgia, rhabdomyolysis, pulmonary edema, and transient aphasia. Of note, however, is that 43% of 14 evaluable patients showed 50% reductions in measurable tumor masses, with 38% persisting at 1 month after treatment (range 1.25–4 months).

Amlot et al. (5) conducted a complementary study, using IgG-RFB4-dgA instead of the Fab' construct. Twenty-six patients with B-cell lymphoma received 2 to 12 infusions over 4 h every 48 h. Again, VLS was the most prevalent toxicity, with the decrease in serum albumin correlating directly with the increase in body weight. Interpretation of the MTD was complicated by the observation that circulating tumor cells in the blood ($>10^{10}$/L) and the presence of splenomegaly were associated with reduced toxicity and apparent shortening of the $T_{1/2}$. However, in the absence of circulating tumor cells or splenomegaly, cumulative doses of <18 mg/M^2 were well tolerated, with toxicity consistently less than Grade III (Grade III toxicity is severe, requiring treatment). At greater than 18 mg/M^2, toxic manifestations increased in frequency, including life-threatening pulmonary edema, hypotension, pleural and pericardial effusions, and a decrease in EKG voltage. Myalgia was observed in 58% of cases, usually Grade II or less in severity, but in two cases with evidence of rhabdomyolysis. Transient aphasia occurred in four patients. There was mild or no hematologic toxicity and no evidence of hepatotoxicity. In patients lacking circulating tumor cells or splenomegaly, the maximal peak serum concentration of IT was 8500 ng/ml at a cumulative dose of 26 mg/M^2, associated with a $T_{1/2}$ of 11.4 $\pm$ 6.5 h, with an AUC of 171.2 $\pm$ 191 µg-h/mL. In contrast, in the presence of circulating tumor cells ($>10^{10}$/L), associated with a total dose of 40 mg/M^2, a maximal peak serum concentration of IT of 7700 ng/mL was achieved, with a $T_{1/2}$ of 5.5 $\pm$ 5.0 h and an AUC of

31.9 ± 30.4 μg-h/mL. These findings provided evidence that both the pharmacology and the MTD of IgG-RFB4-dgA were influenced by the tumor burden. At 1 month following treatment, one complete and five partial responses occurred in 24 evaluable patients. Nine of 24 patients made detectable levels of either human-antimouse antibodies. (HAMA) or human-antiricin antibodies (HARA) within 48 days of treatment.

A major hypothesis to emerge from these studies was that if the peak serum levels were a determining factor for toxicity, the therapeutic index might be improved by administration by a continuous intravenous infusion regimen. This question was explored in a Phase I study employing a continuous infusion (CI) regimen administered over 8 days (6), to mimic the previously intended schedule of total IT exposure in the bolus Phase I studies. Eighteen patients were entered on this study. The MTD was 19.2 mg/M^2/8 d. All toxicities of any import were related to VLS. At 28.8 mg/M^2/8 d, four of 11 evaluable planned 8-day courses of the CI regimen could not be completed due to VLS, as evidenced not only by weight gain and edema, but by pulmonary infiltrates, hypotension, and oliguria. Although one episode of transient aphasia occurred in one of the patients with Grade III VLS, in no patient was there evidence of severe myalgia or rhabdomyolysis. Thus, there was little evidence that a CI schedule of administration markedly affected the therapeutic index or qualitative aspects of toxicities attributable to IgG-RFB4-dgA, with the possible exception that myalgia was a less prevalent complaint in the CI infusion schedule. Notable additional findings of this study included the clear demonstration that the degree of toxicity was related to the serum concentration of IT achieved. Patients with Grade I or II toxicity had in general <500 ng/mL of IT by day 4 of the infusion, whereas patients with Grade IV or V had >1000 ng/mL. No clear change in serum levels of IL-1α, IL-2, IL-4, IL-6, IL-10, sELAM, sICAM, or nitrates were relatable to the occurrence of severe toxicity. Of interest, even in patients treated at or below the MTD, decreases in urine (Na) suggested the occurrence of mild VLS, correlating with minimal decreases in albumin. Four of 16 evaluable patients achieved a partial response (PR) (duration 5–14 months). Although three of the PRs occurred with doses above the MTD, there were also three minor responses (<50% shrinkage for >1 month, one 8 months in duration).

Additional patients treated subsequently with 19.2 mg/M^2/8 d IgG-RFB4-dgA have included one individual with chemotherapy-refractory, EBV-associated B-cell NHL occurring after renal transplant, who has apparently been cured (>3 years without evidence of disease) with retention of the transplanted kidney (7). In addition, however, an individual patient who received this dose and schedule of IgG-RFB4-dgA after high-dose chemotherapy and total-body irradiation experienced prompt onset of fatal hemolytic uremic syndrome; this will be described in detail elsewhere.

III. IgG-HD37-dgA IN NHL

The CD19 determinant, as a treatment target in NHL, has the theoretical advantage that it is expressed on a larger fraction of adult NHL than is CD22. The HD37 Mab is directed against CD19 and offered evidence of activity as a dgA IT in SCID mice with Daudi NHL xenografts (8).

IgG-HD37-dgA was evaluated clinically in Phase I trials (9) that employed both four infusions every 48 h, each infusion lasting 4 h (bolus Phase I), and a CI regimen over 8 days (CI Phase I). Twenty-three patients were treated on the bolus protocol, and ten by CI. The CI regimen produced an MTD of 19.2 mg/M^2/8 d, with VLS defined as the DLT. In addition, one patient on this dose level experienced a Raynaud's-like syndrome of persisting acrocyanosis that progressed to superficial digital necrosis. No evidence of vasculitis was obtained by serologic evaluation; rather, arteriography revealed distal digital filling defects consistent with small clots or a medium vessel arteritis. This side effect occurred in the setting of dramatic concomitant resolution of a large suprascapular tumor mass. There was no evidence of serious myalgia or rhabdomyolysis on the CI regimen. Using the bolus regimen, an MTD of 16 mg/M^2 cumulative dose over 8 days defined the MTD. Two patients treated at 24 mg/M^2 cumulative dose experienced Grade IV elevations of creatine phosphokinase. In one case this was accompanied by transient aphasia, hypoalbuminemia, and hyponatremia; an additional patient experienced aphasia, and two had Raynaud's like phenomenon, with acrocyanosis and superficial digital necrosis resolving within 1 month. The bolus regimen produced one CR, lasting over 40 months, and two PRs (2- and 6-month durations). In patients treated on the bolus regimen at 24 mg/M^2 cumulative dose, three of six experienced stable disease for at least 6 months. At the MTD of the CI and bolus regimens, the peak serum concentrations were 963 ± 473 ng/mL and 1209 ± 430 ng/mL, respectively. In contrast to the behavior of RFB4-dgA, there was a good correspondence between administered dose and serum concentrations. Using data from the CI infusions, 10 of 12 courses analyzed demonstrated a $T_{1/2}$ of 22.8 h (range 24.1–30 h), whereas in 84 courses of the bolus regimen, the $T_{1/2}$ was 18.2 h (range 10–80 h). Interestingly, patients on the CI regimen who experienced Grade I or II toxicity had mean maximal serum concentrations of 560 ± 353 ng/mL, as compared to 1196 ± 477 ng/mL in patients experiencing Grade III toxicity.

A "dose-intense" approach to delivering the IgG-HD37-dgA IT over a 24-h period was pursued by Conry et al. (10), who administered successively increasing doses of IT over 1 h every 4 h for four doses. Cumulative doses of 4, 8, and 12 mg/M^2 were administered. The rationale for this approach was to produce sustained levels of IT over a 36-h period, which might allow penetration of the IT into lymph nodes. VLS was again the dominant toxicity, with hypoalbuminemia detectable within 24 h, and nadir values of albumin reached posttherapy by 6–7 days. The severity of the VLS was clearly relatable to dose, with an average of 2.3% body weight gained by patients at the lowest dose level and 17.2% average weight gain at the highest dose level. At the intermediate and highest dose level there was severe toxicity, with orthostatic hypotension and oliguria. Patients at the highest dose level had severe VLS, in one case complicated by rhabdomyolysis. The maximal concentration of IT achieved was 550 ± 120, 1370 ± 300, and 3730 ± 1910 ng/mL at 4, 8, and 12 mg/M^2, respectively, with $T_{1/2}$'s of 15–18 h. Two of four patients with palpable adenopathy experienced notable regressions, but these had regrown prior to assessment at 28 d. Thus, it is of interest that the only "well-tolerated" dose level on this trial (4 mg/M^2) achieved similar IT concentrations to that achieved in the well-tolerated dose levels of the CI IgG-HD37-dgA or IgG-RFB4-dgA regimens administered over 8 days.

IV. COMBINATION THERAPY WITH ANTI-CD19 + ANTI-CD22 IMMUNOTOXINS IN NHL

Since studies (11) in SCID mice bearing Daudi NHL xenografts had shown enhanced activity by a "cocktail" of the IgG-RFB4-dgA (directed against CD22) and IgG-HD37-dgA (directed against CD19), a Phase I study of a 1:1 mixture of the two ITs given as an 8-day CI was undertaken in 22 patients. The results of this study will not be presented in detail in this chapter. Experience with the initial patient courses on this Phase I trial suggested an unexpected interaction with IT therapy at disease sites with extensive prior radiation. Severe vascular leak with a hemolytic uremic syndrome complicated episodic patient courses even at the lowest dose level tested (E. Sausville and E. Vitetta, unpublished results). However, the magnitude of other toxicities was again influenced by the presence of circulating tumor cells and, in nonirradiated patients, the dose of IT administered. The combination of Ig-RFB4-dgA plus IgG-HD37-dgA will be reexamined using a bolus administration regimen, since extensive analysis of prior experience with bolus administration schedules did not correlate toxicity with prior radiation exposure.

V. IMMUNOTOXIN DIRECTED AGAINST CD25 IN HODGKIN'S DISEASE

RFT5 is a murine Mab directed against CD25, the α-chain of the IL2 receptor (IL2-R). Reed–Sternberg (RS) cells in HD frequently demonstrate staining with anti-CD25 Mabs. Preclinical studies demonstrated that an IT prepared with IgG-RFT5 and dgA potently inhibited protein synthesis in HD RS cells, and the IT was active in SCID mice with subcutaneous HD xenografts (12,13). Engert et al. (14) therefore studied Ig-RFT5-dgA in a Phase I study in 15 patients with relapsed HD. Most patients had been extensively pretreated with an average of five prior chemotherapy regimens; eight had failed prior autologous bone marrow transplants, and 14 had prior extensive radiation therapy. The IT was administered in a bolus regimen over 4 h every 48 h for four doses. The MTD was 15 mg/M^2 cumulative dose, with DLT consisting of VLS with prominent myalgia in one case. Most frequent Grade I or II toxicities included hypoalbuminemia, weight gain, tachycardia, dyspnea, hypotension, and fatigue. Of note, there was no evidence of a hemolytic-uremic syndrome or other coagulopathy. The maximal serum concentration of the IT achieved at the MTD ranged from 2120 to 7940 ng/mL, with a $T_{1/2}$ from 4.9 to 10.5 h. In this very heavily pretreated population, there were two partial and one minor response. One of the partial responses has lasted longer than 18 months. Responses occurred both in nodal and visceral sites. Additional findings included prompt disappearance either by clearance or, more likely, by antigen modulation of CD25(+) peripheral blood CD4 and CD3 subsets. There was no correlation of changes in cytokine levels including IL2, IL6, IFN-γ, TNF-α, or sCD25 and sCD30 with treatment or toxicity. Forty to 50% of the patients made either HAMA or HARA by the fourth course, but all patients were eligible to receive at least two courses of treatment from the point of view of not having formed anti-IT antibodies when eligible to receive a second treatment course.

VI. CONCLUSION

The studies summarized here lead us to the following interim conclusions. First, dgA ITs are very successful in eliminating hepatotoxicity as a potential limitation for the development of immunotoxins. In addition, they have not shown any evidence of notable myelotoxicity, even in heavily pretreated patients. Second, the dominant toxicity encountered irrespective of the targeting antibody is VLS, defined as hypoalbuminemia, weight gain, pulmonary infiltrates, and hypotension. Indeed, it is remarkable that the MTDs from several different Ig-containing ITs administered by several regimens appear to be approximately 15 mg/M^2 cumulative dose, irrespective of whether the dose is administered by CI or by intermittent bolus dosing regimens over an approximate 8-day period. Whether myalgia with ultimate rhabdomyolysis and/or aphasia represent toxicities distinct from VLS or relatable to VLS by reflecting damage to the muscle or cerebral microvasculature, respectively, is not clear. But rhabdomyolysis with or without aphasia are frequent DLTs that closely follow severe VLS. The anti-CD19-directed IT IgG-HD37-dgA has the relative disadvantage that it tends to induce a Raynaud's-like syndrome as part of its spectrum of toxicities. In addition, it has a relatively long $T_{1/2}$ in comparison with the anti-CD22 or -CD25 ITs studied here. That relatively long $T_{1/2}$ may have contributed to excessive toxicity when IgG-HD37-dgA was administered over relatively short administration schedules, as attempted by Conry et al. (10). Third, serum IT concentrations of 500–1000 ng/mL of the IG constructs are well tolerated, whether the ITs are administered by a bolus or by a CI mode of administration. Since CI administration appears to convey no advantage from the standpoint of either response or toxicity, future clinical trials should focus on bolus dose regimens. Fourth, dgA ITs do show evidence of antitumor activity, even in these Phase I experiences in very heavily pretreated patients. In some cases this is clinically valuable, with long-term meaningful responses and, in one case, perhaps a cure (7). The major issue that must be confronted with these agents is how to widen the therapeutic index, for the nature of severe VLS is a difficult toxicity to deal with in routine clinical practice.

The pathophysiology of VLS arising from dgA-containing ITs may involve nontargeted toxicity to the vascular endothelium (15). Initial evidence suggests that ricin A chain can interact with fibronectin, which is required for the normal physiology of vascular endothelial cells (16). Strategies to circumvent this might include blocking this interaction with another agent and/or engineering the dgA molecule to prevent this interaction. Alternatively, a qualitatively different type of toxin might be coupled to these respective targeting molecules.

Despite these concerns, IgG-RFB4-dgA and IgG-RFT5-dgA can achieve therapeutically useful concentrations at safe doses. Thus, a high priority will be to combine these ITs with active chemotherapeutic regimens. Indeed, evidence from SCID mice bearing Daudi xenografts demonstrates that IgG-RFB4-dgA can successfully potentiate the activity of a variety of chemotherapeutic agents when given concomitantly or after chemotherapy (17). Successful demonstration that the clinical toxicities of chemotherapeutic agents are not seriously affected by tolerable doses of IT that produce ~1000 ng/mL of ITs when administered by a bolus schedule would encourage the IT use as an adjuvant to chemotherapy in newly diagnosed patients. The lack of hepatotoxicity of the dgA ITs also favors such an approach.

Thus, initial clinical studies with dgA ITs have been encouraging in that both clinical activity and a basis for further studies have been defined. The challenge for the future will be to design treatment programs that build on the useful features of the molecules while carefully avoiding their toxic features. In particular, empirical dose escalation schemes that produce serum concentrations greater than 1000–1500 ng/mL of dgA IT would not appear to be warranted unless the dgA has been structurally altered to expect loss of its vasculotoxic features.

REFERENCES

1. Ghetie M, Ghetie V, Vitetta ES. The use of immunoconjugates in cancer therapy. Exp Opin Invest Drugs 1996; 5:309–321.
2. Thorpe PE, Detre SI, Foxwell BMJ, Brown ANF, Skilleter DN, Wilson G, Forrester JA, Stirpe F. Modification of the carbohydrate in ricin with metaperiodiate-cyanoborohydride mixtures. Effects on toxicity and in vivo distribution. Eur J Biochem 1985; 147:197–206.
3. Vitetta ES, Stone M, Amlot P, Fay J, May R, Till M, Newman J, Clark P, Collins R, Cunningham D, Ghetie V, Uhr JW, Thorpe PE. Phase I immunotoxin trial in patients with B-cell lymphoma. Cancer Res 1991; 51:4052–4058.
4. Shen G-L, Li JL, Ghetie MA, Ghetie V, May RD, Till M, Brown AN, Relf M, Knowles P, Uhr JW, Janossy G, Amlot P, Vitetta ES, Thorpe PE. Evaluation of four CD22 antibodies as ricin A-chain-containing immunotoxins for the in vivo therapy of human B-cell leukemias and lymphomas. Int J Cancer 1988; 42:792–797.
5. Amlot PL, Stone MJ, Cunningham D, Fay J, Newman J, Collins R, May R, McCarthy M, Richardson J, Ghetie V, Ramilo O, Thorpe PE, Uhr JW, Vitetta ES. A phase I study of an anti-CD22-deglycosylated ricin A chain immunotoxin in the treatment of B-cell lymphomas resistant to conventional therapy. Blood 1993; 82:2624–2633.
6. Sausville EA, Headlee D, Stetler-Stevenson M, Jaffe ES, Solomon D, Figg WD, Herdt J, Kopp WC, Rager H, Steinberg SM, Ghetie V, Schindler J, Uhr J, Wittes RE, Vitetta ES. Continuous infusion of the anti-CD22 immunotoxin IgG-RFB4-SMPT-dgA in patients with B-cell lymphoma: a Phase I study. Blood 1995; 85: 3457–3465.
7. Senderowicz AM, Vitetta E, Headlee D, Ghetie V, Uhr JW, Figg WD, Lush RM, Stetler-Stevenson M, Kershaw G, Kingma DW, Jaffe ES, Sausville EA. Complete sustained response of a refractory, post-transplantation, large B-cell lymphoma to an anti-CD22 immunotoxin. Ann Int Med 1997; 126:882–885.
8. Ghetie MA, May RD, Till M, Uhr JW, Ghetie V, Knowles PO, Relf M, Brown A, Wallace PM, Janossy G, Amlot P, Vitetta ES, Thorpe PE. Evaluation of ricin A chain-containing immunotoxins directed against CD19 and CD22 antigens on normal and malignant human B-cells as potential reagents for in vivo therapy. Cancer Res 1988; 48:2610–2617.
9. Stone MJ, Sausville EA, Fay JW, Headlee D, Collins RH, Figg WD, Stetler-Stevenson M, Jain V, Jaffe ES, Solomon D, Lush RM, Senderowicz A, Ghetie V, Schindler J, Uhr JW, Vitetta ES. A Phase I study of bolus versus continuous infusion of the anti-CD19 immunotoxin, IgG-HD37-dgA, in patients with B-cell lymphoma. Blood 1996; 88:1188–1197.
10. Conry RM, Khazaeli MB, Saleh MN, Ghetie V, Vitetta ES, Liu T, LoBuglio AF. Phase I trial of an anti-CD19 deglycosylated ricin A-chain immunotoxin in non-Hodgkin's lymphoma: effect of an intensive schedule of administration. J Immunotherapy 1995; 18:231–241.
11. Ghetie MA, Tucker K, Richardson J, Uhr JW, Vitetta ES. The antitumor activity of an anti-CD22 immunotoxin in SCID mice with disseminated Daudi lymphoma is

enhanced by either an anti-CD19 antibody or an anti-CD19 immunotoxin. Blood 1992; 80:2315–2320.
12. Engert A, Martin G, Amlot P, Wijdener J, Diehl V, Thorpe P. Immunotoxins constructed with CD25 monoclonal antibodies and deglycosylated ricin A chain have potent anti-tumor effects against human Hodgkin cells in vitro and solid Hodgkin tumors in mice. Int. J. Cancer 1991; 49:450.
13. Winkler U, Gottstein C, Shön G, Kapp U, Wolf J, Hansmann ML, Bohlen H, Thorpe P, Diehl V, Engert A. Successful treatment of disseminated human Hodgkin's disease in SCID mice using deglycosylated ricin A-chain immunotoxins. Blood 1994; 83:466.
14. Engert A, Diehl V, Schnell R, Radszuhn A, Hatwig MT, Drillich S, Schön G, Bohlen H, Tesch H, Hansmann ML, Barth S, Schindler J, Ghetie V, Uhr J, Vitetta E. A Phase I study of an anti-CD25 ricin A-chain immunotoxin (RFT5-SMPT-dgA) in patients with refractory Hodgkin's lymphoma. Blood 1997; 89:403–410.
15. Soler-Rodriguez AM, Ghetie MA, Oppenheimer-Marks N, Uhr JW, Vitetta ES. Ricin A-chain and ricin A-chain immunotoxins rapidly damage human endothelial cells: implications for vascular leak syndrome. Exp Cell Res 1993; 206:227–239.
16. Baluna R, Ghetie V, Oppenheimer-Marks N, and Vitetta ES. Fibronectin inhibits the cytotoxic effect of ricin A chain on endothelial cells. Int J Immunopharmacol 1996; 18:355–361.
17. Ghetie MA, Tucker K, Richardson J, Uhr JW, Vitetta ES. Eradication of minimal disease in severe combined immunodeficient mice with disseminated Daudi lymphoma using chemotherapy and an immunotoxin cocktail. Blood 1994; 84:702–707.

5
Immunotoxin Therapy of Lymphoma: Studies with Anti-B4-Blocked Ricin

Pratik S. Multani and Michael L. Grossbard
Harvard Medical School and Massachusetts General Hospital, Boston, Massachusetts

I. INTRODUCTION

The non-Hodgkin's lymphomas (NHLs) comprise a group of malignancies of B- and T-lymphocytes. Approximately 53,000 patients will be diagnosed with NHL in the United States in 1997 (1). The use of chemotherapy for the treatment of NHL is considered a success story in contemporary oncology. Through the use of combination chemotherapy and modern high-energy radiation therapy, more than 75% of patients can expect an initial remission. Nevertheless many patients will relapse. Even with innovations such as high-dose therapy with autologous stem-cell rescue for the treatment of patients who fail initial therapy, fewer than 25% of these patients will be cured.

Tumor-cell resistance to standard chemotherapy may explain in part the failure of both initial and salvage chemotherapy. Furthermore, conventional cytotoxic therapy carries the risk of significant morbidity and the potential for early mortality, especially in the older patient population. Thus, current research attempts to focus on developing agents with novel mechanisms of action and a lower toxicity profile, simultaneously circumventing the problems of resistance and toxicity.

Monoclonal antibody–based therapies in general, and immunotoxins in particular, hold promise to be such agents. The specificity of the antibody–antigen interaction offers the potential to target cytotoxic therapy to tumor cells with minimal injury to bystander normal tissue, thereby minimizing systemic toxicity. Furthermore, the antibody can be used as a carrier to deliver potent cytotoxic agents that may circumvent the resistance that tumor cells develop to standard chemotherapeutic drugs. Immunotoxins comprise one class of monoclonal antibody–based therapies. These agents combine the specificity of antibodies with the potency of toxins, derived from plants (e.g., ricin, saporin, and pokeweed antiviral protein) as well as from bacteria (e.g., diphtheria toxin and *Pseudomonas* exotoxin A). Despite their varied origins, these toxins all act to inhibit the protein synthetic machinery of cells, typically at picomolar concentrations.

One such toxin is blocked ricin (bR). The bR moiety, a biochemically modified plant-derived toxin, has been conjugated to several monoclonal antibodies, each in an attempt to target a different malignancy. Blocked ricin conjugates have been tested against NHL (2,3), chronic lymphocytic leukemia, multiple myeloma (4), acute myelogenous leukemia (5), acute lymphoblastic leukemia (6), cutaneous T-cell lymphoma (7), and small-cell lung cancer (8–10). Phase I and II studies have demonstrated that the blocked ricin class of immunotoxins can be administered with tolerable and reversible toxicities and that these agents have biologic activity. This chapter will focus on the development and clinical testing of one specific blocked-ricin conjugate, Anti-B4-blocked ricin, used predominantly for the therapy of NHL.

II. BLOCKED RICIN

Ricin is a natural product derived from the castor bean (*Ricinus communis*). It is a heterodimeric protein composed of two chains, an ''A-chain'' and a ''B-chain.'' The cytotoxicity of the heterodimer resides within the A-chain. This portion possesses N-glycosidase activity, which inactivates the 60S ribosomal subunit through hydrolyzing an adenine–ribose linkage within the 23S rRNA component, thus disrupting further protein synthesis (11,12). The B-chain facilitates entry of the A-chain into the cell, by effecting both binding and translocation. After the protein has been taken up through endocytosis, the B-chain binds nonspecifically to galactose residues present on the cell surface of all eukaryotic cells and mediates translocation of the A-chain across the vesicular membrane.

Because of its potent activity as an inhibitor of protein synthesis, unmodified native ricin is lethal to humans in microgram quantities. When incubated at picomolar concentrations in vitro, with either normal or malignant cell lines, native ricin can achieve more than five logs of cell reduction (13). In order to harness this tremendous cytotoxic potency, native ricin has been conjugated to monoclonal antibodies. Phase I clinical studies with native ricin conjugates have demonstrated a maximal tolerated dose (MTD) of 23 µg/m^2 (14). The clinical use of the agent was not explored further, however, because of high toxicity to normal tissues and the absence of a clear therapeutic window. Unfortunately, despite its conjugation to the monoclonal antibody, the presence of the unmodified B-chain allowed nonspecific binding and thus toxicity to bystander cells.

One solution to this dilemma involves utilizing only the ricin A-chain, which is dissociated either through chemical dissociation or produced by recombinant DNA technology. The isolated A-chain then is conjugated to an appropriate monoclonal antibody. Through this approach, any nonspecific binding of the ricin B-chain is prevented, although the membrane translocation capability of the ricin B-chain also is deleted (15). The RFB4 murine monoclonal antibody that recognizes CD22, another B-cell antigen, has been conjugated to ricin A-chain and tested in Phase I trials (16). That approach is the subject of Chapter 4 in this volume.

Another solution to reducing the non-specific toxicity of the ricin-antibody conjugate resides in modifying the B-chain in such a way as to preserve its membrane translocation capacity while subverting its nonspecific binding. Specifically, the B-chain is modified at the two major galactose-binding sites through a covalent linkage with modified glycopeptides containing N-linked oligosaccharides derived from fetuin (13,17). The end result is "blocked ricin," which retains the translocation capacity but not the nonspecific binding ability of native ricin.

III. ANTI-B4-BLOCKED RICIN

A. Introduction

The Anti-B4-blocked ricin immunotoxin comprises the modified, or "blocked," ricin molecule just described conjugated to an IgG1 murine monoclonal antibody, Anti-B4, which binds to the CD19 cell-surface antigen. This cell-surface antigen is an attractive target for antibody-mediated therapy because it is found on a broad range of hematologic malignancies, including 95% of cases of B-cell NHL, acute lymphoblastic leukemia (ALL), and chronic lymphocytic leukemia (CLL) (18,19). The CD19 antigen is the earliest detectable pan-B-cell antigen and is present throughout B-cell development. Conversely, the antigen appears to be restricted to the B-cell lineage, for extensive tissue binding assays fail to demonstrate expression on other normal tissues. Of critical importance is the fact that hematopoietic stem cells also do not express CD19 and thus are potentially spared toxicity from the Anti-B4-blocked ricin (Anti-B4-bR) conjugate, unlike normal B-cells.

B. Single-Agent Studies

1. In Vitro Studies

Cytotoxic cell culture assays using both CD19-positive and CD19-negative cell lines were conducted with the Anti-B4-bR conjugate (3,13,20,21). The cultured cell lines were incubated with the immunoconjugate in growth medium for 24 h at 37°C. The treated cells then were washed and placed into fresh medium, with the surviving fraction determined by a direct cytotoxicity assay, termed the *growth back-extrapolation assay*. Cytotoxicity was measured as the IC_{37} (inhibitory concentration—37%) and the log kill (see Figure 1).

Incubation with the Namalwa cell line, a B4 (CD19)-positive Burkitt's lymphoma cell line, demonstrated that concentrations of the immunotoxin conjugate of 5 nanomolar (nM) could deplete greater than five logs of malignant cells (21). The IC_{37} values ranged from 10.3×10^{-3} nM to 45×10^{-3} nM. The IC_{37} for native ricin is 4×10^{-6} nM. In contrast, incubation with the CD19-negative MOLT-4 cell line, a T-cell line, showed a lack of cytotoxicity, with an IC_{37} ranging from 1.0 to 5.7 nM, about 100-fold greater than for the Namalwa cell line.

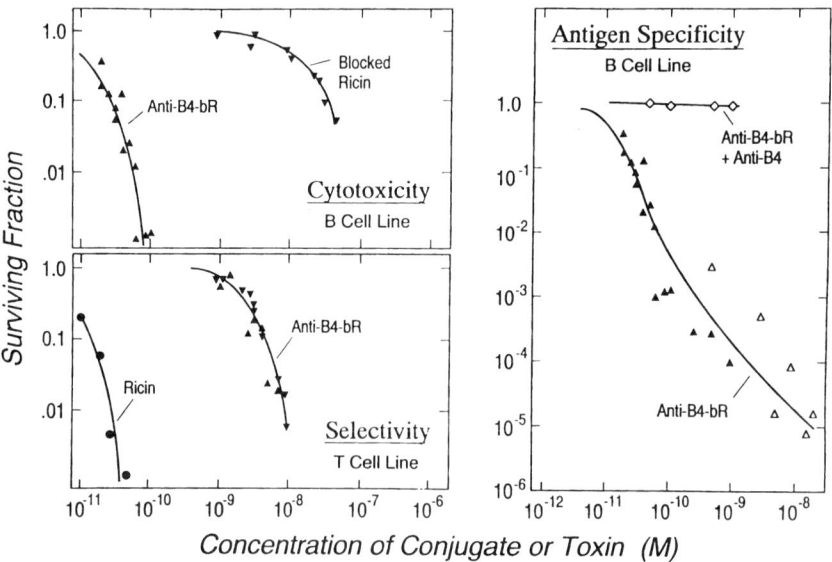

Figure 1 In vitro immunotoxin cytotoxicity. Demonstration of Anti-B4-bR cytotoxicity (upper left), selectivity (lower left), and specificity (right). Cell kill was assessed by determining the fraction of cells surviving after a 24-h incubation with the immunotoxin. (From Ref. 3. Reprinted with permission.)

Exposure of both cell lines to unconjugated blocked ricin showed equal nonspecific cytotoxicity but at concentrations two to three logs higher than the concentration used in the conjugated immunotoxin assays against CD19-positive cells (13).

The same incubation studies were done in the presence of lactose (which blocks B-chain binding to galactose residues) at a concentration of 30 mmol/L, to determine if cytotoxicity was due to residual unblocked ricin mediating nonspecific binding. The IC_{37} would be expected to be higher in the presence of lactose interference if even part of the cytotoxicity were mediated by nonspecific binding of unblocked ricin B-chain. These studies found no increase in the IC_{37} for Anti-B4-bR. Further confirmation that cytotoxicity was mediated through a specific antibody–antigen interaction was obtained by demonstrating that coincubation with excess unconjugated antibody could completely negate the cytotoxicity of the blocked ricin conjugate, such that an IC_{37} could not even be determined.

Immunoperoxidase staining has been used to confirm the tissue specificity of the murine monoclonal Anti-B4 antibody. Comparison of the Anti-B4 monoclonal antibody with the blocked ricin conjugated antibody showed an identical distribution using immunoperoxidase staining (M. Borowitz, Duke University School of Medicine, personal communication, June 1989). The Anti-B4 blocked ricin conjugate bound to all tissues expected to harbor significant numbers of CD19-positive cells, such as lymph nodes, spleen, bone marrow, and thymus. Conversely, epithelial, mesenchymal, and neuroectodermal tissues did not react with Anti-B4-bR. Other tissues that showed no reactivity included liver, specifically hepatocytes, bile ducts, Kupffer cells, and endothelial cells, myocardium, skeletal muscle, gastrointestinal tract, breast, lung, pancreas, and ovaries.

Thus, the coupling of the blocked ricin toxin to a monoclonal antibody confers both increased specificity and potency. The in vitro studies also demonstrated that the degree of cell kill was a function of both the concentration of the immunotoxin and the exposure time. The latter provided rationale for consideration of continuous infusion drug schedules during in vivo testing.

2. Animal Studies

Dose Escalation

Preclinical studies in animals were performed in both murine and simian models (22). Studies in Swiss albino mice were performed using bolus infusion of the Anti-B4-bR conjugate. The drug was given over 60 s at doses ranging from 50 µg/kg to 2000 µg/kg. Doses below 500 µg/kg showed no lethal toxicity. Histopathologic exam revealed minimal periportal inflammation within the liver, bone marrow hyperplasia, and necrosis of germinal centers within the spleen and lymph nodes. At single-bolus doses between 1000 and 2000 µg/kg, all mice were dead within 3 days. Histopathologic exam of these animals revealed multifocal hepatocyte necrosis and hemorrhage. The bone marrow, lymph nodes, and spleen also revealed necrosis.

Studies then were performed giving the drug on five consecutive days at doses of 40 µg/kg/d (total dose 200 µg/kg) and 200 µg/kg/d (total dose 1000 µg/kg). The lower dose resulted in no lethal toxicity, whereas 4 of the 20 mice given the higher dose died. These mice had multifocal hepatocellular necrosis, acute tubular necrosis of the kidney, moderate to severe alveolar edema, and bone marrow and lymphoid hyperplasia.

Similar dose ranging studies were carried out in adult cynomolgus monkeys, again using the schedule of single-day bolus dose over 60 s as well as the schedule of daily dosing for five consecutive days. The single-dose regimen was given at doses ranging from 50 to 1000 µg/kg. Doses under 200 µg/kg resulted in no clinically evident toxicity. As in the murine tests, however, histopathologic examination of the liver revealed mild to moderate hepatocellular vacuolation and hyperplasia of lymphoid tissues and bone marrow. Doses of 500 µg/kg resulted in clinical toxicity, specifically lethargy and anorexia. Histopathologic examination demonstrated superficial hemorrhages within the pancreas, heart, lungs, and kidneys, as well as the hepatic and bone marrow findings seen at the lower doses. The highest dose level, 1000 µg/kg, resulted in death within 5 days. Histopathologic findings were similar to those described earlier.

The 5-consecutive-day dosing schedule was tested at 10 µg/kg/d (total dose 50 µg/kg) and at 100 µg/kg/d (total dose 500 µg/kg). The lower dose resulted in minimal multifocal hepatic necrosis, mild bone marrow hyperplasia, diffuse hyperplasia of lymph nodes, and hyaline deposition within renal tubules. The higher dose level showed similar histopathologic toxicity but of higher degree. Neither dose level, however, was associated with any lethal toxicity.

Continuous infusion toxicity studies were performed in four rhesus monkeys (23). These animals were given a bolus dose of Anti-B4-bR over 60 s (equal to 7.5% of the total administered dose), followed by a continuous infusion to a total dose of either 200, 500, 1000, or 1500 µg/kg over 4–7 days. Pharmacokinetic studies demonstrated that a plateau serum level of 1.8 nm was achieved in the monkey treated at the 200-µg/kg dose level and 5.5 nm at the 1500-µg/kg dose level.

No lethal toxicity was observed. Reversible transaminase elevation was observed in all monkeys, with the AST peaking on day 1 or 2 and returning to near normal by day 15. The AST peaks were fourfold, eightfold, and 13-fold from baseline in the first three animals, but only sevenfold for the animal treated at 1500 µg/kg. The ALT peaked on days 2–5 at two- to fourfold above baseline, and again was reversible. Histopathologic changes in these animals were similar to those found in the cynomolgus monkeys. Day 15 examination of the livers demonstrated hepatocellular changes, ranging from mild fatty changes to mild inflammation with multicellular necrosis. These changes did not appear to be dose dependent. All monkeys also showed evidence of bone marrow and lymphoid hyperplasia.

Taken together, these data clearly show a strong schedule dependence to the toxicity profile of the Anti-B4-blocked ricin immunotoxin, with the liver being the primary site of toxicity. These animal studies provided the rationale for subsequent human Phase I trials in which a continuous dosing schedule was employed.

Efficacy

Therapeutic efficacy studies of the Anti-B4-blocked ricin conjugate also have been tested in vivo, using SCID mouse tumor models (24). In these survival experiments, SCID mice received one of three tumor cell lines: the Namalwa human lymphoma cell line, a human non-T, non-B acute lymphoblastic leukemia cell line (Nalm-6), or a murine B-cell lymphoma cell line transfected with the human CD19 gene (300B4). In the first survival model, SCID mice were given an intraperitoneal injection of 5×10^7 Namalwa or 300B4 cells. One hour later, they received 100 µg/kg of the ricin conjugate, followed by four more doses on successive days for a total dose of 500 µg/kg. In the second survival model, SCID mice were administered an intravenous injection (via the tail vein) of 4×10^6 Namalwa or Nalm-6 cells, followed 7 days later by the ricin conjugate, again 100 µg/kg/d for five successive days.

In both models, there was demonstrable efficacy, with a prolongation of survival in the treated animals. For example, in the group given tumor cells intraperitoneally, the time of survival of 50% of the 300B4 cohort was 9 days for control animals versus 19 days for the Anti-B4-bR-treated animals. Similarly, in the group given Namalwa tumor cells intravenously, the time of survival for 50% of the animals was 27 days for control animals versus 41 days for the treated animals. Furthermore, quantitation of in vivo tumor cell kill demonstrated elimination of up to 3 logs of tumor cells. Thus, efficacy of the immunotoxin could be demonstrated in an in vivo animal model.

C. Combination Studies

1. In Vitro Combination Studies

Preclinical studies also have been performed using Anti-B4-bR in combination with conventional chemotherapy drugs in both in vitro and in animal tumor models. The in vitro studies were performed using the Namalwa cell line and a special *P*-glycoprotein-expressing cell line, Namalwa/*mdr*-1, created by transfecting Namalwa cells with the *mdr*-1 gene (25). Cells were incubated for 3 days with Anti-B4-bR alone, Anti-B4-bR in combination with one of two conventional chemotherapeutic agents, or with one of the chemotherapeutic agents alone. The chemotherapeutic drugs, etoposide and doxorubicin, are known substrates for the transmembrane *P*-glycoprotein pump.

As expected, the *P*-glycoprotein-expressing cell line was sixfold more resistant to etoposide and doxorubicin, confirming the resistance conferred by expression of the *mdr*-1 gene. Interestingly, however, the *P*-glycoprotein-expressing cells were slightly more sensitive to Anti-B4-bR alone than were the Namalwa cells, with IC_{37} values of 4×10^{-3} nM and 8×10^{-3} nM concentrations, respectively.

When the Anti-B4-bR conjugate was combined with either etoposide or doxorubicin, additive or synergistic cell kill of both cell lines was observed. For example, the Namalwa cells were incubated with Anti-B4-blocked ricin at a range of concentrations, from 8×10^{-3} nM to 16×10^{-3} nM, in combination with doxorubicin at 2–12 nM. Additive cytotoxicity was observed; and at the higher ricin conjugate concentrations, synergistic cytotoxicity was observed. The *P*-glycoprotein Namalwa cell line similarly was tested, using Anti-B4-bR concentrations ranging from 10×10^{-3} nM to 20×10^{-3} nM in combination with doxorubicin at 30–90 nM. At all dose combinations, cell kill was synergistic with the two agents. A similar phenomenon was observed with etoposide.

These studies suggest two exciting possibilities. The first is that the ricin immunoconjugate may be a potential therapeutic modality for patients with previously treated disease who are likely to harbor resistant clones. The second is the provocative finding of synergistic interaction with conventional chemotherapy.

2. In Vivo Combination Studies

Xenografts of the Namalwa and Namalwa/*mdr*-1 cell lines in SCID mice also have been used to test the in vivo interaction of the ricin immunoconjugate and conventional chemotherapeutic agents (25). When these animals were treated with either doxorubicin or etoposide alone, at their respective maximum tolerated doses, 3 mg/kg/d every 4 d $\times$ 3 and 15 mg/kg/d every 2 d $\times$ 3, a 26–32% increase in survival was observed for the Namalwa xenograft cohort and no increase in survival for the Namalwa/*mdr*-1 xenograft cohort as compared with untreated control mice. Treatment with five daily bolus doses of Anti-B4-blocked ricin at 50 µg/kg/d resulted in a 43–56% increase in survival in both groups, again suggesting that the expression of *P*-glycoprotein has no bearing on the efficacy of the ricin conjugate. In contrast to the single-agent experiments, combination treatment with Anti-B4-bR followed by one or the other chemotherapeutic agent resulted in a 109–129% increase in survival, again in both the Namalwa and the Namalwa/*mdr*-1 xenograft cohorts. Furthermore, analysis of *P*-glycoprotein expression of Namalwa/*mdr*-1 tumor cells from treated animals demonstrated a subpopulation of tumor cells with lower levels of *P*-glycoprotein expression compared with untreated controls. In contrast, CD19 expression was maintained at high levels in treated animals.

These same researchers extended their findings by examining the efficacy in vivo of Anti-B4-bR conjugate with conventional combination chemotherapy (26). Again SCID mice xenografts were created using either the Namalwa or Namalwa/*mdr*-1 cell lines. Similar results as earlier were obtained with single-agent chemotherapy using etoposide, doxorubicin, and vincristine; that is, these agents increased survival by 22–32% in Namalwa xenografts and 0–4% in Namalwa/*mdr*-1 xenografts. All three drugs are known substrates of the *mdr*-1 gene product. Two other drugs tested, cyclophosphamide and cisplatin, are not *P*-glycoprotein substrates and did demonstrate efficacy in the Namalwa/*mdr*-1 xenografts, increasing survival by 92% and 28%, respectively. Animals treated with the ricin immunoconjugate alone had increased survivals of 65% in the Namalwa xenografts and 72% in the Namalwa/*mdr*-1 xenografts.

Animals with Namalwa/*mdr*-1 xenografts treated with combination chemotherapy regimens alone, either CHOE (cyclophosphamide, doxorubicin, vincristine, and etoposide) or CCE (cyclophosphamide, cisplatin, and etoposide), showed increased survivals of 58% and 129%, respectively. There were no cures. When the CHOE regimen was combined with the Anti-B4-bR, however, efficacy was markedly increased, with survival times increasing 173% and cures achieved in 2 of 10 mice (i.e., disease-free at 180 days). Combination with the CCE regimen was even more efficacious, with long-term cures in 50% of the mice.

These studies represent the closest analog to how immunotoxins could be used in the treatment of human malignancies. The authors suggest that the sequencing of the two modalities may be critical in their synergistic efficacy. The initial administration of the ricin immunotoxin, besides being cytotoxic in its own right, may also sufficiently disrupt the protein synthesis of surviving cells such that *P*-glycoprotein expression is inhibited, permitting greater activity of the conventional chemotherapeutic agents.

D. Phase I/II Studies

1. Relapsed or Refractory Disease

Building on this extensive preclinical testing, the first Phase I trial of Anti-B4-bR was conducted in 25 patients with refractory B-cell neoplasms, including 23 patients with NHL and one each with CLL and ALL (22) (see Table 1). The majority of patients were in resistant relapse, with nine patients being treated after failing bone marrow transplant. Patients were given a daily 1-hour infusion for five consecutive days at doses ranging from 1 µg/kg/d to 60 µg/kg/d. The maximal tolerated dose (MTD) was 50 µg/kg/d (total dose 250 µg/kg).

The dose-limiting toxicity (DLT) was transient, Grade 3 elevations of the AST and ALT, similar to the toxicity in the simian experiments. Transaminase elevation occurred within 24–48 h after beginning treatment, peaked within 48 h

Table 1 Human Studies of Anti-B4-Blocked Ricin

Disease	Setting	No. of patients	Schedule	Total dose (MTD)	Toxicity	HAMA/HARA	Response
Refractory B-cell neoplasms (23)	Phase I	25	IV bolus over 1 h daily × 5 d	250 µg/kg	Transaminase elevations, thrombocytopenia, fever, fatigue, nausea, pleural effusion	9/25	1 CR, 2 PR
Refractory B-cell neoplasms (24)	Phase I	34	Continuous IV infusion × 7 d	350 µg/kg	Transaminase elevations, thrombocytopenia, dyspnea, edema, hypoalbuminemia, capillary leak, fever	24/34	2 CR, 3 PR
B-cell NHL (35)	Phase I adjuvant Rx post-ABMT	12	Continuous IV infusion × 7 d	280 µg/kg	Transaminase elevations, thrombocytopenia, dyspnea, edema, hypoalbuminemia, capillary leak, fever	7/12	7 relapse-free, median F/U 4 yr

Disease	Phase	N	Regimen	Dose	Toxicity	Response	Outcome
B-cell NHL (36)	Phase II adjuvant Rx post-ABMT	49	Continuous IV infusion × 7 d every 14 d	210 μg/LBM	Transaminase elevations, thrombocytopenia, capillary leak, edema	23/49	27 relapse-free, median F/U × yr; 3 died in CR
B-cell NHL[a]	Phase III adjuvant Rx post-ABMT	145	Continuous IV infusion × 7 d	210 μg/LBM	Still under analysis	Still under analysis	Still under analysis
Indolent NHL[a]	Phase II	37	ProMACE-CytaBOM × 6–8 cycles + continuous IV infusion × 7 d every 14 d	210 μg/LBM	Stil under analysis	Still under analysis	Still under analysis
Relapsed AIDS-related NHL (39)	Phase I	9	Continuous IV infusion × 28 d	560 μg/kg	Transaminase elevations	3/9	1 CR, 1 PR
Newly diagnosed AIDS-related NHL (40)	Phase II	47 enrolled; 28 received anti-B4-bR	Low-dose m-BACOD + continuous IV infusion × 7 d with cycles 3 ± 4	140 μg/kg	Transaminase elevations	8/28	14 CR, 12 PR Median survival for all patients 9.1 months

[a] Unpublished

after the day-5 dose, and generally resolved within the next 7 d. Additional liver-associated clinical parameters remained unchanged, including alkaline phosphatase, bilirubin, and prothrombin time. Other toxicities included fever, hypoalbuminemia, and, in three patients, Grade 4 thrombocytopenia. There was no evidence of cardiac or pulmonary toxicity. Twenty of the 25 patients received only one course of immunotoxin, and five patients were retreated.

Pharmacologic studies demonstrated that peak serum levels greater than 2 nM could be achieved at the MTD, a concentration capable of killing up to five logs of tumor cell kill based on in vitro data with the Namalwa cell line. Peak levels on subsequent treatment days did not vary significantly from day 1. Peak levels were achieved within 1–2 h after dosing in all patients. Serum levels rapidly fell, however, decreasing to below 0.5 nM within 4 h after the end of the infusion in patients treated at the MTD.

All patients were tested for the development of human-antimouse antibodies (HAMA) and human-antiricin antibodies (HARA). Nine of the 25 patients developed both HAMA and HARA within 23 and 41 d, respectively, following therapy, in a nondose- and nondisease-associated pattern. Of the five patients who were retreated, only one patient eventually developed a HAMA response. Of note, there were no allergic manifestations associated with HAMA or HARA responses, and no patient was treated after documentation of HAMA response.

Finally, there were one complete response (CR) and two partial responses (PRs) observed in patients with NHL, as well as, eight transient or mixed responses. Thus, the Anti-B4-bR immunotoxin could be delivered safely and had demonstrable clinical efficacy in patients with relapsed resistant disease. The main shortcoming of the study, however, was the use of bolus dosing. Although levels that correlated with significant in vitro cytotoxicity could be achieved, they were not maintained, potentially limiting efficacy.

Because of the concern of insufficient exposure time of tumor to adequate levels of the immunotoxin, the next Phase I trial utilized a continuous infusion dosing schedule (23). Preclinical studies in primates demonstrated that effective plateau levels could be achieved using this regimen. This study enrolled 34 patients with relapsed and refractory B-cell neoplasms, 26 patients with NHL, and the remainder with either CLL or ALL. Sixteen patients had failed bone marrow transplant. Patient cohorts were treated at doses ranging from 10 µg/kg/d to 70 µg/kg/d in 10-µg/kg increments, delivered as a continuous infusion for 7 d. Patients treated at the three lowest dose levels (10, 20, and 30 µg/kg/d) also received an initial loading bolus dose of 20 µg/kg.

The MTD was reached at 50 µg/kg/d × 7 days (total dose 350 µg/kg). The DLTs were reversible Grade 4 elevations in the serum AST and ALT and Grade 4 thrombocytopenia. As with the bolus dosing schedule, transaminase levels rose within 24–48 h, continued to rise during the remainder of the infusion, peaked within 48 h of the end of the infusion, and returned to baseline within

7–14 d. No other clinical parameters of liver function were affected. Almost 80% of patients experienced Grade 2 or greater thrombocytopenia, with six patients experiencing Grade 4 toxicity. Other toxicities included fever, nausea, headaches, and myalgias. All patients experienced some degree of hypoalbuminemia, and more than half of patients experienced peripheral edema and weight gain. Dyspnea occurred in five patients. This last constellation of toxicities was felt to be secondary to a generalized capillary leak syndrome.

Pharmacokinetic studies demonstrated that patients with NHL treated at the MTD achieved a serum level greater than 0.5 nM within 24–48 h, and greater than 1.0 nM within 96 h. These plateau levels then were sustained for the remainder of the 7 d. Again these levels correspond to what would be potentially therapeutic serum levels based on in vitro data. Lower serum plateau levels were obtained in patients with a greater burden of circulating CD19-positive cells, namely, the patients with CLL and ALL. In fact, all eight patients with CLL and ALL failed to achieve serum levels greater than 0.2 nM, regardless of dose.

Analysis of humoral immune responses in all the patients also was performed. Twenty-four patients developed HAMA and/or HARA responses, with 13 developing both. Immune responses developed within 12–92 days of treatment, at a median of 24 days for HAMA and 22 days for HARA. As with the prior Phase I study, no patient experienced any allergic reaction.

Two complete remissions occurred in patients with minimal tumor burdens. Responses also included three PRs and 11 transient responses. These data confirm that the continuous infusion regimen can be delivered safely, permitting the administration of a higher total dose of Anti-B4-bR than the bolus dosing regimen. Unlike the preclinical studies, however, continuous infusion did not decrease the toxicity when tested in humans, although the majority of toxicities were tolerable and reversible. The continuous dosing schedule also did not decrease the rate of formation of HAMA and HARA responses. Although not designed to be an efficacy study, there did not appear to be any increase in clinical response rates with the continuous dosing schedule.

Taken together, the two Phase I trials demonstrate that the Anti-B4-bR immunoconjugate can be given safely and that serum levels corresponding to therapeutically meaningful concentrations can be achieved when using a continuous infusion schedule. All toxicities were reversible and tolerable. The low response rate does raise the question of whether use of the immunoconjugate as a single agent is appropriate in patients with bulk disease, where penetration of the large immunotoxin molecule may be suboptimal. Furthermore, the use of the ricin conjugate in patients with circulating CD19-positive cells results in rapid clearance of the antibody from the circulation, potentially limiting the ability of the antibody to penetrate into tissue sites of disease (27).

This issue was highlighted in a subsequent Phase II study of patients with either relapsed or previously untreated low-grade NHL. Patients were given Anti-

B4-bR at doses of 30–50 µg/kg/d × 7 d at 14-d intervals. One patient experienced Grade 5 (lethal) toxicity, developing nausea, abdominal pain, and subsequent Grade 4 hypotension and thrombocytopenia, all felt to be secondary to severe generalized capillary leak syndrome. Despite the fact that these patients were not heavily pretreated, there were no sustained complete or partial responses. Again this poor response rate was attributed to bulk of disease and poor penetration of the immunotoxin. Furthermore, in vitro studies have demonstrated that bulky tumors can limit diffusion of immunotoxin due to significant interstitial pressures (28).

2. Minimal Residual Disease After BMT

Given the concern that bulk disease posed a barrier to adequate tumor penetration of the ricin conjugate, a series of studies was undertaken in patients likely to harbor only minimal tumor burdens, namely, as a consolidation therapy in patients who had undergone high-dose chemotherapy with autologous bone marrow transplant (HDT-ABMT) for chemotherapy-sensitive relapsed NHL (29–33). This latter procedure has been shown to achieve high rates of complete remission. Unfortunately, 55–85% of these patients will relapse within 24 months following transplant, due either to chemotherapy-resistant tumor cells that survived the conditioning regimen or from the reinfusion of tumor-contaminated bone marrow or peripheral blood stem cells. Such patients would be expected to harbor only minimal residual disease without any of the potential obstacles posed by bulk tumor deposits. Anti-B4-bR immunotoxin therapy would offer an attractive adjuvant treatment, given that previous in vitro data suggest that chemotherapy-resistant cells would retain sensitivity to this alternate therapeutic modality.

In a Phase I trial of 12 patients who had achieved a CR after HDT-ABMT for B-cell NHL, patients received Anti-B4-bR at doses ranging from 20 to 50 µg/kg/d as a 7-d continuous infusion at a median of 83 d after ABMT (34). The observed DLTs were similar to those seen in earlier Phase I studies, namely, reversible Grade 4 transaminase elevations and thrombocytopenia. Of note, these patients had baseline low platelet counts, since they were treated soon after bone marrow engraftment following high-dose conditioning therapy. Evidence of capillary leak syndrome was observed but was not dose-limiting.

The MTD was 40 µg/kg/d for 7 d (total dose 280 µg/kg), lower than that observed in previous investigations conducted in patients with bulk disease. This finding was not surprising given the low tumor burden of these patients and the greater potential for nonspecific exposure of normal tissues to the immunotoxin. Despite the profound immunologic deficit in patients early after ABMT, seven patients still developed HAMA and/or HARA responses, highlighting the significant immunogenicity of the ricin immunoconjugate. At a median follow-up of more than 4 years, seven of 12 patients remained in CR.

A follow-up Phase II trial of Anti-B4-bR as adjuvant treatment following HDT-ABMT in patients with B-cell NHL subsequently was completed (35). In this trial, patients were eligible for retreatment at 14-d intervals rather than the 28-d intervals used in earlier trials, because prior data demonstrated no evidence of HAMA or HARA responses earlier than 21 d. Furthermore, a lower dose level was used in an attempt to decrease toxicity while still achieving potentially therapeutic serum levels. Finally, it became appreciated that Anti-B4-blocked ricin is a lipophobic compound and thus would be more appropriately dosed based upon lean body mass (LBM) rather than actual body weight.

With these changes, 49 patients who were in a CR 30–210 days after HDT-ABMT for B-cell NHL received the Anti-B4-bR immunoconjugate at a dose of 30 µg/kg LBM/d as a 7-d continuous infusion every 14 d. Thirty-four patients received two or more courses of therapy, demonstrating that patients could be retreated safely on the 14-d schedule. Pharmacokinetic data showed that a potentially therapeutic mean plateau serum level of 0.74 nM could be achieved. Only three patients experienced transient Grade 4 thrombocytopenia, and two patients experienced Grade 3 reversible transaminase elevation. Capillary leak syndrome with edema was observed in six patients. HAMA and/or HARA responses occurred in 23 patients at a median of 22 days after the initiation of therapy. After follow-up extending to 38 months, 19 patients relapsed, 27 were alive and in CR, and 3 died while in CR.

These Phase I and II trials of Anti-B4-bR in patients post-HDT-ABMT again demonstrate that the ricin immunotoxin can be delivered safely, with tolerable side effects. Nevertheless, there is a lack of convincing efficacy data. A Phase III national intergroup trial therefore was initiated, under the auspices of the Cancer and Leukemia Group B (CALGB). This randomized, controlled trial was designed to answer the question of efficacy of the immunotoxin in the post-ABMT minimal disease setting and was the first randomized trial to address the issue of the in vivo efficacy of an immunotoxin.

In this study, patients with B-NHL in CR 60–120 days after HDT-ABMT were randomized to no further therapy or to two courses of Anti-B4-blocked ricin at 30 µg/kg LBM/d as a 7-d continuous infusion at 14-d intervals. Over 500 patients were registered to the HDT-ABMT phase of the trial, and 157 patients were randomized. Patients were not randomized after ABMT for several reasons, including refusal of further therapy (82 patients), inadequate engraftment (65 patients), and early relapse after ABMT (47 patients). The immunotoxin could be delivered with tolerable toxicity, and there were few instances of Grade 3/4 toxicity related to Anti-B4-bR alone and not at least partially attributable to the high-dose therapy. However, 15% of patients did develop Grade 3/4 dyspnea after Anti-B4-bR and ABMT. The study was terminated early following an interim data analysis by the Data and Safety Monitoring Board in March 1997 when it was deemed highly unlikely that Anti-B4-bR would demonstrate an improvement in disease-free survival as compared with the observation arm.

There are several potential reasons to explain the failure of this immunotoxin in the adjuvant setting. First, Anti-B4-bR simply may lack sufficient toxicity to overcome tumor-cell resistance. Second, cells that are resistant to chemotherapy also may be resistant to ricin. Finally, selection bias of patients may have contributed to the apparent improved outcome with adjuvant Anti-B4-bR observed in the earlier pilot studies.

The efficacy of the ricin immunotoxin also has been tested in another setting of minimal residual disease. A Phase II trial enrolled patients with advanced indolent NHL who achieved a minimal residual disease state following conventional therapy with ProMACE-CytoBOM, an aggressive third-generation combination chemotherapy regimen shown to achieve high CR rates in previously untreated patients (D. Longo, National Cancer Institute, personal communication, October 1997). After receiving six to eight cycles of chemotherapy, 37 patients received Anti-B4-bR at a dose of 30 µg/kg LBM/d as a continuous 7-d infusion. Patients received up to six courses of immunotoxin at 14-d intervals. Unfortunately, follow-up from that study is lacking at present.

3. Anti-B4-Blocked Ricin in HIV-Related NHL

Other potential clinical settings for the Anti-B4-bR immunoconjugate also have been explored. One of these is in the treatment of AIDS-related NHL (ARL), a disease that poses significant therapeutic obstacles to the use of conventional combination chemotherapy regimens, given the poor tolerance these patients have for myelosuppression and further immunosuppression. Moreover, the incidence of ARL appears to be increasing, at least in part, due to the longer survival enjoyed by these patients secondary to advances in antiretroviral therapy and other supportive measures (36). As many as 30–40% of AIDS patients ultimately may develop NHL, given a long enough survival. Unfortunately, combination chemotherapy regimens have achieved only 50% CR rates and median survival times on the order of 15 months (37,38). The use of the Anti-B4-blocked ricin immunotoxin offers a potentially efficacious, nonmyelosuppressive therapeutic modality for these patients.

In an initial Phase I trial, nine patients with relapsed ARL received escalating doses Anti-B4-bR, ranging from 5 to 20 µg/kg/d, as a 28-d continuous infusion (39). Toxicity included mild to moderate elevations of transaminases in five patients. HAMA and/or HARA responses occurred in three patients. One CR and one PR were observed.

A second Phase I/II trial used Anti-B4-bR in combination with modified m-BACOD (methotrexate, bleomycin, doxorubicin, cyclophosphamide, vincristine, and prednisone) chemotherapy to treat patients with newly diagnosed ARL (40).

Forty-seven patients with previously untreated ARL received low-dose m-BACOD for two cycles beyond CR. Without interrupting the chemotherapy, patients who showed no evidence of progression by cycle 3 received a 7-d continuous infusion of Anti-B4-bR on day 15 of cycle 3. Patients who tolerated this infusion and did not develop HAMA or HARA responses were retreated with the immunotoxin on day 15 of cycle 4.

A total of 28 patients received immunotoxin therapy, with 14 patients receiving a second course. The MTD with this dosing scheme was 20 µg/kg/d. Toxicities included Grade 3 transaminase elevation in 58% of patients, as well as, Grade 3 fevers, myalgias, nausea, vomiting, and fatigue. Again, despite the profound immunosuppression of HIV infection, 29% of patients developed HAMA and/or HARA responses, albeit at a median of 47.5 days posttherapy, a longer interval than observed in previous studies in non-AIDS patients. The response rate for the combined therapy was 68%, with 14 CRs and 12 PRs. The median survival for all patients was 9.1 months from the beginning of the chemotherapy.

Another trial in ARL treated patients with standard-dose CHOP for up to eight cycles. Patients received the Anti-B4-bR immunoconjugate with the third and fifth cycles, delivered as a 28-d continuous infusion. Data from this study are as yet not available. These studies in ARL demonstrate again that Anti-B4-bR can be delivered safely to patients in the setting of concomitant chemotherapy. Further trials will need to be performed to determine whether addition of the immunotoxin improves the efficacy of standard chemotherapy. These trials also underscore the tremendous immunogenicity of the Anti-B4-bR conjugate, given the number of HAMA and HARA responses observed.

4. Anti-B4-Blocked Ricin in Other Hematologic Malignancies

Chronic Lymphocytic Leukemia

The Anti-B4-bR immunoconjugate has been used in patients with CLL. The initial Phase I studies included a limited number of patients with this disease (22,23). The major finding in these trials was the dramatically different pharmacokinetic profile of Anti-B4-bR in patients with CLL. Peak serum levels of the immunoconjugate were much lower in patients with CLL than in the patients with NHL, presumably due to rapid clearance of the immunotoxin by circulating tumor cells. As one might expect, toxicity was similarly decreased, likely because of minimal nontarget tissue exposure to drug. Responses in these patients were transient, and no effect on bone marrow disease could be demonstrated.

A Phase II study subsequently was performed in six patients with refractory B-cell CLL (4). Patients received Anti-B4-bR at a dose of 30 µg/kd/d for 7 d or 50 µg/kd/d for 7 d, by continuous infusion. Patients could be retreated at 14-d intervals. Out of a total of 14 administered courses, nine resulted in a 25% or greater decrease in circulating CLL cells. Similar to the findings in the Phase I trials, peak serum levels of Anti-B4-bR were consistently below the postulated therapeutic level. Two out of six patients developed HAMA/HARA responses. Toxicities included Grade 4 thrombocytopenia in two patients, Grade 3 anemia in one patient, and Grade 3 fevers and rigors in one patient. These data again demonstrate safety and some degree of efficacy, although the circulating tumor cells adversely affect the pharmacokinetics of the immunotoxin, perhaps limiting its ultimate utility in this disease.

Multiple Myeloma

The use of an anti-CD19 immunoconjugate for treatment of multiple myeloma at first seems inappropriate, given that both normal and malignant plasma cells do not express the cell-surface antigen. Nevertheless, the clonogenic myeloma tumor cell arises from an earlier compartment that possibly expresses the antigen. Thus treatment with Anti-B4-bR potentially could target the underlying malignant progenitor cell without being rapidly cleared by an excess of malignant plasma cells.

A Phase II trial of Anti-B4-bR was completed in five patients with multiple myeloma who were treated with a 7-d continuous infusion (4). The first four patients were treated at a dose of 40 µg/kd/d for 7 days, which resulted in intolerable toxicity in two patients. Therefore, the dose was lowered to 30 µg/kd/d for 7 days for the fifth patient. Pharmacokinetic studies demonstrated very high serum levels of the immunotoxin in the two patients who developed intolerable toxicity, with peak levels (that did not plateau) of 2.4 ± 0.48 nM, twofold higher than the levels observed with this dosing regimen in patients with NHL and minimal disease. The other three patients had levels comparable to those achieved in the trials of NHL patients. The high levels in the two patients were attributed to possible nonspecific uptake of the immunotoxin by the reticuloendothelial system in the setting of circulating paraprotein. One patient, however, had a nonsecretory tumor, arguing against this explanation.

Toxicity paralleled that observed in other studies with the immunotoxin, although it was more severe. Two patients developed Grade 4 thrombocytopenia, and three experienced a decline in performance status. One patient died secondary to neurologic toxicity. Although this death was likely the result of the underlying multiple myeloma and hypercalcemia, a contribution from the immunotoxin could not be excluded. HAMA and HARA responses occurred in two of four evaluable patients. No reductions in paraprotein could be demonstrated over the 28 days of follow-up, but such a reduction would be difficult to detect given the long half-life of circulating paraprotein. The one patient with a nonsecretory myeloma remained in complete remission for more than 3 years after completing therapy, but ultimately did develop progressive disease. Because of the toxicity observed, the trial was closed early. This trial demonstrates that an MTD determined in one setting, namely, NHL, does not always translate into the same MTD in other disease settings. A separate Phase I trial with patients with multiple myeloma is needed to define safe dose levels for this group of patients.

IV. CONCLUSION

The Anti-B4-bR immunotoxin remains one of the few biologic agents to complete the Phase I through Phase III clinical testing process. The difficulties encountered demonstrate many of the problems associated with the development of antibody-based therapies. The choice of using an immunotoxin as the cytotoxic mechanism requires the development of methods to limit nonspecific toxicity while not interfering with specific cytotoxicity. The blocked ricin construct was one solution to this challenge.

Furthermore, the toxin must be selectively delivered to the cancer cell. The B4 murine monoclonal antibody takes advantage of the cell-surface molecule CD19 to achieve this specificity. The CD19 molecule appeared to be an ideal choice, for it was present on a vast range of B-cell malignancies but absent on other host tissues. Unfortunately, CD19 may not internalize with sufficient frequency when it binds antibody, thus impairing the ability of the blocked ricin B-chain to translocate the A-chain into the cell cytoplasm. Thus, in retrospect, the CD19 molecule may be a suboptimal target.

Finally, the Anti-B4-bR conjugate proved to be very immunogenic, generating host humoral responses after a single treatment in a majority of patients. Although short interval retreatment was possible, the generation of HAMA and HARA responses would ultimately limit the repeated use of the agent. It is possible that other formulations of ricin may prove to be less immunogenic, and second-generation immunotoxins will need to overcome this obstacle.

Overall, the Anti-B4-bR experience demonstrates that antibody-targeted immunotoxin therapy is feasible. The conjugate could be delivered safely with tolerable toxicity. Importantly, objective responses could be observed in patients with otherwise refractory disease. The next generation of immunotoxins will need to build on this experience and demonstrate greater efficacy while maintaining the relatively modest toxicity profile of the Anti-B4-bR immunotoxin conjugate.

ACKNOWLEDGMENTS

The authors would like to thank Sheeba Koshy for her research assistance in the preparation of this manuscript.

REFERENCES

1. Parker SL, Tong T, Wingo PA. Cancer statistics. CA Cancer J Clin 1997; 47:5–27.
2. Grossbard ML, Press OW, Appelbaum FR, Bernstein ID, Nadler LM. Monoclonal antibody-based therapies of leukemia and lymphoma. Blood 1992; 80:863–878.
3. Grossbard ML, Nadler LM. Immunotoxin therapy of malignancy. In: Devita Jr. VT, Hellman S, Rosenberg SA, eds. Important Advances in Oncology 1992. Philadelphia: Lippincott, 1992:111–135.
4. Grossbard ML, Fidias P, Bernstein ZP, et al. Phase II studies of anti-B4-blocked ricin (anti-B4-bR) in multiple myeloma (MM) and chronic lymphocytic leukemia (CLL). Proc ASCO 1995; 14:422.
5. Roy DC, Griffin JD, Belvin M, Blattler WA, Lambert JM, Ritz J. Anti-MY9-blocked ricin: an immunotoxin for selective targeting of acute myeloid leukemia cells. Blood 1991; 77:2404–2412.
6. Szatrowski TP, Larson RA, George S, et al. Anti-B4-blocked ricin as consolidation therapy for patients with B-lineage acute lymphoblastic leukemia (ALL): A Phase II trial (CALGB 9311). Blood 1995; 86:783a.
7. LeMaistre CF, Rosen S, Frankel A, et al. Phase I trial of H65-RTA immunoconjugate in patients with cutaneous T-cell lymphoma. Blood 1991; 78:1173–1182.
8. Lynch TJ, Jr. Immunotoxin therapy of small-cell lung cancer. N901-blocked ricin for relapsed small-cell lung cancer. Chest 1993; 103:436S–439S.
9. Epstein C, Lynch T, Shefner J, et al. Use of the immunotoxin N901-blocked ricin in patients with small-cell lung cancer. Int J Cancer—Suppl 1994; 8:57–59.
10. Lynch TJ, Jr., Lambert JM, Coral F, et al. Immunotoxin therapy of small-cell lung cancer: a Phase I study of N901-blocked ricin. J Clin Oncol 1997; 15:723–734.
11. Endo Y. Mechanism of action of ricin and related toxins on the inactivation of eukaryotic ribosomes. Cancer Treatment Res 1988; 37:75–89.
12. Endo Y, Tsurugi K. Mechanism of action of ricin and related toxic lectins on eukaryotic ribosomes. Nucleic Acids Symposium Series 1986:187–90.
13. Lambert JM, Goldmacher VS, Collinson, AR, Nadler LM, Blattler WA. An immunotoxin prepared with blocked ricin: a natural plant toxin adapted for therapeutic use. Cancer Res 1991; 51:6236–6242.
14. Fodstad O, Kvalheim G, Godal A, et al. Phase I study of the plant protein ricin. Cancer Res 1984; 44:862–865.
15. Vitetta ES, Fulton RJ, May RD, Till M, Uhr JW. Redesigning nature's poisons to create anti-tumor reagents. Science 1987; 238:1098–1104.
16. Vitetta ES, Stone M, Amlot P, et al. Phase I immunotoxin trial in patients with B-cell lymphoma. Cancer Res 1991; 51:4052–4058.
17. Lambert JM, McIntyre G, Gauthier MN, et al. The galactose-binding sites of the cytotoxic lectin ricin can be chemically blocked in high yield with reactive ligands prepared by chemical modification of glycopeptides containing triantennary N-linked oligosaccharides. Biochemistry 1991; 30:3234–3247.
18. Anderson KC, Bates MP, Slaughenhoupt BL, Pinkus GS, Schlossman SF, Nadler LM. Expression of human B-cell-associated antigens on leukemias and lymphomas: a model of human B-cell differentiation. Blood 1984; 63:1424–1433.

19. Nadler LM, Anderson KC, Marti G, et al. B4, a human B-lymphocyte-associated antigen expressed on normal, mitogen-activated, and malignant B-lymphocytes. J Immunol 1983; 131:244–250.
20. Grossbard ML, Fidias, P. Prospects for immunotoxin therapy of non-Hodgkin's lymphoma. Clin Immunol Immunopathol 1995; 76:107–114.
21. Grossbard ML, Lambert JM, Goldmacher VS, Blattler WA, Nadler LM. Correlation between in vivo toxicity and preclinical in vitro parameters for the immunotoxin anti-B4-blocked ricin. Cancer Res 1992; 52:4200–4207.
22. Grossbard ML, Freedman AS, Ritz J, et al. Serotherapy of B-cell neoplasms with anti-B4-blocked ricin: a Phase I trial of daily bolus infusion. Blood 1992; 79:576–585.
23. Grossbard ML, Lambert JM, Goldmacher VS, et al. Anti-B4-blocked ricin: a Phase I trial of 7-day continuous infusion in patients with B-cell neoplasms. J Clin Oncol 1993; 11:726–737.
24. Shah SA, Halloran PM, Ferris CA, et al. Anti-B4-blocked ricin immunotoxin shows therapeutic efficacy in four different SCID mouse tumor models. Cancer Res 1993; 53:1360–1367.
25. O'Connor R, Liu C, Ferris CA, et al. Anti-B4-blocked ricin synergizes with doxorubicin and etoposide on multidrug-resistant and drug-sensitive tumors. Blood 1995; 86:4286–4294.
26. Liu C, Lambert JM, Teicher BA, Blattler WA, O'Connor R. Cure of multidrug-resistant human B-cell lymphoma xenografts by combinations of anti-B4-blocked ricin and chemotherapeutic drugs. Blood 1996; 87:3892–3898.
27. Kwak LW, Grossbard ML, Urba WJ. Cinical applications of monoclonal antibodies in cancer: B-cell lymphomas. In: DeVita Jr. VT, Hellman S, Rosenberg SA, eds. Biologic Therapy of Cancer. Philadelphia: Lippincott, 1995:553–565.
28. Jain RK. Physiological barriers to delivery of monoclonal antibodies and other macromolecules in tumors. Cancer Res 1990; 50:814s–819s.
29. Takvorian T, Canellos GP, Ritz J, et al. Prolonged disease-free survival after autologous bone marrow transplantation in patients with non-Hodgkin's lymphoma with a poor prognosis. N Eng J Med 1987; 316:1499–1505.
30. Vose JM, Anderson JR, Kessinger A, et al. High-dose chemotherapy and autologous hematopoietic stem-cell transplantation for aggressive non-Hodgkin's lymphoma. J Clin Oncol 1993; 11:1846–1851.
31. Gribben JG, Goldstone AH, Linch DC, et al. Effectiveness of high-dose combination chemotherapy and autologous bone marrow transplantation for patients with non-Hodgkin's lymphomas who are still responsive to conventional-dose therapy. J Clin Oncol 1989; 7:1621–1629.
32. Philip T, Armitage JO, Spitzer G, et al. High-dose therapy and autologous bone marrow transplantation after failure of conventional chemotherapy in adults with intermediate-grade or high-grade non-Hodgkin's lymphoma. N Eng J Med 1987; 316:1493–1498.
33. Freedman AS, Takvorian T, Anderson KC, et al. Autologous bone marrow transplantation in B-cell non-Hodgkin's lymphoma: very low treatment-related mortality in 100 patients in sensitive relapse. J Clin Oncol 1990; 8:784–791.
34. Grossbard ML, Gribben JG, Freedman AS, et al. Adjuvant immunotoxin therapy

with anti-B4-blocked ricin after autologous bone marrow transplantation for patients with B-cell non-Hodgkin's lymphoma. Blood 1993; 81:2263–2271.
35. Grossbard ML, O'Day S, Gribben JG, et al. A phase II study of anti-B4-blocked ricin (anti-B4-bR) therapy following autologous bone marrow transplantation (ABMT) for B-cell non-Hodgkin's lymphoma (B-NHL). Proc ASCO 1993; 13:293.
36. Selik RM, Chu SY, Ward JW. Trends in infectious diseases and cancers among persons dying of HIV infection in the United States from 1987 to 1992. Ann Int Med 1995; 123:933–936.
37. Gill PS, Levine AM, Krailo M, et al. AIDS-related malignant lymphoma: results of prospective treatment trials. J Clin Oncol 1987; 5:1322–1328.
38. Gisselbrecht C, Oksenhendler E, Tirelli U, et al. Human immunodeficiency virus-related lymphoma treatment with intensive combination chemotherapy. French-Italian Cooperative Group. Am J Med 1993; 95:188–196.
39. Tulpule A, Anderson LJJ, Levine AM, et al. Anti-B4 (CD 19) monoclonal antibody, conjugated with ricin (B4-blocked ricin: B4-bR) in refractory AIDS-lymphoma. Proc ASCO 1994; 13:10.
40. Scadden DT, Doweiko J, Schenkein D, et al. A Phase I/II trial of combined immuno-conjugate and chemotherapy for AIDS-related lymphoma. Blood 1993; 82(suppl 1): 386a.

6
Radioimmunoconjugate Therapy of Non-Hodgkin's Lymphoma

Thomas A. Davis and Susan J. Knox
Stanford University, Stanford, California

I. INTRODUCTION

Radioimmunotherapy (RIT) is a promising new therapeutic modality for the treatment of a wide variety of malignancies. It is a form of targeted systemic radiation therapy that combines principles of radiation therapy and chemotherapy. This form of therapy utilizes antibodies to carry radioactivity to disease sites. Antibodies are immunoglobulin protein molecules produced by B-lymphocytes that are capable of binding to specifically targeted antigens. Monoclonal antibodies (MAbs) are produced by a single clone of antibody producing cells and are highly specific for a given antigen. Radionuclides can be chemically linked to MAbs by a variety of techniques, resulting in stable radioimmunoconjugates that can be used for therapy.

Patients with recurrent B-cell lymphoma generally are considered to be incurable with standard chemotherapy (1), and new therapies are needed for this disease. Encouraging results have been obtained in clinical studies using unlabeled anti-idiotype and pan B-cell MAbs for the treatment of this patient population (2–10). Although clinical responses have been observed using unlabeled MAbs (2–10), the frequency and duration of responses have been limited by a number of factors, including (a) heterogeneity of antigen expression on tumor cells, (b) selection for variants (wild-type negative cells) or emergence of antigenic mutants, (c) inaccessibility of tumor cells, (d) circulating antigen, which may preclude localization of MAbs in disease sites, and (e) failure of host effector mechanisms to eliminate MAb-coated cells. The use of radiolabeled MAbs (vs. unlabeled MAbs) may solve some of these problems, since the local emission of ionizing radiation by radiolabeled MAbs may kill cells that are in close proximity to bound antibody whether or not those cells express the targeted antigen. Similarly, the penetrating radiation associated with radiolabeled MAbs may obviate the problem of limited access in bulky or poorly vascularized tumors. In addition, radiolabeled MAbs can be cytotoxic with or without internalization, and host effector mechanisms are not required for tumor cell killing. The aforementioned factors combined with the inherent radiosensitivity of lymphoma cells make lymphoma an ideal disease to treat with RIT and account for the overall increased efficacy of RIT compared with unlabeled MAb therapy.

II. DETERMINANTS OF RIT EFFECTS

Radioimmunotherapy differs from conventional external beam radiation therapy (XRT) in several important ways. Radioimmunotherapy is systemically targeted radiotherapy with both specific and non-specific components. Radiolabeled MAbs specifically bind to targeted tumors, but there is also nonspecific uptake of MAbs by normal tissues, which is determined in part by the presence of reticuloendothelial cells bearing Fc receptors that are capable of binding the constant regions of intact antibody molecules. This nonspecific uptake can be modified by using antibody fragments or constructs. Circulating radiolabeled MAbs also contribute to nonspecific dose distribution and whole-body irradiation. Specific and nonspecific uptake of MAbs are important determinants of both efficacy and toxicity. The antitumor effect of RIT is due primarily to the associated radioactivity of the radiolabeled antibody, which emits continuous, exponentially decreasing, low-dose-rate irradiation with a heterogeneous dose deposition. In some situations, the antibody itself may contribute to tumor cell killing as well. The effective half-life of the radiolabeled MAb is determined by the physical half-life of the radionuclide and the biological half-life of the MAb. In contrast, conventional XRT is delivered in multiple fractions of high-dose-rate irradiation with a relatively homogenous dose distribution within the defined treatment volume. In summary, important determinants of RIT effects include the antibody (specificity, affinity, avidity, dose, and immunoreactivity), the radionuclide (emission properties and chemical stability of the radioimmunoconjugate), the targeted antigen (density, location, heterogeneity of expression, stability, and modulation), and characteristics of the targeted tumor, including the intrinsic radiosensitivity, proliferative rate, volume, blood supply, and the presence or absence of hypoxic areas and necrosis. Other important determinants of efficacy and toxicity include the heterogeneity of dose deposition and dose rate effects, which are determined, in part, by the factors listed previously.

III. RADIOIMMUNOCONJUGATES FOR THE TREATMENT OF NON-HODGKIN'S LYMPHOMA

A variety of MAbs have been used for the RIT of non-Hodgkin's lymphoma. The ideal MAb for therapy should have minimal cross-reactivity with normal tissues and react with a nonmodulating antigen that does not undergo endocytosis and is expressed relatively homogeneously at a high density on targeted tumor cells. The different MAbs utilized to date in clinical trials have been characterized in Table 1 in terms of specificity, expression of the targeted antigen on malignant cells, and the ability of the antibody–antigen complex to undergo endocytosis (11–19). Antigenic modulation is of particular importance for Iodine-131 (^{131}I) labeled MAbs, since tumor-cell-mediated dehalogenation of radiolabeled MAbs can significantly shorten the retention time of the ^{131}I-MAb, and thereby limit the cumulative tumor dose (14,15,20,21,22). The MAbs listed in Table 1 also differ in terms of the expression of the targeted antigen on normal cells (11–13,17,19). Other potential antigenic targets for RIT of B-cell lymphoma include CD19, CD40, and CD45 (11–13).

A number of radionuclides are suitable for use in RIT (11,23,24), and recent improvements in labeling and chelation chemistry have resulted in improved chelate stability (25–27) and radioiodination (28) with less tumor-cell-mediated dehalogenation. RIT studies in non-Hodgkin's lymphoma have utilized ^{131}I, yttrium-

Table 1 Antibodies Used in Clinical Studies

Antibody	Antigen	Expression on targeted malignant cells	Endocytosis
Anti-idiotype	Idiotypic immunoglobulin	>95%	+
LYM-1	HLA Class II (HLA DR)	>95%	+
B1	CD20	>95%	−
1F5	CD20	>95%	−
2B8	CD20	>95%	−
OKB7	CD21	≥50%	+
LL2	CD22	≥70%	+
MB-1	CD37	≥90%	+
T101	CD5	70–90%	+
Anti-TAC	CD25 (IL-2 receptor)	100%	+

Source: Reproduced with permission from Ref. 117.

90 (^{90}Y), and copper-67 (^{67}Cu). The half-life, the type of decay, and the emission properties of these radionuclides are summarized in Table 2. ^{131}I- and ^{90}Y-labeled MAb have been studied the most extensively. ^{131}I has a half-life of 193 h and a large component of γ emissions (81% with an energy of 0.364 MeV). ^{90}Y is a pure β emitter with a half-life of 64 h, a maximum energy of 2.28 MeV, and an average energy of 0.935 MeV. The mean range of the β particles from ^{131}I and ^{90}Y in tissue is approximately 0.4 and 2.5 mm, respectively. The path length over which 90% of the emitted energy is absorbed is 0.8 mm for ^{131}I and 5.3 mm for ^{90}Y (11,29,30). In theory, the emission properties of ^{90}Y should result in relatively higher tumor doses that may be more homogeneous in distribution than obtained with ^{131}I-MAb, but this is entirely speculative, since these two radionuclides have not been directly compared in clinical trials. In order to do so in a meaningful way, patients in a given study should be randomized to receive either ^{131}I- or ^{90}Y-labeled MAbs, using the same MAb and optimal labeling methods for both radionuclides. Other potential advantages of ^{90}Y-MAb include the associated minimal amount of penetrating radiation (Bremsstrahlung), which facilitates outpatient administration of relatively high doses, and decreased contamination hazards because of the reduced urinary excretion compared with ^{131}I-MAb. In addition, if the targeted antigen undergoes modulation, ^{90}Y-MAb is bound internally and is not subject to enzymatic degradation. It is important to note, however, that the recently revised Nuclear Regulatory Commission guidelines will allow for discharge of patients treated with ^{131}I-MAbs earlier than before, where these guidelines are in effect. This will permit outpatient administration of ^{131}I-MAbs in many situations.

Table 2 Radionuclides Used for RIT of Non-Hodgkin's Lymphoma

Radionuclide	Half-life (h)	Type of decay	Emission[a]	Energy (MeV)[b]	Mean range (mm)	Source
Iodine (^{131}I)	193.0	β-	γ	0.364 (81.2%)[c]		Nuclear reactor
			β	0.810 (89.4%)	0.4	
Yttrium (^{90}Y)	64.1	β-	β	2.28	2.5	Generator
Copper (^{67}Cu)	62.0	β-	γ	0.185 (48.7%)		Accelerator
			β	0.577 (55.9%)	0.4	

[a] May include multiple emissions; only the major emissions are shown.
[b] The energy of the β emission is the maximum energy, in MeV.
[c] The percentages in parentheses represent the relative contribution of the major emissions shown to the total γ and β emissions, respectively, for the specified radionuclide.
Source: Reproduced with permission from Ref. 117.

Interestingly, the concept of time dose fractionation has been applied to RIT by Rao and Howell (31). This approach incorporates differences in dose rate, the biological half-life of the antibody, the physical half-life of the radionuclide, and the total dose needed for a given effect, as follows: TDF $= 0.122 r_0^{1.35} \tau_e$, where total dose is proportional to the initial dose rate r_0 and the effective time τ_e. This relationship suggests that high initial tumor dose rates are important determinants of clinical efficacy. However, since clinical studies have demonstrated that initial tumor uptake of radiolabeled MAbs is slow, a high effective time is also necessary for the optimization of therapy. Therefore, it has been suggested that radionuclides with a half-life of one to three times the biological half-life of the MAb in tumor are more likely to be clinically efficacious than radionuclides with longer or shorter half-lives (31).

IV. DETERMINANTS OF RADIOLABELED MONOCLONAL ANTIBODY BIODISTRIBUTION

Sequential imaging studies following administration of MAbs labeled with small quantities of radionuclides (e.g., 5 mCi) allow for study of the biodistribution of the radiolabeled MAb prior to therapy. When possible, imaging studies utilize MAbs labeled with the same radionuclide that will be used for therapy (32). This requires that the emission(s) from the radionuclide be well imaged by gamma cameras. The absence of significant gamma radiation makes imaging with ^{90}Y difficult. Therefore, Indium-111 (^{111}In)-labeled MAbs have commonly been used for imaging prior to administration of therapeutic doses of ^{90}Y-labeled MAbs. ^{111}In has a chemistry similar to ^{90}Y with gamma emissions of 173 and 247 keV. Optimal imaging of known sites of disease generally occurs at 3–6 days after antibody administration. In a review of imaging studies in 173 patients with hematologic malignancies (33), the rate of tumor visualization was 72%. Excellent results also have been reported by Goldenberg et al. (34), with imaging of 49/60 known sites of disease and detection of 41 occult tumor sites. In addition, Kaminski et al. (35,36) have reported imaging of all known disease sites >2 cm with ^{131}I-anti-CD20 MAb. The effective biological half-life of radiolabeled murine MAb is variable and depends, in part, upon the particular antibody, its antigenic specificity, and the method utilized for radiolabeling the MAb. For many antibodies, it has been reported to be in the range of 1.5–3.0 days.

Important determinants of radiolabeled MAb biodistribution include spleen size (11,37), tumor burden (11,38), and the pre- or coinfusion of unlabeled MAb (38,39). Press et al. (11,37) have reported that favorable biodistributions were obtained in 100% of splenectomized patients, 77% of patients with normal-size spleens, and only 12.5% of patients with splenomegaly. In high-dose-RIT studies the Seattle group has excluded patients with splenomegaly or treated such patients only after splenectomy, which improved the biodistribution of ^{131}I-anti-B1. In contrast, the DeNardo group suggests that radiation dose to tumor using ^{131}I-LYM-1 is reduced only in cases of extraordinarily large spleens and have found that there was no relationship between spleen volume and therapeutic response. They argue that splenomegaly should not exclude patients from therapy with B-cell-targeted radioimmunoconjugates (40,41). Press et al. (11,38) also estimated tumor burden using computed tomography and found that only 1/12 patients with >500 cc of tumor had a favorable ^{131}I-MAb biodistribution, whereas 23/31 patients with ≤500 cc of tumor had favorable biodistributions ($p < 0.001$). Several studies have demonstrated marked effects of preinfusion of different doses of unlabeled MAbs on the biodistribution and pharmacokinetics of radiolabeled MAbs (38,39,42). Improvements in biodistribution of radiolabeled MAbs following pre- or coadministration of unlabeled MAbs are presumably secondary, in part, to decreased nonspecific uptake of intact MAb molecules by cells with Fc receptors within the reticuloendothelial system. It therefore has become a widespread practice to predose with unlabeled antibody (35,36).

V. CLINICAL STUDIES

Clinical trials using RIT for B-cell lymphoma and T-cell lymphoma and leukemia have been summarized in Tables 3 (34–36,38,42–57) and 4 (58–62) in terms of general study design (nonmyeloablative vs. myeloablative), radionuclide and antibody utilized, number of treatments, number of treated evaluable patients, and responses to date. The general study design employed for RIT at myeloablative doses is as follows:

Bone marrow or peripheral stem cell collection → Imaging study → Therapy → Reinfusion of bone marrow or peripheral stem cells

These trials differ from one another in several important ways. Myeloablative studies have included bone marrow and/or peripheral stem-cell collection and reinfusion. In some studies, these cells were automatically reinfused at a specified time after treatment, whereas in other studies there were specific criteria that had to be met prior to reinfusion of bone marrow or peripheral stem cells. The trials summarized in Tables 3 and 4 also differed in terms of eligibility criteria, MAbs, and radionuclides (^{131}I, ^{90}Y, or ^{67}Cu) utilized, MAb and radionuclide doses, number of treatments, labeling method, doses of unlabeled MAbs pre- or coinfused, and the biodistribution or dosimetry estimations required for administration of a therapeutic dose of radiolabeled MAb. A variety of dose escalation schemes have been employed. These have included incremental increases

Table 3 Radioimmunotherapy Trials for B-Cell Lymphoma

Radionuclide (cumulative mCi)	Antibody (cumulative mg)	Treatments	No. evaluable patients	Responses[a]	References
Nonmyeloablative					
^{131}I (26–1044)	LYM-1 (8–676)	1–16	57	11 CR, 20 PR	46–48
^{131}I (50.4–266.8)	LYM-1 (30–67.3)	1–2	13	4 PR	43,44
^{131}I (6.2–343)	LL2 (0.2–157)	1–7	12	2 CR, 2 PR, 2 MR	34
^{131}I (14.5–59.1)	LL2 (54.3–138.9)	1	10	1 CR, 1 PR, 1 MR	unpublished data
^{131}I (25–161)	MB-1 (40)	1	10	1 CR, 2 PR, 1 MR	49
^{131}I (38–161)	B1 (15–1565)	1–2	47	16 CR, 18 PR	36,45
^{131}I (90–200)	OKB7 (25)	3–4	18	1 PR, 12 MR	50
^{67}Cu (131–388)	LYM-1 (135–288)	1–4	3	1 CR, 1 PR	46,47
^{90}Y (10–54)	Anti-idiotype (1000–4050)	1–4	9	2 CR, 1 PR, 1 MR	51,52
^{90}Y (13.5–21.6)	B1 (2–110)	1	4	1 CR, 1 PR	42
^{90}Y (19.9–53.4)	2B8 (55–294)	1–2	14	5 CR, 6 PR	42[b]
Myeloablative					
^{131}I (280–785)	B1 (58–1168)	1	29	23 CR, 4 PR	37,38,57
^{131}I (608)	1F5 (274)	1	1	1 PR	38
^{131}I (234–628)	MB1 (275–970)	1	6	6 CR	38,53
^{131}I (232)	Anti-idiotype (1000)	1	1	1 CR	54
^{131}I (145–323)	LL2 (97.3–110.5)	1	7	2 PR, 3 MR	unpublished data[c]
^{90}Y (20)	B1 (N/A)[d]	1	3	1 PR, 1 MR	unpublished data[e]

CR: complete response = no evidence of disease for ≥1 month. PR: partial response = ≥50% decrease from baseline in overall tumor size for ≥1 month. MR: minor response = 25–49% decrease from baseline in overall tumor size for ≥1 month.
[b] A Phase 1 dose escalation trial—two patients required stem-cell reinfusion of four patients treated at the highest dose (50 mCi).
[c] Personal communication from Dr. D. M. Goldenberg.
[d] N/A: not available.
[e] Personal communication from Drs. S. O'Day and L. M. Nadler.
Source: Revised from Ref. 117.

Table 4 RIT Trials for T-Cell Lymphoma and Leukemia

Radionuclide (cumulative mCi)	Antibody (cumulative mg)	No. treatments	No. evaluable patients	Responses[a]	Reference
Nonmyeloablative					
^{131}I (25–50)	T101 (10)	1	4	0[b]	58[c]
^{131}I (100–150)	T101 (10–16)	1[d]	6	2 PR, 4 MR	59
^{90}Y (N/A)[s]	T101 (N/A)[e]	1	6	3 PR	61[f]
^{90}Y (5–15)	Anti-Tac (2–10)	1–9	16	2 CR, 9 PR	62[g]

[a] CR: complete response = no evidence of disease for ≥1 month. PR: partial response = ≥50% decrease from baseline in overall tumor size for ≥1 month. MR: minor response = 25–49% decrease from baseline in overall tumor size for ≥1 month.
[b] No objective clinical responses were observed; however, a transient decrease in peripheral blood lymphocytes was observed in one patient.
[c] CLL (chronic lymphocytic leukemia).
[d] Three patients were subsequently retreated (60), but responses shown are for the first treatment with a single dose of ^{131}I-T101.
[e] N/A: not available.
[f] CTCL (cutaneous T-cell lymphoma)/CLL.
[g] Adult T-cell leukemia.
Source: Revised from Ref. 117.

of 10 mCi in the dose of ^{90}Y-MAb administered (42) and increases in ^{131}I-MAb doses in increments anticipated to increase the whole-body dose by 10 cGy (35,36) or the dose to the normal organ (liver, kidneys, or lungs) expected to receive the highest dose by 1.75–5.0 cGy (37,38).

The results summarized in Tables 3 and 4 are promising and show a relatively high response rate with a number of durable partial responses (PR) and complete responses (CR) for up to 9 years (34–36,38,42–62 and personal communication from Dr. O. Press). The highest overall response and CR rates and the longest remission durations have been reported in patients treated with very high doses of radiolabeled MAbs in single doses in conjunction with autologous bone marrow transplantation (11,37,38,42,53,57). Although higher doses of RIT have tended to be more efficacious, there has not been a direct correlation between dose and response in most reported studies. Dose is only one of several determinants of efficacy, which include antibody specificity, characteristics of the targeted antigen, immunoconjugate stability, tumor burden and bulk, spleen size, and the use of unlabeled MAbs.

These results are particularly encouraging, since all of the patients treated in the RIT trials summarized in Tables 3 and 4 have had recurrent disease following at least one form of conventional therapy. Many of the patients had failed multiple courses of therapy, and some were unable to tolerate additional chemotherapy for a variety of reasons. Although caution should be exerted in the interpretation of these results, given the relatively small numbers of patients, limited follow-up, and predominance of patients with low- or intermediate-grade lymphomas treated on these studies, the results are quite good, and many patients have experienced remissions of longer duration than achieved with previous chemotherapy (11,36,37,42).

The optimal time to use radioimmunotherapy in the course of non-Hodgkin's lymphoma is not defined. An ongoing trial using ^{131}I-MAb as primary therapy for low-grade disease has shown impressive results, with a response rate of 100% and evidence of conversion to molecular negativity by PCR testing for bcl-2 rearrangements (55). It is interesting to note that side effects during antibody infusion are more common in these patients than in patients who have received prior cytotoxic therapy. Response durations are not yet defined. Patients who have failed bone marrow transplantation also have experienced excellent tumor responses to RIT (56).

There are relatively few clinical data comparing the innate clinical activity of unlabeled MAb with the same MAb when radiolabeled. It is assumed that the added radioactivity enhances efficacy, as well as toxicity, particularly to marrow. An ongoing randomized trial is comparing the efficacy and toxicity of unlabeled as compared to ^{131}I-labeled anti-CD20 MAb. Preliminary results suggest that the unlabeled murine antibody does have some innate antitumor activity, but responses are limited and durations are short (70). It is expected that this trial will

Table 5 Ongoing RIT Trials for B-Cell Lymphoma

Labeled MAb	Phase	Histologic grade
Nonmyeloablative		
^{131}I-LYM 1	**III**	**Int/High**
^{67}Cu-LYM 1	II	Int/High
^{131}I-B1	**II/III**	**Low/Transformed**
	II	Low/Transformed
	Hot vs. Cold[a]	
	II	Low
	Primary therapy	
^{90}Y-2B8	II	Any
Myeloablative		
^{131}I-LL2	I/II	Any
^{131}I-B1	**III**	**Any**
	RIT + Chemo	

[a] Radiolabeled vs. unlabeled antibody. Trials shown in boldface are considered pivotal for FDA approval.

confirm the significant contribution of the radioisotope to the production of durable remissions.

A summary of current ongoing trials are listed in Table 5. Those listed in bold type are considered pivotal for FDA approval, and it is anticipated that one or more radiolabeled MAbs may receive approval in the next 2 years.

VI. TOXICITY

The circulation and biodistribution of radiolabeled MAbs outside the targeted area contribute to toxicity, which is determined by the inherent radiosensitivity (tolerance) of nontargeted tissues and organs (63). Without bone marrow or peripheral stem-cell reinfusion, the dose-limiting toxicity of ^{131}I-, ^{90}Y-, and ^{67}Cu-labeled MAbs is myelosuppression (64). As with conventional external beam XRT, erythrocyte progenitors are less sensitive to exponentially decreasing low-dose-rate irradiation than are lymphocyte, granulocyte, and platelet progenitor cells (65). Our experience in trials using nonmyeloablative doses of ^{131}I-B1 suggests that myelotoxicity is quite variable from patient to patient. The onset of peripheral count suppression can occur from 2 to 6 weeks post therapy and last as long as 16 weeks. The myelotoxicity also varies in timing and severity, with nadirs at approximately 6 weeks for WBC and platelets and 9 weeks for hematocrit. ^{90}Y-2B8 also resulted in a similar pattern of marrow suppression. At the maximum tolerated dose of 40 mCi (which did not require stem-cell support), white-cell and platelet nadirs were 1700 cells/mm² and 40×10^3/mm², with durations of 3.8 and 3.5 weeks, respectively, and some of the patients treated at this dose level did require G-CSF and transfusion support (42). In general, increasing doses resulted in nadirs that occurred sooner, were more profound, and lasted longer. Factors likely to affect the degree of count suppression following RIT include the type and dose of radioisotope administered, extent of marrow involvement with lymphoma, absorbed radiation dose to marrow-bearing bones, prior cytotoxic and radiation therapy, and initial blood counts. Prior radiotherapy is relevant in terms of total percent of active bone marrow previously irradiated, and prior chemotherapy must be considered in terms of cumulative dose and the myelotoxicity associated with the individual agents received as well as the time interval between last therapy and RIT. Other determinants of marrow toxicity include tumor burden, spleen size, MAb, targeted antigen distribution, and immunoconjugate stability.

Studies to date demonstrate modest correlation of toxicity with dose parameters and the existence of modifying factors. Several analyses of dose-escalating studies have shown that toxicity increased with administered dose, but patient numbers at each dose level are limited. Analysis of toxicity in a dose-escalation study of ^{131}I-anti-CD20 monoclonal antibody demonstrated that dosing based on lean body mass rather than on actual mass provided a superior correlation between dose and hematologic toxicity, with r values of 0.523 for lean body mass versus 0.430 for actual total mass (67). Breitz et al. (68) found that expressing radioactivity administered relative to body size improved the correlation with marrow toxicity, but that some index compensating for prior therapy was needed to improve predictions of toxicity. A recent analysis of data from RIT studies of solid tumors by Liu et al. (66) has shown that whole-body and bone-marrow radiation dose correlate with toxicity, as does plasma half-life of the radioimmunoconjugate.

Nonhematologic toxicity generally has been mild. It too is partially dependent on the MAb, radionuclide, dose, antigenic target, and presence or absence of circulating antigen. Symptoms (usually Grade I) such as rash, fever, chills, myalgias, nausea, nasal congestion, and hypotension have been reported and usually are related to the MAb infusion. These symptoms frequently are transient and usually respond well to acetaminophen, antihistamines, and nonsteroidal antiinflammatory drugs. More serious side effects, such as rigors, bronchospasm, and laryngeal edema, are rare during or immediately following MAb administration. Delayed nonhematologic toxicity generally is uncommon. In a myeloablative ^{131}I-MAb study using high doses of ^{131}I in 29 patients, infection, presumably secondary to neutropenia, occurred in 41% of patients, with one associated death, and 59% of the patients developed elevated TSH levels, although none displayed overt hypothyroidism. Cardiopulmonary toxicity was reported to be the dose-limiting second organ toxicity. Of note, no cases of myelodysplastic syndrome or leukemia were observed, but two malignancies occurred 3 years after treatment, including one noninvasive transitional cell carcinoma of the bladder and one Stage C colon carcinoma (37,38,57). In a nonmyeloablative trial using the same ^{131}I-MAb, no opportunistic infections or hypothyroidism were noted (35,36). With the use of ^{131}I-MAb, it is customary to saturate the thyroid gland with nonradioactive iodine before, during, and after therapy in order to reduce thyroid uptake of ^{131}I and minimize the risk of hypothyroidism. The dose-limiting second organ toxicity for ^{90}Y-MAb has yet to be defined in patients, but in dogs it is hepatic toxicity (69). No late effects have been reported to date in patients treated with ^{90}Y-MAb.

VII. DOSIMETRY

Dosimetric studies routinely are performed prior to RIT in order to study radiolabeled MAb biodistribution and to calculate the dose to be administered. These studies may help to identify patients who are either unlikely to benefit from therapy or likely to experience unacceptable toxicity. This information is used to determine which patients meet the criteria required to proceed to therapy. These studies utilize sequential gamma camera imaging, as previously described, and are frequently complemented by serial measurements of plasma and urine activity, as well as occasional tumor and bone marrow biopsies. A variety of different dosimetric methodologies have been utilized for RIT (72,73). Most commonly the methods are based upon the MIRD (medical internal radiation dose) model for purposes of calculating estimated doses to tumor and normal tissues and organs (70,71). This model takes into account the cumulative and time-dependent accumulation of activity. The reliability of using imaging studies to predict the dosimetry from a therapeutic RIT dose has not been well characterized, but data from DeNardo et al. (32) suggest that when the same radioimmunoconjugate is used for imaging and therapy, the tracer study can be predictive of total-body, major-organ, and tumor doses. Furthermore, data from Erdi et al. (75) showed good correlation between imaging-based dosimetry and biopsy quantitation from resected specimens. In some trials, dosimetric studies are performed after administration of a therapeutic dose of RIT, and direct determination of estimated doses by imaging can be limited by difficulties that include those associated with imaging Bremsstrahlung from ^{90}Y and high-activity levels of ^{131}I (76).

Most imaging studies use whole-body imaging and counting to account for all activities. Radiation doses can be calculated from the cumulative activity, the equilibrium constant, and the specific absorbed fraction for the target. For dose calculations, the mass of each region of interest is needed and can be calculated by converting volume to mass. Published values of organs of interest from the Medical Internal Radiation Dose Committee of the Society of Nuclear Medicine have been used extensively, and this committee has provided guidance for the development of methodology used to calculate absorbed radiation doses, which has been adapted for RIT (77). SPECT (single photon emission computed tomography) is used widely to normalize time-activity data from planar imaging (78–80), which may increase the accuracy of the planar data, although the quantitative value of SPECT is not fully established. More recently, regions of interest (organ and tumor volumetrics) have been defined by image fusion with CT (81,82) or MRI (81,82) or by deriving volumes from projected shadows of organs or structures (83). Image fusion combines the use of radiolabeled MAb images with conventional imaging modalities utilized for the localization of normal organs and/or tumors (81,82,84). This method may allow for improved determination of the activity distribution and ultimately for more accurate estimation of absorbed dose to regions of interest (81,82). Nevertheless, none of the currently available methods address microdosimetry, which at this time is of unknown clinical significance (74).

An area of increasing interest is bone marrow dosimetry, which can be calculated using the nonpenetrating and penetrating radiation contributions from the whole body (85–87). For example, using ^{131}I-Lym-1, DeNardo et al. (86) reported that nonpenetrating radiation from the blood contributed 0.18 cGy/mCi and penetrating radiation from the total body contributed 0.18 cGy/mCi to the bone marrow. The mean total dose was 0.36 ± 0.14 cGy/mCi, and clearances and marrow doses were remarkably constant among different patients and among different therapy doses for the same patient. Wilder et al. have since applied the linear-quadratic model (88,89) to RIT and bone marrow dosimetry in an effort to further improve the accuracy of these estimations. It must be noted, however, that significant regional variability in marrow dosimetry has been identified (90).

Normal organ doses from RIT have generally ranged from 0.7 to 8.2 cGy/mCi (0.2 to 2.2 mGy/MBq), with considerable interpatient variation in most studies despite differences in MAbs and dosimetric techniques (73). Tumor doses have ranged from approximately 18.5 to 200 cGy/mCi (0.5 to 5.4 mGy/MBq), with a relatively poor correlation between tumor responses and estimated tumor doses (74). In most cases, there is considerable patient-to-patient variation, which demonstrates the importance of performing dosimetry studies in individual patients (74). Nevertheless, the validity of these estimates is limited by a number of factors, including the inherent difficulty in accurately measuring activity in small, irregularly shaped tumor masses or regions of interest using gamma camera imaging (74), and by the inability to visualize all known sites of disease in all patients (85,91).

VIII. BIOLOGY

Clinical responses have occurred with doses as small as 5–10 mCi of ^{131}I-MAb (34,92–94), and complete responses have been reported at estimated tumor doses as low as 8.5 Gy (53). Some of these estimated tumor doses are considerably lower than doses usually required to achieve similar responses using conventional fractionated high-dose-rate external beam XRT. Such observations raise the question of whether or not 1-cGy RIT is as effective as 1 cGy of external beam XRT. The answer to this question is no doubt dependent, in part, on the experimental model utilized, the study design, and the tumor type studied. Nevertheless, animal experiments (95,96) designed to compare the relative efficacy of RIT with equivalent doses of high-dose-rate external beam XRT administered as either a single fraction or multiply fractionated doses have generally shown that tumors characterized by a large shoulder on the radiation survival curve (e.g., solid tumors) or small α/β ratio tend to have a significant dose rate effect (95). In contrast, the dose rate effect is generally minimized for tumors such as lymphoma that have poor repair capability, as evidenced by a small shoulder on the radiation survival curve or large α/β ratio (95), and is probably further modified by the tumor doubling time, as suggested by Fowler (97). When the dose rate effect is minimal, other factors—such as (a) cell cycle redistribution with accumulation of cells in G2/M (98–100); (b) targeting of a rapidly proliferating subpopulation of well-oxygenated and assessable tumor cells (101,102); (c) effects on tumor blood flow (103) or vasculature (104–106); (d) rapid reoxygenation of hypoxic cells during protracted exposure (107,108); (e) effects on repair and repopulation (100); and (f) radiation- (109,110) and antibody (111) -induced apoptosis may explain, in part, the increased efficacy of RIT compared with external beam XRT that has been reported in several tumor models (101,112–114). Both MAbs (111) and low-dose-rate radiation (109,110,115) have been reported to induce apoptosis in human lymphoma cell lines, and apoptosis recently was found to be a predominate mechanism of cell killing following low-dose-rate irradiation (115). Additional data may suggest that the binding of anti-CD20 antibodies is additive in the induction of apoptosis in lymphoma cell lines (116). These factors may be important determinants of RIT-mediated tumor-cell killing, with the relative contribution of apoptosis to overall cell killing dependent upon the particular cell line, antibody, and radiation dose rate studied.

IX. AREAS OF ACTIVE RESEARCH

Low tumor uptake of radiolabeled MAbs, normal tissue toxicity, and the immunogenicity of murine antibodies limit the efficacy of RIT for both lymphoma and solid tumors. Optimization of RIT requires: (a) increased targeting of radiolabeled antibody to tumor, (b) decreased targeting of radiolabeled antibody to normal tissues, (c) less normal tissue toxicity from the emitted radiation, and (d) greater therapeutic efficacy of the radiation in tumor (117,118). In addition to predosing with unlabeled antibody, various avenues of research have been pursued for the purpose of improving the therapeutic ratio of RIT over that achieved with simple intravenous administration of radiolabeled MAbs (23,118–122), including use of genetically engineered antibody constructs; multistep pretargeting strategies; hyperthermia; external beam radiation and other therapies that may increase tumor blood flow and vascular permeability; adjuvant use of radiosensitizers or protectors; cytokines; chemotherapeutic agents such as topoisomerase I inhibitors; and hypoxic cytotoxins; the use of gene therapy to amplify tumor targeting; clearance of unbound radiolabeled MAb; and the use of novel targets for RIT. Areas of active investigation that have been particularly helpful for the RIT of non-Hodgkin's lymphoma include: (a) immunoconjugate chemistry, which has allowed for the study of a variety of radionuclides; (b) the use of growth factors and bone marrow transplantation to accelerate hematopoietic recovery after RIT; and (c) studies of fractionated therapy, which may increase the therapeutic index of RIT by decreasing the severity of myelotoxicity, secondary to repair of sublethal damage and repopulation of bone marrow progenitor cells between treatments (122,123).

Several investigators have reported that fractionated RIT is less toxic and more efficacious than single doses of RIT (123–127). However, careful attention should be paid to selection of the interval between fractions. Prolonged intervals are radiobiologically undesirable, because tumor cells can repair radiation-induced damage and proliferate. The fraction interval should be determined in part by the time required for blood count recovery and the rate of tumor growth. In immunocompetent patients, Vriesendorp et al. (69) have suggested that the duration of a fractionated course of RIT should be less than the time required for development of a human anti-mouse antibody (HAMA) response (usually less than 10 days). The incidence of HAMA in B-cell lymphoma patients is generally in the range of 20–33% (35,36,38,55,64), which is considerably less than that observed in patients with other malignancies. This discrepancy is presumably due to the immunosuppressed status of patients with B-cell lymphoma (127). Chimeric and humanized MAbs are less immunogenic than murine MAbs (128). They may be useful for fractionated RIT in some patients, but the prolonged biological half-life of these MAbs may result in increased nonspecific dose deposition and toxicity. If so, this problem may be obviated by improved clearance of circulating unbound radiolabeled MAbs or free radionuclide. This has been accomplished using EDTA to decrease bone levels of ^{90}Y and facilitate excretion of ^{90}Y or ^{90}Y-MAbs (129), extracorporeal immunoadsorption (130), and second clearing antibodies (131). Similarly, in pretargeting approaches (132–134), clearing reagents are used to remove circulating unlabeled MAbs prior to administration of the radionuclide in order to increase tumor-to-normal-tissue ratios (135).

X. CONCLUSION

Radioimmunotherapy studies using a variety of MAbs, radionuclides, and study designs have resulted in high response rates at both myeloablative and nonmyeloablative doses in patients with recurrent or refractory non-Hodgkin's lymphoma. These results are especially promising, since many of these responses have been durable and have lasted longer than prior remissions from previous chemotherapy. It is too soon to know which RIT regimen(s) will be the most efficacious. Radioimmunotherapy may be useful in a variety of clinical situations, including first-line therapy, relapse following conventional or high-dose therapy, and adjuvant treatment for patients with little or no detectable residual disease after other therapies. Radioimmunotherapy also may be useful as part of conditioning regimens for bone marrow transplantation. Investigators at the University of Washington and the Fred Hutchinson Cancer Research Center currently are studying the potential utility of RIT as a replacement for total-body irradiation used alone or in combination with chemotherapy as a preparatory regimen for autologous bone marrow transplantation. In the future, selection of a specific RIT regimen may be determined by considerations such as patient status (e.g., age, general health, extent of disease, or prior therapy) and cost effectiveness. In order to optimize this form of therapy and use it most effectively in the future, studies should: (a) define better which radionuclides (α vs. β emitters) and antibodies (intact MAbs vs. fragmented constructs) are best suited for radioimmunotherapy of leukemias, microscopic disease, and tumor masses of different sizes; (b) develop and optimize strategies for increasing the therapeutic index of RIT; and (c) determine how to combine RIT optimally with other therapeutic modalities.

ACKNOWLEDGMENTS

The authors would like to thank W. B. Saunders Company, which graciously gave permission for the use of text and tables from a prior publication in *Seminars in Radiation Oncology* 1995; 5(4):331–341 (117), and to the American Association for Cancer Research, Inc., for granting permission to use material presented in a paper published in *Cancer Research* 1995; 55 (suppl):5832S–5836S (120).

The authors also thank Dr. Michael Goris for his advice and consultation regarding RIT dosimetry.

REFERENCES

1. Shipp MA, Mauch PM, Harris NL. Non-Hodgkin's lymphomas. In: DeVita VT, Hellman S, Rosenberg DA, eds. Cancer Principals and Practice of Oncology. 5th ed. Philadelphia: Lippincott, 1997:2165–2219.
2. Maloney DG, Liles TM, Czerwinski DK, et al. Phase I clinical trial using escalating single-dose infusion of chimeric anti-CD20 monoclonal antibody (IDEC-C2B8) in patients with recurrent B-cell lymphoma. Blood 1994; 84:2457–2466.
3. McLaughlin P, Grillo-Lopez AJ, Czuzman C, et al. IDEC-C2B8: clinical activity in clinically chemoresistant low-grade or follicular lymphoma and in patients relapsing after anthracycline therapy or ABMT. ASCO Proc 1997, Abs 55.
4. McLaughlin P, Cabanillas F, Grillo-Lopez AJ, et al. IDEC-C2B8 anti-CD20 antibody: final report on a Phase III pivotal trial in patients with relapsed low-grade or follicular lymphoma. Blood 1996; 88(10 suppl 1):Abs 349.
5. Maloney DG, Levy R, Miller RA. Monoclonal anti-idiotype antibody therapy of lymphoma. In: DeVita VT, Hellman S, Rosenberg SA, eds. Biologic Therapy of Cancer. 2d ed. Philadelphia: Lippincott Healthcare Publications, 1995: 1–10.
6. Dyer MJ, Hale G, Hayhoe FG, et al. Effects of CAMPATH-1 antibodies in vivo in patients with lymphoid malignancies: influence of antibody isotype. Blood 1989; 73:1431–1439.
7. Hale G, Dyer MJ, Clark MR, et al. Remission induction in non-Hodgkin's lymphoma with reshaped human monoclonal antibody CAMPATH-1H. Lancet 1988; 2:1394–1399.
8. Press OW, Appelbaum F, Ledbetter JA, et al. Monoclonal antibody 1F5 (anti-CD20) serotherapy of human B cell lymphomas. Blood 1987; 69:584–591.
9. Meeker TC, Lowder J, Maloney DG, et al. A clinical trial of anti-idiotype therapy for B cell malignancy. Blood 1985; 65:1349–1363.
10. Miller RA, Maloney DG, Warnke R, et al. Treatment of B-cell lymphoma with monoclonal anti-idiotype antibody. N Engl J Med 1982; 306:517–522.
11. Press OW, Eary JF, Appelbaum FR, et al. Radiolabeled antibody therapy of lymphomas. In: DeVita VT, Hellman S, Rosenberg SA, eds. Biologic Therapy of Cancer. Philadelphia: Lippincott Healthcare Publications, 1994:1–13.
12. Horibe K, Nadler LM. Human B cell associated antigens defined by monoclonal antibodies. In: Heise ER, ed. Lymphocyte Surface Antigens. New York: ASHI, 1984.
13. Barclay AN, Birkeland ML, Brown MH. The Leukocyte Antigen Facts Book. New York: Academic Press, 1993.
14. Press OW, Farr AG, Borroz KI, et al. Endocytosis and degradation of monoclonal antibodies targeting human B-cell malignancies. Cancer Res 1989; 49:4906–4912.

15. Press OW, Howell CJ, Anderson S, et al. Retention of B-cell-specific monoclonal antibodies by human lymphoma cells. Blood 1994; 83:1390–1397.
16. Lowenthal JW, MacDonald HR, Iacopetta BJ. Intracellular pathway of interleukin 2 following receptor-mediated endocytosis. Eur J Immunol 1986; 16:1461–1463.
17. Schwarting R, Gerdes J, Stein H. Expression of interleukin 2 receptor on Hodgkin's and non-Hodgkin's lymphomas and macrophages [letter]. J Clin Pathol 1985; 38: 1196–1197.
18. Waldmann TA, Greene WC, Sarin PS, et al. Functional and phenotypic comparison of human T cell leukemia/lymphoma virus positive adult T cell leukemia with human T cell leukemia/lymphoma virus negative Sezary leukemia, and their distinction using anti-Tac. Monoclonal antibody identifying the human receptor for T cell growth factor. J Clin Invest 1984; 73:1711–1718.
19. Wormsley SB, Collins ML, Royston I. Comparative density of the human T-cell antigen T65 on normal peripheral blood T cells and chronic lymphocytic leukemia cells. Blood 1981; 57:657–662.
20. Carrasquillo JA, Mulshine JL, Bunn PJ, et al. Indium-111 T101 monoclonal antibody is superior to iodine-131 T101 in imaging of cutaneous T-cell lymphoma. J Nucl Med 1987; 28:281–287.
21. Rosen ST, Zimmer AM, Goldman LR, et al. Radioimmunodetection and radioimmunotherapy of cutaneous T cell lymphomas using an ^{131}I-labeled monoclonal antibody: an Illinois Cancer Council Study. J Clin Oncol 1987; 5:562–573.
22. Press OW, Shan D, Howell-Clark J, et al. Comparative metabolism and retention of Iodine-125, Yttrium-90, and Indium-111 radioimmunoconjugates by cancer cells. Cancer Res 1996; 56:2123–2129.
23. Buchsbaum DJ. Experimental radioimmunotherapy and methods to increase therapeutic efficacy. In: Goldenberg DM, ed. Cancer Therapy with Radiolabeled Antibodies. Boca Raton, FL: CRC Press, 1995:115–140.
24. Waldmann TA, Pastan IH, Gansow OA, et al. The multichain interleukin-2 receptor: a target for immunotherapy. Ann Intern Med 1992; 116:148–160.
25. Li M, Meares CF, Zhong GR, et al. Labeling monoclonal antibodies with ^{90}yttrium- and ^{111}indium-DOTA chelates: a simple and efficient method. Bioconjug Chem 1994; 5:101–104.
26. Safavy A, Buchsbaum DJ, Khazaeli MB. Synthesis of N-[tris[2-[[N-[benzyloxy)amino]carbonyl]ethyl]methyl]succinamic acid, trisuccin. Hydroxamic acid derivatives as a new class of bifunctional chelating agents. Bioconjug Chem 1993; 4: 194–198.
27. Brechbiel MW, Gansow OA. Backbone-substituted DTPA ligands for ^{90}Y radioimmunotherapy. Bioconjug Chem 1991; 2:187–194.
28. Zalutsky MR, Noska MA, Colapinto EV, et al. Enhanced tumor localization and in vivo stability of a monoclonal antibody radioiodinated using N-succinimidyl 3-(tri-n-butylstannyl)benzoate. Cancer Res 1989; 49:5543–5549.
29. Simpkin DJ, Mackie TR. EGS4 Monte Carlo determination of the beta dose kernel in water. Med Phys 1990; 17:179–186.
30. Prestwich WV, Nunes J, Kwok CS. Beta dose point kernels for radionuclides of potential use in radioimmunotherapy [published erratum appears in J Nucl Med 1989 Oct; 30(10):1739–1740]. J Nucl Med 1989; 30:1036–1046.

31. Rao DV, Howell RW. Time-dose-fractionation in radioimmunotherapy: implications for selecting radionuclides. J Nucl Med 1993; 34:1801–1810.
32. DeNardo DA, DeNardo GL, Yuan A, et al. Prediction of radiation doses from therapy using tracer studies with iodine-131 labeled antibodies. J Nucl Med 1996; 37: 1970–1975.
33. Press OW, Eary JF, Appelbaum FR, et al. Radiolabeled antibody therapy of lymphoma. In: Dana B, ed. Malignant Lymphomas, Including Hodgkin's Disease: Diagnosis, Management and Special Problems. Boston: Kluwer Academic Publishers, 1993:127.
34. Goldenberg DM, Horowitz JA, Sharkey RM, et al. Targeting, dosimetry, and radioimmunotherapy of B-cell lymphomas with iodine-131-labeled LL2 monoclonal antibody. J Clin Oncol 1991; 9:548–564.
35. Kaminski MS, Zasadny KR, Francis IR, et al. Radioimmunotherapy of B-cell lymphoma with [^{131}I]anti-B1 (anti-CD20) antibody. N Engl J Med 1993; 329:459–465.
36. Kaminski MS, Zasadny KR, Francis IR, et al. Iodine-131-anti-B1 radioimmunotherapy for B-Cell lymphoma. J Clin Oncol 1996; 14:1974–1981.
37. Press OW, Eary JF, Appelbaum FR, et al. Phase II trial of ^{131}I-B1 (anti-CD20) antibody therapy with autologous stem cell transplantation for relapsed B cell lymphomas. Lancet 1995; 346:336–340.
38. Press OW, Eary JF, Appelbaum FR, et al. Radiolabeled-antibody therapy of B-cell lymphoma with autologous bone marrow support. N Engl J Med 1993; 329:1219–1224.
39. Bunn PJ, Carrasquillo JA, Keenan AM, et al. Imaging of T-cell lymphoma by radiolabelled monoclonal antibody (letter). Lancet 1984; 2:1219–1221.
40. Shen S, DeNardo GL, O'Donnell RT, et al. Impact of splenomegaly on I-131-LYM-1 dosimetry and response for RIT in patients with B-lymphocytic malignancies. Tumor Targeting 1996; 2:175.
41. Shen S, DeNardo GL, O'Donnell RT, et al. Impact of splenomegaly on therapeutic response and I-131-LYM-1 dosimetry in patients with B-lymphocytic malignancies. Cancer 1997; 80(12):2553–2557.
42. Knox S, Goris M, Trisler K, et al. ^{90}Y-labeled anti-CD20 monoclonal antibody therapy of recurrent B cell Lymphoma. Clin Cancer Res 1996 (March); 2:457–470.
43. Kuzel T, Rosen ST, Zimmer AM, et al. A Phase I escalating-dose safety, dosimetry and efficacy study of radiolabeled monoclonal antibody Lym-1. Cancer Biother 1993; 8:3–16.
44. Meredith RF, Khazaeli MB, Plott G, et al. Comparison of diagnostic and therapeutic doses of ^{131}I-Lym-1 in patients with non-Hodgkin's lymphoma. Antib Immunoconjug Radiopharm 1993; 6:1–11.
45. Kaminski MS, Zasadny KR, Mili AW, et al. Updated results of a Phase I trial of ^{131}I-anti-B1 (anti-CD20) radioimmunotherapy (RIT) for refractory B-cell lymphomas. Blood 1993; 82:332a.
46. DeNardo GL, DeNardo SJ. Treatment of B-lymphocyte malignancies with ^{131}I-Lym-1 and ^{67}Cu-2IT-BAT-Lym-1 and opportunities for improvement. In: Gold-

enberg DM, ed. Cancer Therapy with Radiolabeled Antibodies. Boca Raton, FL: CRC Press, 1994:217–227.
47. Lewis JP, DeNardo GL, DeNardo SJ. Radioimmunotherapy of lymphoma: a UC Davis experience. Hybridoma 1995; 14(2):115–120.
48. DeNardo GL, DeNardo SJ, O'Grady LF, et al. Fractionated radioimmunotherapy of B-cell malignancies with ^{131}I-Lym-1. Cancer Res 1990; 50(3 Suppl.):1014s–1016s.
49. Kaminski MS, Fig LM, Zasadny KR, et al. Imaging, dosimetry, and radioimmunotherapy with iodine 131-labeled anti-CD37 antibody in B-cell lymphoma. J Clin Oncol 1992; 10:1696–1711.
50. Czuczman MS, Straus DJ, Divgi CR, et al. Phase I dose-escalation trial of iodine 131-labeled monoclonal antibody OKB7 in patients with non-Hodgkin's lymphoma. J Clin Oncol 1993; 11:2021–2029.
51. Parker BA, Vassos AB, Halpern SE, et al. Radioimmunotherapy of human B-cell lymphoma with ^{90}Y-conjugated antiidiotype monoclonal antibody. Cancer Res 1990; 50(3 Suppl.):1022s–1028s.
52. White CA, Halpern SE, Parker B, et al. Radioimmunotherapy of relapsed B-cell lymphoma with yttrium-90 anti-idiotype monoclonal antibodies. Blood 1996; 87(9):3640–3649.
53. Press OW, Eary JF, Badger CC, et al. Treatment of refractory non-Hodgkin's lymphoma with radiolabeled MB-1 (anti-CD37) antibody. J Clin Oncol 1989; 7: 1027–1038.
54. Badger CC, Eary J, Brown S, et al. Therapy of lymphoma with I-131-labeled antiadiotype antibodies (anti-id). Proc AACR 1987; 28:388.
55. Kaminski M, Estes M, Regan J, et al. Frontline treatment of advanced B cell lowgrade lymphoma with radiolabeled anti-B1 antibody; initial experience. ASCO Proc 1997:abstr 51.
56. Vose J, Colcher D, Bierman P. I-131-LL2 (anti-CD22) radioimmunotherapy of refractory non-Hodgkin's lymphoma: results of a repetitive dosing trial. J Nucl Med, 1997; 38(5): #211.
57. Liu S, Eary J, Press O, et al. Long-term follow-up of patients with relapsed B cell lymphomas treated with iodine-131-labeled anti-CD20 (B1) antibody and autologous stem cell rescue. ASCO Proc 1997: abstr 45.
58. Zimmer AM, Kaplan EH, Kazikiewicz JM, et al. Pharmacokinetics of I-131 T101 monoclonal antibody in patients with chronic lymphocytic leukemia. Antib Immunoconj Radiopharm 1988; 1:291–303.
59. Rosen ST, Zimmer AM, Goldman LR, et al. Progress in the treatment of cutaneous T cell lymphomas with radiolabeled monoclonal antibodies. Int J Rad Appl Instrum [b] 1989; 16:667–668.
60. Zimmer AM, Rosen ST, Spies SM, et al. Radioimmunotherapy of patients with cutaneous T-cell lymphoma using an iodine-131-labeled monoclonal antibody: analysis of retreatment following plasmapheresis. J Nucl Med 1988; 29: 174–180.
61. Raubitschek AA. Yttrium-90 labeled T101 in the treatment of hematologic malignancies. Proceedings of the Fifth International Conference on Monoclonal Antibody Conjugates for Cancer, 1990.
62. Waldmann TA, White JD, Carrasquillo JA, et al. Radioimmunotherapy of Interleu-

kin-2Ra-expressing adult T-cell leukemia with yttrium-90-labeled anti-tac. Blood 1995; 86(11):4063–4075.
63. Stein R, Sharkey RM, Goldenberg DM. Haematological effects of radioimmunotherapy in cancer patients. Br J Haematol 1992; 80:69–76.
64. DeNardo GL, DeNardo SJ, Macey DJ, et al. Overview of radiation myelotoxicity secondary to radioimmunotherapy using ^{131}I-Lym-1 as a model. Cancer 1994; 73(3 Suppl.):1038–1048.
65. Tubiana M, Frindel E, Croizat H, et al. Effects of radiations on bone marrow. Pathol Biol (Paris) 1979; 27:326–334.
66. Liu T, Meredith RF, Saleh MN, et al. Correlation of toxicity with treatment parameters for ^{131}I-CC49 radioimmunotherapy in three Phase II clinical trials. Cancer Biother Radiopharm 1997; 12(2):79–87.
67. Zasadny KR, Gater VL, Fisher SJ, et al. Correlation of dosimetric parameters with hematologic toxicity after radioimmunotherapy of non-Hodgkin's lymphoma with I-131-anti-B1. Utility of a new parameter: "Total body dose-lean." J Nucl Med 1995; 36:214P.
68. Breitz HB, Fisher DR, Wesels B. Correlation of bone marrow absorbed dose estimates with marrow toxicity. Tumor Targeting 1996; 2:173.
69. Vriesendorp HM, Shao Y, Blum JE, et al. Fractionated intravenous administration of ^{90}Y-labeled B72.3 GYK-DTPA immunoconjugate in beagle dogs. Nucl Med Biol 1993; 20:571–578.
70. Knox SJ, Goris ML, Davis TA, et al. Randomized controlled study of 131-I-anti-B1 versus unlabeled anti-B1 monoclonal antibody in patients with chemotherapy refractory low grade non-Hodgkin's lymphoma. Int J Rad Bio Onc Phys 1997; 39(Suppl.):326.
71. Dillman LT, Van der Lage FC. Radionuclide decay schemes and nuclear parameters for use in radiation-dose estimation. Soc Nuc Med 1975; MIRD pamphlet #10.
72. Snyder WS, Ford MR, Warner GG, et al. "S" absorbed dose per unit cumulated activity for selected radionuclides and organs. Soc Nuc Med 1975; MIRD pamphlet #11.
73. Strand SE, Jonsson BA, Ljungberg M, et al. Radioimmunotherapy dosimetry-a review. Acta Oncol 1993; 32:807–817.
74. Siegel JA, Goldenberg DM, Badger CC. Radioimmunotherapy dose estimation in patients with B-cell lymphoma. Med Phys 1993; 20(suppl):579–582.
75. Erdi AK, Wessels BW, DeJager R, et al. Tumor activity confirmation and isodose curve display for patients receiving iodine-131-labeled 16.88 human monoclonal antibody. Cancer 1994; 73:932–944.
76. Pollard KR, Bice AN, Eary JF, et al. A method for imaging therapeutic doses of iodine-131 with a clinical gamma camera. J Nucl Med 1992; 33:771–776.
77. Watson EE, Stabin MG. MIRD formulation. Med Phys 1993; 20(2)pt 2:511–514.
78. Koral KF, Zasadny KR, Swailem FM, et al. Importance of intra-therapy single-photon emission tomographic imaging in calculating tumour dosimetry for a lymphoma patient. Eur J Nucl Med 1991; 18:432–435.
79. Strand SE, Ljungberg M, Tennval J, et al. Radiotherapy dosimetry with special emphasis on SPECT quantification extracorporeal immunoabsorption. Med Biol Engineering Computing 1994; 32(5):551–561.

80. Fisher DR. Radiation dosimetry for radioimmunotherapy. An overview of current capabilities and limitations. Cancer 1994; 73(suppl 3):905–911.
81. Larson SM, Macapinlac HA, Scott AM, et al. Bone marrow dosimetry: regional variability of marrow localizing antibody. J Nucl Med 1996; 37(4):695–698.
82. Folbert KS, Sgouras G, Larson GM. Implementation and evaluation of patient specific three dimensional internal dosimetry. J Nucl Med 1997; 38(2):301–308.
83. Goris ML, Knox SA, Nielsen KR, et al. Organ modeling in the quantitation of planar images for distribution studies. Cancer 1994; 73(suppl):919–922.
84. Koral KF, Zasadny KR, Kessler ML, et al. CT-SPECT fusion plus conjugate views for determining dosimetry in iodine-131-monoclonal antibody therapy of lymphoma patients. J Nucl Med 1994; 35:1714–1720.
85. Eary JF, Press OW, Badger CC, et al. Imaging and treatment of B-cell lymphoma. J Nucl Med 1990; 31:1257–1268.
86. DeNardo GL, Mahe MA, DeNardo SJ, et al. Body and blood clearance and marrow radiation dose of ^{131}I-Lym-1 in patients with B-cell malignancies. Nucl Med Commun 1993; 14:587–595.
87. Siegel JA, Wessels BW, Watson EE, et al. Bone marrow dosimetry and toxicity for radioimmunotherapy. Antib Immunoconjug Radiopharm 1990; 3:213–233.
88. Fowler JF. The linear-quadratic formula and progress in fractionated radiotherapy. Br J Radiol 1989; 62:679–694.
89. Wilder RB, DeNardo GL, Sheri S, et al. Application of the linear quadratic model to myelotoxicity associated with radioimmunotherapy. Eur J Nucl Med 1996; 23:953–957.
90. Sgouros G, Jureidini IM, Scott AM, et al. Bone marrow dosimetry: regional variability of marrow-localizing antibody. J Nuc Med 1996; 37(4):695–698.
91. Meredith RF, Buchsbaum DJ, Knox SJ. Radionuclide dosimetry and radiotherapy of cancer. In: Abrams PG, Fritzberg AR, eds. Radioimmunotherapy of Cancer. New York: Marcel Dekker. In press.
92. DeNardo SJ, DeNardo DL, O'Grady LF, et al. Pilot studies of radioimmunotherapy of B-cell lymphoma and leukemia using I-131 Lym-1 monoclonal antibody. Antib Immunoconj Radiopharm 1988; 1:17–33.
93. DeNardo SJ, DeNardo DL, O'Grady LF, et al. Treatment of B-cell malignancies with ^{131}I Lym-1 monoclonal antibodies. Int J Cancer 1988; 3(suppl):99–101.
94. Kaminski MS, Fig L, Zasadny K, et al. Phase I evaluation of 131-I-MB-1 antibody radioimmunotherapy of B-cell lymphoma. Blood 1990; 76(suppl):355a.
95. Knox SJ, Goris ML, Wessels BW. Overview of animal studies comparing radioimmunotherapy with dose equivalent external beam irradiation. Radiother Oncol 1992; 23:111–117.
96. Buchsbaum DJ, Roberson PL. Experimental radioimmunotherapy: biological effectiveness and comparison with external beam radiation. In: Wannenmacher M, Bihl H, eds. Recent Results in Cancer Research, 1995; 141:9–18.
97. Fowler JF: Radiobiological aspects of low dose rates in radioimmunotherapy. Int J Radiat Oncol Biol Phys 1990; 18:1261–1269.
98. Knox SJ, Sutherland W, Goris ML. Correlation of tumor sensitivity to low-dose-rate irradiation with G2/M-phase block and other radiobiological parameters. Radiat Res 1993; 135:24–31.

99. Williams JR, Zhang YG, Dillehay LE. Sensitization processes in human tumor cells during protracted irradiation: possible exploitation in the clinic. Int J Radiat Oncol Biol Phys 1992; 24:699–704.
100. Wong JY, Williams LE, Demidecki AJ, et al. Radiobiologic studies comparing Yttrium-90 irradiation and external beam irradiation in vitro. Int J Radiat Oncol Biol Phys 1991; 20:715–722.
101. Wessels BW, Vessella RL, Palme DF, et al. Radiobiological comparison of external beam irradiation and radioimmunotherapy in renal cell carcinoma xenografts. Int J Radiat Oncol Biol Phys 1989; 17:1257–1263.
102. Rostock RA, Klein JL, Leichner PK, et al. Distribution of and physiologic factors that affect ^{131}I-antiferritin tumor localization in experimental hepatoma. Int J Radiat Oncol Biol Phys 1984; 10:1135–1141.
103. Sands H, Jones PL, Shah SA, et al. Correlation of vascular permeability and blood flow with monoclonal antibody uptake by human Clouser and renal cell xenografts. Cancer Res 1988; 48:188–193.
104. Bale WF, Spar IL. Studies directed toward the use of antibodies as carriers of radioactivity for therapy. Adv Biol Med Phys 1957; 5:285–356.
105. Rostock RA, Kopher KA, Bauer TW, et al. Factors that affect antiferritin localization in four rat hepatoma models. Cancer Drug Deliv 1985; 2:139–145.
106. Song CW, Levitt SH. Effect of X-irradiation on vascularity of normal tissues and experimental tumor. Radiology 1970; 94:445–447.
107. Hall EJ. Radiobiology for the Radiologist. 3d ed. Philadelphia: Lippincott, 1988.
108. Langmuir VK, Fowler JF, Knox SJ, et al. Radiobiology of radiolabeled antibody therapy as applied to tumor dosimetry. Med Phys 1993; 20:601–610.
109. Macklis RM, Beresford BA, Palayoor S, et al. Cell cycle alterations, apoptosis, and response to low-dose-rate radioimmunotherapy in lymphoma cells. Int J Radiat Oncol Biol Phys 1993; 27:643–650.
110. Macklis RM, Beresford BA, Humm JL. Radiobiologic studies of low-dose-rate ^{90}Y-lymphoma therapy. Cancer 1994; 73(suppl):966–973.
111. Valentine MA, Licciardi KA. Rescue from anti-IgM-induced programmed cell death by the B cell surface proteins CD20 and CD40. Eur J Immunol 1992; 22:3141–3148.
112. Neacy WP, Wessels BW, Bradley EW, et al. Comparison of radioimmunotherapy (RIT) and 4 MV external beam radiotherapy of human tumor xenografts in athymic mice. J Nucl Med 1986; 27:902–903.
113. Wessels BW, Neacy WP, York ED, et al. External beam and radioimmunotherapy dosimetry comparison of colorectal xenografts. In: Watson EE, Schlafke-Stelson AT, eds. Proceedings of the Fifth International Radiopharmaceutical Dosimetry Symposium, 1991:66–76.
114. Knox SJ, Levy R, Miller RA, et al. Determinants of the antitumor effect of radiolabeled monoclonal antibodies. Cancer Res 1990; 50:4935–4940.
115. Murtha A, Rupnow B, Knox S. Low dose rate radiation favors apoptosis as a mechanism of cell death. Int J Rad Bio Onc Phys 1997; 39(Suppl.):242.
116. Illidge T, Cragg M, Glennie M. Cell cycle alterations, apoptosis and response to RIT in lymphoma cells. ASCO Proc 1997, abs 1964.

117. Knox SJ. Radioimmunotherapy of the non-Hodgkin's lymphomas. Sem Rad Onc 1995; 5(4)331–341.
118. Wahl RL. Experimental radioimmunotherapy. A brief overview. Cancer 1994; 73(suppl):989–992.
119. Buchsbaum DJ, Langmuir VK, Wessels BW. Experimental radioimmunotherapy. Med Phys 1993:551–567.
120. Buchsbaum DJ, Lawrence TS. New trends in the use of radioimmunoconjugates for the therapy of cancer. Targeted Diagn Ther 1990; 3:215–255.
121. Knox SJ. Overview of studies of experimental radioimmunotherapy. Cancer Res 1995; 55(suppl 23):5832S–5836S.
122. Schlom J, Milenic DE, Roselli M, et al. New concepts in monoclonal antibody based radioimmunodiagnosis and radioimmunotherapy of carcinoma. Int J Rad Appl Instrum [b] 1991; 18:425–435.
123. Schlom J, Molinolo A, Simpson JF, et al. Advantage of dose fractionation in monoclonal antibody-targeted radioimmunotherapy. J Natl Cancer Inst 1990; 82:763–771.
124. Beaumier PL, Venkatesan P, Vanderheyden JL, et al. ^{186}Re radioimmunotherapy of small cell lung carcinoma xenografts in nude mice. Cancer Res 1991; 51:676–681.
125. Schlom J, Siler K, Milenic DE, et al. Monoclonal antibody-based therapy of a human tumor xenograft with a ^{177}lutetium-labeled immunoconjugate. Cancer Res 1991; 51:2889–2896.
126. Meredith RF, Khazaeli MB, Liu T, et al. Dose fractionation of radiolabeled antibodies in patients with metastatic colon cancer. J Nucl Med 1992; 33:1648–1653.
127. Sutcliffe SB. Immunotherapy of the Lymphomas. Boca Raton, FL: CRC Press, 1985.
128. LoBuglio AF, Wheeler RH, Trang J, et al. Mouse/human chimeric monoclonal antibody in man: kinetics and immune response. Proc Natl Acad Sci USA 1989; 86:4220–4224.
129. Rowlinson BG, Snook D, Epenetos AA. ^{90}Y-labeled antibody uptake by human tumor xenografts and the effect of systemic administration of EDTA. Int J Radiat Oncol Biol Phys 1994; 28:1257–1265.
130. Norrgren K, Strand SE, Nilsson R, et al. A general, extracorporeal immunoadsorption method to increase the tumor-to-normal tissue ratio in radioimmunoimaging and radioimmunotherapy. J Nucl Med 1993; 34:448–454.
131. Sharkey RM, Blumenthal RD, Hansen HJ, et al. Biological considerations for radioimmunotherapy. Cancer Res 1990;964s–969s.
132. Paganelli G, Magnani P, Fazio F. Pretargeting of carcinomas with the avidin-biotin system. Int J Biol Markers 1993; 8:155–159.
133. Paganelli G, Riva P, Deleide G, et al. In vivo labelling of biotinylated monoclonal antibodies by radioactive avidin: a strategy to increase tumor radiolocalization. Int J Cancer 1988; 2:121–125.
134. Goodwin DA, Meares CF, McCall MJ, et al. Pre-targeted immunoscintigraphy of murine tumors with indium-111-labeled bifunctional haptens. J Nucl Med 1988; 29:226–234.
135. Sinitsyn VV, Mamontova AG, Checkneva YY, et al. Rapid blood clearance of biotinylated IgG after infusion of avidin. J Nucl Med 1989; 30:66–69.

7
Monoclonal Antibody-Based Therapy of Cutaneous T-Cell Non-Hodgkin's Lymphoma

Timothy M. Kuzel and Steven T. Rosen
Northwestern University Medical School, Chicago, Illinois

I. INTRODUCTION

Antibody-based therapies have been utilized in an attempt to treat human disease for over five decades. Early trials used unconjugated polyclonal antibodies or radiolabeled polyclonal antibodies developed by immunization of an intermediate species of animal with the target antigen. Since the late 1970s, however, new cell culture and molecular techniques have allowed the use of purified monoclonal antibodies with desired specificity. Still, most investigators would concede that in early trials with unconjugated antibodies the clinical benefits for patients were limited (1). As these trials were often Phase I in design, there was great interest in feasibility, toxicity, pharmacokinetics, and biodistribution of the antibodies, including binding to tumor tissues. Thus, tumors that readily were accessible for biopsy prior to therapy, to ensure tumor antigen presence for targeting, and again easily biopsied after therapy, to assess in vivo targeting, were sought eagerly for these initial trials. Mycosis fungoides was, therefore, an excellent disease choice for many investigators.

Mycosis fungoides and the related Sezary syndrome are the most common of a family of non-Hodgkin's lymphomas termed *cutaneous T-cell lymphomas* (CTCL). These lymphomas involve the skin predominantly, but eventually disseminate widely to involve lymph nodes, spleen, or other internal organs (2). The Sezary syndrome is a leukemic variant of mycosis fungoides, with generalized skin involvement and circulating neoplastic T-lymphocytes. Mycosis fungoides and the Sezary syndrome can be discriminated from other cutaneous T-cell lymphomas by the characteristic epidermotropism and the lack of retroviral elements (in most investigators' experience) (3). This characteristic skin involvement allows ready access to neoplastic cells to assess tumor antigen expression, to assess in vivo targeting by the infused monoclonal antibody, and to assess antitumor effects. Additionally, mycosis fungoides and the Sezary syndrome are relatively indolent diseases, which allows investigators some comfort when using investigational agents, since there is no proven curative therapy for this disease. Finally, the cell of origin has been characterized to be a mature T-helper lymphocyte (4), and the surface antigen expression usually is predictable in patients. Skin biopsy prior to treatment allows the investigator to confirm each patient's extent of target antigen expression.

II. UNCONJUGATED MONOCLONAL ANTIBODY THERAPY OF T-CELL MALIGNANCY

As noted in earlier chapters, unconjugated monoclonal antibodies can be used to eradicate human neoplastic cells via several different mechanisms (5). These include antibody-dependent cellular cytotoxicity through complement activation or by aiding in phagocytosis of tumor cells. They may be able to regulate cellular proliferation by binding to growth factor receptors or to the growth factor directly or by binding to tumor antigens that might trigger intracellular events leading to apoptosis. Finally, strategies utilizing the immunogenicity of these molecules to generate vaccine-type responses are being explored.

A. Results of Clinical Trials

The neoplastic T-lymphocyte in mycosis fungoides expresses a 65,000-dalton protein termed CD-5, which is recognized by several monoclonal antibodies, including T-101 and Leu-1 (6). This antigen also is expressed on the neoplastic B-lymphocyte in chronic lymphocytic leukemia. A number of early reports of clinical use of monoclonal antibodies targeting this antigen suggested biological activity, measured as clearing of circulating malignant blood cells, or even transient partial remissions in a patient with mycosis fungoides (7–9). Several studies subsequently were reported that used a variety of dosage schemes to administer T-101. In these trials, six of fourteen patients with mycosis fungoides manifested significant but short responses (several months' duration) (10,11). A decrease in circulating neoplastic cells was observed in all patients. Binding to tumor cells was demonstrated in vivo in skin, bone marrow, blood, and lymph nodes. Toxicity consisted of fevers and chills; up to 30% of patients manifested allergic-type reactions with pruritus and urticaria. When rapid infusion schedules were utilized, anaphylactoid reactions occurred, manifested as wheezing and hypotension. Pretreatment with steroids or diphenhydramine hydrochloride controlled or prevented many of these side effects.

B. Limitations of Monoclonal Antibody-Based Therapy

Although few clinical responses were observed in these early trials, significant knowledge was gained as to the mechanisms of resistance or treatment failure. Major limitations to monoclonal antibody therapy were identified. It was recognized that the CD-5 antigen modulated (was internalized) from the cell surface after antibody binding, usually within several hours of drug administration. The antigen was not reexpressed for several days, preventing host effector cells from attacking the neoplastic cell. In some patients, circulating neoplastic cells or shed circulating antigen adsorbed most of the infused antibody, limiting efficacy in tissues. Identified clones of the original neoplastic cells were antigen-negative before therapy; this antigen heterogeneity predicted failure of a targeted therapy that had to bind to the cell surface of individual cells to be effective.

Finally, and most significantly, the inherent immunogenicity of the infused monoclonal antibodies (because they were murine derived and hence a foreign protein) has been a major ongoing limitation with this form of therapy. Patients with mycosis fungoides are not inherently immunosuppressed (as compared to many patients with B-cell non-Hodgkin's lymphomas). Hence, human antimouse antibodies (HAMA) developed in approximately 50% of the mycosis fungoides patients in these early trials. It was recognized that high levels of the HAMA were associated with lower peak T-101 serum levels and a lack of clinical response. Thus, multiple cycles of therapy were of no benefit in a large number of the treated patients.

A strategy employed to minimize an HAMA response has been to use "chimeric" monoclonal antibodies. These antibodies retain the variable portion of a murine monoclonal antibody for antigen binding specificity but replace much of the rest of the antibody with a human antibody. This altered structure markedly reduces the immunogenicity of the antibody. Knox et al. have reported several trials using chimeric antibodies directed against the CD-4 antigen in mycosis fungoides patients (12,13). In Phase I trials they have treated fifteen patients. Of note, only three of fifteen developed low levels of HAMA. Significant depletion of peripheral blood CD-4 positive cells suggested targeting of the antigen, which lasted as long as 22+ weeks. No evidence of clinical immunosuppression was noted. Additionally, the researchers observed a number of partial responses, although they tended to be short-lived (median 21 weeks freedom from progression).

C. Vaccine Therapy Based on Antimurine Antibodies Response

Because of these limitations, most investigators chose to abandon unconjugated murine monoclonal antibodies for the therapy of CTCL. However, some investigators chose to exploit the immunogenicity of murine monoclonal antibodies with therapeutic intent. In this instance, the antibody served as an anti-idiotype vaccine, resembling a restricted target antigen on the malignant T-cell. Foon and his colleagues administered a murine monoclonal antibody (4DC6), an anti-idiotype antibody raised against a monoclonal antibody that targets a highly restricted T-lymphocyte antigen expressed on neoplastic T-cells, to four patients with mycosis fungoides or the Sezary syndrome (14). A host anti-idiotype antibody response to this murine monoclonal antibody could cross-react with the tumor antigen and theoretically enhance the host antitumor response. One of four patients experienced a major reduction in tumor masses persisting for 11 months. Humoral and cell-mediated responses to the antibody were noted in all patients

III. CONJUGATED MONOCLONAL ANTIBODY THERAPY OF T-CELL MALIGNANCY

Although occasional dramatic successes are observed in the therapy of B-cell lymphomas with unconjugated monoclonal antibodies, the same has not been true for T-cell disorders. To enhance the cytotoxicity of such agents, investigators have formed immunoconjugates of monoclonal antibodies bound to chemotherapeutic drugs, radionuclides, or bacterial and plant toxins. The monoclonal antibody acts as a carrier for the delivery of these toxic agents to neoplastic cells, ideally sparing normal tissues. Attempts using antibodies to carry various chemotherapeutic agents have been studied least in humans. At doses of drug adequate to achieve the desired clinical response, problems with precipitation of the complex, polymerization, or loss of immunoreactivity (specificity of binding) were noted (15). Therefore, most clinical trials with immunoconjugates have utilized conjugates of monoclonal antibodies and radioisotopes or plant and bacterial protein toxins.

For cutaneous T-cell lymphomas, the most extensively studied class of immunoconjugate is the radioimmunoconjugate. Early trials were conducted primarily with iodine-131, for several reasons: It is an inexpensive isotope, the labeling techniques available were ideal for this isotope, and both imaging (gamma emission) and therapeutic benefit (beta emission) were achievable with the same isotope. The long range of penetration, however, has limited the use of agents with significant gamma emission. The use of these agents creates radiation safety concerns when utilized in high doses. Patients require strict isolation to prevent harm to family members, other patients, and allied health care professionals. In addition, dehalogenation (disintegration of linkage of antibody to isotope) occurs despite the standard conjugating methods, and elimination in urine or feces is seen.

As radiochemistry methodology has become more advanced, other isotopes have been evaluated for use as immunoconjugates. Alpha-emitting radionuclides, which have a linear energy transfer but a short range (astatine-211 or bismuth-212) are being investigated, but their gamma irradiation may have disadvantages similar to those of iodine-131. Iodine-125 produces a low-energy gamma irradiation from its Auger electron decay. These Auger electrons have very short ranges (10 μm) and may best be utilized in conjunction with antibodies that are internalized into cells (16). Finally, isotopes with isolated beta emissions are increasingly utilized for radioimmunotherapy. These isotopes can have cytotoxic effects over a longer range without the troublesome gamma decay. An example of a beta-emitting isotope is yttrium-90, which has a half-life of 64 hours and an effective path length of 5.4 mm (radius of a sphere in which 90% of radiation is deposited). This allows effective tumor irradiation, even if substantial numbers of neoplastic cells are antigen negative. However, uptake into small tumor deposits may result in undesirable normal tissue irradiation, and the avidity of yttrium-90 for bone also contributes to its toxicity. Improved radiochemistry techniques to conjugate antibodies to yttrium-90 may reduce in vivo separation and resultant myelosuppression.

To avoid toxicity to normal organs associated with radioimmunoconjugates, especially the bone marrow, plant or bacterial toxins increasingly are being used as the toxic moiety conjugated to an antibody. However, these immunoconjugates have very short half-lives, thus requiring continuous infusions or high doses to achieve satisfactory tumor cell exposure times. Immune responses against these constructs can be brisk, directed against not only the antibody but also the toxin moiety. Antibodies can be either neutralizing or non-neutralizing (which can increase circulating half-life). Toxicity is related to hepatic scavenging of the immunoconjugate with resultant, nonspecific side effects (elevated liver function tests and hypoalbuminemia) and a poorly understood capillary leak-like syndrome.

A. Radioimmunoconjugate Therapy of T-Cell Malignancy

Since much of the early work with unconjugated monoclonal antibodies utilized the antibody T-101 for therapy of T-cell lymphomas, this antibody was used in the initial radioimmunoconjugate trials as well. In several trials, the antibody was conjugated to either indium-111 or iodine-131 intravenously, intralymphatically, or subcutaneously (17–19). The investigators were able to demonstrate specific cutaneous and nodal localization. Unfortunately, these imaging studies also confirmed the low percentage of administered antibody that actually targeted tumor (approximately 0.01% in these studies). Intralymphatic injection in the feet decidedly increased the administered dose that could be detected in pelvic or periaortic nodes. Thus, despite the significant dehalogenation observed with the iodine-131 construct, therapy trials were designed.

Rosen et al. administered 5.6–13.1 mCi of iodine-131 conjugated to 9.6–10.5 mg of antibody to six patients to assess the biodistribution of the radiolabeled monoclonal antibody and to predict radiation-absorbed doses to specific tumor or organ sites (20). Inguinal and axillary adenopathy could be detected by gamma scintigraphy during the imaging phase. Five patients subsequently received therapeutic doses of 100.5–150 mCi of iodine-131 conjugated to 9.6–16.9 mg of antibody. Two partial remissions which lasted 2 months were observed. Regression of skin lesions and enlarged lymph nodes were observed, and all patients reported diminished pruritus after treatment. These responses were observed despite dosimetry calculations that suggested that responding skin lesions received only modest doses of radiation (40–510 cGy). Additionally, whole-body radiation exposures ranged from 28 to 89 cGy. Thus, this study illustrated the difficulty in determining microdosimetry calculations of radiation-absorbed doses at the cellular level. It demonstrated that the relationship of time of exposure, as well as total radiation dose, to tumor response needed to be explored. External planar imaging via a gamma camera may not be the ideal way to define the dosimetry; there are now preliminary data suggesting that single-photon emission computed tomography (21) or positron emission tomography (22) may be preferable. The interested reader should seek out additional information in other chapters of this text or from an excellent review of radioimmunoconjugates for speculation on mechanisms whereby radioimmunotherapy exerts its cytotoxic effects despite lower theoretic radiation effectiveness (23). Mild reversible myelosuppression was the only toxicity observed in this trial. Dehalogenation of the antibody was witnessed clearly, based on bladder and thyroid imaging and the measurement of free iodine-131 in blood and urine. The benefit ascribed to direct tumor targeting by antibody versus whole-body radiation exposure could not be determined definitely.

Trials of radiolabeled (yttrium-90) anti-Tac monoclonal antibodies, directed against the interleukin-2 receptor alpha chain also have been performed in patients with adult T-cell leukemia/lymphoma. The target antigen (CD2T) is expressed ubiquitously in patients with this HTLV1 (human T-cell lymphotropic virus type 1) associated malignancy. Waldmann and colleagues have reported results of a Phase I/Phase II trial involving eighteen patients (24). Responses (seven partial and two complete) were observed at doses of yttrium-90 of 5–15 mCi. The duration of response was comparable to those seen with aggressive chemotherapeutic approaches utilized previously (median 9 months), with several dramatic durable responses lasting more than 2 years. When these results were compared to their own historic data using the unconjugated anti-Tac, monoclonal antibody, the group felt that the yttrium-90-labeled antibody was superior. Toxicity, as expected, was greater in the radiolabeled cohort, but was limited to the hematopoietic system.

B. Immunotoxin Therapy of Cutaneous T-Cell Malignancy

Fewer clinical studies utilizing immunotoxins for the therapy of cutaneous T-cell malignancies have been reported. The results with immunotoxins have been less imposing than those with radioimmunoconjugates. An early trial in mycosis fungoides patients used a murine antibody against CD-5 conjugated to the A-chain of ricin (25). Patients received ten daily infusions. There were four partial responses, with a median response duration of 3.5 months. Toxicity in this trial consisted of dyspnea at rest with higher doses, fatigue, fever, and chills. A particular syndrome of toxicity seen with immunotoxins was noted in this trial—a vascular leak–like syndrome characterized by hypoalbuminemia, weight gain, and pedal edema. The exact etiology of this side effect is not yet understood. Ten of twelve patients evaluated developed anti-immunotoxin antibodies (either to the antibody itself or to the toxin component). Seven of the ten had blocking antibodies, which interfere with binding.

IV. LIGAND FUSION TOXIN THERAPY OF T-CELL MALIGNANCY

Because of the relatively low efficacy noted against established tumors with immunotoxins and the high rate of host immune responses against the constructs, investigators began to experiment with alternative targeting systems. With the development of recombinant DNA technology, the production of ligands covalently linked to toxins became feasible. The first such toxins to enter clinical trials were $DAB_{486}IL$-2 and $DAB_{389}IL$-2. These fusion toxins bind to the IL-2 receptor and consist of nucleotide sequences of the enzymatically active and membrane-translocating domains of diphtheria toxin and the sequence for human interleukin-2 (26). $DAB_{389}IL$-2 is a second-generation molecule characterized by a deletion of ninety-seven amino acids from the diphtheria toxin translocating domain of $DAB_{486}IL$-2, thereby creating a fusion toxin with a more favorable pharmacokinetic profile (27). Both fusion toxins bind to high-affinity interleukin-2 receptors, are internalized by receptor-mediated endocytosis, and subsequently inhibit protein synthesis by translocation of the active portion of the diphtheria toxin into the cytosol, where it inhibits ADP-ribosylation of elongation factor-2 (26,28,29). Cytotoxic activity of both $DAB_{486}IL$-2 and $DAB_{389}IL$-2 has been limited to neoplastic lymphocytes or cell lines bearing the high-affinity (p55, p75, p64) interleukin-2 receptor complex, while those cells expressing only a partial form of the receptor (p55, p64 or p75, p64) are less sensitive to the toxins.

Although initial Phase I/II studies with these fusion toxins included patients with Hodgkin's disease, B-cell non-Hodgkin's lymphomas, and mycosis fungoides, the activity of the agents appeared greatest in the patients with cutaneous T-cell lymphomas. Twenty percent of patients with mycosis fungoides or the Sezary syndrome treated in various Phase I studies with $DAB_{486}IL-2$ responded, including one patient with tumor stage disease who had a complete response of 36+ months duration (30–33). A Phase II study conducted at the National Cancer Institute accrued fourteen patients with advanced or refractory mycosis fungoides and the Sezary syndrome (34). One patient with extensive plaque stage disease had a partial response, and two patients with the Sezary syndrome had responses that fell just short of the required overall improvement to be considered partial responses. Interleukin-2 receptor expression was measured in skin and on circulating Sezary cells in the treated patients, and no patient who lacked expression of the high-affinity receptor responded to therapy.

A Phase I clinical trial with $DAB_{389}IL-2$ the second-generation IL-2 fusion toxin has been completed for patients with IL-2 receptor expressing lymphomas, including mycosis fungoides, Hodgkin's disease, and relapsed B-cell non-Hodgkin's lymphomas (35). Immunohistochemical analysis of tumor tissue for interleukin-2 receptor expression was a prerequisite for entry to this study. Interleukin-2 receptor positivity was dependent on histology: 45% of B-cell lymphomas, 60% of cutaneous T-cell lymphomas, and 81% of Hodgkin's disease biopsy specimens were positive for p55 expression. In this large trial, 22% of patients achieved a response. Histology was an important predictor for response. No patient with Hodgkin's disease responded, 17% of patients with B-cell lymphomas responded, and 34% of patients with cutaneous T-cell lymphomas responded. The median duration of response in this heavily pretreated population was approximately 9 months. Toxicities included mild and reversible elevations of hepatic transaminases, mild hypoalbuminemia, fever, and hypersensitivity reactions. Immunologic assessment of the non-Sezary patients demonstrated no change in total numbers of peripheral CD-4+, CD-8+, or CD-4/CD-25+ lymphocyte populations, suggesting that there should be no secondary immunosuppressive effects associated with this therapy.

CONCLUSION

At the present time, a number of novel approaches exist for targeted therapy of cutaneous T-cell lymphomas. Our ability to manipulate antibodies, engineer new chimeric constructs, or develop ligand fusion proteins has improved. It is hoped that these more sophisticated and effective constructs will provide oncologists with new weapons to target this family of hematologic malignancies. In addition, the nonoverlapping toxicity spectrum of these agents should allow for new combination approaches with chemotherapeutics or biologic response modifiers.

REFERENCES

1. Grossbard ML, Press OW, Appelbaum FR, et al. Monoclonal antibody–based therapies of leukemias and lymphomas. Blood 1992; 80:863–878.
2. Broder S, Bunn PA. Neoplasms of T-cell origin. Immunological aspects and therapy. Semin Oncol 1980; 7:310–331.
3. Kuzel TM, Rosen ST, Roenigk HH Jr. Mycosis fungoides and the Sezary syndrome: a review of pathogenesis, diagnosis, and therapy. J Clin Oncol 1991; 9:1298–1313.
4. Haynes BF, Metzgar RS, Minna JD, Bunn PA. Phenotypic characterization of cutaneous T-cell lymphoma. Use of monoclonal antibodies to compare with other malignant T-cells. N Engl J Med 1981; 304:1319–1323.
5. Houghton A, Scheinberg D. Monoclonal antibodies in the treatment of hematopoietic malignancies. Semin Oncol 1988; 25(suppl):23–29.
6. Royston I, Majda Baird SM, et al. Human T cell antigens defined by monoclonal antibodies: the 65,000-dalton antigen of T cells (T65) is also found on chronic lymphocytic leukemia cells bearing surface immunoglobulin. J Immunol 1980; 125:725–731.
7. Miller RA, Levy R. Response of cutaneous T-cell lymphoma to therapy with hybridoma monoclonal antibody. Lancet 1981; II:226–229.
8. Miller RA, Maloney DG, McKillop J, Levy R. In vivo effects of murine hybridoma monoclonal antibody in a patient with T-cell leukemia. Blood 1981; 58:78–86.
9. Bunn PA, Foon Ka, Schroff RW, et al. T101 monoclonal antibody therapy for T-cell lymphomas (abstr). Blood 1983; 62:210a.
10. Dillman RO, Shawler DL, Killman JB, et al. Therapy of chronic lymphocytic leukemia and cutaneous T-cell lymphoma with T-101 monoclonal antibody. J Clin Oncol 1984; 2:881–891.
11. Dillman RO, Beauregard J, Shawler DL, et al. Continuous infusion of T-101 monoclonal antibody in chronic lymphocytic leukemia and cutaneous T-cell lymphoma. J Biol Resp Mod 1986; 5:394–410.
12. Knox SJ, Levy R, Hodgkinson S, et al. Observations on the effect of chimeric anti-CD4 monoclonal antibody in patients with mycosis fungoides. Blood 1991; 77:20.
13. Knox S, Hoppe RT, Maloney D, et al. Treatment of cutaneous T-cell lymphoma with chimeric anti-CD4 monoclonal antibody. Blood 1996; 87(3):893–899.
14. Foon KA, Oseroff AR, Vaic Kus L, et al. Immune responses in patients with T-cell lymphoma treated with an anti-idiotype antibody mimicking a highly restricted T-cell antigen. Clin Cancer Res 1995; 1:1285–1294.
15. Dillman RO, Johnson DE, Shawler DL. Comparisons of drug and toxin immunoconjugates. Antibody Immunoconj Radiopharm 1988; 1:65–77.
16. Vriesendorp HM, Quadari SM, Williams JR. Radioimmunoglobulin therapy. In: Armitage JO, Antman KH, eds. High-Dose Cancer Therapy, Pharmacology, Hematopoietins, Stem Cells. Baltimore: Williams & Wilkins, 1992.

17. Carrasquillo JA, Bunn PA Jr, Keenan AM, et al. Radioimmunodetection of cutaneous T-cell lymphoma with in-111 T-101 monoclonal antibody. N Engl J Med 1986; 315: 673–680.
18. Carrasquillo JA, Mulshine JL, Bunn PA, et al. Indium111 T-101 monoclonal antibody is superior to iodine-131 T-101 in imaging of cutaneous T-cell lymphomas. J Nucl Med 1987; 28:281–287.
19. Keenan AM, Weinstein JN, Carrasquillo JA, et al. Immunolymphoscintigraphy and the dose-dependence of indium-111 labeled T101 monoclonal antibody in patients with cutaneous T-cell lymphoma. Cancer Res 1987; 47:6093–6099.
20. Rosen ST, Zimmer AM, Goldman-Leiken R, et al. Radioimmunodetection and radioimmunotherapy of cutaneous T-cell lymphomas using an iodine-131 labeled monoclonal antibody: an Illinois Cancer Council Study. J Clin Oncol 1987; 5:562–573.
21. DeNardo GL, Macey DJ, DeNardo SJ, et al. Quantitative SPECT of uptake of monoclonal antibodies. Semin Nucl Med 1989; 19:22–32.
22. Daghighian F, Pentlow KS, Larson SM, et al. Development of a method to measure kinetics of radiolabeled monoclonal antibody in human tumour with applications to microdosimetry; positron emission tomography studies of iodine-124 labeled 3F8 monoclonal antibody in glioma. Eur J Nucl Med 1993; 20:402–409.
23. Wilder RB, DeNardo GL, DeNardo SJ. Radioimmunotherapy; recent results and future directions. J Clin Oncol 1996; 14:1383–1400.
24. Waldmann TA, White JD, Carrasquillo JA, et al. Radioimmunotherapy of interleukin-2R alpha-expressing adult T-cell leukemia with yttrium-90-labeled anti-Tac. Blood 1995; 86(11):4063–4075.
25. LeMaistre CF, Rosen S, Frankel A, et al. Phase I trial of H65-RTA immunoconjugate in patients with cutaneous T-cell lymphoma. Blood 1991; 78:1173–1182.
26. Williams D, Snyder C, Strom T, et al. Structure/function analysis of interleukin-2 toxin. J Biol Chem 1990; 285:11,885–11,889.
27. Bacha PA, Forte SE, McCarthy DM, Estis L, Yamada G, Nichols JC. Impact of interleukin-2 receptor targeted cytotoxins on a unique model of murine interleukin-2 receptor expressing malignancy. Int J Cancer 1991; 49:96–101.
28. Bacha P, Williams D, Waters C, et al. Interleukin-2 receptor mediated action of a diphtheria toxin related interleukin-2 fusion protein. J Exp Med 1988; 167:612–622.
29. Williams D, Parker K, Bacha P, et al. Diphtheria Toxin receptor binding domain substitution with interleukin-2; genetic reconstruction and properties of a Diphtheria toxin-related interleukin-2 fusion protein. Prot Eng 1987; 1:493–498.
30. LeMaistre CF, Craig F, Rosenblum M, et al. Phase I trial of an interleukin-2 fusion toxin ($DAB_{486}IL-2$) in hematologic malignancies expressing the IL-2 receptor. Blood 1992; 79:2547–2554.
31. LeMaistre CF, Craig F, Meneghetti C, et al. Phase I trial of a 90-minute infusion of the fusion toxin DAB486IL-2 in hematologic malignancies. Cancer Res 1993; 53:3930–3934.
32. Kuzel TM, Rosen ST, Gordon LI, et al. Phase I trial of the diphtheria toxin/interleukin-2 fusion protein $DAB_{486}IL-2$: efficacy in mycosis fungoides and other non-Hodgkin's lymphomas. Leukemia Lymphoma 1993; 11:369–377.

33. Hesketh P, Caguioa P, Koh H, et al. Clinical activity of a cytotoxic fusion protein in the treatment of cutaneous T-cell lymphoma. J Clin Oncol 1993; 11:1682–1690.
34. Foss F, Borkowski T, Gilliom M, et al. Chimeric fusion protein toxin $DAB_{486}IL$-2 in refractory mycosis fungoides and the Sezary syndrome: correlation of activity and IL-2 receptor expression in a phase II study. Blood 1994; 84:1765–1774.
35. Kuzel TM, Foss F, LeMaistre CF, et al. Phase I trial of the diphtheria toxin fusion protein (DAB_{389}-IL2) for the treatment of interleukin-2 receptor expressing hematologic neoplasms. Blood 1995; 86(suppl 1):274a.

8
Antibody-Based Therapies for Hodgkin's Disease

H. L. Morein and R. P. Junghans
Harvard Medical School and Beth Israel Deaconess Medical Center, Boston, Massachusetts

I. INTRODUCTION

Hodgkin's disease (HD) is diagnosed in 8000 Americans each year (1), with a cure rate of approximately 80%, by chemotherapies (primarily) and radiotherapies (2). It is among the most cited examples of the advances offered by cancer therapies in a disease that was 100% fatal 40 years ago. Still, despite the most aggressive interventions, 1600 patients die each year from Hodgkin's disease. The impetus to find new therapies is partly to ameliorate these deaths, typically occurring in early adulthood, and partly because this disease previously has served as a highly successful model for developing new therapies and may do so again.

As in other settings, antibody therapies start with known biologic differences, then strategies are devised to exploit those differences. These differences are often quantitative in nature, such as levels of expression of cellular proteins in tumors versus normal tissues (e.g., CA125, CEA, Tac, MAGE), and only infrequently represent genuinely unique features (e.g., lymphoma idiotypes). These therapies are then regarded as "targeted" because one can attack the trait that was "different" and, by concentration of effect paralleling this difference, attack the tumor. The first part of this chapter discusses the differences that are inherent to the HD tumor versus normal tissues that can be considered as targets for attacking the tumor. In the remainder of the chapter, preclinical and clinical data are presented on different antibody therapeutic modalities in HD.

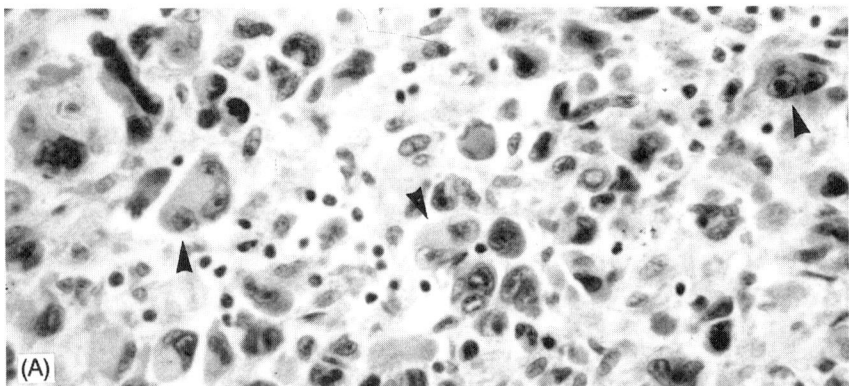

Figure 1 Antigen expression on Reed-Sternberg and Hodgkin's cells. (A) Hodgkin's tumor section with H&E staining. Arrowhead indicates one of several RS/H cells in the field. (Magnification ×600). (B) Immunohistochemical staining of tumor section for CD25 expression with positivity of RS and H cells. (Magnification ×400). (C) Immunohistochemical staining of tumor section for CD30 expression with positivity of RS and H cells. (Magnification ×200). No sclerotic regions are present in the photos; nonstaining areas are the excess of non-RS/H cells in the tumor, which are negative for antigen expression. Tumors selected for abundant RS/H cell presence, which exceeds typical findings. Photographs kindly provided by Dr. S.-M. Hsu, National Taiwan University and University of Arkansas.

A. Cell of Origin

The hallmark of malignancy is the monomorphic expansion of a clonal population of cells. Hodgkin's disease is atypical among malignancies due to its cellular heterogeneity, a feature shared by other disorders of proto- or quasi-malignant status, such as AILD, histiocytosis X, and Castleman's disease. Further, Hodgkin's tumors are characterized by a minor population of Reed-Sternberg/Hodgkin (RS) cells, the presumed malignant population, that is surrounded by a much larger, diverse population of clonally unrelated lymphocytes, macrophages, and granulocytes (see Figure 1A). The basis for the recruitment of normal cells into the tumor is unknown, but it is presumed to be due to cytokines or factors that are released by the malignant cells, including IL6, IL9, IL10, and TNFα and β (3,4).

The mystery surrounding the architecture of these tumors is only part of the picture. The origin of the RS cell has been debated actively for 20 years, variously favoring B-cell, T-cell, monocytic, histiocytic, and interdigitating reticulum (IR) dendritic cell, with evidence for and against each. This judgment is complicated by possible errors in diagnosis, in which some tumors called Hodgkin's may instead be large-cell anaplastic lymphoma, true histiocytic lymphoma,

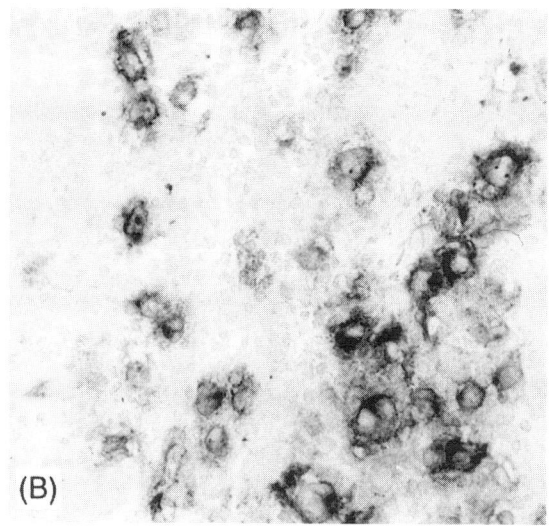

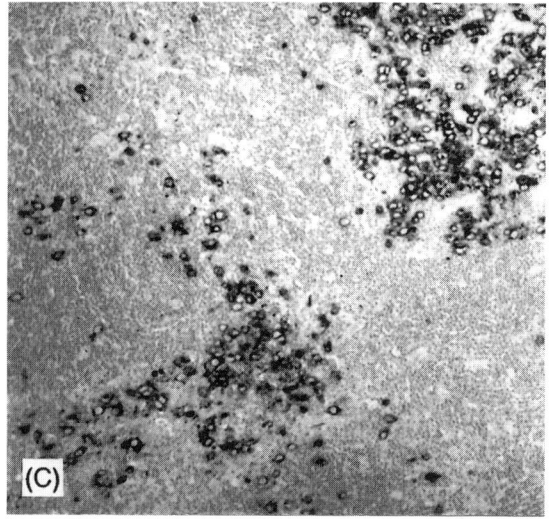

or other disorders. Furthermore, the definitions of HD change: the lymphocyte-predominant (LP) subset of HD is no longer considered HD but a separate entity—germinal center B-cell lymphoma. Reed-Sternberg cells themselves are notoriously difficult to purify or to culture from Hodgkin's tumors, which makes study of pure primary populations of malignant cells problematic. Until recently, it has not been possible to do molecular studies on single RS cells, and these studies must be carefully controlled for contamination by adjacent normal cells in the tumor.

It is beyond the scope of this chapter to review the diverse data on cell of origin, which we present only in outline (for review, see Refs. 4–6). Reed-Sternberg cells are typically negative for B- and T-cell markers, are frequently positive for T-200 (panleukocyte antigen), Leu-M1 (CD15), DR (class II MHC), transferrin receptor (T-9), Ki-1 (CD30), and Tac (CD25). Interestingly, all but T-200 and Leu-M1 are activation antigens, yet none of these is lineage specific. Leu-M1 is a myeloid marker and is also present on some T-cell lymphomas but not on B-cell lymphomas. Leu-M1 is absent on macrophages and IR cells but is revealed with neuraminidase digestion, indicating normal expression of sialylated Leu-M1 on these cells. Lectin binding patterns of RS cells are similar to monocyte-macrophages. Like IR cells, the RS cells bind T-cells. The RS cell shares binucleate morphology with follicular dendritic reticulum cells. Several HD cell lines have been derived, all of which express CD30 and express B-cell or T-cell markers that correlate with B- and T-cell gene rearrangements (3,7–9). Yet the relevance of any of these cell lines to the RS cell is uncertain in the absence of proof of the same rearrangements in individual RS cells from the original tumors. These cell lines have, for the most part, been dismissed as only "possibly" relevant (4,10).

With the advent of advanced PCR techniques, allowing single cell analysis, it recently became possible to address the somatic events within single RS cells. This effort has most recently led to a conclusion of clonal rearrangements of Ig H and L chain in 9/10 tumors tested (10,11). These authors present a cogent discussion of the stringent controls that must be concurrently applied to generate credible data in this setting (10). Barring some developments that invalidate this study, it is probable that the conclusions of Kanzler et al. (11) will stand, that the RS cell is "derived from (crippled) germinal center B cells," making Hodgkin's disease a B cell derived tumor—as long as we assign Ig gene rearrangements and mutation as the exclusive province of B cells. While these PCR studies may possibly settle the question of origin, it does nothing to explain the unique biology, histology and immunophenotypic pattern of Hodgkin's disease. Finally, for a credible HD cell line, one would wish to see the same gene rearrangements in the cell line as in single RS cells in the tumor from which the line was derived.

The cause of Hodgkin's disease is unknown. A role for EBV has been suggested: approximately 30–50% of cases are associated with EBV infection, but rarely in lymphocyte predominant subtype (12), which as stated above, is now considered to be a germinal center B cell lymphoma. When present, the EBV genome is clonally integrated, indicating that the infection took place prior to the malignant transforming event (13). In the 30–50% of HD cases where the genome is present, all of the RS cells are EBV-positive and express LMP1 viral protein. The seroprevalence of EBV is 90% among the general population, but only $1:10^5$ B cells is LMP1-positive in such individuals. Thus, the likelihood of a tumor arising in the EBV-positive B cell is much higher than random. On the other hand, EBV is clearly not a necessary requirement for transformation since at least half of patients have RS cells that are EBV negative. It is likely that EBV infection has a facilitating role, but the nature of that role is unclear. Although chromosomal rearrangements and oncogene overexpression have been observed in HD, these tend to be noted late in the course of the disease and are not reproducible, suggesting these observations are epiphenomena rather than causative in the malignant transformation. This contrasts with other tumors where primary chromosomal abnormalities are thought to have a causal relationship to the disease, such as Burkitt's lymphoma, nodular poorly differentiated lymphoma, chronic myelogenous leukemia, and small cell lung cancer (14).

B. Hodgkin's Disease Markers

The essence of therapy with antibodies is to have a surface marker for targeting with the antibody. Table 1 lists possible markers. Each is discussed in turn. Although ≈50% are LMP1+ from EBV gene expression, this is not a surface antigen, and therefore is not listed (see Refs. 5 and 6 for reviews).

The T-200 antigen is expressed on most hematopoietic cells, including B- and T-lymphocytes, granulocytes, monocytes, and macrophages. As a widely expressed antigen, broad immunosuppression would likely accompany an effective

Table 1 Potential Target Antigens for Antibody Therapy of Hodgkin's Disease

Marker	Synonym	RS cells
T-200	CD45	++
Leu-M1	CD15	++
Transferrin receptor, T9	CD71	++
Class II MHC	DR	++
Tac, IL2 receptor	CD25	++
Ki-1	CD30	++
C3d/EBV receptor	CD21	+

therapy. Nevertheless, T-200 is a late antigen, and stem cells would not be harmed if this antigen were targeted by an effective therapy.

Leu-M1, like T-200, is also a late antigen, but it is less broadly reactive, expressed mainly on mature granulocytes and monocytes. An effective therapy against this antigen would induce neutropenia and predispose the patient to bacterial and fungal infections during treatment. However, it is not expressed on stem cells, and irreversible immune impairment should not be encountered.

Transferrin receptor is expressed on activated B-cells, T-cells, macrophages, and other proliferating cells in order to provide iron to dividing cells. This, like other activation antigens, represents a more selective target, by preserving the resting memory B- and T-cells from harm that are essential for subsequent normal immune responses.

Class II MHC is expressed widely on activated cells, but also on dendritic cells (DC) that are important to antigen presentation and education to new antigens.

Tac, or T activation antigen, is the alpha chain of the IL2 receptor, and is present with high frequency on RS cells (see Figure 1B). It is expressed on activated B- and T-cells and on activated macrophages, but not on normal resting cells.

The Ki-1 antigen first was described on RS cells (see Figure 1C), but has since come to be recognized as a lymphocyte activation antigen that is typically coexpressed with Tac. It is not expressed on normal resting cells. The ligand of CD30 has been described (15), but the biological function of CD30 remains unknown.

C3d is the complement component that is expressed on mature B-cells and follicular dendritic cells. It also serves as the EBV receptor. It is expressed on RS cells in approximately 40% of HD tumors.

Hodgkin's disease is a potentially favorable target for antibody-directed therapies for several reasons: (a) RS cells express large numbers of lymphocyte activation antigens, which are present only in small numbers in normal human tissue; (b) there is a small number of RS cells to be killed; (c) HD tumors tend to be well vascularized, allowing ready access to malignant cells; and (d) HD responds well to conventional therapies, allowing reduction in tumor burden before administration of antibody that could increase its effectiveness.

II. PASSIVE ANTIBODY THERAPY

Passive antibody therapy refers to antibody administered without modification by attachment to cytotoxic agents. This modality seeks to exploit natural immune system interactions against antibody-coated tumor cells. We include in this group the humanized antibodies: these genetically engineered antibodies retrieve some of the activities that may be compromised with mouse antibodies in human therapies. Humanized antibodies also better escape the antiglobulin responses that lead to destruction of rodent antibodies in humans. We exclude from this category the bifunctional antibodies, which are considered separately later.

A. Mechanisms and Toxicities

Passive antibody therapy relies on the native capabilities of antibody to interact and suppress target tumor cells. The possible mechanisms are myriad: complement-dependent cytotoxicity (CDC), antibody-dependent cellular cytotoxicity (ADCC), apoptosis, blockade of a receptor for cytokine that is essential to the tumor cell, and phagocytosis of opsonized tumor cells by phagocytic cells. On the whole, however, passive antibody therapy has met with limited success, with few documented cures in any setting. Of these mechanisms, the most plausible for the in vivo responses obtained are receptor blockade that leads to starvation of tumor cells for an essential ligand or growth factor (16); and ADCC, by which tumor cells are killed by Fc receptor-bearing cytotoxic effectors (17–21). An in vivo role for the other mechanisms has been harder to demonstrate (see Ref. 22 for discussion).

Principles for directed therapy are somewhat different via these two mechanisms. Cell killing by ADCC is proportional to the amount of antibody bound to the cells (23), whereas blockade of an essential growth factor for its receptor may not show a significant suppression until >90% of the receptor is saturated (23,24). Thus, although ADCC may yield tumor killing well below saturation binding of the target antigen, the saturation of such antigen is the proper goal when suppression of its receptor action is the proposed antitumor mechanism. Correspondingly, the higher the expression of antigen, the more antibody that can be bound and the greater the likelihood that the target cell will be killed by ADCC. No such relationship is expected for antigen as receptor. In fact, it may be that higher expression of receptor makes it more difficult to prevent the minimum threshold binding of cytokine or ligand needed for cell proliferation. In general, ADCC is improved by activation of effectors via cytokines.

On the whole, unmodified antibodies against tumor antigens are only rarely associated with toxicity in human therapies, and that has been the case in HD therapies as well.

B. Preclinical Data

1. CD25

The Anti-CD25 murine anti-Tac antibody has an affinity of 10^{10} M^{-1} for antigen and blocks the IL2-binding site of the receptor. It mediates suppression of IL2-dependent proliferation of activated T-cells at concentrations above 1 µg/mL (6 nM), with 50% suppression achieved only after 90% saturation of Tac and 90% suppression of proliferation only after 97% saturation of receptor. The humanized Anti-Tac (Anti-Tac-H) antibody has an affinity of 3×10^9 M^{-1} and essentially identical suppression curves (23). By contrast, the murine Anti-Tac was inactive in ADCC against CD25+ T-cell tumor targets, whereas the humanized version showed significant killing activity that was maximal at 1 μg/mL or higher concentrations. This ADCC killing increased linearly with the amount of antibody bound (23). No testing of RS cell lines was performed, but a similar susceptibility to ADCC would be expected.

2. CD30

The Ber-H2 antibody has played a prominent role in the CD30 studies with Hodgkin's disease, as unmodified antibody, as immunotoxin, and as bispecific antibody. In its available form, it is a murine antibody, which has not been humanized. Its affinity for CD30 antigen is approximately 10^9 M^{-1}. It does not mediate ADCC with human effectors against antigen-expressing targets, and Ber-H2 has no directly suppressive effect upon tumor cell lines in vitro (R. Schwarting, pers. comm.). Recent studies with two other anti-CD30 antibodies, HeFi-1 and M44, curiously had contrary effects on tumor cell growth, depending on the cell line: they suppressed proliferation of ALCL cell lines but were agonistic for (stimulated) proliferation in HD cell lines (25,26). As stated previously, the relationship of HD cell lines to the RS cell in vivo is still unclear, and it may not be possible to extrapolate from the proliferative results of these antibodies in vitro to what would occur in in vivo therapies. The HeFi-1 and M44 antibodies were noted to block CD30-CD30 ligand (CD30L) interactions, but appeared to substitute directly for these interactions, in that effects with these antibodies directly paralleled that of CD30L in stimulation or suppression (25). By contrast, Ber-H2 binds to a non-cross-reactive epitope of CD30. These newer antibodies are unusual in directly mediating toxicity against immortal expressor cell lines in the absence of cytotoxic effector cells, but they would have to be shown to be suppressive in credible HD tumor models (see Section I.A., Cell of Origin) before they could be considered for use in HD therapies. Preclinical studies are summarized in Table 2.

B. Clinical Data

1. CD25

Phase II studies currently are under way, applying anti-Tac-H humanized antibody in clinical trials with advanced-stage Hodgkin's disease (our unpublished results). Bolus infusions of 0.5–1 mg/kg were applied to maintain >5 μg/mL plasma concentrations continuously over a 1-month period, with continuation of

Table 2 Preclinical Passive Antibody Studies

Antibody	Target	Results	Refs.
Anti-Tac-H	CD25, IL2R	In vitro: blocks IL2-dependent proliferation of T-cells; mediates ADCC with human NK cells against CD25+ cells; increased killing with IL2 activation of NK cells	23
Ber-H2	CD30	In vitro: does not block CD30L binding, no ADCC In vivo: does not suppress tumor growth in mice	25, 26

therapy permitted for additional months if there was a response. Several patients had their first dose of antibody tagged with radioactive indium (^{111}In) for imaging and pharmacokinetics. Tumor localization was seen in seven of nine patients, with masses down to 1.2 cm being visualized. Nonspecific uptake in liver and spleen were documented. Four minor responses (not meeting PR criteria of >50% tumor reduction) in the first thirteen evaluable patients have been documented. Interestingly, five of eight patients with B symptoms had marked or total abatement of symptoms, with a general improvement in quality of life measures. Whether this B-symptom suppression is due to a direct effect on the tumor or an indirect effect on other cells responding to tumor factors was not possible to discern. No side effects of therapy have been noted.

Given that antibody was maintained at high levels continuously for 1 month, it is likely that adequate saturation of tumor antigen was achieved as to mediate suppression of an IL2-dependent tumor. The lack of a consistent response pattern and the lack of stimulation of tumor proliferation with IL2 therapies in HD (27,28) suggest that the HD tumor is not IL2-dependent, despite high IL2Rα levels. There is no cytoplasmic domain of Tac that could be implicated in an apoptotic pathway. The minor responses that were seen accordingly are plausibly due to ADCC activity, and are compatible with the in vitro ADCC activity of this antibody.

2. CD30

Six patients were administered Ber-H2 murine antibody in single doses of 0.5–50 mg (approximately 0.01–1 mg/kg) (29). Radioimaging of ^{131}I-tagged antibody showed tumor localization in approximately 50% of tumors, with better results in larger tumors and in tumors with higher fractions of RS cells. An important control test was performed with an irrelevant antibody of the same IgG isotype that showed no tumor uptake. Nonspecific uptake in liver and spleen were apparent, as for the CD25 studies just discussed. Biopsies showed apparent tumor

Table 3 Clinical Passive Antibody Studies

Trial Type	No. patients	Administration	Lab results/ toxicity	Clinical results	Refs.
Humanized anti-Tac-H Ab (CD25)	10 with refractory HD	1 mg/kg, then 0.5 mg/kg; q wk × 4	No toxicity	4/13 minor responses	Junghans et al., unpublished data
Murine Ber-H2 Ab (CD30)	6 with refractory HD	0.01–1 mg/kg; × 1	No toxicity	0/6 responses	29

CD30 saturation at the 30–50 mg doses. No patients showed any type of response in this limited single-dose study. A summary of clinical studies is presented in Table 3.

D. Conclusion

The pattern of responses with unmodified antibodies suggests borderline activity against HD with anti-CD25 humanized antibody during prolonged therapy; prolonged therapy was not applied with the only anti-CD30 therapy reported. This relative lack of potency with unmodified antibodies parallels the results that are typical of such therapies in most tumor settings. Preliminary analysis suggests that the responses that have been seen may be due to ADCC activity. In this regard, there are strong data in animal models that activation of effector cells with cytokines such as IL2 and/or IL12 to enhance ADCC can induce dramatic improvements in the therapeutic potency of unmodified antibodies (27,28). The apparent lack of IL2 responsiveness of the HD tumors could permit such cytokine applications in conjunction with passive antibody therapies that might improve their therapeutic profile.

III. BISPECIFIC ANTIBODY THERAPY

Unconjugated monoclonal antibody therapies, although associated with low toxicity and effective targeting, have had little clinical success (22). This is most likely due to the inability of mAbs to recruit effectively host cytotoxic mechanisms. Investigators have worked to combine the specificity of monoclonal antibodies with the cytotoxicity of immune effector cells in order to eliminate clinically measurable tumor (30). Bispecific monoclonal antibody (bi-mAb), an antibody with two different specificities combined in one molecule, has evolved out of this work (see Figure 2). Bispecific monoclonal antibodies link target cells directly to killer cells via cytotoxic trigger molecules such as the T-cell receptor (TcR) or Fc receptor that trigger lysis and/or phagocytosis by the effector cells (31). Bispecific monoclonal antibodies have the potential to enrich effector cells at the tumor site and to activate tumor-bound effector cells by mediating cross-linking between effector and target cells (32). Bispecific monoclonal antibodies are produced in a variety of ways (for review see Ref. 31), mediating cellular cytotoxicity by various effector cells, including phagocytic cells, natural killer (NK) cells, and T-lymphocytes.

A. Mechanisms and Toxicities

Although representing only about 4% of peripheral blood cells, NK cells are cytotoxic lymphocytes that are an important line of cellular, non-MHC-restricted defense against pathogens for the immune system. Natural killer cells lack the CD3/TcR complex and express CD56 and CD16 (FcγRIII) surface molecules (33). Unless activated by IL2 or via the FcγRIII receptor, NK cells are inefficient in killing most tumor cell lines. Therefore, most Bi-mAb studies using NK cells have been mediated through FcγRIII. FcγRIII binding by IgG or mAb induces triggering of NK-cell cytolytic activity via ADCC and lymphokine secretion. With Bi-mAbs, a high-affinity anti-FcR:FcR interaction is substituted for the low-affinity Fc:FcR interaction of monoclonal antibodies, with a consequent decrease in competition by circulating IgG for FcR binding. This yields a higher efficiency of tumor targeting in vivo. Initial studies using Bi-mAb specific to

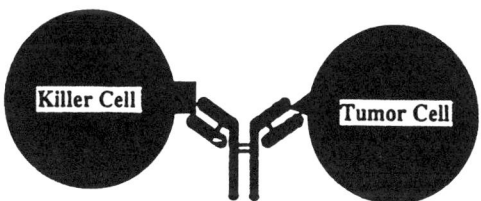

Figure 2 Bispecific antibody-mediated destruction of tumor cells. In bispecific antibody therapy, an antibody with two different specificities combined in one molecule can mediate the conjugation of targets (tumor cells) with appropriate host killer (effector) cells. Triggering of the effector cell cytolytic mechanism(s) by the bispecific antibody results in target cell destruction. (From Ref. 31.)

FcγRIII mediated tumor cell killing by NK cells in vitro and in vivo, and cytotoxicity also was enhanced by the addition of IL2 (31). The presence of FcγRIII on the surface of PMNs and of soluble FcγRIII in the blood did not appear to decrease the effectiveness of Bi-mAb-mediated NK killing (34).

T-lymphocytes have also been targeted to tumor cells by Bi-mAbs. T-cell receptor (TcR) recognition is dependent on two mechanisms: (a) MHC presentation by an antigen-presenting cell, and (b) costimulatory signals for proliferation and effector function. Killing through the T-cell CD3 complex via Bi-mAbs is not MHC-dependent and may involve both CD4+ and CD8+ T-cells. Investigators have taken advantage of the possibility of stimulating resting T-cells by combined triggering of TcR and costimulatory molecule CD28 (33). CD28 activates the lytic potential and proliferative capacities of cytotoxic T-cells (31). Crosslinking of tumor antigens and T-cell markers CD3 and CD28 can increase IL2 secretion, which induces proliferation and upregulates cytotoxicity in resting T-cells (35).

Toxicities are due mainly to effects of crosslinking TCRs by antibody, generating a cytokine-release syndrome. Crosslinking of CD16 (FcγRIII) on NK cells has no similar effect.

B. Preclinical Data

1. CD16-CD30

Hombach et al. (32) used Bi-mAb CD16-CD30 (naming by the antigens targeted) to investigate NK cell lysis of Hodgkin's-derived cell line L540. Bispecific monoclonal antibody CD16-CD30 induced lysis of L540 cells by NK cells, whereas no activity was observed using either mAb alone or in combination. Bispecific monoclonal antibody–mediated killing was not observed with a CD30-negative cell line. Treatment of SCID mice bearing xenografted human Hodgkin's tumors 4–6 mm in diameter with 100 mg of Bi-mAb CD16-CD30 and 10^7 human peripheral blood lymphocytes (PBLs) induced 10/10 complete responses. Sixty percent of the mice had relapse of tumors, but the 40% cure rate after one administration of human PBLs and Bi-mAbs represents one of the most effective immunotherapy demonstrations to date (33). Hombach et al. stated that tumor regression by Bi-mAb CD16-CD30 was at least, if not more, effective than that achieved with ricin-A-chain immunotoxins prepared from the same CD30 mAb by the same research group (see next section) (see Ref. 65).

Hartmann et al. (33) suggested the concurrent administration of IL12 to increase NK activation during Bi-mAb therapy. Stimulation of resting NK cells with IL12 increases the number of cytotoxic granules undergoing exocytosis (36), and IL12 acts as a chemotactic factor for NK cells, increasing NK cell recruitment in tissues (37). It also has been shown that a variety of NK-resistant tumor cell lines are sensitive to IL12-activated NK cells (38). A study of IL2 and IL12 activation of NK cells during CD16-antigen-triggering Bi-mAb administration was conducted by Sahin et al. (39). They reported that a combination of CD16-antigen-triggering-Bi-mAb and low doses of IL12 induced significantly higher tumor cell death than with Bi-mAb or IL12 alone. Tumor cell death was achieved equivalently with IL12 or IL2. It was also found that IL12 or IL2 reduced the antibody concentrations needed to induce tumor cell lysis. This is relevant, in that the expense of Bi-mAb and toxicity associated with them, such as cytokine-release syndrome, may be reduced.

2. CD3-CD30 and CD28-CD30

To test the ability of Bi-mAbs to activate and induce proliferation of T-cells, Renner et al. (40) studied CD3-CD30 and CD28-CD30 Bi-mAbs in comparison with monospecific mAbs to CD3, CD28, and CD30 in vitro. It was determined that a combination of CD3-CD28 and CD3-CD30 Bi-mAbs induced stronger proliferation of CD3+ cells in the presence of L540 (CD30+) Hodgkin's cells than did a combination of monoclonal antibodies or either Bi-mAb alone. The cytotoxic activity of resting human T-cells, however, did not increase unless the T-cells were previously activated.

Carrying out the same testing in SCID mice with xenografted human tumor and activated human T-cells yielded results similar to the in vitro studies (40). All animals that received a combination of Bi-mAbs CD3-CD30 and CD28-CD30 with previously stimulated T-cells were cured of xenografted human tumor. All other mice died by 80 days, due to progressing tumor (see Figure 3). Using pre-stimulated human T-cells labeled with ^{3}H-uridine, the investigators showed that Bi-mAbs mediate trafficking of effector cells into the tumor, compared to control antibodies. Biopsies taken at 96 hours after human T-cell injection showed CD4+ and CD8+ T-cells present. The same group demonstrated the long persistence of T-lymphocytes at the tumor in vivo, suggesting that stimulatory signals for the T-cells could be provided by the tumor cells themselves, eliminating the need to prestimulate T-cells in vitro (33). Accordingly, resting human peripheral blood lymphocytes and the combination of CD3-CD30 and CD28-CD30 Bi-mAbs achieved a 100% cure rate of SCID mice grafted with Hodgkin's tumor cell lines (41). Preclinical studies are summarized in Table 4.

C. Clinical Data

A Phase I/II clinical trial of Bi-mAb CD16-CD30 in relapsed Hodgkin's disease opened in July 1995 (see Table 5). Patients were treated with Bi-mAb CD16-CD30 for 1-hour infusions four times a day every 3–4 days (33). Toxicity has been low, and human anti-mouse antibodies (HAMAs) have been detected in one

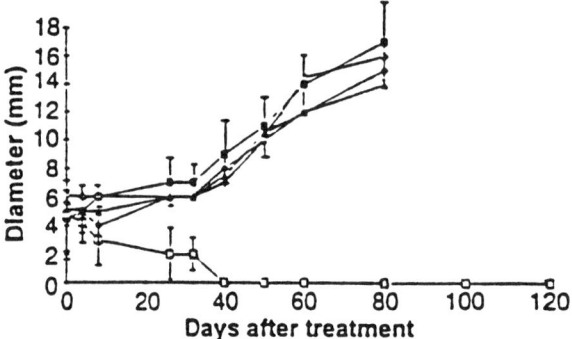

Figure 3 Bispecific monoclonal antibody treatment of xenografted human Hodgkin's tumor. SCID mice injected with Bi-mAbs CD3-CD30 and CD28-CD30 were cured (□). Animals injected with Bi-mAb CD3-CD30 (◆), Bi-mAb CD28-CD30 (▲), or mAb to CD3, CD28, or CD30 (■) died by day 80. (From Ref. 40.)

Table 4 Preclinical Bi-mAb Studies

Bi-mAb	Effector (1) and Target (2)	Results	Refs.
CD16-CD30	1. NK cells 2. CD30+ L540 HD cell line	In vivo: 10/10 CRs in SCID mice; 4/10 long-term (cure)	32
CD3-CD28 + CD3-CD30	1. T-cells (CD4+, CD8+) 2. CD30+ L540 HD cell line	In vitro: Cytotoxic activity with activated T-cells when previously stimulated by CD30+ cells In vivo: 100% cure in SCID mice	40, 41

Table 5 Clinical Bi-mAb Studies

Trial type	No. patients	Administration	Lab results/ toxicity	Clinical results	Ref.
CD16-CD30	11 patients with refractory HD	1–128 mg/m^2, q4d × 4	No toxicity at doses below 16 mg/m^2, MTD not yet reached	Not yet published	33

of four patients tested. No clinical trials using CD3 Bi-mAb alone or in combination with CD28 Bi-mAb have been started so far. Preliminary studies determining the ability of this method to activate lymphocytes from cancer patients have been promising. T-cells from Hodgkin's and non-Hodgkin's lymphoma patients were activated, and conferred cytotoxicity as effectively as healthy control donors against autologous tumor cells or tumor cell lines (41).

D. Conclusion

In theory, anti-CD16 Bi-mAb therapy bypasses problems of unmodified antibody for ADCC, which must compete for binding by the receptor FcRIII on NK cells in IgG-containing plasma. T-cell Bi-mAbs recruit an entirely new class of cells to antibody-dependent killing. Early studies show that Bi-mAbs can bring together the effector and target cells, with improved cytotoxic efficacy in vitro and in vivo.

Bispecific monoclonal antibody therapy has been shown to be very effective with T-cells when added with costimulatory molecules in preclinical studies, but the T-cell Bi-mAbs are presently without clinical data to judge their value for human therapy. A future direction of Bi-mAb therapy would be to use Bi-mAbs to redirect T-cells to the tumor target in a clinical setting. This remains a very promising area for clinical therapies for Hodgkin's disease.

Obstacles in Bi-mAb therapy include the difficulty in producing Bi-mAbs in sufficient quantity and quality for use in clinical settings. HAMA responses are also of concern, because they will cause the formation of immune complexes and rapid clearance of the Bi-mAb from circulation (41), although this problem will be relieved with conversion to use of human or humanized antibodies. Also, treatment with T-cell-specific Bi-mAbs may yield systemic immune activation because of TCR crosslinking. However, modification of the Fc of the antibody so it will not interact with FcR via Fc would minimize this problem (42).

IV. IMMUNOTOXINS

In order to limit the extent of nonspecific toxicity characteristic of current chemotherapy regimens, toxic substances can be selectively delivered to malignant cells through the use of immunotoxin therapy. Immunotoxins (ITs) consist of an antibody or other cell-binding moiety chemically or genetically linked to a potent toxin.

A. Mechanisms and Toxicities

Several toxins have been tested in preclinical and in vivo animal studies. One major group are ribosome-inactivating proteins (RIPs). The RIPs have adenosine nucleosidase activity specific to rRNA that irreversibly damages ribosomes and inhibits protein biosynthesis. Two types of RIPs have been tested against HD. Type I RIPs include saporin and are single-chain proteins. Type II RIPs include ricin and consist of two to four polypeptide chains, one being an A-chain, which executes RNA N-gylcosidase activity, and another, a B-chain, which binds to cells via galactose-containing glycoproteins and glycolipids. Both of these toxins are plant-derived. A second major group of immunotoxins are the ADP-ribosylators that include diphtheria toxin and *Pseudomonas* exotoxin. Diphtheria toxin is comprised of two chains, of which one mediates binding and the other the enzymatic activity. *Pseudomonas* exotoxin contains both functions in a single chain.

Unmodified native ricin coupled to tumor-specific mAbs results in substantial nonspecific toxicity to nontarget cells (43). The B-chain that mediates cell binding was later omitted, leaving only the enzymatically active A-chain. This increased the specific cytotoxicity of the IT in vitro but not in vivo (44). To increase antitumor activity, A-chains were deglycosylated, thereby abolishing binding by liver and RES cells (45). Deglycosylated A-chain (dgA) ITs have increased blood survival times in vivo (46). A new crosslinker, SMPT, was added that greatly extended stability and half-life in vivo (47).

Saporin has similar enzymatic activity to the ricin A-chain (43). The half-life of its conjugates is longer compared to the same mAbs linked to ricin A-chain (48). Saporin is one of the most potent but also one of the most toxic type I RIPs. Linkage to a monoclonal antibody prolongs its survival in vivo and amplifies its toxicity, with hepatotoxicity one of the major side effects (49).

Diphtheria toxin (DT) is produced by *Corynebacterium diphtheriae* carrying a lysogenic β-phage (50). The native cell-binding domain of diphtheria toxin was replaced with interleukin-2 (IL2) rather than antibody in the studies cited below.

Similarly, truncated forms of *Pseudomonas* exotoxin (PE) have been developed into another class of immunotoxins using PE38 or PE40, in which the cell-binding domain is deleted and genetically fused to antibody constructs (51).

All of the foregoing toxins, either in their native state or conjugated to mAb, are capable of killing five or more logs of normal or diseased cells (52). A single molecule of any of these toxins in the cytoplasm may kill the cell. As a result, nonspecific toxicity to liver and muscle often is associated with therapies involving immunotoxins. However, in the discussed clinical trials, the immunotoxins were administered safely to patients with tolerable reversible toxicities.

B. Preclinical Data

1. CD25

Twenty-three anti-CD25 mAbs were tested in indirect in vitro assays against Hodgkin's-derived cell lines in order to determine their potential use as ITs. The assay treated cells with dilutions of the antibodies followed by a secondary antibody coupled to ricin A-chain. The five with the highest potency were linked to deglycosylated ricin A-chain (dgA) (53,54). The most potent of the five, RFT5-SMPT-dgA, inhibited protein synthesis at levels identical to that of native ricin without cross-reactivity of normal tissues seen with unmodified ricin (see Table 6) (55). In vivo studies with the same IT had a 78% cure rate in triple-beige nude mice (55). Size of the tumor appeared to be important, with better response in smaller tumors. This was confirmed in another study. In a SCID mouse model, cures were observed in 95% of the animals when animals were treated with RFT5-SMPT-dgA 1 day after tumor challenge with L540 Hodgkin's cells (56). However, when mice were treated with IT 12 days after tumor challenge, allowing extra time for tumor cell growth, cure rates were decreased to 46%.

Anti-Tac(sFv)PE40 has been shown to kill the cell line HUT-102 (57) as well as activated human T-cells and fresh malignant cells from ATL patients, all of which express CD25 (58). Anti-Tac(sFv)-PE40 also demonstrated antitumor activity against CD25 positive subcutaneous tumors in nude mice (59). Anti-Tac(Fab)-PE40 was shown to have a significantly longer beta phase (430 min vs. 30 min) and a cytotoxic activity 50% greater than that of anti-Tac(sFv)-PE40, without a significant increase in toxicity (60). At this time, PE40-derived immunotoxins have not been tested against Hodgkin's cell lines.

Because CD25 is a growth factor receptor, it can also be targeted by ligand-toxin constructs. The high-affinity IL2 receptor (IL2R) is composed of three subunits: alpha (CD25), beta, and gamma. Expression of CD25 on malignant cells is necessary for the antibody therapies discussed earlier, but alone may not be sufficient to achieve tumor response in diphtheria toxin therapy due to its low affinity for IL2. Unless all three subunits are present, internalization of IL2 or IL2 toxin is not efficient, and the effectiveness of diphtheria-containing immunotoxins thus depends on high-affinity IL2R.

Two diphtheria-containing immunotoxins have been studied. $DAB_{486}IL2$, the first IT tested, binds to and kills only cells that possess the high-affinity IL2R (61). In vitro observations suggest that cytotoxicity is dependent not only upon dose but also upon length of exposure of $DAB_{486}IL2$ to the tumor cell (62). Bacha et al. (63) state that the minimum contact time required for killing target cells in vitro is 15–30 minutes. $DAB_{389}IL2$, constructed by deleting amino acids 389–485, binds with fivefold-higher affinity, with a correspondingly higher potency (~10-fold) than $DAB_{486}IL2$ (64). Drug localization studies in rats suggest that the liver is the major site of uptake and clearance of $DAB_{486}IL2$ (63).

2. CD30

Ricin A-chain immunotoxins have been linked to the CD30 antibodies HRS-1, HRS-3, HRS-4, Ber-H2, and Ki-1, and the cytotoxic activity of the resulting ITs

Table 6 Preclinical Immunotoxin Studies

Immunotoxin	IC$_{50}$, M^a	Cross-reactivity	Response	Refs.
RFT5-SMPT-dgA (CD25)	7×10^{-12}	No major cross-reactivity	In vivo: triple beige nude mice, 78% CR (big tumors 37.5%, small tumors 100%), SCID mice 95% CR	56
Anti-Tac(Fab)-PE40 Anti-Tac(Fv)-PE40	2.3×10^{-12}	No major cross-reactivity	In vitro: cytotoxic to cells expressing CD 25 In vivo: effective antitumor agent in mice	57–60
DAB$_{486}$IL-2, DAB$_{389}$IL-2 (IL2R)	1×10^{-11}, high-affinity IL2R only	No major cross-reactivity at concentrations used	In vitro: cytotoxic only to cells expressing high-affinity IL2R	61, 64
HRS-3-SMPT-dgA (CD30)	9×10^{-11}	Large mononuclear cells in human bone marrow, liver, lymph nodes, skin, spleen, thymus	In vivo: triple-beige nude mice, 69% CR	65
Ber-H2-SMPT-dgA (CD30)	2×10^{-10}	Large mononuclear cells in human bone marrow, liver, lymph nodes, skin, spleen, thymus	In vivo: triple-beige nude mice, 38% CR	65
Ki-4-SMPT-dgA (CD30)	6×10^{-11}	No major cross-reactivity in 29 normal human organs	In vivo: SCID mice had 3-fold longer survival after administration of IT	66
Ber-H2-saporin (CD30)	5×10^{-14} to 5×10^{-12}	No major cross-reactivity	In vitro: superior cytotoxicity compared to ricin A-chain to 3 different cell lines In vivo: 80% CR in SCID mice 24 h postadministration	67, 68

^{a} IC$_{50}$ = concentrations giving 50% of protein inhibition in comparison to control values.

has been determined in vitro (see Table 6). HRS-3-SMPT-dgA and Ber-H2-SMPT-dgA had high binding specificity, reacting with only a few large mononuclear cells in the bone marrow, liver, lymph nodes, skin, spleen, and thymus (43). Triple-beige nude mice challenged with subcutaneous Hodgkin's tumors and injected with either IT showed complete remission in 69% (HRS-3-SMPT-dgA) and 38% (Ber-H2-SMPT-dgA) of the experimental animals (65).

Schnell et al. (66) linked six anti-CD30 mAbs (Ki-2 to Ki-7) to deglycosylated ricin A-chain. Ki-4.dgA was reported to be fivefold more potent than previously reported CD30 ricin A-chain ITs against Hodgkin's cells in vitro. SCID mice challenged with L540Cy cells were given a single injection of Ki-4.dgA 1 day later. Median survival time of controls was 41 days. Therapy resulted in a threefold increase in median survival and a cure rate of 50% with no relapses after 100 days.

When Ber-H2 was linked to saporin, the resulting IT was highly potent in vitro (49), with superior cytotoxicity compared to ricin A-chain linked to the same antibody under the same experimental conditions (see Figure 4) (67). It has been suggested that the higher potency of saporin ITs may be due to easier uptake by the target cell or to differences in intracellular routing of the toxins (49). Thus, type 2 RIPs may be subject to inactivation by lysosomal enzymes from which type I RIPs are relatively spared. The Ber-H2-saporin immunotoxin inhibited

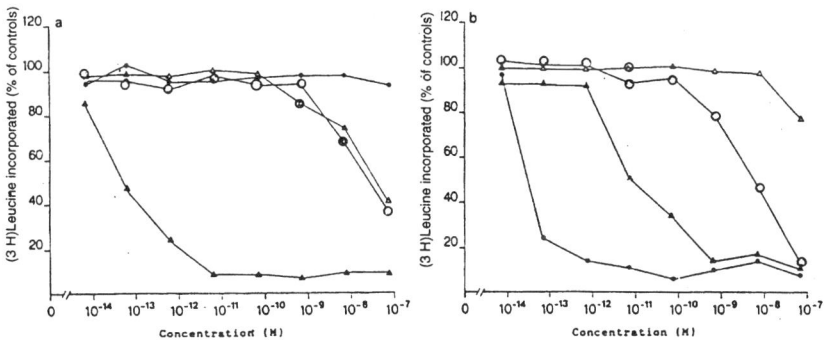

Figure 4 Cytotoxicity of ITs containing Ber-H2 and either saporin or ricin A-chain. (a) Saporin constructs: Ber-H2-saporin (▲), Ber-H2 (●), saporin (○), and Ber-H2 + saporin (△). (b) Ricin constructs: Ber-H2-ricin A-chain (▲), ricin A-chain (○), Ber-H2 + ricin A-chain (△), and ricin (●). All ITs were tested on the L428 HD-derived cell line. The IC_{50} of Ber-H2-saporin is lower than that of Ber-H2-ricin A-chain, and the difference between the toxic and therapeutic doses is larger. Complete ricin toxin is much more nonspecifically toxic than ricin A-chain, illustrating the need for modification of toxins. (From Ref. 49.)

protein synthesis by the L428, Co, and L540 Hodgkin's cell lines. A CD30 negative control cell line was not affected. CD34+ bone marrow stem cells were also not affected by Ber-H2-saporin immunotoxin, indicating that major bone marrow toxicity would not be a problem in either in vivo or ex vivo treatment, such as bone marrow purging (49). An in vivo study showed that Ber-H2-saporin induced cures in 80% of mice when administered 24 hours after tumor challenge (68).

Ber-H2 also has been linked to two other Type I RIPs, momordin (MOM) and pokeweed antiviral protein from seeds (PAP-S), neither of which cross-react with saporin or each other. Both toxins inhibited protein synthesis by the HD CD30+ target cell line L540 (69). Ber-H2–PAP-S inhibited protein synthesis at levels comparable to Ber-H2-saporin (49). Ber-H2–MOM was less potent but was also less toxic in mice. In a SCID mouse model of CD30+ human anaplastic large-cell lymphoma, a 3-day treatment of nontoxic doses of Ber-H2–MOM 24 hours posttumor challenge prevented tumor development in 40% of the mice and delayed tumor growth in others (69). IC_{50} levels with Ber-H2–MOM were slightly lower than those of Ber-H2-saporin. Death of experimental mice treated with Ber-H2-saporin was due to liver toxicity. Ber-H2–MOM appears to be less toxic to liver than Ber-H2-saporin, but more toxic to muscle. Table 6 summarizes these data.

As discussed previously, the RS cell may have nonuniform expression of surface antigens such as CD25 and CD30. By targeting different surface antigens at the same time, subpopulations that are deficient in one surface antigen but abundant in another would not be "overlooked." For this reason, "cocktails" of different combinations of ITs may be suitable in future therapies. The possibility of treating lymphomas expressing both CD25 and CD30 with anti-CD25 and anti-CD30 immunotoxins simultaneously has been suggested (43,49). Engert et al. (70) tested a "cocktail" of three different ITs, BB10-dgA (CD25), HRS3-dgA (CD30), and IRac-dgA, each of which reduced protein synthesis to 8.8%, 3.3%, and 7.1% of control, respectively (IRac recognizes a 70-kDa antigen on RS cells). All three ITs were toxic to Hodgkin's cells in vitro but combined had a stronger cytotoxic effect than a combination of two or any of the three alone. The combination of all three ITs reduced protein synthesis to 0.7%. The same superior antitumor effect of "cocktail" ITs was demonstrated in vivo in nude mice. Single intravenous injection of BB10.dgA, HRS3.dgA, or IRac.dgA had a 60% complete response rate, but 15–20% subsequently relapsed. All animals treated with all three ITs were cured.

C. Clinical Data

Responses to immunotoxin therapy in clinical trials are often short and partial. One reason for this is the inability to readminister ITs because of the formation of antibodies against the toxin, which is typically a potent immunogen. HAMAs frequently develop against murine elements of the antibody component of the IT. Trials conducted with immunotoxins have been mainly Phase I/II studies designed to determine maximum tolerated dose and dose-limiting toxicities and are summarized in Table 7. Few complete responses have been observed to date, probably reflecting the massive tumor volumes in the studied patients.

1. CD25

RFT5-SMPT-dgA (Anti-CD25) was studied in a Phase I dose escalation trial in fifteen patients with refractory Hodgkin's disease. The IT was administered intravenously over 4 hours, and serum half-life of the IT was 6 hours, on average (71). Seven of the fifteen patients produced human antiricin Abs, and six of the fifteen patients developed human antimouse Abs. Clinical responses included two partial and one minor response. This study is being continued in a Phase II clinical trial.

Studies with Anti-Tac(sFv)PE38, a shorter form of PE40, are presently in a Phase I dose escalation trial at the National Cancer Institute, with no dose-limiting toxicity at 40 μg/kg × 3 doses, showing only transaminase elevations that are reversible. Among five HD patients treated so far, initial encouraging results have been obtained, but it is too early to describe response rates (72; R. Kreitman and I. Pastan, pers. commun.).

LeMaistre et al. (61) conducted a clinical study of the ligand-fusion toxin $DAB_{486}IL2$ in eighteen patients with IL2Rα positive malignancies. When administered by bolus infusion, the in vivo half-life was about 5 minutes. Even with such a short half-life, six of eighteen patients had antitumor activity. However, the three Hodgkin's patients treated had no tumor response. In this study, $DAB_{486}IL2$ was well tolerated at all dose levels, and patients received multiple doses of IT even in the presence of anti-$DAB_{486}IL2$ antibodies. About 50% of the patients developed an antibody response to the therapy, but the presence of these antibodies did not interfere with antitumor activity, for four of the six responders had detectable antibody titers during treatment. It was assumed that antibodies directed against epitopes of diphtheria toxin distinct from the binding region will not interfere with IT efficacy (73).

In a later study of non-Hodgkin's lymphoma (no Hodgkin's patients were included), LeMaistre et al. (74) administered $DAB_{486}IL2$ over 90 minutes, with good tolerance by patients, and active IT levels were achieved for the duration of the infusion. No difference in response rate was noted (6/15) but the one complete remission lasted more than 2 years (75). In order to predict the antitumor activity of $DAB_{486}IL2$ or its shorter form, $DAB_{389}IL2$, better screening for high-affinity IL2R is required. In general, the recombinant fusion cytokine toxins have had weaker antitumor potency. One reason for this might be their short half-lives compared to IgG-based ITs or the smaller number of high-affinity IL2Rs compared to other tumor antigens.

Table 7 Clinical Immunotoxin Studies

Trial type	No. patients	Administration	Lab results/toxicity	Clinical results	Refs.
RFT5-SMPT-dgA (CD25)	12 with refractory HD	i.v. infusion over 4 h on days 1, 3, 5, and 7	Significant decrease in CD25+ PBMCs by FACS analysis, vascular leak syndrome, decrease in serum albumin, edema, weight gain	2/15: PR (2 mo. and 10+ mo.) 1/15: minor 3/15: stable 9/15: progressive	71
$DAB_{486}IL2$	18 with CD25+ malignancies, includes NHL and HD	i.v. bolus infusions daily on days 1–10	Rapid serum clearance, half-life of 5 min, elevations of hepatic transaminases	0/3, 0/4, 1/4 (PR), 0/17	61
Ber-H2-saporin (CD30)	12 with refractory HD	i.v. infusion over 4 h	4–5-fold increase in liver enzymes	4/12: PR 3/12: minor Avg. duration: 2 mo.	76, 77

2. CD30

After treatment with Ber-H2 chemically linked to saporin, tumor reduction in three of four patients with refractory Hodgkin's disease was reported by Falini et al. (76). Recently, eight further patients have been reported. Of the twelve patients treated, four had partial responses, and three had minor responses that were short-lived, with an average duration of 2 months (77). These patients developed antimouse antibody responses, preventing treatment beyond 2–3 weeks.

D. Conclusion

When used against RS-associated antigens, immunotoxins have shown initial promise in the treatment of Hodgkin's disease. These studies have demonstrated that immunotoxins can be safely administered to patients with acceptable toxicities. However, due to decreased therapeutic effectiveness when tumor burden is large, it appears that IT therapy would be most useful once tumor burden has been decreased by other forms of therapy. The large size of immunotoxins coupled with lower vascularization and high interstitial pressure associated with larger tumors may limit the quantity of immunotoxin reaching the malignant cells inside the tumor (78). The clinical application of immunotoxins may also be hindered by their immunogenicity. In all the discussed trials, multiple doses of immunotoxins were associated with the development of antitoxin and/or antiglobulin antibody responses. Humanization of mAbs and the sequential application of different immunotoxins, such as Ber-H2/MOM or Ber-H2/PAP-S may help to bypass problems of immunogenicity.

It is difficult to compare the efficacies of the different immunotoxins discussed above because in many cases different target cell lines were used to compare the various immunotoxins. The binding affinity and number of targeted receptors are not constant from one cell line to the next as well as the number of toxins internalized by the cell membrane. Terenzi et al. (49) did do direct comparisons between of Ber-H2-saporin and Ber-H2-ricin A-chain using two different cell lines (see Figure 4). As stated earlier, Ber-H2-saporin was more cytotoxic than Ber-H2-ricin A-chain. The same group also compared Ber-H2-saporin (CD30) and BB-10-saporin (CD25) and found that although CD30 expression determined by FACS analysis was greater than CD25 expression, the potency of the two immunotoxins was similar. This would suggest the CD25 is internalized easier than CD30, but there were no data on the amount of immunotoxin bound to the cell and internalized to make a valid conclusion.

Pharmacokinetic evaluation in most of the above studies demonstrated that bolus injections of ITs achieved therapeutic serum levels for only short periods of time. Studies have been proposed to determine whether continuous infusions of ITs have a more advantageous pharmacokinetic profile without increased toxicity (79). Searching for new toxins with greater cytotoxic potency is also important. Tonevitsky et al. (80) recently reported that immunotoxins containing the A-chain of mistletoe lectin I, a toxin similar in structure and mechanism of action as other type II RIPs, are more cytotoxic than immunotoxins with ricin A-chain, thus warranting further investigation for possible clinical use.

V. RADIOIMMUNOTHERAPY

Few patients with relapsed lymphomas of any type are curable with conventional radiotherapy or chemoradiotherapy. Massive doses of chemoradiotherapy coupled with bone marrow transplantation can salvage 10–50% of relapsed patients, but many others expire due to transplant-related complications (81). Normal organ toxicity might be avoided if radiation could be selectively delivered to tumor sites using monoclonal antibodies against tumor-associated antigens. Radioimmunotherapy (RIT) involves the combination of a radioisotope conjugated to an antibody.

A. Mechanisms and Toxicities

Theoretically, this treatment approach has inherent advantages over direct (passive) and toxin-based antibody immunotherapies. Radioimmunotherapy cytotoxicity is not dependent on the direct cytotoxicity or internalization of the antibody. The cytotoxic effects of radiolabeled antibodies result from DNA damage due to electron or alpha-particle emissions (22). Radiolabeled antibody has the ability to induce lethal DNA damage to neighboring cells not expressing the antigen target because of the range and random direction of radioactive emissions by "cross-fire." The range is determined by energy, charge, and mass of the emission. The range is approximately 3 cell layers for alpha emissions and between 10 and 500 cell layers for beta emissions.

Potency is influenced by the type of radioisotope administered to the patient. Gamma, or photon, emitters include indium-111, and they deposit very little energy within tissue, thereby exerting little cytotoxic effects. Photon emissions of an appropriate energy (100–400 keV) can be imaged externally, using nuclear scanners to gather antibody targeting and diagnostic information. Gamma emissions are not used for therapeutic effect in radioantibody therapies. Beta or electron emitters such as yttrium-90 are more potent than gamma emitters in local energy deposition. Iodine-131 produces beta and gamma emissions. Only the beta emission is therapeutically useful; it has a weaker beta emission than yttrium-90 and deposits its energy over a shorter range. Alpha emitters, such as bismuth-212, are high linear energy transfer isotopes and are far more cytotoxic per decay than beta or gamma emitters, but have the shortest range of activity (22).

Toxicities associated with radioimmunotherapy are most often caused by radiation of bone marrow cells, resulting in myelosuppression (76). Autologous bone marrow harvesting/transplantation is sometimes used to reverse the effects of severe myelosuppression. Other nonhematologic radiation toxicities, such as hypothyroidism, nausea, vomiting, pulmonary fibrosis, and heptotoxicity are rarely observed.

B. Preclinical Data

Hodgkin's tumors, as stated previously, are characterized by the presence of a small number of the Reed-Sternberg cells and numerous benign inflammatory cells such as lymphocytes, histiocytes, and eosinophils. If the antigenic target were on the Reed-Sternberg cell, such as CD25 or CD30, the concentration of the dose in the tumor would be expected to be low due to low concentration of positive cells in the tumor. To overcome this obstacle, researchers have directed efforts at identifying targets that are abundant in Hodgkin's tumors although not necessarily present on the surface of the malignant cell. Two such targets have been identified.

1. Eosinophil Peroxidase

Extracellular deposits of eosinophil peroxidase, an enzyme that catalyzes the production of hypohalous acids from hydrogen peroxide, have been reported in mixed-cellularity and nodular sclerosis Hodgkin's tumors (83). While this enzyme is normally found only in intracellular granules within eosinophils, it is released into the extracellular space in some malignancies (84). Eosinophil peroxidase has a high avidity for cell membranes and does not circulate in the blood, theoretically making it an excellent target for radiotherapy because it concentrates diffusely in the tumor tissues. ^{111}In-labeled mAb EOS directed against eosinophil peroxidase was studied by Samoszuk et al. (85) and was shown to yield excellent tissue localization in mice injected with human eosinophils. As few as 10^6 eosinophils could be imaged in vivo.

2. Ferritin

The other target for radioimmunotherapy of relapsed Hodgkin's disease is ferritin, an iron (Fe) storage protein that accumulates in normal bone marrow and liver. It is also a tumor-associated protein in Hodgkin's tumors. Although ferritin is present in normal tissue, relatively selective tumor targeting has been demonstrated in clinical scanning (86). A study by Klein et al. (87) tested radiolabeled polyclonal antiferritin against an experimental human hepatoma in athymic nude mice, which accumulates ferritin. Mice treated with 400 µCi of ^{131}I-antiferritin had prolonged survival, but there were no cures. ^{90}Y-antiferritin-treated mice had

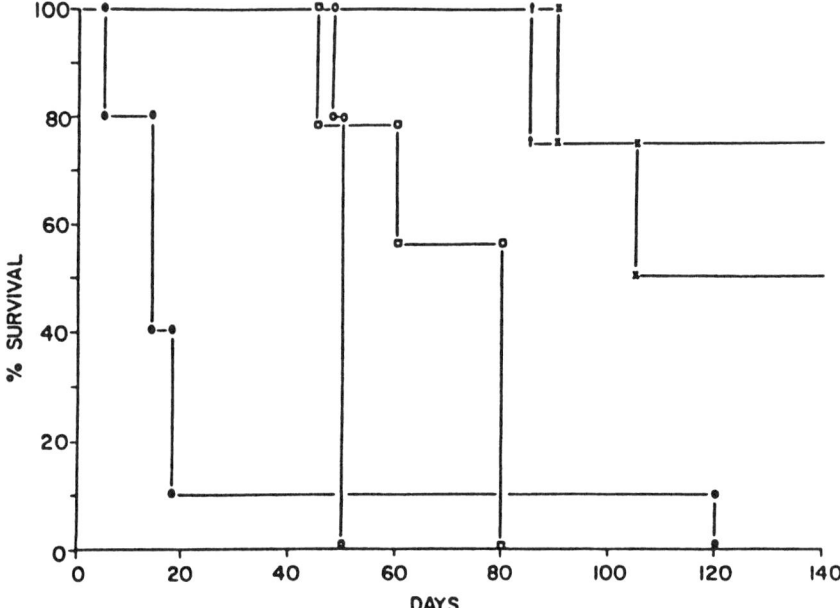

Figure 5 Radioantibody dose optimization with ^{90}Y-antiferritin and survival of tumor-bearing animals following therapy. Mice treated with 100 μCi (□), 200 μCi (×), 300 μCi (+), or 400 μCi (●) of ^{90}Y-antiferritin. Optimal survival occurs at doses of 200 μCi and 300 μCi of ^{90}Y-antiferritin. Specific targeting of 200 μCi of ^{90}Y-antiferritin versus 200 μCi of ^{90}Y-nonspecific labeled antibody (○) results in a doubling of the survival rate, with a significant fraction of cures. (From Ref. 87.)

significantly prolonged survival, and 50% and 75% of mice treated with 200 μCi and 300 μCi, respectively, had no evidence of disease after 140 days (see Figure 5). Klein et al. (87) showed that ^{90}Y-labeled antibodies delivered up to 7.3 times the radiation dose to tumor as that delivered by the same antibodies labeled with ^{131}I (see Figure 6), correlating with the improved cure rate. Monoclonal antibodies reactive with ferritin were of higher curative potential in mice than polyclonal antibodies reactive with ferritin.

C. Clinical Data

Trials using ^{131}I- or ^{90}Y-labeled monoclonal antibodies against lymphoid activation antigens have reported encouraging data in NHL treatment. Targeted antigens include HLA class II molecules, B-cell immunoglobulin idiotype, CD5,

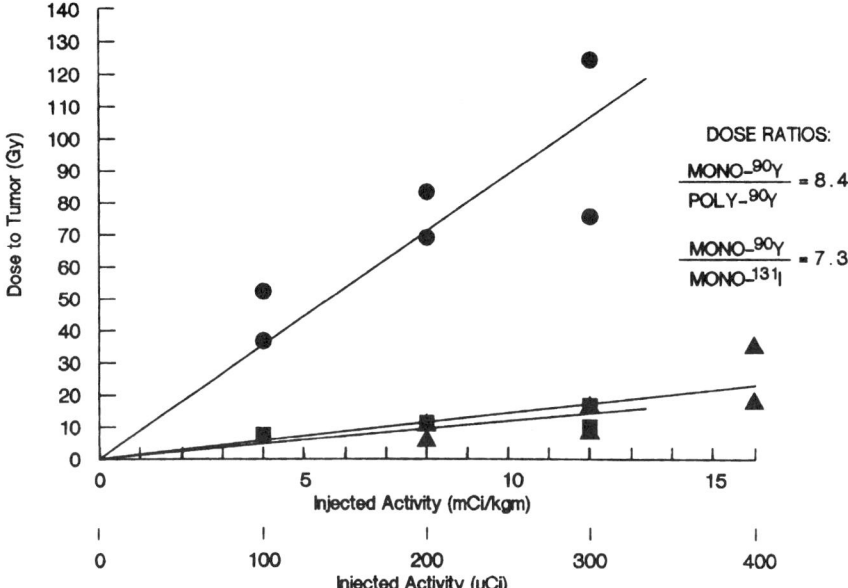

Figure 6 Dose delivered to tumors by monoclonal or polyclonal antiferritin antibodies conjugated with iodine-131 or with yttrium-90. The two symbols at each data point represent the maximum dose calculated at the edge of the tumor (lower symbol) or at the center of the tumor. Antiferritin monoclonal antibody labeled with ^{90}Y (●) delivered a much higher radiation dose to tumor compared to ^{131}I-antiferritin (▲) or ^{90}Y-labeled polyclonal antiferritin (■). (From Ref. 97.)

CD20, CD22, CD25, CD33, and CD37 (22,81,88). Overall, 42% of the patients with refractory hematologic malignancies treated with low doses of radiolabeled antibodies in these trials achieved partial or complete remissions lasting from 2 to 15 months (89).

Studies involving radioisotopes have been applied in Hodgkin's disease for imaging and staging purposes. Carde et al. (90) used ^{123}I- or ^{131}I-labeled mAb HRS-1 (CD30) to image patients. Although positive imaging was seen in six of eight patients, significant accumulation of radioisotope was also seen in the spleen. Similar nonspecific accumulation of mAbs in the spleen has been observed in other studies. Junghans et al. [ongoing trial] used ^{111}In-anti-CD25 to image Hodgkin's patients in conjunction with a passive antibody trial discussed earlier in the chapter. Positive imaging has been seen with seven of nine patients. Radioantibodies against surface antigens have not been applied therapeutically in Hodgkin's disease.

1. Eosinophil Peroxidase

Samoszuk et al. (91) administered ^{111}In conjugated to EOS to ten patients. Nonspecific accumulation by the spleen and bone marrow was low. Nonspecific uptake by the liver was reported in all of the patients, but the investigators concluded that eosinophil peroxidase is a suitable in vivo target for imaging and therapy in Hodgkin's patients who experience eosinophil degranulation. The balance of efficacy versus toxicity with this antigenic target awaits clinical studies with cytotoxic isotopes.

2. Ferritin

Polyclonal antiferritin immunoglobulin obtained from rabbits, pigs, or baboons was radiolabeled and administered to HD patients in two different studies (92,93). Lenhard et al. (92) administered ^{131}I-antiferritin intravenously to 37 patients. Patients were initially given 30 mCi of ^{131}I-antiferritin followed by a further 20 mCi 5 days later. Fifteen of the 37 patients (40%) demonstrated a measurable response to treatment (1 CR, 14 PR). Seventy-seven percent of patients suffering from B symptoms related to Hodgkin's disease showed an improvement or complete clearing of their symptoms. However, treatment was limited because of prolonged bone marrow toxicity. The authors indicated that selective tumor targeting was demonstrated by diagnostic scans, but a data breakdown was not included.

In a later study by Herpst et al. (93), 39 patients deemed eligible after imaging positive with ^{111}In-antiferritin were treated with ^{90}Y-antiferritin antibody (doses ranging from 10 to 50 mCi). ^{90}Y has more energetic beta emissions with larger ranges than ^{131}I (94). Vriesendorp et al. state that higher and more homogeneous doses were delivered to the tumor by yttrium-labeled antibodies than iodine-labeled antibodies. In accordance with preclinical studies, ^{90}Y-labeled antibody appeared more effective in the patient setting than ^{131}I-labeled antibodies for equivalent marrow toxicity (89) (see Tables 8 and 9). Of the 39 patients infused with ^{90}Y-labeled antiferritin, none developed antiglobulin antibodies, presumably due to radiation exposure superimposed on the immunosuppression inherent to patients with Hodgkin's disease. Myelosuppression, the expected toxicity, was severe at doses of 20 mCi or greater of ^{90}Y. However, the 20-mCi dosing schedule of this trial was better tolerated than the 50-mCi schedule of the previous ^{131}I-antiferritin trial. Only 29 of the 39 patients were evaluable and a 62% response rate (9 CRs and 9 PRs lasting 2–26 months) was demonstrated amongst them. A significant positive correlation was found between blood radioactivity 1 hour after administration and subsequent response of the patient (93). Patients with lower fractional blood radioactivity were hypothesized to have a larger apparent volume of distribution, whether it be due to larger tumor volume or a vascular leak phenomenon due to the presence of B symptoms (93).

Using 20 mCi as a dividing line, 41% of patients receiving high-dose ther-

Table 8 Clinical Radioimmunotherapy Studies

Radioantibody	No. patients	Administration	Lab results/ toxicity	Clinical results	Ref.
^{131}I-antiferritin	37 patients	Bolus injection, 30 mCi on day 0, 20 mCi on day 5	Bone marrow depression, with thrombocytopenia greater than leukopenia	15/37 responses (40%); 1 CR, 14 PRs	92
^{90}Y-antiferritin	39 patients (29 evaluable)	Bolus injection, 10, 20, 30, 40, or 50 mCi	Bone marrow toxicity	18/29 responses (62%); 9 CRs, 9 PRs	93

Table 9 Radiolabeled Anti-Ferritin Antibody in End-Stage Hodgkin's Disease

	Isotope		χ^2	P^a
	^{131}I	^{90}Y		
Response rate	15/37	18/29	3.01	<.1
CR	1/37	9/29	—	<.02
PR	14/37	9/29	0.3	>.5

[a] Fisher's exact test.
Source: Ref. 96.

apy of ^{90}Y-antiferritin achieved complete responses, compared to 17% of patients on the low-dose protocol using the same radioisotope, but survival differences were not demonstrated. Single-massive-dose therapy appears to achieve more favorable response rates and durations than repetitive administration of low doses of radioisotope. However, data showed variable tumor uptake of ^{90}Y-antiferritin independent of the injected activity. In this study (93), a dose–effect escalation could not be established. In a subsequent study (96), patients receiving higher activities (0.4 or 0.5 mCi ^{90}Y-labeled antiferritin per kilogram) had higher response rates than patients receiving 0.3 mCi/kg. As with immunotoxin therapy, responses were more commonly observed after ^{90}Y-antiferritin therapy in patients with small tumors (<30 cm^3), as opposed to patients with large tumors (>500 cm^3). The volumes given are the median tumor volumes of responsive and nonresponsive patients, respectively.

D. Conclusion

Initial results of the few clinical studies using radioimmunotherapy for the treatment of Hodgkin's disease have been encouraging. Extracellular protein deposits appear to be a better target for therapy than RS cell antigens because of the small number of Reed-Sternberg cells. The malignant cells are destroyed by radiation crossfire.

The identification of the preferred or optimal radioisotopes for human treatment has been investigated with Hodgkin's disease. According to the foregoing studies, ^{131}I-labeled mAbs inhibit tumor growth for only short periods of time. Other problems with ^{131}I may include occasional dehalogenation. ^{90}Y-labeled mAbs have also shown a superior therapeutic potential overall. Outpatient therapy is possible, but is limited by bone marrow toxicity (97). Vriesendorp et al. (96) used a bifunctional diethylenetriamine pentaacetic acid ligand for the chelate in ^{90}Y-antiferritin studies. This and newer conjugates, such as MX, are much more stable and have reduced the problems associated with free ^{90}Y (98). ^{212}Bismith (^{212}Bi) labeled mAb, an alpha emitter, has a 60-minute half-life, which limits its therapeutic use because of the time required following intravenous administration to achieve effective tumor:normal tissue ratios of radioactivity (93). ^{212}Bi has many emission cascades including beta, gamma, and alpha. Stable chelation for ^{212}Bi or other alpha emitters remains to be defined. It has been suggested that ^{67}copper (^{67}Cu) offers some advantages over other radioisotopes because it emits both beta particles for therapy and gamma rays for imaging studies. It has been difficult, however, to attach it stably to mAbs, limiting its in vivo study. ^{67}Cu is a low-energy beta emitter and has a localized energy deposition. In situations where treatment of very small tumors is necessary, most of the radioactive dose would be deposited in the tumor area, compared to ^{90}Y, for which long-range beta emissions would deposit outside of the area of interest. ^{67}Cu showed effective biodistribution characteristics in animal studies using nude mice (100). Welch et al. (97) succeeded in inhibiting tumor cell growth in an animal model using both ^{64}Cu- and ^{67}Cu-labeled anticolorectal-cancer mAbs at nontoxic doses.

One of the major obstacles to the advancement of radioimmunotherapy is the low accumulation of the radioisotope in human tumors, in the range of 0.001–0.01% of injected dose (82). Low tumor uptake could be the result of antibody dilution after administration, slow rate of diffusion across the vascular endothelium, and/or restricted vascular access to the tumor sites. Tumor size also influences the effectiveness of radioimmunotherapy. Generally, small tumors are more sensitive to radioisotope than are large tumors because of a larger fractional uptake of bioavailable mAb per unit mass and faster penetration of antibody into the tumor (101). Larger tumors require larger doses of radioisotope for saturation, thereby increasing toxicity in patients. Studies are needed to increase the rate of uptake of radioisotope by larger tumors to decrease this problem.

Alternative routes of delivery have been studied. Different approaches have included subcutaneous injection (102) and administration of interleukin-2 prior to treatment with radiolabeled mAbs to induce vascular leak syndrome, by which it was hypothesized that the uptake of radiolabeled mAbs would be enhanced. An increase by a factor of 2 was demonstrated in tumor uptake of Lym-1 mice coadministered IL2 (103).

Other methods to deliver radioactivity to malignant cells have been developed to decrease bone marrow toxicity. Two-stage targeting involves injecting the antibody and radioactivity separately, to join at the tumor site through a ligand/receptor interaction (104). First, antibody–avidin conjugate is injected and allowed time to saturate the tumor cells, after which excess free antibody is removed by clearing agents. Next, biotinylated radioisotope is injected and rapidly distributes to the pretargeted antibody or is eliminated in the urine. This method permits high tumor doses of radioactivity, with six to seven times the maximum tolerated dose of conventional radioimmunotherapies. Preliminary studies of refractory colon and ovarian cancers with two-stage deliveries have been encouraging (104).

VII. Summary

Despite the unique architectural features of Hodgkin's tumors, with a minor fraction of malignant cells, the picture of monoclonal antibody therapies in Hodgkin's disease has, in large measure, mirrored that in other hematologic malignancies. There have been marginal effects in unmodified antibody treatments, intriguing preclinical data for immunotoxins and bispecific antibodies, but as yet little clinical impact, and a more important clinical impact for radioantibodies, particularly with use of ^{90}Yttrium conjugates of anti-ferritin antibodies. Particular areas of promise lie in the co-application of cytokines in unmodified and bispecific antibody therapies, the cointroduction of CD3- and CD28-bispecific antibodies under conditions that avoid systemic activation, sequential or concurrent use of immunotoxins with different toxin moieties with humanized antibody domains, and the application of two-stage targeting procedures and use of improved chelate molecules for retaining radioactivity on radioantibodies. Many of these improvements will be developed and applied concurrently in a variety of different malignancies, with important hoped-for positive impact on the ability of antibodies to mediate target cell destruction with minimal toxicity to the patients. As these technologies advance and as our growing experience with these therapies stimulate modifications to their application, the profile of clinical responses with antibodies in Hodgkin's disease and other cancers is likely to improve.

REFERENCES

1. Parker SL, Tong T, Bolden S, Wingo PA. CA Cancer Stat 1997; 47:5–27.
2. DeVita VT, Hellman S, Jaffe ES. Hodgkin's disease. In: DeVita VT, Hellman S, Rosenberg SA, eds. Cancer: Principles and Practice of Oncology. Philadelphia: Lippincott 1993: 1819–1858.
3. Klein S, Jücker M, Diehl V, Tesch H. Production of multiple cytokines in Hodgkin's disease derived cell lines. Hematol Oncol 1992; 10:319–329.
4. Hsu S, Hsu P. The nature of Reed-Sternberg cells: phenotype, genotype and other properties. Crit Rev Oncog 1994; 5:213–245.
5. Strauchen JA. Immunopathology of Hodgkin's disease. Pathol Immunopathol Res 1986; 5:253–264.
6. Perkins SL, Kjeldsberg CR. Immunophenotyping of lymphomas and leukemias in paraffin-embedded tissues. Am J Clin Pathol 1993; 99:362–373.
7. Newcom SR, Ansari AA, Gu L. Interleukin-4 is an autocrine growth factor secreted by the L-428 Reed-Sternberg cell. Blood 1992; 79:191–197.

8. Tesch H, Günther A, Abts H, Jücker M, Klein S, Krueger GRF, Diehl V. Expression of interleukin-2Rβ in Hodgkin's disease. A J Pathol 1993; 142:1714–1720.
9. Gruss HJ, Brach MA, Drexler HG, Bross KJ, Herrmann F. Interleukin 9 is expressed by primary and cultured Hodgkin and Reed-Sternberg cells. Cancer Res 1992; 52:1026–1031.
10. Küppers R, Kanzler H, Hansmann ML, Rajewsky K. Single cell analysis of Hodgkin/Reed-Sternberg cells. Ann Oncol 1996; 7(suppl 4):27–30.
11. Kanzler H, Küppers R, Hansmann ML, Rajewsky K. Hodgkin and Reed-Sternberg cells in Hodgkin's disease represent the outgrowth of a dominant tumor clone derived from (crippled) germinal center B cells. J Exp Med 1996; 184:1495–1505.
12. Niedobitek G. The role of Epstein-Barr virus in the pathogenesis of Hodgkin's disease. Ann Oncol 1996; 7(suppl 4):11–17.
13. Stein H, Herbst H, Anagnostopoulos I, Niedobitek G, Dallenbach F, Kratzsch HC. The nature of Hodgkin and Reed-Sternberg cells, their association with EBV, and their relationship to anaplastic large-cell lymphoma. Ann Oncol 1991; 2(suppl 2): 33–38.
14. Rowley JD, Mitelman F. Principles of molecular cell biology of cancer: chromosome abnormalities in human cancer and leukemia. In: DeVita VT, Hellman S, Rosenberg SA, eds. Cancer: Principles and Practice of Oncology. Philadelphia: J.B. Lippincott, 1993:67–91.
15. Gruss HJ, Duyster J, Herrmann F. Structural and biological features of the TNF receptor and TNF ligand superfamilies: interactive signals in the pathobiology of Hodgkin's disease. Ann Oncol 1996; 7(suppl 4):19–26.
16. Waldmann TA, Pastan I, Gansow OA, Junghans RP. The multichain interleukin-2 receptor: a target for immunotherapy. Ann Intern Med 1992; 116:148–160.
17. Bernstein I, Tamm M, Nowinski RC. Mouse leukemia: therapy with monoclonal antibodies against a thymus differentiation antigen. Science 1980; 207:68–71.
18. Kodama K, Ghanta VK, Hiramoto NS, Hiramoto RN. Regression of MOPC 104E plasmacytoma with monoclonal anti-idiotype antibodies. J Biol Response Med 1989; 8:385–396.
19. Buschbaum DJ, Wahl RL, Normolle DP, Kaminski MS. Therapy with unlabeled and I^{131}-labeled pan-B cell monoclonal antibodies in nude mice bearing Raji Burkitt's lymphoma xenografts. Cancer Res 1992; 52:6476–6481.
20. Hamblin TJ, Cattan AR, Glennie MJ, MacKenzie MR, Stevenson FK, Watts HF, Stevenson GT. Initial experience in treating human lymphoma with a chimeric univalent derivative of monoclonal anti-idiotype antibody. Blood 1987; 69:790–797.
21. Dyer MJ, Hale G, Hayhoe FG, Waldmann H. Effects of CAMPATH-1 antibodies in vivo in patients with lymphoid malignancies: influence of antibody isotype. Blood 1989; 73:1431–1439.
22. Junghans RP, Sgouros G, Scheinberg DB. Antibody-based immunotherapies for cancer. In: Chabner BA, Longo DL, eds. Cancer Chemotherapy and Biotherapy: Principles and Practice. Philadelphia: Lippincott, 1996:655–689.
23. Junghans RP, Waldmann TA, Landolfi NF, Avdaloric NM, Scheider WP, Queen C. Anti-Tac-H, a humanized antibody to the interleukin 2 receptor with new features of immunotherapy in malignant and immune disorders. Cancer Res 1990; 50:1495–1502.

24. Begley CG, Metcalf D, Nicola NA. Proliferation of normal human promyelocytes and myelocytes after a single pulse simulation by purified GM-CSF or G-CSF. Blood 1988; 71:640–645.
25. Gruss HJ, Pinto A, Gloghini A, Wehnes E, Wright B, Boiani N, Aldinucci D, Gatei V, Zagonel V, Smith CA, Kadin ME, von Shilling C, Goodwin RG, Herrmann F, Carbone A. CD30 ligand expression in nonmalignant and Hodgkin's disease-involved lymphoid tissues. Am J Pathol 1996; 149:469–481.
26. Tian ZG, Longo DL, Funakoshi S, Asai O, Ferris DK, Widmer M, Murphy WJ. In vivo antitumor effects of unconjugated CD30 monoclonal antibodies on human anaplastic large-cell lymphoma xenografts. Cancer Res 1995; 55:5335–5341.
27. Bernstein N, Levy R. Treatment of a murine B cell lymphoma with monoclonal antibodies and IL-2. J Immunol 1987; 139:971–976.
28. Gill I, Agah R, Hu E, Mazumder A. Synergistic antitumor effects of interleukin 2 and the monoclonal Lym-1 against human Burkitt's lymphoma cell in vitro and in vivo. Cancer Res 1989; 49:5377–5379.
29. Falini B, Flenghi L, Fedeli L, Broe MK, Bonino C, Stein H, Durkop H, Bigerna B, Barbabietola G, Venturi S, Aversa F, Pizzolo G, Bartoli A, Pileri S, Sabattini E, Palumbo R, Martelli MF. In vivo targeting of Hodgkin and Reed-Sternberg cells of Hodgkin's disease with monoclonal antibody Ber-H2 (CD30): immunohistological evidence. Br J Haematol 1992; 82:38–45.
30. Hwu P, Rosenberg SA. The genetic modification of T-cells for cancer therapy: An overview of laboratory and clinical trials. Cancer Detect Prev 1994; 18:43–50.
31. Fanger MW, Morganelli PM, Guyre PM. Use of bispecific antibodies in the therapy of tumors. In: Rosen ST, Kuzel TM, eds. Immunoconjugate Therapy of Hematologic Malignancies. Kluwer Academic, 1993:181–194.
32. Hombach A, Jung W, Pohl C, Renner C, Sahin U, Schmits R, Wolf J, Kapp U, Diehl V, Preundschuh M. A CD16/CD30 bispecific monoclonal antibody induces lysis of Hodgkin's cells by unstimulated natural killer cells in vitro and in vivo. Int J Cancer 1993; 55:830–836.
33. Hartmann F, Renner C, Jung W, Sahin U, Pdreundschuh M. Treatment of Hodgkin's disease with bispecific antibodies. Ann Oncol 1996; 7 Suppl 4:143–146.
34. Weiner LM, Gercel-Taylor C, Ketson J, Garcia dePalazzo IE. Bispecific antibodies and targeted cellular cytotoxicity. Romet-Lemonne JL, Fanger MW, Segal DM. 1991: p. 33–36.
35. Pohl C, Denfeld R, Renner C, Jung W, Bohlen H, Sahin U, Hombach A, van Lier R, Schwonzen M, Diehl V, Pfreundschuh M. CD30-antigen-specific targeting and activation of T cells via murine bispecific monoclonal antibodies against CD3 and CD28: Potential use for the treatment of Hodgkin's lymphoma. Int J Cancer 1993; 54:820–827.
36. Bonnema JD, Rivlin KA, Ting AT, Schoon RA, Abraham RT, Leibson PJ. Cytokine enhanced NK cell-mediated cytotoxicity: positive modulatory effects of IL-2 and IL-12 on stimulus-dependent granule exocytosis. J Immunol 1994; 152:2098.
37. Allavena P, Paganin C, Zhou D, Bianchi G, Sozzani S, Mantovani A. Interleukin-12 is chemotactic for natural killer cells and stimulates their interaction with vascular endothelium. Blood 1994; 84:2261–2268.

38. Aste-Amezaga M, D'Andrea A, Kubin M, Tinchieri G. Cooperation of natural killer cell stimulatory factor/interleukin 12 with other stimuli in the induction of cytokines and cytotoxic cell-associated molecules in human T and NK cells. Cell Immunol 1994; 156:480–492.
39. Sahin U, Kraft-Bauer S, Ohnesorge S, Pfreundschuh M, Renner C. Interleukin-12 increases bispecific-antibody-mediated natural killer cell cytotoxicity against human tumors. Cancer Immunol Immunother 1996; 42:9–14.
40. Renner C, Jung W, Sahin U, Denfeld R, Pohl C, Trumper L, Hartmann F, Diehl V, van Lier R, Pfreundschuh M. Cure of xenografted human tumors by bispecific monoclonal antibodies and human T cells. Science 1994; 264:833–835.
41. Renner C, Pfreundschuh M. Tumor therapy by immune recruitment with bispecific antibodies. Immunol Rev 1995; 145:179–209.
42. Junghans RP. Next-generation Fc chimeric proteins: avoiding immune system interactions. Trends Biotechnol 1997; 15:155.
43. Barth S, Schnell R, Diehl V, Engert A. Development of immunotoxins for potential clinical use in Hodgkin's disease. Ann Oncol 1996; 7(suppl 4):135–141.
44. Byers VS, Baldwin RW. Therapeutic strategies with monoclonal antibodies and immunoconjugates. Immunology 1988; 65:329–335.
45. Thorpe PE, Detre SI, Foxwell BMJ, Brown AN, Skilleter DN, Wilson G, Forrester JA, Stirpe F. Modification of the carbohydrate in ricin with metaperiodate-cyanoborohydride mixtures. Effects on toxicity and in vivo distribution. Eur J Biochem 1985; 147:197–206.
46. Fulton RJ, Uhr JW, Vitteta ES. *In vivo* therapy of BCL_1 tumor: effect of immunotoxin valency and deglycosylation of the ricin A-chain. Cancer Res 1988; 48:2626–2631.
47. Thorpe PE, Wallace PM, Knowles PP, Relf MG, Brown AN, Watson GJ, Blakely DC, Newell DK. Improved anti-tumor effects of immunotoxins prepared with deglycosylated ricin A-chain and hindered disulfide linkages. Cancer Res 1988; 48:6396–6403.
48. Thorpe PE, Brown ANF, Bremmer JAG, Foxwell BMJ, Stirpe F. An immunotoxin composed of monoclonal anti-Thy 1.1 antibody and a ribosome-inactivating protein from *Saponaria officinalis:* potent antitumor effects in vitro and in vivo. J Natl Cancer Inst 1985; 19:157–162.
49. Tazzari PL, Bolognesi A, De Totero D, Falini B, Lemoli RM, Soria MR, Pileri S, Gobbi M, Stein H, Flenghi L, Martelli MF, Stripe F. Ber-H2 (anti-CD30)-saporin immunotoxin: a new tool for the treatment of Hodgkin's disease and CD30+ lymphoma: *in vitro* evaluation. Br J Haematol 1992; 81:203–211.
50. Greenfield L, Bjorn MJ, Horn G, Fong D, Buck GA, Collier RJ, Kaplan DA. Nucleotide sequence of the structural gene for diphtheria toxin carried by corynebacteriophage beta. Proc Natl Acad Sci USA 1983; 80:6853–6857.
51. Kondo T, Fitzgerald D, Chaudhary VK, Adhya S, Pastan I. Activity of immunotoxins constructed with modified Pseudomonas exotoxin A lacking the cell recognition domain. J Biol Chem 1988; 263:9470–9475.
52. Grossbard ML, Nadler LE. Immunotoxin therapy of lymphoma. In: Rosen ST, Kuzel TM, eds. Immunoconjugate Therapy of Hematologic Malignancies. Kluwer Academic, 1993:111–131.

53. Diehl V, Kirchner HH, Schaadt M, Fonatsch C, Stein H, Gerdes J, Boie C. Hodgkin's disease: Establishment and characterization of four in vitro cell lines. J Cancer Res Clin Oncol 1981; 101:111–124.
54. Casellas P, Brown JP, Gros O, Gros P, Hellström I, Jansen FK, Poncelet P, Roncucci R, Vidal H, Hellström KE. Human melanoma cells can be killed in vitro by an immunotoxin specific for melanoma-associated antigen p97. Int J Cancer 1982; 30:237–243.
55. Engert A, Martin G, Amlot P, Wijdenes J, Diehl V, Thorpe P. Immunotoxins constructed with anti-CD25 monoclonal antibodies and deglycosylated ricin A-chain have potent anti-tumor effects against human Hodgkin's cells in vitro and solid Hodgkin's tumors in mice. Int J Cancer 1991; 49:450–456.
56. Winkler U, Gottstein C, Schon G, Kapp U, Wolf J, Hansmann ML, Bohlen H, Thorpe P, Diehl V, Engert A. Successful treatment of disseminated human Hodgkin's disease in SCID mice with deglycosylated ricin A-chain immunotoxins. Blood 1994; 82:466–475.
57. Chaudhary VK, Queen C, Junghans RP, Waldmann TA, Fitzgerald DJ, Pastan I. A recombinant immunotoxin consisting of two antibody variable domains fused to *Pseudomonas* exotoxin. Nature 1989; 339:394–397.
58. Kreitman RJ, Chaudhary VK, Waldmann TA, Hanchard B, Cranston B, Fitzgerald DJ, Pastan I. Cytotoxic activities of recombinant immunotoxins composed of Pseudomonas toxin or diphtheria toxin toward lymphocytes from patients with adult T-cell leukemia. Leukemia 1993; 7:553–562.
59. Kreitman RJ, Bailon P, Chaudhary VK, Fitzgerald DJ, Pastan I. Recombinant immunotoxins containing anti-Tac(Fv) and derivatives of *Pseudomonas* exotoxin produce complete regression in mice of an interleukin-2-receptor-expressing human carcinoma. Blood 1994; 83:426–434.
60. Kreitman RJ, Chang CN, Hudson DV, Queen C, Bailon P, Pastan I. Anti-Tac(Fab)-PE40, a recombinant double-chain immunotoxin which kills interleukin-2-receptor-bearing cells and induces complete remission in an in vivo tumor model. Int J Cancer 1994; 57:856–864.
61. LeMaistre CF, Meneghetti C, Rosenblum M, Reuben J, Parker K, Shaw J, Deisseroth A, Woodworth T, Parkinson DR. Phase I trial of interleukin-2 (IL-2) fusion toxin ($DAB_{486}IL-2$) in hematologic malignancies expressing the IL-2 receptor. Blood 1992; 79:2547–2554.
62. Touw I, Delwel R, VanZanen G, Lowenberg B. Acute lymphoblastic leukemia and non-Hodgkin's lymphoma of T lineage: colony forming cells retain growth factor (interleukin-2) dependence. Blood 1986; 67:1714–1720.
63. Bacha P, Forte S, Kassam N, Thomas J, Akiyoshi O, Waters C, Nichols J, Rosenblum M. Pharmacokinetics of the recombinant fusion protein $DAB_{486}IL-2$ in animal models. Cancer Chemother Pharmacol 1990; 26:409–414.
64. Williams DP, Snider CE, Strom TB, Murphy JR. Structure/function analysis of interleukin-2 toxin ($DAB_{486}IL-2$). J Biol Chem 1990; 265:11885–11889.
65. Engert A, Martin G, Pfreundschuh M, Amlot P, Hsu SM, Diehl V, Thorpe P. Antitumor effects of ricin A-chain immunotoxins prepared from intact antibodies and Fab fragments on solid human Hodgkin's disease tumors in mice. Cancer Res 1990; 50:2929–2935.

66. Schnell R, Linnartz C, Katouzi AA, Schon G, Bohlen H, Horn-Lohrens O, Parwaresch RM, Kange H, Diehl V, Lemke H, Engert A. Development of new ricin A-chain immunotoxins with potent anti-tumor effects against human hodgkin cells in vitro and disseminated Hodgkin tumors in SCID mice using high-affinity monoclonal antibodies directed against the CD30 antigen. Int J Cancer 1995; 63:238–244.
67. Engert A, Burrows F, Jung W, Tazzari PL, Stein H, Pfreundschu M, Diehl V, Thorpe P. Evaluation of ricin A-chain-containing immunotoxins directed against the CD30 antigen as potential reagent for the treatment of Hodgkin's disease. Cancer Res 1990; 50:84–88.
68. Pasqualucci L, Wasik M, Teicher BA, Flenghi L, Bolognesi A, Stirpe F, Polito L, Falini B, Kadin ME. Antitumor activity of anti-CD30 immunotoxin (Ber-H2/saporin) in vitro and in severe combined immunodeficiency disease mice xenografted with human CD30+ anaplastic large-cell lymphoma. Blood 1995; 85:2139–2146.
69. Terenzi A, Bolognesi A, Pasqualucci L, Flenghi L, Pileri S, Stein H, Kadin M, Bigerna B, Polito L, Tazzari PL, Martelli MF, Stirpe F, Falini, B. Anti-CD30 (Ber-H2) immunotoxins containing the type-1 ribosome-inactivating proteins momordin and PAP-S (pokeweed antiviral protein from seeds) display powerful antitumor activity against CD30+ tumour cells in vitro and in SCID mice. Br J Haematol 1996; 92:872–879.
70. Engert A, Gottstein C, Bohlen H, Winkler U, Schon G, Manske O, Schnell R, Diehl V, Thorpe P. Cocktails of ricin A-chain immunotoxins against different antigens on Hodgkin and Reed-Sternberg cells have superior anti-tumor effects against RS cells in vitro and solid Hodgkin tumors in mice. Int J Cancer 1995; 63(2):304–309.
71. Engert A, Diehl V, Schnell R, Radszuhn A, Hatwig MT, Drillich S, Schon G, Bohlen H, Tesch H, Hansmann ML, Barth S, Schindler J, Ghetie V, Uhr J, Vitetta E. A phase I study of an anti-CD25 ricin A-chain immunotoxin (RFT5-SMPT-dgA) in patients with refractory Hodgkin's lymphoma. Blood 1997; 89, 2:403–410.
72. Krietman RJ, White JD, Pearson D, Top LE, Waldmann TA, Pastan I. Phase I clinical trial with recombinant immunotoxin anti-Tac(Fv)-PE38 (LMB-2) in patients with hematologic malignancies. Proc Am Assoc Cancer Res 1997; 38:4089.
73. Zucker DR, Murphy JR. Monoclonal antibody analysis of diphtheria toxin-I. Localization of epitope and neutralization of cytotoxicity. Molec Immunol 1984; 21:785–793.
74. LeMaistre CF, Craig FE, Meneghetti C, McMullin B, Parker K, Reuben J, Boldt DH, Rosenblum M, Woodworth T. Phase I trial of a 90-minute infusion of the fusion toxin daB$_{486}$IL-2 in hematological cancers. Cancer Res 1993; 53:3930–3934.
75. Tepler I, Schwartz G, Parker K, Charette J, Kadin ME, Woodworth TG, Schnipper LE. Phase I trial of an interleukin-2 fusion toxin (DAB$_{486}$IL-2) in hematologic malignancies: Complete response in a patient with Hodgkin's disease refractory to chemotherapy. Cancer 1994; 73:1276–1285.
76. Falini B, Bolognesi A, Flenghi L, Tazzari PL, Broe MK, Stein H, Durkop H, Aversa

F, Cornell P, Pizzolo G, Barbabietola G, Sabattini E, Pileri S, Martelli MF, Stirpe F. Response of refractory Hodgkin's disease to monoclonal anti-CD30 IT. Lancet 1992; 339:1195–1196.
77. Falini B, Pasqualucci L, Flenghi L et al. Anti-CD30 immunotoxins: Experimental and clinical studies. In: Fourth International Symposium on Immunotoxins 1995: 160.
78. Jain RK. Physiological barriers to the delivery of monoclonal antibodies and other macromolecules in tumors. Cancer Res 1990; 50(suppl):s814–s819.
79. Sausville E, Headlee D, Jaffe E, Stetler-Stevenson M, Cooper M, Ghetie V, Thorpe P, Uhr J, Wittes R, Vitetta E. Continuous infusion IgG-RFB4-SMPT-dgA in CD22+ B cell lymphoma. In: Third International Symposium on Immunotoxins, Orlando, FL 1992:127.
80. Tonevitsky AG, Agapov II, Shamshiev AT, Temyakov DE, Pohl P, Kirpichnikov MP. Immunotoxins containing A-chain of mistletoe lectin I are more active than immunotoxins with ricin A-chain. FEBS Lett 1996; 392:166–168.
81. Press OW, Eary J, Badger CC, Appelbaum FR, Wiseman G, Matthews D, Martin PJ, Bernstein ID. High-dose radioimmunotherapy of lymphomas. In: Rosen ST and Kuzel TM, eds. Immunoconjugate Therapy of Hematologic Malignancies. Kluwer Academic, 1993:13–22.
82. Kuzel TM, Rosen ST. Radioimmunotherapy of lymphoma. In: Rosen ST and Kuzel TM, eds. Immunoconjugate Therapy of Hematologic Malignancies. Kluwer Academic, 1993:1–12.
83. Samoszuk MK, Nathwani BN, Lukes RJ. Extensive deposition of eosinophil peroxidase in Hodgkin's and non-Hodgkin's lymphomas. Am J Pathol 1986; 125:426–428.
84. Samoszuk MK, Petersen A, Gidanian F, Rieltveld C. Cytophilic and cytotoxic properties of human eosinophil peroxidase plus major basic protein. Am J Pathol 1988; 132:455–460.
85. Samoszuk MK, Fang M, Anderson ALJ. Radioimmuno-detection of degranulated human eosinophils in mice: a potential model for imaging Hodgkin's disease and other pathologic conditions. J Nuc Med 1991; 32:89–94.
86. Rostock RA, Klein JL, Leichner P, Kopher KA, Order SE. Selective tumor localization in experimental hepatoma by radiolabeled antiferritin antibody. Int J Radiat Oncol Biol Phys 1983; 9:1345–1350.
87. Klein JL, Nguyen TH, Laroque P, Kopher KA, Williams JR, Wessels BW, Dillehay LE, Frincke J, Order SE, Leichner PK. Yttrium-90 and Iodine-131 radioimmunoglobulin therapy of an experimental human hepatoma. Cancer Res 1989; 49:6383–6389.
88. Waldmann TA, White J, Goldman CK, Top L, Grant A, Bamford R, Roessler E, Horak I, Zaknoen S, Kasten-Sportes C, England R, Horak E, Mishra B, Dipre M, Hale P, Fleisher T, Junghans RP, Jaffe ES, Nelson DL. The interleukin 2 receptor: a target for monoclonal antibody treatment of human T cell lymphotropic virus-I induced T cell leukemia. Blood 1993; 82:1701–1712.
89. Grossbard ML, Press OW, Appelbaum FR, Bernstein ID, Nadler L. Monoclonal antibody based therapies of leukemia and lymphoma. Blood 1992; 80:863–878.
90. Carde P, Manil L, de Costa L et al. Hodgkin's disease immunoscintigraphy: Use

of the anti Reed-Sternberg cells H-RS-1 monoclonal antibody in 9 patients. Proc Am Soc Clin Oncol 1988; 7:227.
91. Samoszuk M, Anderson AL, Wang F, Braunstein P, Majmundar H, Ravel J, Ramzi E, Slater L. Phase I imaging study of Hodgkin's disease of non-Hodgkin's lymphomas with radiolabeled antibody to eosinophil peroxidase. Cell Biophys 1993; 21: 53–60.
92. Lenhard RE, Spunberg J, Order SE, Asbell SO, Leibel SA. Isotopic immunoglobulin: A new systemic therapy for advanced Hodgkin's disease. J Clin Oncol 1985; 3:1296–1300.
93. Herpst JM, Klein JL, Leichner PK, Quadri SM, Vriensendorp HM. Survival of patients with resistant Hodgkin's disease after polyclonal Yttrium-90-labeled antiferritin treatment. J Clin Oncol 1995; 13:2394–2400.
94. Vriensendorp HM, Herpst RN, Leichner PK, Klein JL, Order SE. Polyclonal ^{90}Yttrium labeled antiferritin for refractory Hodgkin's disease. Int J Radiation Oncol Biol Phys 1989; 17:815–821.
95. Vriensendorp HM, Quadi SM, Stinson RL, Onyekwere OC, Shao Y, Klein JL, Leichner PK, Williams JR. Selection of reagents for human radioimmunotherapy. Int J Radiation Oncol 1991; 22:37–45.
96. Vriesendorp HM, Herpst JM, Germack MA, Klein JL, Leichner PK, Loudenslager DM, Order SE. Phase I-II studies of yttrium-labeled antiferritin treatment for end-stage Hodgkin's disease, including radiation therapy oncology group 87-01. J Clin Oncol 1991; 9:918–928.
97. Connett JM, Anderson CJ, Guo LW, Schwarz SW, Zinn KR, Rogers BE, Siegel BA, Philpott GW, Welch MJ. Radioimmunotherapy with a ^{64}Cu-labeled monoclonal antibody: A comparison with ^{67}Cu. Proc Natl Acad Sci USA 1996; 93:6814–6816.
98. Kozak RW, Raubitschek A, Mirzadeh S, Brechbiel MW, Junghans RP, Gansow OA, Waldmann TA. The nature of the bifunctional chelating agent used for radioimmunotherapy with yttrium-90 monoclonal antibody is a critical factor in determining in vivo survival and organ toxicity. Cancer Res 1989; 49:2639–2644.
99. Hartmann F, Horak EM, Garmestani K, Wu C, Brechbiel MW, Kozak RW, Tso J, Kosteiny SA, Gansow OA, Nelson DL, Waldmann TA. Radioimmunotherapy of nude mice bearing a human interleukin 2 receptor alpha-expressing lymphoma utilizing the alpha-emitting radionuclide-conjugated monoclonal antibody ^{212}Bi-anti-Tac. Cancer Res 1994; 54:4362–4370.
100. Desphande SV, DeNardo SJ, Meares CF, McCall MJ, Adams GP, Moi MK, DeNardo GL. Copper-67 labeled monoclonal antibody Lym-1, a potential radiopharmaceutical for cancer therapy labeling and biodistribution in RAJI tumor mice. J Nucl Med 1988; 29:217–225.
101. Sharkey R, Pykett M, Siegel J, Alger E, Primus F, Goldenberg D. Radioimmunotherapy of the GN-39 human colonic tumor zenograft with ^{131}I-labeled murine monoclonal antibody to carcinoembryonic antigen. Cancer Res 1987; 47:5672–5677.
102. Mulshine JL, Carrasquillo JA, Weinstein JN, Keenan AM, Reynolds JC, Herdt J, Bunn PA, Sausville E, Eddy J, Cotelingham JD. Direct intralymphotic injection of

radiolabeled ^{111}In-T101 in patients with cutaneous T-cell lymphoma. Cancer Res 1991; 51:688–695.
103. DeNardo GL, DeNardo SJ, Lamborn KR, Van Hoosear KA, Kroger LA. Enhancement of tumor uptake of monoclonal antibody in nude mice with PEG-IL2. Antibody Immunocon Radiopharm 1991; 4:859–870.
104. Abrams PG. Pre-targeted radiotherapy of solid tumors: Results of phaseI/II clinical trials. Abstract, Antibody-Based Therapeutics Conference, IBC, Boston, MA. June 5, 1997.

9
Antibody-Based Therapies for the Treatment of Acute Leukemia

Pratik S. Multani
Harvard Medical School and Massachusetts General Hospital, Boston, Massachusetts

David J. Flavell
University of Southampton and Southampton General Hospital, Southampton, England

I. INTRODUCTION

Enormous progress has been made within the past 30 years in the successful treatment of acute leukemia in both adults and children. Large multicenter national randomized clinical trials of chemotherapy regimens coordinated by bodies such as the United Kingdom Childhood Cancer Study Group (UKCCSG) in Britain and the Pediatric Oncology Group (POG) in the United States have resulted in continual improvements until today over three-quarters of children with low-risk common acute lymphoblastic leukemia (cALL) are curable with carefully defined multidrug chemotherapy regimes. Similar, though less impressive, improvements have been achieved with acute myeloid leukemia in both adults and children. Such successes have come about entirely as a result of meticulous randomized clinical trials with large cohort sizes. Despite the successes, it is becoming increasingly clear that there are significant subgroups of acute leukemia patients that are not curable with today's conventional chemotherapy regimens and for whom additional new therapeutic approaches may be required.

Cytotoxic antibodies, alone (i.e., unconjugated) or conjugated to toxins or radioisotopes, may provide one such new therapeutic approach. If this new modality can be made to work, it will hold distinct advantages: (a) leukemia cells would be selectively killed without normal tissue damage, and (b) the mechanism of cytotoxicity would be completely different from conventional chemotherapy, thus possibly overcoming any acquired drug resistance. Antibodies are also being used to treat autologous bone marrow ex vivo to purge contaminating malignant cells, the subject of Chapter 11 in this book. This chapter will discuss the potential role of antibody-based therapies for the in vivo treatment of acute leukemias, review the preclinical and clinical data that already have been obtained in this area, and discuss the problems that have thus far limited the success of this therapeutic modality. It will also express the authors' views on how some of these limiting problems will eventually be overcome and the most realistic way in which antibody-based therapy is likely to be applied in the treatment of acute leukemia in the foreseeable future.

II. ACUTE LEUKEMIA AS A TARGET DISEASE FOR ANTIBODIES

Acute leukemias are characterized by an outpouring from the bone marrow into the blood of clonally derived immature neoplastic leukemic blast cells, which can rapidly increase in numbers in the peripheral blood, replacing normal blood elements and becoming the dominant cell category seen. In the bone marrow itself, where the clonal leukemia stem cell arises following a neoplastic transformation event, normal marrow hematopoietic elements are crowded out and eventually replaced by rapidly proliferating leukemic blast cells, a process that if left unchecked will result in bone marrow failure and the eventual death of the patient. Acute leukemia can be divided broadly into two distinct categories: those arising from lymphoid precursors, resulting in acute lymphoblastic leukemia (ALL of B- or T-cell lineage) and those arising from myeloid precursors, resulting in acute myeloid leukemia (AML).

In general, leukemias are liquid tumors, and therefore the bulk of disease should be much more accessible to antibody-based therapies than solid tumors, where penetration into the tumor interior by large-molecular-weight unconjugated antibodies and radioimmunoconjugates and even larger immunotoxin molecules can be problematic (1). Such an advantage, however, can also be the source of significant pharmacologic disadvantage. Studies with both conjugated and unconjugated antibodies in leukemic patients have documented markedly shortened serum half-lives, presumably due to rapid clearance of the administered therapeutic agent after binding circulating antigen-bearing cells (2). The ability to achieve sustained therapeutic serum levels is therefore compromised and may limit the ability of the antibody to penetrate into other sites of disease, namely, bone marrow, lymph nodes, and possibly soft tissue sanctuaries.

III. PRECLINICAL STUDIES

Several studies detail the preclinical evaluation of antibody-based therapies with potential clinical applications in acute leukemia. Early investigations with unconjugated antibodies against granulocytic and monocytic antigens were able to demonstrate selective cytotoxicity in vitro against both normal and leukemic cells in the presence of rabbit complement without toxicity to CFU-GM or BFU-E cells (3–5). Other studies of antibodies targeting the common ALL antigen (CD10) in conjunction with complement demonstrated their ability to inhibit colony formation of peripheral blood or bone marrow cells from 15 patients with ALL (6). Similarly, in vivo studies with an unconjugated monoclonal antibody against the T-cell differentiation antigen, Thy 1.1, demonstrated that selective cytotoxicity could be achieved in experimental animal leukemia models (7–9).

Selectivity has also been demonstrated with a number of immunotoxins, particularly those with Anti-CD19 (10,11) and Anti-CD7 (12,13) specificities, intended for use in B-and T-lineage leukemias, respectively. Such preclinical studies have demonstrated that immunotoxins are capable of selectively delivering toxin only to targeted leukemia cells that express the relevant antigen. Selective immunotoxin potency has been demonstrated in vitro in clonogenic and protein synthesis inhibition assays and in vivo in severe combined immune-deficient (SCID) mice bearing xenografts of human leukemia cell lines. In the latter studies, immunotoxin treatment has been shown to prolong survival significantly compared with sham-treated control animals. Preclinical studies in a SCID mouse model of CNS leukemia also have shown that immunotoxins may have a role in the treatment of CNS leukemia (14).

Other preclinical studies have demonstrated the selective potency of Anti-CD2 (15), -CD5 (16), -CD10 (17), CD38 (18), -CD40 (19), -CD22 (20), -CD24 (21), -CD33 (22), and -CD72 (23) immunotoxins, all with potential for the treatment of acute leukemia. Indeed, recombinant immunotoxins and growth factor–*Pseudomonas* exotoxin fusion proteins are now available for clinical use (24,25). There also is preclinical evidence showing that immunotoxins synergize with conventional cytotoxic drugs (26–28), yielding significantly better therapeutic effects when used in combination. Such observations are of potentially great importance to the way in which these new therapeutics are likely to be employed clinically in the future.

IV. POTENTIAL CLINICAL APPLICATIONS

There are at least three potential clinical applications for antibody-based therapies in leukemia:

1. To treat (purge) bone marrow ex vivo prior to autologous transplantation in an attempt to eliminate residual leukemia cells in the graft
2. To deplete T-cells ex vivo from allogeneic bone marrow prior to host infusion in order to reduce the incidence of graft-versus-host disease (GVHD) or alternatively in vivo administration to deplete donor T-cells in patients with life-threatening steroid-resistant GVHD
3. To deliver antibodies to patients with minimal residual disease, either alone or in combination with conventional cytotoxic therapies

The idea of eliminating leukemia cells ex vivo from bone marrow prior to autografting, utilizing single or cocktails of unconjugated antibodies or immunotoxin conjugates, has been developed for many years (29). Unconjugated antibodies can be employed with complement as a cytotoxic effector (30,31), or immunomagnetic beads may be utilized (32,33). Immunotoxins have been used for a similar purpose, with the advantage that one avoids the potential host or bystander toxicity observed when these agents are administered in vivo. Typically, a reduction of several logs of leukemia cell numbers from bone marrow is achievable following ex vivo treatment with unconjugated antibodies (34) or immunotoxins (35). Bone marrow purging of patient bone marrow is discussed more fully in Chapter 11.

Early studies also demonstrated that ex vivo depletion of T-cells from donor marrow can result in a significant reduction in the incidence of GVHD. Both unconjugated Anti-pan-T-cell antibody with complement (36), as well as immunotoxins, such as an Anti-CD5 immunotoxin (37,38), have been demonstrated to reduce the risk of serious GVHD. However, removal of donor T-cells from the graft prior to transplant can compromise engraftment (39,40) and reduce the graft-versus-leukemia (GVL) effect that plays an important role in the curative benefits of allogeneic bone marrow transplantation (41). Again, the use of this approach is detailed in Chapter 10 of this book.

V. THERAPEUTIC USE OF ANTIBODY-BASED THERAPIES

Leukemia cells express a wide variety of well-characterized molecules on their surface that may act as potential targets for antibody therapy. Some of these molecules already have been investigated in preclinical studies and are detailed in Table 1. None are leukemia specific, all being expressed to varying degrees on normal lymphoid or myeloid counterparts. This fact alone does not exclude them from use, provided that the recognized target molecule is not expressed by a life-sustaining tissue (e.g., heart, liver, brain) or by a stem-cell population that supplies and replenishes a normal hematologic population. It can be expected that antibody-based therapies directed against normal tissue-differentiation anti-

Table 1 Potential Target Molecules for Antibody-Based Treatment of Acute Leukemia

Target molecule	Normal expression	Indicated disease	Mean reactivity (%)[a]		
			c-ALL	T-ALL	AML
CD2	T-cells, NK cells, thymocytes	T-ALL	18	60	<10
CD5[b]	Mature T-cells, thymocytes, subset B-cells	cALL, T-ALL	21	<10	<10
CD7[b]	Early and late T-cells	T-ALL	<5	50	<10
CD10[b]	Early B- and T-cell precursors, stromal cells, kidney, and gut	cALL	66	14	<10
CD19[b]	All B-cells, follicular dendritic	cALL	78	<5	<10
CD22[b]	Subset of mature B-cells; cytoplasmic in pro-B and pre-B cells	cALL	26	0	<10
CD24	Early and late B-cells; absent from plasma cells	cALL	78	<5	<10
CD33[b]	Myeloid precursors in bone marrow; not on pluripotent stem cell	AML	<5	<5	40
CD38	Early B- and T-cells, activated B- and T-cells, myeloid precursors	Myeloma, cALL, T-ALL, AML	52	72	50
CD40	All mature B-cells; absent from plasma cells	cALL	32	<5	16
CD72	All B-cells; absent from plasma cells	cALL	30	<5	<10

[a] Data from Leukocyte Typing IV (Boston workshop).
[b] Studied clinically.

gens will likely result in complete or partial ablation of normal cellular counterparts, although this is not necessarily important if these populations can be replenished from a parental stem cell. The presence of normal lymphoid or myeloid cells that express such target molecules is a potential disadvantage in one very important respect: These cells will compete for antibody binding along with the malignant clone, thus reducing the amount available for delivery to the leukemic cell population.

There are thus three absolute requirements for potential leukemia target molecules to be of real practical value: (a) homogeneous expression on the target cell surface, (b) lack of expression by life-sustaining normal tissue or stem cells, and (c) modulation characteristics appropriate to the type of antibody-based therapy being used. Specifically, unconjugated antibodies appear to work best if the antigen does not internalize after binding antibody, thus allowing the exposed Fc portion to trigger complement or antibody-dependent cellular cytotoxicity (ADCC) (42). Immunotoxins, on the other hand, are generally more cytotoxic if the antigen–antibody complex does undergo internalization (43–45), allowing ready access of the toxin moiety to the ribosomal complex. In all cases, shed antigen can interfere with binding of the antibody to its intended target (46).

Given the pharmacologic limitations of antibody treatment in patients with excess circulating antigen, many have logically concluded that the optimal therapeutic use of antibody-based therapy would be in the setting of minimal residual disease. Only rare studies, however, have been done in such a patient population, while the vast majority have been conducted as Phase I/II clinical trials in patients with active acute leukemia. In order to group these many studies into a coherent structure, they will be discussed based upon the target cell-surface antigen, since the characteristics of the antigen are one of the most important, if not the most important, determinant of the success of any antibody-based therapy.

A. CD10

CD10, the common acute lymphoblastic leukemia antigen, or CALLA is, as its name suggests, expressed by a large proportion of cALL cells (>65%). This antigen was the target of the unconjugated J-5 antibody (42). Four patients with relapsed ALL were treated with three to eight infusions of the anti-CALLA monoclonal antibody at doses ranging from 3 mg to 170 mg. The three patients with circulating cells did experience immediate and rapid falls in the number of circulating CALLA+ blasts, but a population of CALLA− blasts persisted. Furthermore, once serum levels of J-5 fell below detectable levels, CALLA+ lymphoblasts reemerged, suggesting that the CALLA antigen had undergone modulation or downregulation in the presence of antibody (47). Of more concern was the observation that there appeared to be no impact on bone marrow cellularity or differential, despite evidence of J-5 binding in one patient.

Immunotoxins have also been constructed with anti-CD10 antibodies. Two anti-CD10 monoclonal antibodies, each directed against a different epitope on the CD10 antigen, were conjugated to ricin A-chain (17). The researchers found each to be more potent than their unconjugated counterparts both in vitro against NALM-6 cells and in vivo in SCID mouse models. Unfortunately CD10 expression by normal tissues, particularly kidney, severely limits its value for in vivo use.

B. CD19

CD19 is a pan-B-lineage–restricted differentiation antigen expressed on the surface of the earliest pre-B-cell through to the mature B-cells (expression is lost by plasma cells). Levels of expression of CD19 on malignant B-cells tend to be high and homogeneous, which makes this molecule very attractive for targeting purposes; in fact, CD19 has been the most extensively utilized marker for targeting malignant B-cells. A number of immunotoxins, including Anti-B4-blocked ricin, target the CD19 antigen.

In a Phase I study, 25 patients with B-lineage leukemia and lymphoma were treated with bolus infusions of an Anti-CD19-blocked ricin immunotoxin (Anti-B4-bR) (48). While one patient with B-cell lymphoma had a complete response in this study, none of the patients with leukemia had a sustained response to therapy. The toxicities encountered included reversible hepatotoxicity in most patients, thrombocytopenia, fevers, fatigue, and capillary leak syndrome. In an attempt to achieve more favorable pharmacokinetics and steady serum levels of immunotoxin, a second Phase I study was undertaken with Anti-B4-bR in which the agent was given as a continuous infusion over 7 days to 43 patients with B-lineage CD19+ leukemia and lymphoma (2). In this study, two B-cell lymphoma patients had complete responses, but none of the ALL patients showed any marked response. Anti-B4-bR has been further evaluated in a minimal residual disease setting where patients receiving autografts for B-cell lymphoma received the immunotoxin following transplant (49).

A Phase I study by Uckun and colleagues treated patients with refractory B-cell ALL with an Anti-CD19 immunotoxin (B43-PAP) using the single-chain-ribosome–inactivating protein pokeweed antiviral protein (50). In preclinical studies B43-PAP was shown to be highly effective at eliminating the cALL cell line NALM-6 from SCID mice (11). B43-PAP was given to 17 patients over 5 days as one or three courses of treatment, and four complete and one partial responses were observed. This was a dose escalation study, with doses ranging from 0.5 to 1250 µg/kg, and the primary endpoint was the determination of the maximum tolerated dose. The occurrence of four complete responses in this type of study is encouraging. None of the patients developed human antimouse antibody (HAMA) or HAPA (human Anti-PAP antibody) responses. Toxicities included capillary leak syndrome and myalgia, but there were no significant hepatic, renal, cardiac, or neurological toxicities. A Phase II study with this immunotoxin is currently in progress.

We ourselves have a Phase I study in progress in B-cell lymphoma patients with the anti-CD19 immunotoxin BU12-saporin, which utilizes the single-chain-ribosome–inactivating protein saporin from the soapwort plant (*Saponaria officinalis*). This immunotoxin has been shown to have significant therapeutic activity both in vitro and in vivo against the cALL cell line NALM-6 (10). This dose escalation study is ongoing, with no toxicities encountered to date (current dose level 120 µg/m^2/day × 7d). While we have no plans to treat ALL patients with BU12-saporin as a single agent, we are planning a trial with a combination of three immunotoxins in ALL patients that will include BU12-saporin as one of the three components (51).

C. CD22

A number of therapies have been developed based upon the CD22 antigen, another true B-lineage–restricted differentiation antigen. Toxin conjugates with these antibodies have proven to be considerably more potent than the immunotoxins directed against CD19 described earlier. This finding probably reflects differences between the two molecules in their internalization and trafficking characteristics (52). Unfortunately, CD22 is expressed very heterogeneously by malignant B-cells populations, with many cells within the tumor often expressing surface antigen at low levels or not at all. Moreover, B-lineage ALL blasts express CD22 in their cytoplasm but not on their surface membrane. This severely limits the value of CD22 as a target molecule in ALL, although there may be a role in B-cell lymphoma, where surface membrane expression of this antigen does occur.

Phase I dose escalation studies have been undertaken with the Anti-CD22 immunotoxin RFB4-dgA, which uses a deglycosylated ricin A-chain as the toxin component. This immunotoxin has been studied in Phase I clinical trials for therapy of resistant B-cell lymphoma as an intact antibody conjugate and as a Fab′ fragment conjugate, in order to improve penetration into tumor masses (53,54). In neither study were complete responses obtained in any of the treated patients, and the toxicities included pulmonary edema, aphasia, rhabdomyolysis, renal failure, and severe vascular leak syndrome.

D. CD38

CD38 is a potentially interesting and valuable target molecule, expressed by small normal subpopulations of B- and T-cells, plasma cells, and myeloid progenitors. CD38 also is expressed by some lymphoid malignancies of B- and T-cell origin, by myeloma cells, and by some myeloid leukemias. Approximately 50% of B-lineage leukemias express CD38. A mouse/human chimeric Anti-CD38 unconjugated antibody has been demonstrated to mediate ADCC in preclinical work (55). We currently are developing the Anti-CD38 immunotoxin OKT10-saporin for use in Phase I/II trials in multiple myeloma, B-cell lymphoma, and ALL of both B- and T-cell origin (56,57). Concerns have been raised about the expression of CD38 by normal myeloid progenitor cells and the likely problems this may pose if targeted by an immunotoxin (58). However, studies have shown that while committed myeloid progenitors do express CD38, the primitive hematologic stem cell does not (59). As part of the toxicological workup of OKT10-saporin for clinical studies, we have demonstrated that this Anti-CD38 IT does indeed possess toxicity for late progenitors, which give rise to CFU-GEMM, CFU-G, CFU-M, and BFU-E, but not for the primitive long-term-culture–initiating cell (LTCIC), which is capable of reestablishing all of the above CFU progenitors in long-term culture (Gibson, unpublished observations). Thus, we can expect treatment with Anti-CD38 immunotoxins to induce transient reversible myelosuppression.

E. CD40

CD40 is another potential target molecule restricted to the surface of B-cells and monocytes. CD40 is an important signaling molecule that plays a role in driving antigen-specific B-cell responses. As yet, there is no information on its clinical use in humans, and it is therefore largely unknown what effects its targeting might have. We currently are evaluating CD40 immunotoxins in preclinical studies.

F. CD5

Specific T-cell antigens, such as CD5 (Leu-1), have also been targeted for the treatment of T-cell leukemias. Eight patients with T-cell ALL were treated with an unconjugated anti-Leu-1 antibody alone or in combination with two or three other T-cell-specific monoclonal antibodies (60,61). As with most other studies, there were transient decreases in the number of circulating blasts but no sustained responses.

A number of immunotoxins have been investigated in Phase I studies in T-cell malignancies. An anti-CD5 ricin A-chain immunotoxin was administered in escalating doses to 11 patients with chronic lymphocytic leukemia (CLL) or T-cell ALL, but no significant clinical responses were observed. Side effects included fever, rash, and nausea (62).

G. CD25 (IL-2 Receptor)

The IL-2 receptor can also serve as a T-cell-specific target for antibody therapy, based on the observation that expression is increased in lymphoblasts of adults with HTLV-1 induced T-cell ALL (63–65). The Anti-TAC antibody recognizes the p55 chain of the IL-2 receptor (CD25). This unconjugated murine antibody was used to treat 19 patients with adult T-cell ALL (66,67). They received multiple doses of 20–100 mg per dose over a period of 8–445 days. There were six responses, of which two were complete responses, lasting from 2 months to 3 years. Given the significant T-cell depletion and the immunocompromised nature of the treated patients, it is not surprising that immunosuppression-related complications were seen, including Kaposi's sarcoma in one patient and pneumocystis pneumonia in another.

A humanized version of the Anti-TAC antibody, Anti-TAC-H, has been developed (68). A trial of a yttirum-90 Anti-TAC-H radioimmunoconjugate was conducted in 17 patients with HTLV-1-associated adult T-cell ALL at doses of 5, 10, and 15 microCi (67). Of these, 11 patients achieved a sustained partial or complete remission. Thus, for this particular disease, targeting the IL-2 receptor either with unconjugated or conjugated antibodies may offer patients a new therapeutic option.

H. CD33

The CD33 molecule is expressed by myeloid precursors in the bone marrow and also on the surface membrane of some cases of AML but is not expressed by the pluripotent stem cell. While in theory, treatment with an Anti-CD33 antibody would result in ablation of CD33+ myeloid progenitors, these would be replenished by the stem-cell compartment. An Anti-CD33 unconjugated murine antibody, M195, was used to treat 10 patients with AML (69). Although no responses were observed, detailed pharmacologic and imaging studies with trace-iodine-labeled M195 demonstrated rapid uptake into bone marrow.

These localization studies formed the basis for a Phase I radioimmunoconjugate trial of iodine-131-conjugated M195 in 25 patients with relapsed or refractory leukemia (16 with AML, five with advanced MDS, two with secondary AML, and one with blast transformation of CML) (70). Decreases in peripheral blasts were seen in 23 patients, while 89% of patients demonstrated a significant reduction on the number of blasts in the bone marrow. There were three complete responses, and eight patients went on to bone marrow transplant. Few nonmyeloid toxicities were observed except for one patient who experienced hepatic toxicity, and the maximal tolerated dose was not reached. Finally, 37% of assessable patients developed HAMA responses. Two of these patients were retreated with the M195 antibody, but adequate serum levels could not be maintained, and no therapeutic effect resulted.

A humanized version of the M195 antibody has been constructed and has been demonstrated to be significantly less immunogenic than the parent murine antibody (71–73). An iodine-131 conjugate of this humanized antibody has undergone Phase I testing in patients with AML. One study treated 19 patients with the iodine conjugate in combination with cyclophosphamide and busulfan as a preparative regimen for bone marrow transplant (74). The combination was well tolerated, and 18 patients achieved a complete remission. A second trial examined its use in seven patients with relapsed acute promyelocytic leukemia who had achieved a second remission and thus were in a minimal residual disease state after treatment with all-trans retinoic acid (75). The drug could be safely given with myelotoxicity as its major side effect. Of six patients who were PCR positive for the PML/RAR-alpha mRNA transcript, two became transiently negative. Median overall survival exceeded 21 months. Finally, an immunotoxin composed of gelonin and the humanized M195 antibody is undergoing preclinical testing (22).

An immunotoxin based upon a different Anti-CD33 antibody (Anti-My9-bR) was used in a Phase I clinical trial to treat patients with relapsed AML but fatal dose-limiting capillary leak syndrome led to a termination of clinical development of the agent. This toxicity likely was related to the blocked ricin toxin rather than the Anti-CD33 antibody, My9. No sustained clinical responses were observed in more than 20 patients treated (Grossbard ML, personal communication, 1998).

Anti-CD33 immunotoxin conjugates are also being tested with another promising "toxin," calicheamicin. This antitumor antibiotic produces double DNA-strand breaks at less than picomolar concentrations, which can be directed toward antigen-bearing cells when conjugated to an appropriate monoclonal antibody (76,77). A humanized version of the murine P67.6 Anti-CD33 antibody conjugated to a calicheamicin derivative is undergoing Phase I testing in patients with AML (78,79). Thus the CD33 antigen may prove to be a critical target for future, more refined therapies for AML.

I. CD52

The CAMPATH-1 family of rat antibodies (80–82) recognize CD52, a highly expressed cell-surface antigen found on virtually all normal lymphocytes, most lymphoid malignancies, and some cases of AML (83). Three isoforms exist—IgM, IgG2a, and IgG2b—all of which fix complement, but only the IgG2b also mediates ADCC activity. Five patients with ALL were treated with the IgG2b isoform; in all cases, circulating normal lymphocytes and neoplastic lymphoblasts were cleared from the circulation (84). All patients also demonstrated reduction in marrow infiltration, with three patients showing completely cleared marrow. Repeated treatment was limited by the development of human antirat antibodies (HARA). Toxicities were minimal, except for a transient rise in transaminases in all patients up to three times the upper limit of normal. Although these results suggest good penetration of the antibody, patients with other lymphoproliferative disorders, such as B-cell lymphoma, were also treated as part of this study, and few lymph node or extranodal responses were seen, arguing against full access of the antibody to all sites of disease.

A humanized version of the IgG1 isoform, CAMPATH-1H, has since been developed by grafting the rat hypervariable regions of the parent monoclonal antibody onto a human IgG framework. No experience with this humanized unconjugated antibody in the treatment of acute leukemia has yet been reported, but the compiled toxicity data from multiple Phase I trials, composed of more than 160 patients with either non-Hodgkin's lymphoma or CLL, is informative (85). Patients received doses ranging from 0.5 to 240 mg from one to five times a week. Almost all patients experienced an acute reaction with the first dose, with a significant fall in incidence with subsequent doses. Such reactions consisted of fever, rigors, hypotension, rash nausea/vomiting, headache, and dyspnea. Most patients experienced rapid and profound falls in lymphocyte numbers, again resulting in a significant number of immunosuppression-related toxicities. There were two documented cases and three suspected cases of pneumocystis pneumonia. There were three cases of CMV-related disease, as well as multiple cases of *Herpes zoster* and *Herpes simplex* recurrence. Thus, even this unconjugated antibody has a significant toxicity profile, highlighting the potential complications of ablating, even temporarily, a normal hematologic subpopulation.

J. Uncharacterized Targets

Not all therapeutic antibodies recognize well-characterized antigens. Some antibodies were selected based on their ability to identify selectively certain neoplastic cell subsets, although the particular antigen and its normal function remains to be elucidated. Despite this gap in information, some of these antibodies have proven to be active agents in the clinical setting.

An early Phase I study treated three patients with AML with one or more murine antibodies, identified through their ability to recognize granulocytes and/or monocytes as well as specific subtypes of AML blasts in vitro with relative selectivity. Three of these antibodies were IgMs (PM-81, PMN-29, and PMN-6), reactive against cell-surface glycolipids, while the fourth was an IgG2b (AML-2-23) (3–5), directed against a protein antigen. The patients received a cocktail of one or more of these antibodies, and in each case the number of circulating cells decreased significantly but transiently (86). Minimal toxicity was observed, and one patient developed a HAMA response.

VI. FACTORS LIMITING EFFICACY OF ANTIBODY-BASED THERAPIES: PROBLEMS AND SOLUTIONS

The principle behind the selective cytotoxicity of an unconjugated antibody or the targeted delivery of a potent toxin or radioisotope to an unwanted cell population such as leukemia is very attractive, but its potential success is jeopardized by a variety of factors that limit the therapeutic effect that can be achieved. Some of the early clinical trials just described were plagued by these problems, particularly the short duration of response and, in the case of immunotoxins, the occurrence of life-threatening vascular leak syndrome (87). Strategies aimed therefore at improving antibody penetration in general and improving the therapeutic index of immunotoxin-based therapies in particular would be a welcome advance.

Unconjugated antibodies and immunotoxins (but not most radioisotope conjugates) have no bystander effect, and it is therefore essential that antibody bind to all cells within the leukemia cell population. Failure to achieve this will result in therapy failure due to regrowth of leukemia cells that did not bind active agent. It is thus of vital importance to ensure that the selected target antigen is expressed by the leukemic stem cell and not just by daughter leukemia cells in the peripheral circulation that have a limited proliferative capacity. Heterogeneity of target antigen expression by the leukemic stem cell may result in therapy failure due to lack of expression of any single target molecule by a small number of cells. The use of cocktails directed against multiple target molecules may provide the solution here, as demonstrated recently in SCID mouse models of B-cell lymphoma and T-cell leukemia (51,56).

Another vitally important issue is the occurrence of human antimouse antibody (HAMA) and human antitoxin antibody (HATA) responses in patients treated with xenoantibodies. These serologic reactions make retreatment of patients problematic once they have mounted such a response. While it is possible to overcome the HAMA problem by replacing the murine antibody with a fully human or "humanized" antibody, there is no easy solution to the HATA problem. One possible, though cumbersome, way of circumventing the HATA problem would be to change to a different, immunologically distinct toxin with each treatment.

Immunotoxins face still further obstacles of their own. The major dose-limiting toxicity with immunotoxins, which prevents the administration of therapeutically effective doses in the patient, is vascular leak syndrome (VLS). Ways aimed at preventing or suppressing VLS following immunotoxin treatment need to be explored. There is some suggestion that administration of fibronectin to immunotoxin-treated patients may limit the development of VLS (88).

Other strategies relating to the internalization and intracellular routing of immunotoxins also could be adopted to improve their therapeutic index. The translocation of toxin from endosome to cytosol is an inefficient process, possibly relying on a nonspecific leakage of toxin across the endosomal membrane. Furthermore, different antigens vary in their efficiency at delivering toxin to the appropriate intracellular compartment in the target cell. This probably represents the differing abilities of target antigens to route the immunotoxin to the appropriate intracellular compartment or to a lysosomal compartment, where degradation of immunotoxin would take place. Ways to improve the efficiency of the endosome-to-cytosol translocation process and appropriate intracellular trafficking could come from including trafficking signals and/or membrane-disruptive peptide sequences into the immunotoxin molecule. In unpublished work we have demonstrated that the coupling of a 16-mer membrane fusogenic peptide sequence derived from influenza virus hemagglutinin 2 (89) into the Anti-CD19 immunotoxin BU12-saporin increases the in vitro toxicity of this immunotoxin for CD19+ B-cell lymphoma cell lines almost one log and also significantly improves its therapeutic efficacy in SCID mouse models of human B-cell lymphoma. There is also preclinical experimental evidence that conventional cytotoxic drugs used in combination with immunotoxins act in an additive or synergistic fashion, and this aspect needs to be explored in clinical trials.

Exploiting other cytotoxic mechanisms or growth regulatory signals in conjunction with antibody-based therapy also may yield therapeutic effects that are more than additive in outcome. In this context Ghetie et al. have shown that the growth-inhibitory signal exerted by Anti-CD19 antibodies against a human B-cell lymphoma cell line acts in conjunction with an Anti-CD22-ricin A-chain immunotoxin to give a significantly better therapeutic outcome in SCID mice bearing this tumor than that obtained with each therapeutic used alone (90). Similarly, Shen et al. have shown that a bispecific ricin A-chain immunotoxin capable of targeting toxin via its Anti-CD22 arm to a B-cell lymphoma cell line and of recruiting cytotoxic T-cells via its Anti-CD3 arm has enhanced cytotoxicity compared to toxin delivery alone (91). We ourselves have recently demonstrated that the in vivo therapeutic potency of an anti-CD7 saporin immunotoxin is significantly enhanced when NK cells are also directed to the target T-ALL cell surface via the Fc portion of antibody (92). Abrogation of NK cell activity significantly reduced the therapeutic potency of the immunotoxin, demonstrating that both mechanisms contributed to the therapeutic efficacy.

It might therefore be envisaged that future generations of antibody therapies will be comprised of a fully human antibody component. Immunotoxins will be constructed so as to include molecular structures that assist their internalization and intracellular routing. The same molecule will recruit host cytotoxic effector cells (i.e., NK, CTL) and provide growth-inhibitory signals via the cells own signal transduction machinery. The rationale for such a multimodal attack on the target cell is soundly based in recent experimental evidence, the challenge now being to translate this into new therapeutics that will fulfill their experimental promise.

VII. FUTURE PROSPECTS

All the clinical studies that have been undertaken with antibody-based therapies have of necessity been conducted in patients with heavily pretreated and advanced disease that has become refractory to conventional therapy. This is far from the ideal patient group in which to make an assessment of response data. The fact that there have been responses at all in this patient group is encouraging. The use of antibodies as single agents in these studies has also been of limited value for the reasons discussed previously, and a move to undertake clinical studies with combinations of antibodies should take high priority. Acute leukemias should provide a promising test system in which the real therapeutic value of antibody-based treatment can be tested. There is clearly some way to go before any definitive judgments can be made in this regard.

REFERENCES

1. El-Kareh AW, Braunstein SL, Secomb TW. Effect of cell arrangement and interstitial volume fraction on the diffusivity of monoclonal antibodies in tissue. Biophysical 1993; 64:1638–1646.
2. Grossbard ML, Lambert JM, Goldmacher VS, et al. Anti-B4-blocked ricin: a phase I trial of 7-day continuous infusion in patients with B-cell neoplasms. J Clin Oncol 1993; 11:726–737.
3. Ball ED, Graziano RF, Shen L, Fanger MW. Monoclonal antibodies to novel myeloid antigens reveal human neutrophil heterogeneity. Proc Natl Acad Sci USA 1982; 79: 5374–5378.
4. Ball ED, Fanger MW. The expression of myeloid-specific antigens on myeloid leukemia cells: correlations with leukemia subclasses and implications for normal myeloid differentiation. Blood 1983; 61:456–463.
5. Ball ED, Graziano RF, Fanger MW. A unique antigen expressed on myeloid cells and acute leukemia blast cells defined by a monoclonal antibody. J Immunol 1983; 130:2937–2941.
6. Marie JP, Choquet C, Perrot JY, et al. In vitro depletion of clonogenic cells in adult acute lymphoblastic leukemia with a CD10 (anti-calla) monoclonal antibody. Eur J Cancer Clin Oncol 1987; 23:1181–1187.
7. Badger CC, Bernstein ID. Therapy of murine leukemia with monoclonal antibody against a normal differentiation antigen. J Exper Med 1983; 157:828–842.
8. Bernstein ID, Tam MR, Nowinski RC. Mouse leukemia: therapy with monoclonal antibodies against a thymus differentiation antigen. Science 1980; 207:68–71.

9. Kirch ME, Hammerling U. Immunotherapy of murine leukemias by monoclonal antibody. I. Effect of passively administered antibody on growth of transplanted tumor cells. J Immunol 1981; 127:805–810.
10. Flavell DJ, Flavell SU, Boehm DA, et al. Preclinical studies with the anti-CD19-saporin immunotoxin BU12-SAPORIN for the treatment of human-B-cell tumors. B J Cancer 1995; 72:1373–1379.
11. Uckun FM, Manivel C, Arthur D, et al. In vivo efficacy of B43 (anti-CD19)-pokeweed antiviral protein immunotoxin against human pre-B-cell acute lymphoblastic leukemia in mice with severe combined immunodeficiency. Blood 1992; 79:2201–2214.
12. Flavell DJ, Boehm DA, Okayama K, Kohler JA, Flavell SU. Therapy of human T-cell acute lymphoblastic leukaemia in severe combined immunodeficient mice with two different anti-CD7-saporin immunotoxins containing hindered or non-hindered disulphide cross-linkers. Int J Cancer 1994; 58:407–414.
13. Jansen B, Vallera DA, Jaszcz WB, Nguyen D, Kersey JH. Successful treatment of human acute T-cell leukemia in SCID mice using the anti-CD7-deglycosylated ricin A-chain immunotoxin DA7. Cancer Res 1992; 52:1314–1321.
14. Gunther R, Chelstrom LM, Tuel-Ahlgren L, Simon J, Myers DE, Uckun FM. Biotherapy for xenografted human central nervous system leukemia in mice with severe combined immunodeficiency using B43 (anti-CD19)-pokeweed antiviral protein immunotoxin. Blood 1995; 85:2537–2545.
15. Press OW, Martin PJ, Thorpe PE, Vitetta ES. Ricin A-chain containing immunotoxins directed against different epitopes on the CD2 molecule differ in their ability to kill normal and malignant T cells. J Immunol 1988; 141:4410–4417.
16. Better M, Bernhard SL, Lei SP, et al. Potent anti-CD5 ricin A chain immunoconjugates from bacterially produced Fab' and F(ab')2. Proc Natl Acad Sci USA 1993; 90:457–461.
17. Luo Y, Seon BK. Marked difference in the in vivo antitumor efficacy between two immunotoxins targeted to different epitopes of common acute lymphoblastic leukemia antigen (CD10). Mechanisms involved in the differential activities of immunotoxins. J Immunol 1990; 145:1974–1982.
18. Goldmacher VS, Bourret LA, Levine BA, et al. Anti-CD38-blocked ricin: an immunotoxin for the treatment of multiple myeloma. Blood 1994; 84:3017–3025.
19. Uckun FM, Gajl-Peczalska K, Myers DE, Jaszcz W, Haissig S, Ledbetter JA. Temporal association of CD40 antigen expression with discrete stages of human B-cell ontogeny and the efficacy of anti-CD40 immunotoxins against clonogenic B-lineage acute lymphoblastic leukemia as well as B-lineage non-Hodgkin's lymphoma cells. Blood 1990; 76:2449–2456.
20. Ghetie MA, Richardson J, Tucker T, Jones D, Uhr JW, Vitetta ES. Antitumor activity of Fab' and IgG-anti-CD22 immunotoxins in disseminated human B lymphoma grown in mice with severe combined immunodeficiency disease: effect on tumor cells in extranodal sites. Cancer Res 1991; 51:5876–5880.
21. Schnell R, Katouzi AA, Linnartz C, et al. Potent anti-tumor effects of an anti-CD24 ricin A-chain immunotoxin in vitro and in a disseminated human Burkitt's lymphoma model in SCID mice. Int J Cancer 1996; 66:526–531.
22. Xu Y, Xu Q, Rosenblum MG, Scheinberg DA. Antileukemic activity of recombinant

humanized M195-gelonin immunotoxin in nude mice. Leukemia 1996; 10:321–326.
23. Myers DE, Uckun FM. An anti-CD72 immunotoxin against therapy-refractory B-lineage acute lymphoblastic leukemia. Leukemia Lymphoma 1995; 18:119–122.
24. Francisco JA, Kiener PA, Moran-Davis P, Ledbetter JA, Siegall CB. Cytokine activation sensitizes human monocytic and endothelial cells to the cytotoxic effects of an anti-CD40 immunotoxin. J Immunol 1996; 157:1652–1658.
25. Kreitman RJ, Pastan I. Targeting *Pseudomonas* exotoxin to hematologic malignancies. Sem Cancer Biol 1995; 6:297–306.
26. O'Connor R, Liu C, Ferris CA, et al. Anti-B4-blocked ricin synergizes with doxorubicin and etoposide on multidrug-resistant and drug-sensitive tumors. Blood 1995; 86:4286–4294.
27. Ghetie MA, Tucker K, Richardson J, Uhr JW, Vitetta ES. Eradication of minimal disease in severe combined immunodeficient mice with disseminated Daudi lymphoma using chemotherapy and an immunotoxin cocktail. Blood 1994; 84:702–707.
28. Uckun FM, Chelstrom LM, Finnegan D, et al. Effective immunochemotherapy of CALLA + C mu+ human pre-B acute lymphoblastic leukemia in mice with severe combined immunodeficiency using B43 (anti-CD19) pokeweed antiviral protein immunotoxin plus cyclophosphamide. Blood 1992; 79:3116–3129.
29. Vallera DA, Ash RC, Zanjani ED, et al. Anti-T-cell reagents for human bone marrow transplantation: ricin linked to three monoclonal antibodies. Science 1983; 222:512–515.
30. Freedman AS, Takvorian T, Nadler LM, Anderson KC, Sallan SE, Ritz J. Autologous bone marrow transplantation in acute leukemia and lymphoma following ex vivo treatment with monoclonal antibodies and complement. Cancer Treat Res 1988; 38:265–283.
31. Kersey JH, Weisdorf D, Nesbit ME, et al. Comparison of autologous and allogeneic bone marrow transplantation for treatment of high-risk refractory acute lymphoblastic leukemia. N Engl J Med 1987; 317:461–467.
32. Trickett AE, Ford DJ, Lam-Po-Tang PR, Vowels MR. Immunomagnetic bone marrow purging of common acute lymphoblastic leukemia cells: suitability of BioMag particles. Bone Marrow Transpl 1991; 7:199–203.
33. Kvalheim G, Sorensen O, Fodstad O, et al. Immunomagnetic removal of B-lymphoma cells from human bone marrow: a procedure for clinical use. Bone Marrow Transpl 1988; 3:31–41.
34. Gribben JG, Freedman AS, Neuberg D, et al. Immunologic purging of marrow assessed by PCR before autologous bone marrow transplantation for B-cell lymphoma. N Engl J Med 1991; 325:1525–1533.
35. Uckun FM, Ramakrishnan S, Houston LL. Immunotoxin-mediated elimination of clonogenic tumor cells in the presence of human bone marrow. J Immunol 1985; 134:2010–2016.
36. Herve P, Cahn JY, Flesch M, et al. Successful graft-versus-host disease prevention without graft failure in 32 HLA-identical allogeneic bone marrow transplantations with marrow depleted of T cells by monoclonal antibodies and complement. Blood 1987; 69:388–393.

37. Filipovich AH, Vallera DA, Youle RJ, et al. Graft-versus-host disease prevention in allogeneic bone marrow transplantation from histocompatible siblings. A pilot study using immunotoxins for T cell depletion of donor bone marrow. Transplantation 1987; 44:62–69.
38. Filipovich AH, Vallera DA, Youle RJ, Quinones RR, Neville DM, Jr., Kersey JH. Ex-vivo treatment of donor bone marrow with anti-T-cell immunotoxins for prevention of graft-versus-host disease. Lancet 1984; 1:469–472.
39. Blazar RR, Filipovich AH, Kersey JH, et al. T-cell depletion of donor marrowgrafts effects on graft versus host disease and engraftment. In: Gale RP, Champlin R, eds. Progress in Bone Marrow Transplantation. New York: Alan R. Liss, 1987:381–397.
40. Kernan NA, Bordignon C, Heller G, et al. Graft failure after T-cell-depleted human leukocyte antigen identical marrow transplants for leukemia: I. Analysis of risk factors and results of secondary transplants. Blood 1989; 74:2227–2236.
41. Weisdorf DJ, Nesbit ME, Ramsay NK, et al. Allogeneic bone marrow transplantation for acute lymphoblastic leukemia in remission: prolonged survival associated with acute graft-versus-host disease. J Clin Oncol 1987; 5:1348–1355.
42. Ritz J, Pesando JM, Sallan SE, et al. Serotherapy of acute lymphoblastic leukemia with monoclonal antibody. Blood 1981; 58:141–152.
43. van Horssen PJ, van Oosterhout YV, de Witte T, Preijers FW. Cytotoxic potency of CD22-ricin A depends on intracellular routing rather than on the number of internalized molecules. Scandinavian J Immunol 1995; 41:563–569.
44. Preijers FW, Tax WJ, De Witte T, et al. Relationship between internalization and cytotoxicity of ricin A-chain immunotoxins. Brit J Haematol 1988; 70:289–294.
45. Vitetta ES, Fulton RJ, May RD, Till M, Uhr JW. Redesigning nature's poisons to create anti-tumor reagents. Science 1987; 238:1098–1104.
46. Press OW, Howell-Clark J, Anderson S, Bernstein I. Retention of B-cell-specific monoclonal antibodies by human lymphoma cells. Blood 1994; 83:1390–1397.
47. Ritz J, Pesando JM, Notis-McConarty J, Schlossman SF. Modulation of human acute lymphoblastic leukemia antigen induced by monoclonal antibody in vitro. J Immunol 1980; 125:1506–1514.
48. Grossbard ML, Freedman AS, Ritz J, et al. Serotherapy of B-cell neoplasms with anti-B4-blocked ricin: a phase I trial of daily bolus infusion. Blood 1992; 79:576–585.
49. Grossbard ML, Gribben JG, Freedman AS, et al. Adjuvant immunotoxin therapy with anti-B4-blocked ricin after autologous bone marrow transplantation for patients with B-cell non-Hodgkin's lymphoma. Blood 1993; 81:2263–2271.
50. Uckun FM. Immunotoxins for the treatment of leukaemia. Brit J Haematol 1993; 85:435–438.
51. Flavell DJ, Noss A, Pulford KA, Ling N, Flavell SU. Systemic therapy with 3BIT, a triple combination cocktail of anti-CD19, -CD22, and -CD38-saporin immunotoxins, is curative of human B-cell lymphoma in severe combined immunodeficient mice. Cancer Res 1997; 57:4824–4829.
52. Ghetie MA, May RD, Till M, et al. Evaluation of ricin A chain-containing immunotoxins directed against CD19 and CD22 antigens on normal and malignant human B-cells as potential reagents for in vivo therapy. Cancer Res 1988; 48:2610–2617.

53. Vitetta ES, Stone M, Amlot P, et al. Phase I immunotoxin trial in patients with B-cell lymphoma. Cancer Res 1991; 51:4052–4058.
54. Amlot PL, Stone MJ, Cunningham D, et al. A phase I study of an anti-CD22-deglycosylated ricin A chain immunotoxin in the treatment of B-cell lymphomas resistant to conventional therapy. Blood 1993; 82:2624–2633.
55. Stevenson FK, Bell AJ, Cusack R, et al. Preliminary studies for an immunotherapeutic approach to the treatment of human myeloma using chimeric anti-CD38 antibody. Blood 1991; 77:1071–1079.
56. Flavell DJ, Boehm DA, Noss A, Emery L, Flavell SU. Therapy of human T-cell acute lymphoblastic leukaemia in severe combined immunodeficient mice with a combination of anti-CD7- and anti-CD38-saporin immunotoxins. In preparation.
57. Flavell DJ, Boehm DA, Emery L, Noss A, Ramsay A, Flavell SU. Therapy of human B-cell lymphoma bearing SCID mice is more effective with anti-CD19- and anti-CD38-saporin immunotoxins used in combination than with either immunotoxin used alone. Int J Cancer 1995; 62:337–344.
58. Vooijs WC, Schuurman HJ, Bast EJ, de Gast GC. Evaluation of CD38 as target for immunotherapy in multiple myeloma. Blood 1995; 85:2282–2284.
59. Terstappen LW, Huang S, Safford M, Lansdorp PM, Loken MR. Sequential generations of hematopoietic colonies derived from single nonlineage-committed CD34+ CD38− progenitor cells. Blood 1991; 77:1218–1227.
60. Miller RA, Maloney DG, McKillop J, Levy R. In vivo effects of murine hybridoma monoclonal antibody in a patient with T-cell leukemia. Blood 1981; 58:78–86.
61. Levy R, Miller RA. Biological and clinical implications of lymphocyte hybridomas: tumor therapy with monoclonal antibodies. Annu Rev Med 1983; 34:107–116.
62. Laurent G, Pris J, Farcet JP, et al. Effects of therapy with T101 ricin A-chain immunotoxin in two leukemia patients. Blood 1986; 67:1680–1687.
63. Greene WC, Leonard WJ, Depper JM, Nelson DL, Waldmann TA. The human interleukin-2 receptor: normal and abnormal expression in T cells and in leukemias induced by the human T-lymphotropic retroviruses. Ann Int Med 1986; 105:560–572.
64. Waldmann TA, Pastan IH, Gansow OA, Junghans RP. The multichain interleukin-2 receptor: a target for immunotherapy. Ann Int Med 1992; 116:148–160.
65. Waldmann TA, White JD, Goldman CK, et al. The interleukin-2 receptor: a target for monoclonal antibody treatment of human T-cell lymphotrophic virus I–induced adult T-cell leukemia. Blood 1993; 82:1701–1712.
66. Waldmann TA, Goldman CK, Bongiovanni KF, et al. Therapy of patients with human T-cell lymphotrophic virus I–induced adult T-cell leukemia with anti-Tac, a monoclonal antibody to the receptor for interleukin-2. Blood 1988; 72:1805–1816.
67. Waldmann TA. Anti-IL-2 receptor monoclonal antibody (anti-Tac) treatment of T-cell lymphoma. Important Adv Oncol 1994:131–141.
68. Junghans RP, Waldmann TA, Landolfi NF, Avdalovic NM, Schneider WP, Queen C. Anti-Tac-H, a humanized antibody to the interleukin 2 receptor with new features for immunotherapy in malignant and immune disorders. Cancer Res 1990; 50:1495–1502.
69. Scheinberg DA, Lovett D, Divgi CR, et al. A Phase I trial of monoclonal antibody

M195 in acute myelogenous leukemia: specific bone marrow targeting and internalization of radionuclide. J Clin Oncol 1991; 9:478–490.
70. Schwartz MA, Lovett DR, Redner A, et al. Dose-escalation trial of M195 labeled with iodine 131 for cytoreduction and marrow ablation in relapsed or refractory myeloid leukemias. J Clin Oncol 1993; 11:294–303.
71. Caron PC, Co MS, Bull MK, Avdalovic NM, Queen C, Scheinberg DA. Biological and immunological features of humanized M195 (anti-CD33) monoclonal antibodies. Cancer Res 1992; 52:6761–6767.
72. Caron PC, Jurcic JG, Scott AM, et al. A Phase 1B trial of humanized monoclonal antibody M195 (anti-CD33) in myeloid leukemia: specific targeting without immunogenicity. Blood 1994; 83:1760–1768.
73. Caron PC, Schwartz MA, Co MS, et al. Murine and humanized constructs of monoclonal antibody M195 (anti-CD33) for the therapy of acute myelogenous leukemia. Cancer 1994; 73:1049–1056.
74. Jurcic JG, Caron PC, Nikula TK, et al. Radiolabeled anti-CD33 monoclonal antibody M195 for myeloid leukemias. Cancer Res 1995; 55:5908s–5910s.
75. Jurcic JG, Caron PC, Miller WH, Jr., et al. Sequential targeted therapy for relapsed acute promyelocytic leukemia with all-trans retinoic acid and anti-CD33 monoclonal antibody M195. Leukemia 1995; 9:244–248.
76. Hinman LM, Hamann PR, Wallace R, Menendez AT, Durr FE, Upeslacis J. Preparation and characterization of monoclonal antibody conjugates of the calicheamicins: a novel and potent family of antitumor antibiotics. Cancer Res 1993; 53:3336–3342.
77. Hinman LM, Hamann PR, Beyer CF, Smith FO, Flowers DA, Bernstein ID. Calicheamicin conjugates of the anti-CD33 antibody, p67, show potent, selective antitumor effects in models of acute myeloid leukemia (AML) and against human leukemic bone marrow cells (meeting abstr). Proc Annu Meet Am Assoc Cancer Res 1994; 35:A3025.
78. Hamann PR, Hinman LM, Hollander IJ, et al. Anti-CD33 calicheamicin hybrid conjugates for the treatment of acute myelogenous leukemia (meeting abstr). Proc Annu Meet Am Assoc Cancer Res 1996; 37:A3213.
79. Hollander IJ, Hamann PR. Preparation of monoclonal antibody-calicheamicin conjugates (meeting abstr). Proc Annu Meet Am Assoc Cancer Res 1996; 37:A3187.
80. Hale G, Hoang T, Prospero T, Watt SM, Waldmann H. Removal of T cells from bone marrow for transplantation. Comparison of rat monoclonal anti-lymphocyte antibodies of different isotypes. Molecular Biology Med 1983; 1:305–319.
81. Hale G, Bright S, Chumbley G, et al. Removal of T cells from bone marrow for transplantation: a monoclonal antilymphocyte antibody that fixes human complement. Blood 1983; 62:873–882.
82. Hale G, Cobbold SP, Waldmann H, Easter G, Matejtschuk P, Coombs RR. Isolation of low-frequency class-switch variants from rat hybrid myelomas. J Immunological Methods 1987; 103:59–67.
83. Hale G, Swirsky D, Waldmann H, Chan LC. Reactivity of rat monoclonal antibody CAMPATH-1 with human leukaemia cells and its possible application for autologous bone marrow transplantation. Br J Haematol 1985; 60:41–48.
84. Dyer MJ, Hale G, Hayhoe FG, Waldmann H. Effects of CAMPATH-1 antibodies

in vivo in patients with lymphoid malignancies: influence of antibody isotype. Blood 1989; 73:1431–1439.
85. Clendeninn NJ, Nethersell AB, Scott JE, Offenhauser KO, Collier MA. Early safety and efficacy results using Campath-1H (CP-1H), a humanized antilymphocyte monoclonal antibody (MAB), in non-Hodgkin's lymphoma (NHL) and chronic lymphocytic leukemia (CLL) (meeting abst). Proc Annu Meet Am Soc Clin Oncol 1993; 12:A1286.
86. Ball ED, Bernier GM, Cornwell GGd, McIntyre OR, O'Donnell JF, Fanger MW. Monoclonal antibodies to myeloid differentiation antigens: in vivo studies of three patients with acute myelogenous leukemia. Blood 1983; 62:1203–1210.
87. Vitetta ES, Thorpe PE, Uhr JW. Immunotoxins: magic bullets or misguided missiles? Immunol Today 1993; 14:252–259.
88. Baluna R, Ghetie V, Oppenheimer-Marks N, Vitetta ES. Fibronectin inhibits the cytotoxic effect of ricin A chain on endothelial cells. Int J Immunopharmacol 1996; 18:355–361.
89. Skehel JJ, Bizebard T, Bullough PA, et al. Membrane fusion by influenza hemagglutinin. Cold Spring Harbor Symposia Quantitative Biol 1995; 60:573–580.
90. Ghetie MA, Tucker K, Richardson J, Uhr JW, Vitetta ES. The antitumor activity of an anti-CD22 immunotoxin in SCID mice with disseminated Daudi lymphoma is enhanced by either an anti-CD19 antibody or an anti-CD19 immunotoxin. Blood 1992; 80:2315–2320.
91. Shen GL, Li JL, Vitetta ES. Bispecific anti-CD22/anti-CD3-ricin A chain immunotoxin is cytotoxic to Daudi lymphoma cells but not T cells in vitro and shows both A-chain-mediated and LAK-T-mediated killing. J Immunol 1994; 152:2368–2376.
92. Flavell DJ, Noss A, Warnes S, Flavell SU. Host-mediated antibody dependent cellular cytotoxicity (ADCC) contributes to the therapeutic outcome obtained following immunotoxin therapy of human T-ALL in severe combined immunodeficient mice. Blood. In press.

10
Immunotoxin Therapy of Graft-Versus-Host Disease

Carlos R. Bachier and Charles F. LeMaistre
South Texas Cancer Institute, San Antonio, Texas

I. INTRODUCTION

High-dose chemotherapy with allogeneic stem-cell transplant (SCT) has been used for the treatment of hematologic malignancies now for over 30 years. Graft-versus-host disease (GVHD) continues to be the most problematic complication associated with allogeneic SCT. Despite advances in histocompatibility testing and the introduction of cyclosporine and its analogs for prophylaxis, GVHD is still the most frequent cause of morbidity and mortality associated with allogeneic SCT.

In this chapter, we will summarize the pathophysiology and clinical features of GVHD, with special emphasis on recent discoveries on the role of the different components of the immune system. We will then discuss new advances in the treatment and prevention of GVHD, including the use of immunotoxin conjugates.

II. GRAFT-VERSUS-HOST DISEASE: THE IMMUNE SYSTEM

Graft-versus-host disease occurs when alloreactive donor T-cells recognize and interact with major and minor histocompatibility antigens in the host. These interactions activate effector cells and initiate the release of cytokines that results in the clinical manifestations of GVHD (see later). Billingham defined the essential requirements for the development of GVHD more than 30 years ago:

1. Donor cells must contain immunologically competent cells.
2. The recipient must have isoantigens not present in the donor so that the recipient is recognized as antigenically foreign by the donor's immune system.
3. Host cells should be immunodeficient enough to allow donor cells to mount an antigenic reaction (1).

Although the details on the etiology of GVHD remain elusive, new information is now available on the afferent and efferent arms of the immune system and the role of cytokines in immune activation and tissue destruction. GVHD is now viewed as a three-step process (Figure 1):

A. Damage to Host Tissues

Animal models of GVHD implicate preparative-regimen-induced cytokine release as important mediators of immune activation (2,3). In the P→F1 allogeneic bone marrow transplant murine model, parental (P) splenic lymphocytes are transplanted into unirradiated adult's (F1) hosts. Three to four weeks after transplantation, recipient animals show approximately 85% donor-derived lymphohematopoietic cells. These transplanted mice develop T- and B-cell dysfunction and lymphocytic infiltrates in visceral organs and are at risk of infections. Nevertheless, they rarely develop the clinical symptoms of acute GVHD (aGVHD). Interestingly, animal models transplanted in a similar fashion but with the administration of radiation or chemotherapy develop the clinical spectrum of aGVHD and have a high mortality.

The administration of chemotherapy and radiation therapy induces tissue damage to, among other sites, the gastrointestinal tract, the liver, and blood vessels. Damage to these tissues induces an inflammatory reaction, with secondary release of cytokines, including IL-1 and TNF-α (4). These cytokines in turn cause the overexpression of cytoadhesion molecules and MHC class II antigens (5–9). These changes enhance the activation and alloreactivity of donor T-cells against host tissues. Finally, damaged tissues can produce endotoxins that mediate the release of inflammatory cytokines involved in tissue damage during GVHD (see later).

B. Donor T-Cell Activation

Donor T-lymphocytes play a central role in the pathogenesis of GVHD. Furthermore, manipulation of donor T-cells in the graft and their production of IL-2 has been the most common mode of treatment and prevention of aGVHD. Most T-lymphocytes express the CD3 antigen and the T-cell receptor $\alpha\beta$. Within this population of T-lymphocytes, CD4+ lymphocytes interact with the major histo-

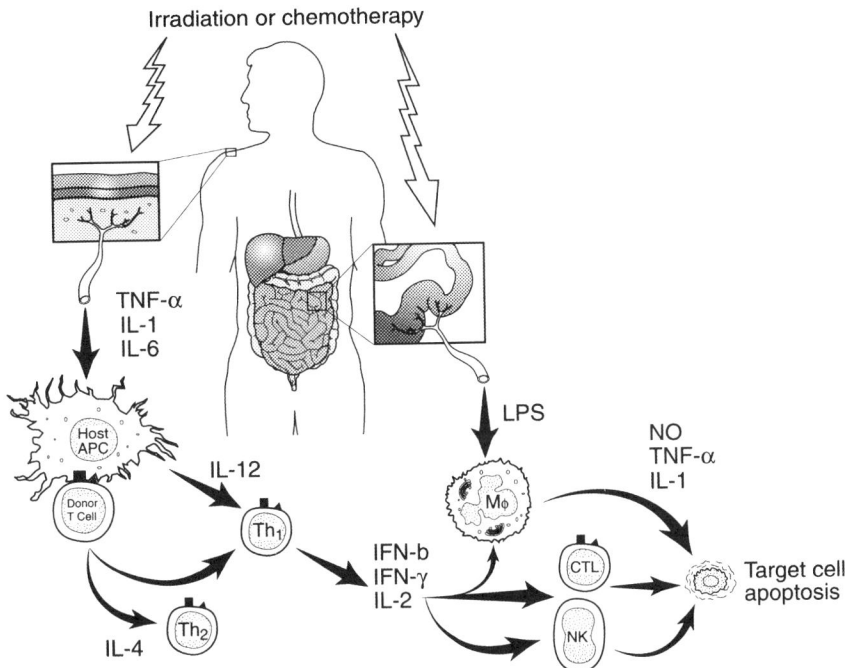

Figure 1 Immune activation during aGVHD. A. Chemotherapy and radiation therapy induce tissue damage, with secondary release of cytokines, including IL-1, IL-6, and TNF-α. These cytokines increase the expression of cytoadhesion molecules and MHC class II antigens. Endotoxins released during tissue damage promote the secondary release of inflammatory cytokines from macrophages. B. Th1-like cells expand after tissue-damage-induced T-lymphocyte activation. IL-12 plays an important role in differentiation of T-lymphocytes into a Th1 pathway. C. Release of IFN-γ and IL-2 from Th1 cells and lipopolysaccharide from chemoradiation-induced tissue damage activate phagocytes to secrete inflammatory cytokines, including TNF-α, IL-1, and nitric oxide. The combined effect of these inflammatory cytokines and cytotoxic T-lymphocytes mediates damage to target tissues during GVHD reactions.

compatibility complex (MHC) class II antigens and CD8+ lymphocytes interact with MHC class I antigens.

Newer discoveries suggest different roles for T-cell subtypes and other cytokines as mediators of the activation and effector arms of GVHD. Murine models have identified two subtypes of CD4+ T-cells based on their cytokine secretion (10). T-helper 1 (Th1) cells secrete predominantly IL-2, IFN-γ, TNF-α, and TNF-β, whereas T-helper 2 (Th2) cells produce IL-4, IL-5, IL-6, IL-10, and IL-13

(11). T-cells can be driven to differentiate into either Th1 or Th2 cells by in vitro incubation with IL-12 or IL-4, respectively (12). Th1- and Th2-like T-cells are also seen among human T-cells, although the pattern of cytokine production is not as clearly demarcated as in the murine model (13). A similar pattern of cytokine secretion has been demonstrated among CD8+ T-cells (14,15). The importance of these findings on the in vivo differentiation of T-cells and its relevance to GVHD are unknown. The general hypothesis is that Th1 responses are associated with cell-mediated immune processes, including the activation of aGVHD reactions, whereas Th2 responses are associated with humoral responses and protection against aGVHD.

Animal studies have shown the potential application of these concepts in the prevention of GVHD. Mice transplanted with splenocytes driven to differentiate into Th2 cells by injections with IL-2 and IL-4 protected recipient mice from the development of lipopolysaccharide-induced GVHD (16).

C. Effector Phase: Immune-Mediated End Organ Damage

Secretion of IL-2 and IFN-γ by Th1 cells, together with endotoxin released during the preparative regimen, activate mononuclear phagocytes to secrete proinflammatory cytokines, including TNF-α, IL-1, and nitric oxide (17–19). These cytokines are important mediators of organ damage during graft-versus-host reactions in animal models and in humans.

Thus, by the selective removal of specific populations, GVHD may be prevented or treated. Immunotoxins should be well suited for this type of targeted therapy.

III. CHRONIC GRAFT-VERSUS-HOST DISEASE

The production of autoreactive lymphocyte autoantibodies characterizes the pathogenesis of chronic graft-versus-host disease (cGVHD). The immune dysregulation seen in cGVHD leads to increased collagen deposition, resulting in clinical symptoms similar to those seen in patients with autoimmune disorders, including scleroderma and Sjogren's disease. Whereas tissue necrosis is the pathologic hallmark of acute GVHD, cGVHD is associated with organ deposition of collagen.

Animal models identified two important factors needed for the development of graft-versus-host reactions. First, the development and maintenance of cGVHD is dependent on the continued presence of host-reactive T-cells that, unlike aGVHD, fail to become tolerant of the host (20). Second, and also different from aGVHD, the cytokine production in cGVHD is characterized by a Th2 pattern

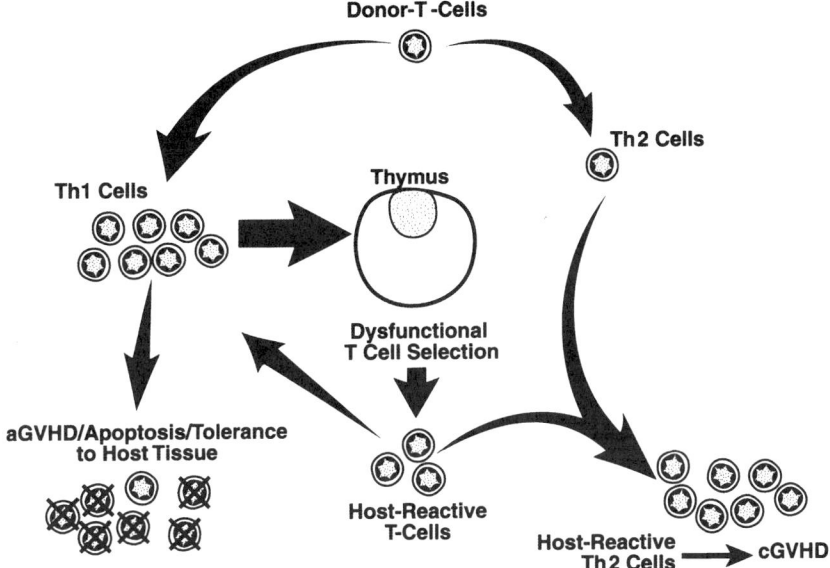

Figure 2 Immune dysregulation during cGVHD. Th1 cells and cytokines originating from donor T-cells mediate the inflammatory reaction seen in aGVHD. These cells eventually undergo clonal deletion, either by apoptosis or by becoming anergic to host tissues. Thymic damage occurring during aGVHD alters host reactivity. Th2 cells emerging from the donor or maturing from the host in a dysfunctional thymus increase in numbers and predominate as Th1 cells become deleted. These Th2 cells and their cytokine production are then responsible for the clinical spectrum of chronic GVHD.

(21). These Th2 cytokines are important for both the pathology and the immune dysregulation seen in cGVHD.

Based on the foregoing findings, the following hypothesis has been proposed (Figure 2). Initially, Th1 cells and cytokines originating from donor T-cells mediate the inflammatory reaction seen in aGVHD. These cells eventually undergo clonal deletion either by apoptosis or by becoming anergic to host tissues. Thymic damage occurring during aGVHD alters host reactivity. Th2 cells emerging from the donor or maturing from the host in a dysfunctional thymus increase in numbers and predominate as Th1 cells become deleted. These Th2 cells and their cytokine production are then responsible for the clinical spectrum of chronic GVHD.

IV. GRAFT-VERSUS-HOST DISEASE: CLINICAL MANIFESTATIONS AND TREATMENT

An inflammatory reaction involving the skin, liver, gastrointestinal tract, and lymphoid organs characterizes acute graft-versus-host disease. The onset of symptoms occurs 2–3 weeks (and usually within the first 2 months) after allogeneic bone marrow transplantation (22). The first manifestations of aGVHD are usually an erythematous and pruritic skin rash. Initially, it may involve the palms and soles, but it can progress to involve the whole body, with bullae formation and denudation of the skin. Liver involvement is manifested by elevation of liver function tests and usually occurs concomitant with or after the development of skin GVHD. Gastrointestinal symptoms of aGVHD include nausea, vomiting, abdominal pain, and diarrhea. In aGVHD's severe form, patients develop voluminous bloody diarrhea or paralytic ileus. Finally, aGVHD causes significant cellular and humoral dysfunction and increases the risk of infections. Different grading systems have been formulated to evaluate the severity of aGVHD (Table 1).

As previously discussed, cGVHD is considered an autoimmune process, with clinical features similar to scleroderma and Sjogren's. It develops after the third month following allogeneic bone marrow transplantation and usually follows aGVHD. cGVHD also can occur de novo in patients with no previous history of aGVHD. Skin manifestations include lichenoid papules, areas of local erythema, and hyper- or hypopigmentation. With progression of skin involve-

Table 1 Grading of aGVHD

	Extent of organ involvement		
Stage	Skin	Liver	Gut
1	Rash on <25%	Bilirubin 2–3 mg/dL	Diarrhea >500 mL/day
2	Rash on 25–50%	Bilirubin 3.1–6 mg/dL	Diarrhea >1000 mL/day
3	Rash on >50%	Bilirubin 6.1–15 mg/dL	Diarrhea >1500 mL/day
4	Generalized erythroderma with bullous formation	Bilirubin >15 mg/dL	Severe abdominal pain with or without ileus
	Overall grading of aGVHD		
Grade	Skin	Liver	Gut
I	Stage 1–2	None	None
II	Stage 3 or	Stage 1 or	Stage 1
III	—	Stage 2–3 or	Stage 2–4
IV	Stage 4 or	Stage 4	—

ment, patients develop skin and subcutaneous fibrosis. Liver manifestations of cGVHD are similar to aGVHD and include an increase in liver function tests. Gastrointestinal manifestations include abdominal pain, diarrhea, and mouth ulcers.

Without prophylaxis, most patients undergoing allogeneic stem cell transplantation will develop severe graft-versus-host disease. The use of cyclosporine-based immunosuppression decreases the incidence of GVHD to approximately 40% in HLA-matched sibling stem-cell transplantation. Other strategies to decrease the incidence of GVHD, especially in matched unrelated and HLA-mismatched transplants include the depletion of T-cells from the graft and the use of other immunosuppressive drugs, including tacrolimus, antithymocyte globulin, and immunotoxins.

V. GRAFT-VERSUS-HOST DISEASE: IMMUNOTOXIN THERAPY

Despite the use of potent immunosuppressive drugs, including cyclosporine and its analogs, GVHD is still a major cause of morbidity and mortality in allogeneic bone marrow transplantation. This complication is even more prevalent now as the bone marrow donor pool is increasing with the use of matched unrelated and mismatched related donors.

The agents presently available for prevention or treatment of GVHD are nonspecific and cause broad immunosuppression. As we increase our knowledge of the pathogenesis of GVHD, immunotoxin conjugates will provide the potential advantage of targeted therapy to subsets of T-cells involved in graft-versus-host reactions. These advances may allow removal from the grafts of T-cells involved in graft-versus-host disease, as well as prevention and treatment GVHD posttransplant by the systemic administration of these immunotoxin conjugates.

A. Targets

Immunotoxin conjugates were initially directed at the pan T-lymphocyte antigen CD-5. Preclinical in vitro studies showed significant reductions in alloreactivity as measured by phytohemagglutinin responses (23). Animal studies demonstrated a decrease in the incidence of GVHD when CD-5 immunotoxins were used for T-cell depletion of grafts or in the prevention and treatment of animal models of GVHD posttransplant (see later). Responses in these models were usually transient. An explanation for these transient responses may be the T-cell activation achieved by the known CD5 costimulatory effect of the CD72 molecule on B-cells (24).

Other CD antigens also have been evaluated as potential targets. More potent Anti-GVHD responses were achieved when immunotoxin conjugates were targeted to the CD3 antigen (25). Several factors made the CD3 antigen a more attractive target for the treatment of GVHD: (a) the CD3 antigen is more broadly expressed in different T-cell subsets (26), (b) immunotoxin conjugates are more rapidly and completely internalized when directed against the CD3 antigen (26), (c) Anti-CD3 immunotoxins can deplete up to 3 logs of CD3-expressing cells (27). In preclinical and clinical studies the Fc component of the intact Anti-CD3 antibody molecule was removed to avoid the toxicities associated with T-cell activation (28). Immunotoxin targets also have been directed against other T cell antigens, including CD2 and CD18 (29,30).

B. Toxins

Initial studies used ricin-A toxin immunoconjugates for the treatment and prevention of graft-versus-host disease (31–33). Both animal and human studies showed occasional allergic reactions, including dyspnea, wheezing, hoarseness, and swelling (34,35). Other side effects included weight gain, edema, and capillary leak syndrome with pulmonary infiltrates. These prompted the analysis of diphtheria toxins (DT) as candidate for conjugation with antibased immunotoxins T-cell monoclonal antibodies (36). At least in animal models, the use of DT has not been associated with capillary leak syndromes. Their effectiveness and toxicity in humans await the results of clinical trials.

C. Animal Studies

Murine models have allowed the preclinical evaluation of immunotoxin conjugates' effectiveness and toxicity profiles, giving insight into their potential clinical application to humans. In one of these models, mice are lethally irradiated and then transplanted with bone marrow and increasing doses of lymphocytes. Donor and host combinations are used that differ at MHC class I, II, or minor antigens (37,38). Another murine model of GVHD is the P→F1 discussed earlier. Irradiated F1 hosts develop aGVHD, whereas unirradiated F1 hosts develop immune deficiencies and signs of cGVHD (2).

Initial evaluation of immunotoxins for T-cell purging in murine models of GHVD included pretreatment with Anti-Thy-1.2 conjugated to intact ricin administered in the presence of exogenous lactose to block the B-chain galactose binding sites (39). Mice receiving marrow treated with α Thy-1.2 immunotoxin were protected against GVHD, compared to untreated controls, in which mortality was greater than 90%. Mice treated with unconjugated antibody had only transient protection against GVHD, with a 72% mortality from GVHD. Importantly, there was no evidence of toxicity to the stem-cell compartment. Others studies corroborated initial studies showing protection against GVHD by the use of immunotoxin conjugates. Follow-up studies compared the intact ricin complexes with A-chain hybrids. Antibody linked to intact ricin was 20–117-fold more inhibitory to PHA reactions than A-chain conjugates, suggesting that the B-chain increased the conjugate's effectiveness by facilitating the entry of the toxin into target cells (40). Again, no effect on stem cells was seen until high levels of immunotoxin conjugates were reached.

Animal studies also showed protection against GVHD when immunotoxin conjugates were administered systemically for prevention or treatment of established GVHD. Initial studies with Anti-CD5 ricin A-chain immunotoxins significantly prevented the development of GVHD in the SCID C57B6 model (31). More recently, Vallera and collaborators evaluated the effectiveness of targeting the CD3 antigen with diphtheria and ricin-A-toxin-based immunoconjugates. They evaluated the protection against GVHD, both by the ability to purge T-cells and by the systemic administration of Anti-CD3 immunoconjugates. A fusion protein was produced from a construct made by splicing sFv cDNA from a hybridoma to a truncated form of the diphtheria toxin gene (DT_{390}). DT_{390} encodes a molecule that retains full enzymatic activity. The DT_{390}-Anti-CD3sFv immunotoxin conjugate showed potent in vitro inhibition against PHA-stimulated and alloantigen-stimulated T-cells. Furthermore, when tested in the C.B.-17scid ($H-2^d$) GVHD model, DT_{390}-Anti-CD3sFv showed a survival advantage, with 86% of mice alive compared to 43% of mice receiving DT_{390}-Fc fusion toxin, and to 17% of mice receiving phosphate-buffered saline (36).

D. Human Studies

Immunotoxin conjugates have been used in clinical trials for the depletion of T-cells in allografts, as prophylaxis, and for treatment of established GVHD (Table 2).

1. T-Cell Depletion

There are significant preclinical and clinical data demonstrating that the removal of T-lymphocytes from the donor graft reduces or prevents GVHD. The depletion of donor T-lymphocytes from the graft also has the deleterious effects of delaying or preventing engraftment, affecting immune reconstitution, and increasing the relapse rate posttransplant.

Initial pilot studies of T-cell depletion with immunotoxin conjugates demonstrated a decrease in the incidence of aGVHD (41–43). Conjugates in these trials included Anti-CD3 and Anti-CD5 ricin immunotoxins. Greater than 90% T-cell depletion was achieved, with minimal effect to the progenitor compartment. Unfortunately, as in other T-cell depletion trials, the rate of engraftment failure and relapse was unacceptable.

Table 2 Results of Clinical Studies

Immunotoxin therapy	Type of BMT	No. pts.	GHVD Prophylaxis	GVHD	Survival
T-cell depletion (OKT3)/CD5-ricin-A (P) (44)	MUD/1 Ag mismatch—sib	10	CSA/methylpred/CD5 ricin A	5/9	3/10
T-cell depletion (T10B9+C')/CD5-ricin-A (P) (45)	Mismatched—related	40	Methylpred vs. methylpred/CD5 ricin A	92 vs. 19%	18 vs. 40
CD5-ricin-A (P) (46)	Matched—sib	6	Methylpred/CD5 ricin A	6/6	4/6
CD5-ricin-A (P) (48)	MUD	31	Methylpred or MTX + CD5 ricin A	9/15 (a) 6/8 (c)	4/22
T-cell depletion (T10B9+C')/CD5-ricin-A (P) (49)	MUD	8	Methylpred/CD5 ricin A	2/8	4/8
CD5-ricin-A (T) (steroid resistant) (51)	Matched—sib	34	—	CR = 9/34 PR = 7/34	—
CD5-ricin-A vs. ATG (T) (steroid resistant) (52)	Matched—sib	75	—	CR = 24% PR = 28% RR = 52% vs. 31%	—
CD5-ricin-A/steroid vs. steroid (T) (53)	Matched—sib	243	—	CR = 40 vs. 25% (@ 4 wks) PR = 44 vs. 38% (@ 6 wks) SR = 49 vs. 45% (@ 1 yr)	—

P = prophylaxis, T = treatment, ATG = antithymocyte globulin, MUD = matched unrelated donor, Ag = antigen, CSA = cyclosporine, MTX = methotrexate, a = acute, c = chronic, CR = complete response, PR = partial response, SR = survival rate.

More recently, T-cell depletion with immunotoxin conjugates has been used in allogeneic bone marrow transplants where there is high risk for GVHD, including matched unrelated and haploidentical, partially mismatched transplants. Henslee and collaborators evaluated the role of in vitro and in vivo T-cell depletion in haploidentical mismatched related transplants using an Anti-T-cell (T10B9-1A-31) monoclonal antibody for T-cell depletion and systemic administration of Anti-CD5 ricin A immunotoxin posttransplant (44). Anti-T-cell monoclonal antibody plus complement achieved a 1–2 log reduction in T-cells, as measured by limiting dilution analysis. The incidence of GVHD was reduced from 92% to 19% when patients undergoing bone marrow transplant with T-cell depletion and posttransplant immunotoxin therapy were compared to historical control patients undergoing bone marrow transplant with T-cell purging only. The rate of engraftment was 100%. The only side effect of Anti-CD5 ricin immunotherapy was hypoalbuminemia, which was corrected by albumin replacement.

A similar approach was used by Przepiorka et al. in pediatric patients undergoing allogeneic bone marrow transplant from antigen mismatched related and matched unrelated adult donors (45). Bone marrow grafts underwent T-cell depletion by immunomagnetic purging using a CD3 antibody. The median T-cell content after purging was 1.4×10^6 CD3+ cells/kg. Of ten patients treated, five developed severe (GR III, IV) GVHD. All patients engrafted, and no patient developed renal failure or capillary leak syndromes.

2. GVHD Prophylaxis

Only small series have been reported using immunotoxin therapy for the prophylaxis of GVHD in HLA identical-sibling transplant. In pediatric patients, the use of Anti-CD5 ricin immunotoxin along with methylprednisolone was unable to prevent the incidence of severe GVHD (46). Additional studies are needed to evaluate the use of posttransplant immunotherapy in combination with cyclosporine analogs as prophylaxis for GVHD.

Immunotoxin therapy also has been used for the prevention of GVHD in patients undergoing matched unrelated bone marrow transplants. The addition of Anti-CD5 ricin immunotoxins to either cyclosporine/methylprednisolone or cyclosporine/methotrexate was associated with an incidence of severe GVHD (grade $\geq$ II) of 33% (5/15) (47). Of eight evaluable patients, six developed extensive cGVHD (47). In another study, thirty-one patients underwent matched unrelated transplant with Anti-CD5 ricin immunotoxin in combination with cyclosporine and methotrexate as prophylaxis for GVHD (48). Severe (grade III, IV) aGVHD was seen in seven of twenty-nine patients. In both of these studies, an increased incidence of renal toxicity was seen, particularly in patients receiving cyclosporine/methotrexate in combination with the immunotoxin conjugate. Finally, Koehler and collaborators incorporated Anti-CD5 ricin A toxin for GVHD prophylaxis in conjunction with partial depletion of donor T-cells in patients undergoing matched unrelated bone marrow transplant. Only one of eight patients developed severe GVHD, but there was a high mortality from viral infections associated with a slow CD4 and CD8 immune reconstitution (49).

The incidence of severe GVHD in all of these small series is similar to that found with the use of current GVHD prophylactic regimens using cyclosporine-based therapy. Larger, randomized studies may show benefits in favor of immunotoxin conjugate combination therapy.

3. Treatment of Established GVHD

The treatment of established GVHD with immunotoxin conjugates was based on favorable results seen in in vitro and in vivo studies. Clinical trials also were sparked by the success of treatment with Anti-CD5 ricin immunotoxin in a patient with steroid-resistant grade IV GVHD (50). That patient had complete resolution of GVHD, with minimal secondary side effects associated with administration of H65-RTA.

Based on these results, Phase I studies were conducted to evaluate the efficacy and schedule of administration of immunotoxins for the treatment of resistant GVHD. In the first of these studies, patients with steroid-resistant GVHD received escalating doses of the H65-RTA Anti-CD5 ricin immunotoxin (51). Complete responses were seen in nine of thirty-four patients, with partial responses seen in another seven. Responses were sustained, and no patient responding died of GVHD or a GVHD-associated complication. Higher response rates were seen in patients with skin GVHD. Side effects were typical of immunotoxins and included depression, lethargy, hypoalbuminemia, weight gain, and renal insufficiency. Some patients developed HAMA, but these antibodies did not interfere with binding of H65 monoclonal antibodies to the CD5 antigen and were not associated with allergic reactions. Follow-up studies corroborated the results of initial trials. Lomen and collaborators treated 75 patients with steroid refractory GVHD with H65-RTA and compared them with historical matched control subjects receiving antithymocyte globulin (52). The response rate was 52%, with 24% complete and 28% partial responses. Responses were seen in patients with GVHD of the skin, gastrointestinal tract, and liver, but higher response rates were again seen in patients with skin GVHD. The response rate was higher than in historical controls treated with ATG (52% vs. 31%). Median survival also favored patients treated with H65-RTA (148 vs. 80 days).

The concomitant therapy of steroids and the H65-RTA immunotoxin was evaluated as initial therapy of aGVHD. Patients (243) were randomized to receive methylprednisolone and H65-RTA versus methylprednisolone and placebo (53). After 4 weeks, 40% of patients in the immunotoxin group had complete responses, compared to 25% in the steroid/placebo group. These differences became nonsignificant at 6 weeks (CR = 44% vs. 38%). Furthermore, the incidence of chronic GVHD or survival at 1 year were not statistically different.

VI. CONCLUSION

Clinical studies have shown that some patients with steroid-resistant GVHD will have resolution of clinical signs and symptoms of GVHD after administration of immunotoxin conjugates. The benefits of immunotoxin conjugates for prophylaxis of GVHD in matched siblings, partially mismatched, or unrelated bone transplant are at best marginal. As we learn more about the T-cell subsets involved in graft-versus-host reactions, we may be able to target those T-cells both in vivo and in vitro and decrease the incidence of GVHD without affecting the graft-versus-tumor effects.

REFERENCES

1. Bellingham T. The biology of graft versus host reaction. Harvey Lecture. 1966; 21.
2. Hakim FT, Sharrow SO, Payne S, Shearer GM. Repopulation of host lymphohematopoietic systems by donor cells during graft versus host reaction in unirradiated adult F1 mice injected with parental lymphocytes. J Immunol 1991; 146:2108.
3. Johnson BD, Drobyski WR, Truitt RL. Delayed infusion of normal donor cells after MHC—matched bone marrow transplantation provides and antileukemia reaction without graft versus host disease. Bone Marrow Transplantation 1993; 11:329.
4. Xun CQ, Thompson JS, Jennings CD. Effect of total body irradiation, busulfan—cyclophosphamide, or cyclophosphamide conditioning on inflammatory cytokine release and development of acute and chronic graft versus host disease in H2 incompatible transplanted SCID mice. Blood 1994; 83:2360.
5. Cavender DE, Haskard DO, Joseph B, et al. Interleukin 1 increases the binding of human B and T lymphocytes to endothelial cell monolayers. J Immunol 1986; 136: 203.
6. Thornhill MH, Wellicome SM, Mahiouz DL, et al. Tumor necrosis factor combines with IL-4 or IFN-γ to selectively enhance endothelial cell adhesiveness for T cells. J Immunol 1991; 146:592.
7. Pober JS, Gimbrose MA, Lapierre LA, et al. Overlapping patterns of activation of human endothelial cell by interleukin 1, tumor necrosis factor, and interferon. J Immunol 1986; 137:1893.
8. Leeuwenberg JF, Van Damme J, Maeger, et al. Effects of tumor necrosis factor on the interferon γ induced major histocompatibility complex class II antigen expression by human endothelial cells. Eur J Immunol 1988; 18:1469.
9. Chang RJ, Lee SH. Effects of interferon γ and tumor necrosis factor α on the expression of an Ia antigen on a murine macrophage cell line. J Immunol 1986; 137:2853.
10. Mosmann TR, Cherwinski H, Bond MW, et al. Two types of murine helper T cell

clones. I. Definition according to profiles of lymphokine activities and secreted proteins. J Immunol 1986; 136:2348.
11. Mosnann TR, Coffman RL. Heterogeneity of cytokine secretion patterns and functions of helper T cells. Adv Immunol 1989; 46:111.
12. Seder RA, Paul WE. Acquisition of lymphokine-producing phenotype by CD4+ T cells. Ann Rev Immunol 1994; 21:635.
13. Del Prete G, Maggi E, Romagnani S. Human Th1 and Th2 cells: functional properties, mechanisms of regulation, and role in disease. Lab Invest 1994; 70:299.
14. Croft M, Carter L, Swain SL, et al. Generation of antigen-specific CD 8 effector populations: reciprocal action of interleukin (IL)-4 and IL-12 in promoting type 2 versus type 1 cytokine profiles. J Exp Med 1994; 180:1775.
15. Seder RA, Boulay JL, Finkelman FD, et al. CD 8+ T cells can be primed in vitro to produce IL-4. Immunology 1992; 148:1652.
16. Fowler DH, Kurasawa K, Husebekk A, et al. Cells of the Th2 cytokine phenotype prevent LPS-induced lethality during murine graft-versus-host reaction. J Immunol 1994; 152:1004.
17. Piguet, PF. Tumor necrosis factor and graft-versus-host disease. In: Burakoff SJ, Deeg HJ, Ferrera JLM, Atkinson K, eds. Graft-vs.-Host Disease. New York: Marcel Dekker, 1990:258.
18. Abhyankar S, Gilliland DG, Ferrera JLM. Interleukin 1 is a critical effector molecule during dysregulation in graft-versus-host disease to minor histocompatibility antigens. Transplantation 1993; 53:1518.
19. Hoffman RA, Langrehr JM, Wren SM, et al. Characterization of the immunosuppressive effects of nitric oxide in graft versus host disease. J Immunol 1995; 155:15.
20. RozendaalL. Pals ST, Gleichmann E, Melief CJ. Persistence of allospecific helper T cells is required for maintaining autoantibody formation in lupus-like graft versus host disease. Clin Exp Immunol 1990; 82:527.
21. Garlisi CG, Pemmline KJ, Smith SR, et al. Cytokine gene expression in mice undergoing chronic graft versus host disease. Mol Immunol 1993; 30:669.
22. Thomas ED, Storb R, Clift RA, et al. Bone marrow transplantation. N Engl J Med 1975; 292:832.
23. Jackman R, Nowicki S, Anaeshansley D, Eisner T. Anti T cell reagents for human bone marrow transplantation: ricin linked to three monoclonal antibodies. Science 1983; 222:512.
24. Van de Velde, von Hoegen I, Luo W, Parnes JR, Thielemans K. The B-cell surface protein CD72/Jyb-2 is the ligand for CD5. Nature 1991; 351:662.
25. Vallera DA, Tailor PA, Panoskaltsis-Mortari A, Blazar BR. Therapy of ongoing graft versus host disease induced across the major or minor histocompatibility barrier in mice with anti-CD3F (ab')$_2$-RTA (ricin toxin A chain) immunotoxin. Blood 1995; 86:4367.
26. Press OW, Vitetta ES, Farr AG, Hansen JA, Martin PJ. Evaluation of ricin A-chain immunotoxins directed against human T cells. Cellular Immunol 1986; 102:10.
27. Martin PJ, Hansen JA, Torok-Storb B, Moretti L, Press O. Effects of treating marrow with a CD3 specific immunotoxin for prevention of acute graft versus host disease. Bone Marrow Transplant 1989; 4:215.
28. Blazar BR, Hirsch R, Gress RE, Carroll SF, Vallera DA. In vivo administration of

anti-CD3 monoclonal antibodies or immunotoxins in murine recipients of allogeneic T-cell depleted marrow for the promotion of engraftment. J Immunol 1991; 147: 1492.
29. Jackman R, Nowicki S, Anaeshansley D, Eisner T. Anti-T-cell reagents for human bone marrow transplantation: ricin linked to three monoclonal antibodies. Science 1983; 222:512.
30. Unkun F, Azemove S, Myers D, Vallera D. Anti-CD2 (t, p50) intact ricin immunotoxins for GVHD-prophylaxis in allogeneic bone marrow transplantation. Cancer Res 1986; 10:3154.
31. Vallera DA, Carroll SF, Snover D, Carlson GJ, Blazar BR. Toxicity and efficacy of anti-T-cell ricin toxin A chain immunotoxins in a murine model of established graft versus host disease induced across the major histocompatibility barrier. Blood 1991; 77:182.
32. Cavazzana-Calvo M, Stephan JL, Sarnacki S, Cheveret S, Fromont C, de Coene C, Le Deist F, Guy-Grand D, Fischer A. Attenuation of graft versus host disease and graft rejection by ex vivo immunotoxin elimination of alloreactive T cells in an H-2 haplotype disparate mouse combination. Blood 1994; 83:288.
33. Byers VS, Henslee J, Kernan N, Blazar BR, Gingrich R, Phillips GL, LeMaistre CF, Gilliland G, Antin JH, Vogelsang G, Martin P, Tutschka PJ, Trown P, Ackerman SK, O'Reilly RJ, Scannon PJ. Use of anti pan T lymphocyte ricin A chain immunotoxin as targeted immunotherapy in steroid resistant acute graft versus host disease. Blood 1990; 75:1426.
34. Weisdorf D, Filipovich A, McGlave P, Ramsay N, Kersey J, Miller W, Blazar B. Combination graft versus host disease prophylaxis using immunotoxin (anti CD5 RTA (Xomazyme-CD5) plus methotrexate and cyclosporine of prednisone after unrelated donor marrow transplantation. Bone Marrow Transplant 1993; 12:531.
35. Krance R, Heslop HE, Mahmoud H, Ribeiro R, Douglass E, Hurwitz C, Santana V, Kun L, Horowitz MM, Brenner MK. Anti pan T lymphocyte ricin A chain immunotoxin (H65p TRA) and methylprednisolone for acute GHVD prophylaxis following allogeneic BMT, from HLA-identical sibling donors. Bone Marrow Transplant 1993; 11:33.
36. Vallera DA, Panoskaltsis-Mortari A, Jost C, Ramakrishnan S, Eide CR, Kreitman RJ, Nicholls J, Pennell C, Blazar BR. Anti-graft versus host disease effect of DT_{390}-anti-CD3sFv, a single-chain Fv fusion immunotoxin specifically targeting the CD3ε moiety of the T-cell receptor. Blood 1996; 88:2342.
37. Moser M, Sharrow SO, Shearer GM. Role of $L3T4^+$ and $Lyt\ 2^+$ donor cells in graft versus host immune deficiency induced across a class I, class II, or whole H-2 difference. J Immunol 1988; 140:2600.
38. Hakim FT, Mackall CL. The immune system: effector and target of graft versus host disease. In: Ferrarar LM, Deeg HJ, Burakoff SJ, eds. Graft Versus Host Disease. New York: Marcel Dekker, 1996:258–259.
39. Vallera D, Yould R, Neville D, Kersey J. Bone marrow transplantation across major histocompatibility barriers. J Exp Med 1982; 155:949.
40. Vallera D, Yould R, Neville D, Soderling C, Kersey J. Monoclonal antibody toxin conjugates for experimental graft versus host disease prophylaxis. Transplantation 1983; 36:73.

41. Martin P, Hansen J, Torok-Storb B, Moretti L, Storb R, Thomas D, Weiden P, Vitetta E. Effects of treating marrow with a CD3 specific immunotoxin for prevention of acute graft versus host disease. Bone marrow Transplant 1988; 3:437.
42. Laurent G, Maraninchi D, Gluckman E, Derocq J, Gaspare M, Roi B, Michalet M, Reiffers J, Dreyfus F, Casellas P, Schneider P, Blythaman H, Bouloux C, Jansen F. Donor bone marrow treatment with T101 Rab fragment-ricin A chain immunotoxin prevents graft versus host disease. Bone Marrow Transplant 1989; 4:367.
43. Filipovich A, Vallera D, McGlave P, Gajl-Peczalska K, Haake R, Lasky L, Blazar B, Ramsay J, Weisdorf D. T cell depletion with anti-CD5 immunotoxin in histocompatible bone marrow transplantation. Transplantation 1990; 50:410.
44. Henslee PJ, Parrish RS, Macdonald JS, Romond EH, Maciniack E, Coffey C, Ciocci G, Thompson JS. Combined in vitro and in vivo T lymphocyte depletion for the control of graft versus host disease following haploidentical marrow transplant. Transplantation 1996; 61(5):738.
45. Przepiorka D, Chan KW, Champlin RE, Culberr SJ, Petropoulos D, Ippoliti, Khouri I, Huh YO, Vriesendorp H, Deisseroth AB, Bleyer WA. Prevention of graft versus host disease with anti CD5 ricin A chain immunotoxin after CD3 depleted HLA nonidentical marrow transplantation in pediatric leukemia patients. Bone Marrow Transplantation 1995; 16:737.
46. Krance R, Heslop HE, Mahmoud H, Ribeiro R, Douglass E, Hurwitz C, Santana V, Kun L, Horowitz MM, Brenner MK. Anti-pan T lymphocyte ricin A chain immunotoxin (H65-TRA) and methylprednisolone for acute GVHD prophylaxis following allogeneic BMT from HLA-identical sibling donors. Bone Marrow Transplantation 1993; 11:33–36.
47. Wiesdorf D, Filipovich A, Mcglave P, Ramsay N, Kersey J, Miller W, Blazar B. Combination graft versus host disease prophylaxis using g immunotoxin (anti CD5 RTA (Xomazyme CD5) plus methotrexate and cyclosporine or prednisone after unrelated donor marrow transplantation. Bone Marrow Transplantation 1993; 12:531.
48. Phillips GL, Nevill TJ, Spinelli JJ, Nantel SH, Klingemann HG, Barnerr MJ, Sheperd JD, Chan KW, Meharchand JM, Sutherland HJ, Reece DE, Messner HA. Prophylaxis for acute graft versus host disease following unrelated donor bone marrow transplantation. Bone Marrow Transplantation 1995; 15:213.
49. Koehler M, Hurwitz CA, Krance RA, Coustan E, Williams LL, Santana V, Ribeiro RC, Brenner MK, Heslop HE. Xomazyme CD5 immunotoxin in conjunction with partial T cell depletion for prevention of graft rejection and graft versus host disease after bone marrow transplantation from matched unrelated donors. Bone Marrow Transplantation 1994; 13:571.
50. Kernan N, Byers V, Scannon P, Mischak R, Brochstein J, Flomenberg N, Dupont B, O'Reilly R. Treatment of steroid resistant acute graft versus host disease by in vitro administration of an anti T cell ricin A chain immunotoxin. JAMA 1988; 259:3154.
51. Byers V, Henslee J, Kernan N, Blazar B, Gingrich R, Phillips G, LeMaistre CF, Gilliand G, Antin J, Martin P, Tutscha Pk Trown P, Ackerman S, O'Reilly R, Scannon P. Use of an anti-pan T-lymphocyte ricin A chain immunotoxin in steroid resistant acute graft versus host disease. Blood 1990; 75:1426.
52. Lomen PL, Steward KK, Saks SR. Xoma Bone Marrow Transplantation Study

Group. Safety and efficacy of H65-RTA in the treatment of steroid-resistant acute graft versus host disease after allogeneic bone marrow transplantation. Blood 1991; 78(suppl 1):230.
53. Martin PJ, Nelson BJ, Appelbaum FR, Anasetti C, Deeg HJ, Hansen JA, McDonald GB, Nash RA, Sullivan KM, Witherspoon RP, Scannon PJ, Friedmann N, Storb R. Evaluation of a CD5 specific immunotoxin for treatment of acute graft versus host disease after allogeneic marrow transplantation. Blood 1996; 88(3):824.

11
Hematopoietic Progenitor-Cell Graft Processing and Treatment

Nadine Beauger and Denis Claude Roy
University of Montreal and Maisonneuve-Rosemont Hospital, Montreal, Quebec, Canada

I. INTRODUCTION

Autologous progenitor-cell transplantation (PCT) relies on high doses of chemotherapy with or without irradiation for the elimination of patient malignant cells. The delivery of such excessive amounts of toxic agents destroys both normal and malignant cells simultaneously. Thus, patient survival depends on the capacity of hematopoietic stem cells collected before this intensive therapy to reconstitute hematologic and immunologic function. Strategies to promote the movement of these stem cells into the peripheral blood have increased stem-cell availability and decreased the pain and other complications associated with bone marrow (BM) harvesting. However, this major breakthrough, combined with recent critical findings about the nature of the hematopoietic stem cell, has caused the field of transplantation and particularly hematopoietic cell processing to explode. Major improvements in the identification, characterization, and storage of hematopoietic progenitor cells have almost trivialized standard progenitor-cell harvesting. The impetus is now toward the engineering of grafts to obtain high-quality, specifically designed grafts (devoid of malignant contaminating cells) and replenished in normal progenitors, demonstrating enhanced hematopoietic reconstituting ability. Selected individual cell populations can be manipulated to alter their proliferation, differentiation, or other characteristics in order to induce desired hematologic or immunologic roles. Monoclonal antibodies (mAbs) have been key players in each of these exciting steps, representing the cornerstone of hematopoietic cell graft therapies.

In this chapter, we will address the most important issues in progenitor-cell processing: progenitor-cell collection and ex vivo manipulation. We will focus primarily on strategies involving mAbs to eliminate neoplastic cells from hematopoietic grafts, to select normal progenitor cells, and to improve their engraftment potential, through a review of the principal malignancies where these crucial developments are currently occurring.

A. Quality of Stem-Cell Grafts

Cells with the capacity to engraft and to induce hematologic as well as immunologic reconstitution can be obtained from bone marrow and/or peripheral blood. In contrast to peripheral blood, the bone marrow is remarkably enriched in hematopoietic progenitor cells and, when sufficient numbers are collected (greater than 10^8 BM cells/kg), most collections are sufficiently homogeneous to obviate the need for extensive quality control. While circulating peripheral blood cells can support short- and long-term reconstitution, a finding documented several years ago in patients with chronic myelogenous leukemia (CML) (1,2), it is impossible to ensure that adequate numbers of progenitor cells are harvested by performing cell counts alone.

Short- and long-term colony-forming assays, particularly long-term culture-initiating cells (LTCICs) can be used to measure the progenitor-cell content of such grafts (3,4), but delays in the generation of results prompted a search for more accurate and immediate markers. The identification of the CD34 antigen on hematopoietic progenitor cells came as a blessing (5–7). The CD34 antigen is a 115-kDa heavily glycosylated type I transmembrane protein that is a member of the sialomucins (8,9). It is expressed on only a few bone marrow cells (less than 3%), including committed progenitors, but is of major importance because of its presence on the earlier primitive progenitors (LTCIC) (8,10). CD34 was also found on small-vessel endothelial cells (6,11) and embryonic fibroblasts (12), but these cells do not interfere with hematopoietic cell monitoring. The number of CD34 molecules seems particularly high ($CD34^{bright}$) on LTCIC, CFU-blast, and CFU-GEMM, a meaningful finding for the detection of these relatively rare cell populations (7,13,14). CFU-G, CFU-GM, BFU-E, and CFU-megakaryocytes usually display intermediate fluorescence intensity, while $CD34^{dim}$ represent the most mature lineage-committed progenitors (15,16).

Further characterization of CD34+ cells by studying coexpression of other antigens, such as CD38 and HLA-DR, enabled the identification of distinct clonogenic subpopulations. Indeed, CD34+CD38+DR+ cells, which comprise the overwhelming majority of CD34+ cells, express lineage-specific markers, such as CD33, CD19, and CD14, and generate mostly myeloid colonies. They cannot induce second-generation progeny (17), but the detection of circulating hematopoietic cells from the graft as early as a few days posttransplant suggests that the more mature progenitors are involved in early hematopoietic reconstitution after transplantation (18). CD34+CD38− cells are usually scarce, comprising only 3% of CD34+ cells, and do not express differentiation antigens (lin−), but can reconstitute long-term hematopoiesis, both in long-term cultures and in SCID mice (7,19,20). These cells can generate lymphoid and myeloid colonies and express the Thy-1 antigen (present on early undifferentiated progenitors) (17).

The low numbers of CD34+ cells circulating in the periphery (21,22) can be enhanced by the administration of a single high dose of cyclophosphamide (23,24) or of growth factors such as G-CSF, GM-CSF, PIXY321, IL-3, and IL-6 (25–27). However, when intensive chemotherapy is followed by cytokine administration, the yield of CD34+ cells is potentiated, reaching 100-fold higher CD34 counts and enabling the collection of CD34+ cells in numbers sufficient for stable engraftment after a single collection only (28–31).

CD34 positivity can be used to assess the quality of the graft and, when performed in peripheral blood on a daily basis, to predict even 1 day in advance the optimum time for leukopheresis (32,33). Complete hematopoietic engraftment is usually attained by infusing a minimum of 2 million CD34+ mobilized blood cells/kg patient weight (34–36). Nevertheless, in most instances, the percentage of CD34+ cells is so low that their monitoring involves extremely delicate flow-cytometric conditions and underlines the need for developing standardized procedures and quality control assessment tools. This is becoming particularly urgent, since engraftment characteristics may be better defined by measuring subsets of CD34+ cells, particularly CD38 expression (20,37).

B. Tumor-Cell Contamination in Stem-Cell Grafts

In most hematologic malignancies and several solid tumors, malignant cells infiltrate the bone marrow and can also be detected in peripheral blood. However, after patients are treated and attain a complete remission, it is unclear whether residual neoplastic cells in hematopoietic progenitor grafts can cause disease relapse. To address this question, the *neo* resistance gene was inserted via a retroviral vector into a portion of marrow grafts and administered to patients with acute myeloid leukemia and neuroblastomas. This and a similar study in patients with CML demonstrated that relapsing cells had the *neo* gene marker (38,39). These landmark studies clearly indicate that malignant cells from the infused graft can contribute to disease relapse. These findings come as logical conclusions to previous clinical studies showing that patients with acute myeloid leukemia (AML) (40) who received marrow grafts purged of their malignant cells had a significantly better disease-free survival (DFS) than those infused with unmanipulated cells. However, not all clinical studies arrive at the same conclusion (41), underlining the need for efficient and standardized purging methods as well as for a better characterization of patient and disease populations, particularly of the tumor-cell load in progenitor-cell grafts. At the same time, several approaches involving other monoclonal antibodies (mAbs) (42,43), cell culture (44,45), or the polymerase chain reaction (PCR) (46–50) were developed to identify malignant cells within stem-cell grafts. Such methods are able to detect malignant cells in the bone marrow of patients in complete clinical remission, whether they have leukemia, lymphoma, or solid tumors, such as neuroblastoma and breast cancer. In patients with active disease, the peripheral blood is often less infiltrated than bone marrow, and one wonders if this is also true at the time of stem-cell harvest. Some studies have suggested that, at the time of transplant, PCR and culture-detectable malignant cells are found in fewer patients' peripheral blood (PB) than in bone marrow (BM), suggesting that PB may be a better source of stem cells (51,52). In contrast, other studies found that malignant cells were detectable as often in PB as in BM (53–55). Moreover, effective progenitor-cell mobilization strategies may adversely affect the circulating tumor load, as observed in patients with multiple myeloma, breast cancer, and small-cell lung cancer (56–58), by releasing into the PB clonogenic malignant cells that previously adhered to BM stroma.

In order to determine differences in malignant-cell levels between BM, PB, and mobilized PB, we have developed a quantitative competitive PCR assay for the bcl-2/IgH rearrangement in patients with NHL (59). With this approach, we demonstrated that steady-state peripheral blood is, indeed, favored with fewer lymphoma cells than BM but that the difference is of less than 1 log of cells. Moreover, we could not identify a difference in the proportion of lymphoma cells present in BM and mobilized PB grafts. This suggests that mobilized PB progenitor-cell grafts, which usually contain more cells than do BM grafts, may actually harbor even more malignant cells than do BM grafts. These results argue strongly that the choice of the harvesting site should not be based primarily on concerns about tumor-cell infiltration, but rather on practical considerations regarding the accessibility of normal progenitors, time to hematologic reconstitution, and the potential presence of T-cells, NK cells, and other cells with antitumor activity in the stem-cell graft. In this context, contamination by tumor cells must be addressed separately. Tools such as quantitative competitive PCR may help identify the few patients in whom tumor cell infiltration may vary by several logs differences between BM and PB (59), yet the major impact of these methodologies will be in the evaluation of clinical trials, where they will provide an accurate measurement of the tumor-cell load before and after treatment. Quantitative PCR will also play a determining role in the design of informative clinical trials aimed at identifying the role of purging of progenitor-cell grafts. This will enable the randomization of patients based not only on clinical parameters, but on direct measurement of the number of malignant cells in progenitor-cell grafts, and provide a precise evaluation of the purging approach used. Indeed, a few studies have already demonstrated, using indirect or nonquantitative assays, that patients transplanted with either low numbers of or no leukemia cells in their grafts had an improved outcome (43,60,61). These results seem to indicate that more effective purging leads to better survival following autologous progenitor-cell transplantation. However, the persistence of malignant cells following purging may also reflect a higher tumor burden in these patients and failure of the preparative regimen to eradicate cells in the host rather than in the graft. Knowing that malignant cells both in the graft and in the host can contribute to relapse, we now need to address both issues. Interestingly, progenitor-cell manipulation may offer therapeutic options to both problems.

II. STRATEGIES TO GENERATE TUMOR-FREE PROGENITOR-CELL GRAFTS

Purging strategies have been available for close to 20 years, but this field has taken a major leap forward in the last few years with the development of highly effective and noninvasive strategies to harvest hematopoietic progenitors, of accurate monoclonal-antibody–based approaches to monitor these collections, and of readily available purging agents. Among purging strategies, physical methods are among the first developed and include albumin density gradients (62), counterflow elutriation (63,64), the use of lectins, such as soybean agglutinin, for T-cell depletion (65), and peanut agglutinin, for the depletion of myeloma cells (66), and hyperthermia with or without lipids (67). However, it is with agents such as 4-hydroperoxycyclophosphamide or mafosfamide, that purging was first performed on a broad scale and generated particularly encouraging results (68–71). Other classes of purging agents include: cortivazol, an unusual steroid with activity against lymphoid malignant cells (72), and photosensitizers (73–75). Cytokines such as IL-2 and IL-12 can potentiate the cytotoxic activity of T-cells and NK cells and enable the elimination of autologous malignant cells in stem-cell grafts (76–78). Molecular approaches using antisense oligonucleotides are also being used to eradicate leukemia cells in vitro (79). Finally, mAbs represent the most favored intermediate to generate tumor-cell-free grafts.

Indeed, mAbs, which were among the first agents used for in vitro purging (80), remain impressively appropriate for in vitro manipulation of progenitor-cell grafts. While the initial use of mAbs was limited to the specific elimination of neoplastic cells from stem-cell grafts, recent immunologic advances have enabled their use for the positive selection of normal hematopoietic stem cells. For the negative selection of malignant cells, these methods rely on the basic principle of antigen–antibody recognition. Different antigenic determinants on a tumor cell can lead to the development of multiple mAbs, which can then be selected according to their specificity for the target cell and absence on normal hematopoietic progenitor cells. In addition, the almost constant, simultaneous expression of antigens on both normal and malignant cells of the same lineage can usually be circumvented by replacement from earlier normal hematopoietic ontogeny. However, mAbs are not capable of either positive or negative selection by themselves, and they must rely on intermediate effector molecules.

Immunologic selection relies principally on the following mechanisms: (a) mAb-mediated complement (C) lysis: with complement originating either from animals (rabbits) or, in rare cases, humans (81–83); (b) toxin-mediated cytotoxicity in immunotoxins (ITs) (84,85); (c) radioisotopes (RIs) for radioimmunotherapy; (d) immunomagnetic beads, or microspheres (86,87); absorption substrates in columns or flasks (58), and (f) high-speed flow sorting (see Table 1). The first three approaches can be used for negative selection only, while the latter three combine the potential for both positive and negative selection. Several factors limiting the efficacy of mAb-mediated purging include: antigen density of the cell surface, affinity of the mAb for its ligand, nonspecific binding of the lytic component to other normal cells, antigenic heterogeneity on the surface of malignant cells between different patients and also within individual subjects, and, finally, antigenic modulation and internalization. Nevertheless, when these methods are used for the negative selection of malignant cells or positive selection of normal hematopoietic progenitor cells, most strategies result in tumor-cell depletions in the range of 3–6 logs.

Methodological limitations also vary according to the effector moiety involved. For example, the level of nonspecific toxicity against tumor cells varies from low (with immunomagnetic beads) to very high (with radionuclides). Complement-mediated purging requires only short incubation periods but is associated with higher levels of nonspecific toxicity, and variations in efficiency observed between different C lots imply the need for elaborate standardization procedures (83). In addition, relative resistance to C-mediated lysis has previously been documented (88,89). Purging with immunotoxins usually relies on very small amounts of immunoconjugates, which, at saturating concentrations, result in high levels of malignant-cell depletion (90,91). Immunotoxins are not harmful if inadvertently administered to patients, and could even add to the benefit of the procedure, since immunotherapy can act in synergy with conventional chemotherapeutic agents (92,93). Immunomagnetic beads and absorption columns distinguish themselves by the short time needed to reach high levels of efficacy, even with low target antigen density and while preserving high levels of progenitors (94). These versatile methodologies enable either the subtraction of malignant cells or the positive selection of normal hematopoietic progenitors from stem-cell grafts or their combination (95). However, both are limited by nonspecific cell trapping. Flow cytometry is probably the most specific selection process, enabling the sorting of cells assessed for the simultaneous presence and/or absence of various cell-surface antigens, but practical concerns about the number of cells necessary for engraftment necessitate sophisticated, high-speed apparatus. In addition, mAbs, usually of murine origin, that coat sorted cells are also administered to

Table 1
Characteristics of Selection Strategies

	Complement	Immunotoxins	Radionuclides	Immunomagnetic beads	Absorption substrates	High-speed flow sorting
Mechanism of selection	Negative	Negative	Negative	Positive and negative	Positive and negative	Positive and negative
Efficacy	High (3–4 logs)	High (3–5 logs)	High	High (3–6 logs)	High (3–4 logs)	High (3–4 logs)
Level of nonspecific toxicity	Moderate	Low	High	Low	Low	Low
Mechanism of nonspecificity or toxicity	C activation	Binding of toxin moiety	Irradiation of bystander cells	Trapping (parachute effect)	Trapping	Processing
Stability	Short (hours)	Long (months to years)	Short (hours)	Long (months to years)	Long (months to years)	Long (months to years)
Availability	Moderate	Wide	Limited	Wide	Wide	Limited
Standardization	Difficult	Easy	Difficult	Easy	Easy	Intermediate
Regulatory concerns	mAb and C of animal source	mAb and toxin delivery	mAb and radionuclide delivery	mAb and bead escape	mAb escape	Conjugated mAb delivery

patients. Finally, radioimmunotherapy implies emissions contained within a short range to prevent nonspecific elimination of normal cells but of sufficient depth to eliminate malignant cells from cell-surface binding sites or internalized vacuoles. These delicate considerations, added to the restricted availability and extensive standardization and confinement requirements, justify the preferential implementation of these agents in vivo rather than in vitro. Overall, mAbs are burdened by a number of obstacles related either to the characteristics of antigen expression on malignant cells or to mechanisms of toxicity or elimination through effector molecules. Nevertheless, their specificity remains the prominent feature, which, along with their high reliability and broad availability, justifies their foremost position as stem-cell processing agents.

III. PRINCIPAL CLINICAL APPLICATIONS

A. Acute Myelogenous Leukemia

The role of autologous PCT in front-line therapy of acute myelogenous leukemia (AML) is a subject of debate. A large, multicenter, randomized trial has demonstrated that patients undergoing autologous PCT have an improved disease-free survival (DFS) over those treated with conventional-dose chemotherapy. Yet when patients in the latter group relapsed and were treated with autologous PCT, their prognosis reached that of the former group of patients, indicating the high salvage potential of transplantation and the possibility of delaying autologous PCT until relapse (96,97). In addition, recent improvements in the therapy of patients with a t(8;21), t(15;17) or inv(16) imply that these low-risk patients should probably not be subjected initially to autologous PCT. In contrast, for patients with relapsed disease, conventional chemotherapy or autologous PCT with unpurged grafts rarely results in long-term cure unless marrow grafts are collected during the first complete remission or extensive chemotherapeutic approaches are used to purge leukemia cells in vivo. Thus, the high DFS of second- or subsequent-remission patients undergoing autologous 4-hydroperoxycyclophosphamide-purged PCT were particularly supportive of the benefit of purging (68). In addition, a comparison of outcomes for first-remission AML patients treated with autologous PCT showed that those receiving mafosfamide-purged grafts had a disease-free survival superior to those receiving unmanipulated grafts (40,98). This is consistent with previous studies indicating that patients with the highest levels of elimination of myeloid progenitors benefited most from the purging procedure (60). Altogether, these studies underline variations in purging efficacy not only between purging methods, but also between individuals, and, not surprisingly, suggest that effective elimination of malignant cells is important for optimal results. These findings are also in line with the observation that patients transplanted in the first 6 months postremission benefit most from purging

(40), since those are the highest-risk patients and those most likely to harbor the highest levels of tumor-cell infiltration. However, as interesting and compelling as they are, these results mandate confirmation in large, well-controlled, randomized trials. As shown in Table 2, several clinical studies using 4-HC or mafosfamide purging generated interesting survival characteristics. Unfortunately, such chemotherapeutic purging procedures are complicated by the need to adjust carefully for red blood cell number, the nature and concentration of nucleated cells, as well as plasma concentration (99). In addition, optimal protection of normal hematopoietic progenitors necessitates the addition of another agent, amifostine (100). Because purging mandates the development of easy and standardizable methodologies, efforts were made to take advantage of the specificity of mAbs to direct cytotoxic reagents toward antigens found on AML cells.

Acute myeloid leukemia is a logical target for mAb-mediated purging, since the antigens found on the cell surface are well characterized and since AML progenitor cells can be evaluated in vitro. Immunization strategies resulted in the production of mAbs directed at CD14 (AML-2-23) and CD15 (PM-81) (101), which react with the overwhelming majority of total AML cells (more than 76%) and clonogenic AML cells (30 and 65% for each antigen, respectively) (102). The CD14 antigen is found primarily on AML cells of monocyte lineage (FAB-M4 and -M5) and is usually considered a relatively mature antigen. CD15 is recognized through its particularly immunogenic lacto-N-fucopentose III (LNF) moiety, an epitope with increased expression following neuraminidase treatment (103). Interestingly, the latter procedure increases LNF expression on malignant but not normal progenitors, resulting in improved purging efficacy and sustained engraftment (104).

Bone marrow transplantation with a single Anti-CD15 mAb and C-purged autologous graft was evaluated in seven patients and resulted in relatively rapid neutrophil engraftment (median of 20 days) (105). In this study, relapsing AML cells in two patients were found to lack expression of CD15, a finding that reinforces efforts to target antigens found on clonogenic AML progenitor cells. Autologous PCT using a combination of Anti-CD14 and -CD15 mAb and complement purging was used in 63 patients with various stages of AML, ranging from first to third remission and first relapse. Engraftment occurred at a median of 37 days for neutrophils and 44 days for platelets (106). The long-term DFS was 31% for patients in second or third complete remission (CR), 71% for patients in CR1, and even a 41% DFS in patients with relapsed disease. These interesting results persist in an update reporting on a total of 115 patients (107).

Robertson et al. rather targeted AML cells through CD33, a 67-kDa surface molecule, homologous to sialoadhesin and a member of the immunoglobulin superfamily (108–113). This sialic acid–dependent adhesion molecule is expressed on more than 80% of AML cells (109) and on most leukemic progenitors in at least 95% of AML patients (102). MY9, the Anti-CD33 mAb, with complement

Table 2 Autologous Bone Marrow Transplantation in AML

Group	Purging	n	Median age (range)	CR or Rel	Reparative regimen	Median no. infused (cells × 10^8/kg)	Days to neutrophils (0.5 × 10^9/L)	Days to platelets (20 × 10^9/L)	Relapse (2–8 yrs)	Overall survival (2–8 yrs)	DFS (2–8 yrs)
Lowenberg et al (135)	No	32	40 (16–58)	1	CY + TBI	1.5	39	63	60%	37%	35%
Sierra et al (286)	No	43	25 (6–51)	1/2/3	CY + TBI		27	47	48 ± 11%		48 ± 11%
									54 ± 14%		28 ± 11%
Mitus et al (287)	No	27	42 (17–62)	1	BU + CY		31 (allo + auto)	32* (allo + auto)	38%		45%
McMillan et al (288)	No	76 [26]	40 (16–55)	1	BDCYAT		22 [27]	34* [38]*	47% [30%]	55% [73%]	50% [67%]
Mehta et al (289)	No	74	31 (5–53)	1	Mel + TBI	2.2	32	59*	53%		34%
Stein et al (290)	No	44	39 (16–55)	1	TBI + VP-16 + Y	2.3 BM 4.2 PB	28	87*	33%		61%
Petersen et al (291)	4-HC	21		Rel1	BU + CY ± TBI	4.3	28	55	30 ± 26%	48%	45 ± 22%
	No	26		CR2		2.7	29	74	44 ± 23%	35%	32 ± 18%
Linker et al (292)	4-HC	35	39 (17–59)	1	BU + VP-16	2.4	31	69*	19 ± 8%		79 ± 8%
		27	38 (15–58)	2			37	180*	23 ± 10%		42 ± 10%
Laporte et al (293)	Maf	64	36 (16–53)	1	CY + TBI		30	90	25%		58%
	Maf	20	32 (17–53)	2					48%		34%
Selvaggi et al (106)	PM-81 + AML-2-23 + C	7	42 (35–52)	1	CY ± TBI ± BU	0.4	33	50		71%	71%
		45	36 (11–57)	2/3		0.3	37	42		58%	31%
		11	27 (16–53)	Rel1		0.4	41	49		35%	45%
Ball et al (107)	PM-81 + AML-2-23 + C	8		1	CY + TBI					71%	71%
		13		1	BU + VP-16					58%	50%
		44		2/3	BU + CY					50%	41%
		27		2/3	CY + TBI					33%	26%
		23		Rel1	BU + CY					37%	29%
Robertson et al (112)	Anti-My9 + C	12	40 (25–49)	1/2/3	CY + TBI ± BU	0.4	43	92			33 ± 14%
Roy et al (241)	Anti-My9-bR	11	40 (18–58)	1	BU + CY	0.5	42	66		64%	62%
		14		2/3						33%	33%

Abbreviations—*n*: number of patients; CR: complete remission; Rel: relapse; TBI: total-body irradiation; Maf: mafosfamide; BU: busulfan; DFS: disease-free survival; C: complement; 4-HC: 4-hydroperoxycyclophosphamide; CY: cyclophosphamide; BDCYAT: BCNU+doxorubicin+cyclophosphamide+cytarabine+6-thioguanine; Mel: melphalan; *: days to 50 × 10^9 platelets/L.

resulted in 3.6 logs of depletion of the HL-60 AML cells but almost all normal CFU-GM progenitors (99%) and half of CFU-GEMM (109,111). Twelve AML patients had their marrow purged with MY9 + C; 10 of these patients were in CR2 (112,113). Neutrophils engrafted at a median of 43 days, and platelets at a median of 92 days following autologous PCT. These patients had a 33% DFS, with four patients remaining in continuous CR 3–5 years post-PCT. Results from clonogenic assays suggest that it is possible to eliminate clonogenic AML progenitors and that the few normal progenitors infused were capable of hematologic reconstitution. These results also suggest that engraftment originated mostly from CFU-GEMM escaping elimination or from earlier progenitors, where CD33 is not expressed.

In order to increase the efficacy of purging, the addition of chemotherapeutic agents such as 4-hydroperoxycyclophosphamide (4-HC) and VP-16 (92), and ara-C and VP-16 (114), or of an anti-CD55 mAb directed at the decay-accelerating factor were studied. These combinations potentiate cytotoxicity and, in the latter case, protect host cells from damage by autologous complement (115). Complement-mediated cytotoxicity is, however, complicated by its limited availability, variable efficacy, and nonspecific toxicity, which mandate extensive quality control (83), and by its animal origin, implying important regulatory issues (116). Immunoconjugates could offer an interesting alternative, by providing efficient, standardized, and pharmaceutical-grade reagents. Radioactive immunoconjugates incorporating the Anti-CD33 mAb and iodine-131 can bind to and eliminate AML cells in vivo (117). However, implementation of such antigens for in vitro progenitor cell graft purging would be difficult, since the irradiation reaches 50 cell diameters and would inexorably destroy stem cells in its path. Another option is the conjugation of mAbs such as Anti-CD33, Anti-CD13, and Anti-CD14 to cytotoxic molecules such as ricin and gelonin (111,118).

The ricin molecule consists of two chains, A and B, the former chain being the cytotoxic moiety with 60S ribosome-inactivating potential, and the latter chain essentially representing a galactose-binding molecule (119,120). Since galactose is a ubiquitous residue, several strategies were devised to obviate nonspecific binding and toxicity through the toxin. Such strategies include the selection of single-chain toxins without galactose-binding sites (e.g., saporin) and linkage to mAbs specific for myeloid lineage antigens, as performed for mAbs LAM3 and LAM7 (121). Alternatively, lactose can be added in vitro to block ricin-binding competitively while enabling specific mAb attachment and elimination of AML cells (118). This technically simple and effective approach limits such ITs to in vitro use. Removal of the ricin B-chain, to eliminate nonspecific binding, with linkage of the A-chain to the desired mAb can result in highly effective purging (122). However, the activity of the conjugate then depends on the intrinsic internalization potential of the mAb. Because few mAbs show effective spontaneous internalization and because ricin B-chain is also involved in the translocation potential of ITs, galactose binding sites on native ricin were chemically blocked (123,124). Conjugation of blocked-ricin to the CD33 mAb, resulting in an Anti-MY9 blocked ricin (Anti-MY9-bR), can eliminate more than 4 logs of AML cell lines and 3 logs of primary AML cells (111). Approximately 10% of normal CFU-GM, which also express CD33, were spared, along with half of CFU-GEMM, corresponding to the proportion of cells with CD33 surface expression. Interestingly, the IT conjugate, which incorporates the same Anti-CD33 mAb as that used for C purging, eliminated more AML cells and fewer normal progenitors than its C counterpart. This raises the possibility of internalization kinetics favorable to the IT approach. Moreover, ITs are easy to use, stable, can be standardized, do not imply sophisticated equipment and could have in vivo therapeutic potential.

Purging with Anti-MY9-bR was used in a clinical Phase I/II study at Maisonneuve-Rosemont Hospital, Montreal, and Dana-Farber Cancer Institute, Boston. Twenty-five patients with a median age of 40, (range 18–58 years) underwent a bone marrow harvest just prior to the autologous PCT and Anti-MY9-bR purging. Most patients enrolled were in second or subsequent CR (14 patients), while 11 patients were in first CR. The preparative regimen consisted of busulfan and cyclophosphamide. As predicted, the IT treatment eliminated a majority of myeloid progenitors. Nevertheless, myeloid engraftment occurred 42 days after PCT (range 17–64 days) and platelet engraftment 66 days after PCT (range 16 to 307). Patients receiving IT-treated grafts had a more gradual recovery of myeloid cells than did patients receiving C-purged grafts, with an earlier time to a neutrophil count greater than $0.1 \times 10^9/L$ ($p = 0.0005$) (113). Five of 13 patients transplanted in CR2 or 3, and 7 of the 11 patients in CR1 are in continuous unmaintained remission more than 2 years after transplantation.

For patients in first remission, autologous unpurged marrow transplantation seems to generate survival and DFS rates either better or comparable to conventional chemotherapy (96,125). Thus, the issue of purging of progenitor cell grafts in a disease where malignant cells infiltrate primarily the marrow and where molecular markers substantiate their contribution to relapse is a major one, which should have been clarified by now. While high-risk patients can now be identified, the selection of the most appropriate target antigen to eliminate leukemic progenitors still represents an important obstacle. Indeed, surface antigen on AML cells usually vary according to FAB subtype, with few preponderant antigens (126,127). Even AML cells from a single patient can be heterogeneous in terms of antigen expression (128–131). The identification of antigens on clonogenic cells is even more difficult and is further complicated by sharing of several antigens on leukemic and normal progenitors (102,131). The identification of AML clonogenic precursors among the very early CD34+CD38− cells also further complicates the issue (132–134). The number of cells infused will also be an important factor to monitor, for a limited number of persistent AML precursors could probably be eradicated by the immune system.

It is possible that purging of stem-cell grafts may impair their myeloid engraftment potential, but this may also be related to underlying disease and treatment characteristics (135). In addition, the earlier-mentioned clinical studies clearly indicate that mAb-mediated purging not only is feasible but usually results in improved DFS. Such interesting results warrant confirmatory randomized double-blind clinical studies to evaluate purging. Unfortunately, such large efforts will be possible and justified only when pathophysiologic and practical concerns about the nature of AML cells and their manipulation are resolved.

B. Chronic Myelogenous Leukemia

Chronic myelogenous leukemia (CML) originates from the clonal expansion of a pluripotent hematopoietic stem cell and can easily be identified by the presence of a Philadelphia chromosome (Ph) with a *bcr-abl* fusion gene resulting from a reciprocal translocation between the long arms of chromosome 22 (*bcr*) and chromosome 9 (*abl*). In patients with CML, complete remissions are uncommon, and both normal and Ph+ hematopoietic stem cells are present in the bone marrow (BM) as well as in peripheral blood (PB) (136–138). In addition, infusions of retrovirally marked progenitor cells were found to contribute to disease relapse after autologous PCT (39). Thus, attempts to purge Ph+ cells from CML patient grafts seem justified.

In vivo purging consists of intensive chemotherapy induction and/or interferon-alpha therapy followed by harvesting of peripheral blood stem cells or bone marrow (139–144). This approach usually promotes the collection of normal progenitors, mostly in patients in the early stages of their disease. Unfortunately, stem-cell grafts remain contaminated by CML cells, even when obtained from patients with favorable risk characteristics, substantiating efforts to develop in vitro purging methodologies. Bone marrow or PB harvests can be treated ex vivo with chemotherapeutic agents such as mafosfamide (145), 5-fluorouracil (146), and eilatin (147), with gamma interferon (148), with photosensitizing agents (75), with anti-sense oligonucleotides (149), or with long-term culture systems (150–152).

Cytogenetic analysis has revealed that normal early progenitors (long-term culture-initiating cells or LTCICs) are present in the PB and BM of patients in chronic phase at diagnosis (153). Podesta et al. showed that in six out of eight newly diagnosed CML patients, the number of normal LTCICs far exceeded the number of leukemic LTCICs and was, in addition, much higher than the corresponding number of LTCICs present in normal individuals (153). However, both normal and leukemic LTCICs were CD34+CD71−, and CD38 or Thy-1 expression could not discriminate between the two cell populations (154). These findings are in agreement with previous immunophenotypic characterization of LTCICs in normal BM (155). On the other hand, Verfaillie et al. demonstrated that selection of the CD34+DR− population yields primarily Ph− LTCICs, especially in patients at the early stages of the disease (156). In fact, long-term BM cultures of CD34+DR− cells yielded secondary colony-forming cells (CFCs) similar in numbers and phenotype to CD34+DR− cells from normal BM. This group demonstrated further that purification of normal LTCICs can be achieved on both experimental and clinical scales, thus providing an important source of normal cells for future autografts in chronic-phase CML patients. Moreover, while normal (Ph−) and leukemic (Ph+) cells from chronic-phase CML patients repopulate the BM of sublethally irradiated severe combined immunodeficient (SCID) mice, 30–90 days after transplantation, the majority (70%) of progenitors found in the engrafted SCID BM are normal (Ph−) and of human origin (132). This preferential engraftment and expansion of normal hematopoietic progenitors in vivo provides additional arguments for autologous PCT, even in instances where purging cannot completely eradicate CML cells from grafts.

While long-term culture conditions can select for normal progenitor cells ex vivo, another appealing option, which involves only short-term culture methods, has been recently identified. This strategy takes advantage of the capacity of cytokines, such as macrophage inflammatory protein-1 alpha (MIP-1α), to inhibit selectively the proliferation of normal, but not CML, progenitors (157,158). Normal CD34+ cells are thus sequestered into the compartment of cytokine nonresponsive (CNR) cells, a small population of cells that do not respond to cytokine activation, remain quiescent, continue to express CD34, and are enriched in LTCICs (159). Based on these studies, Veena et al. immunomagnetically selected CD34+ cells from chronic-phase CML patients and, following 10-day cultures with MIP-1α, induced the preferential sequestration of *bcr-abl* negative hematopoietic progenitor cells among CNR cells (160). Moreover, upon seeding of these CNR cells in secondary long-term cultures, the percentage of *bcr-abl*+ progenitors went from 100% to below 20% from day 0 to day 28. Therefore, cytokines can be used in combination with immunologic selection of CD34+ cells to modify the differential kinetics of proliferation of normal and malignant progenitors and to decrease tumor-cell contamination levels.

Finally, selection of normal progenitor cells based on CD34 expression and other immunologic markers, along with ex vivo expansion of this very small cell population, can lead to the production of clinical-scale autologous grafts. Indeed, when CD34+DR− selected cells from CML patients are cultured for 2 weeks in stroma-conditioned medium + IL-3 with or without stem-cell factor, there is a significant expansion of normal CFU-GM and LTCICs along with maintenance of natural killer progenitor cells (161). Similarly, the selection of CD34+CD38− cells followed by their expansion in a serum-free medium containing FLT3L,

Steel Factor, IL-3, IL-6, and G-CSF led to the preferential decrease of Ph+ LTCICs (151).

Autologous PCT for CML has been performed for many years, but in a relatively limited number of institutions. A compilation of data from eight major transplant centers has shown that autologous transplantation leads to prolonged survival (3–7.5 years post-PCT) in patients transplanted in first chronic phase, with low procedure-related toxicity and adequate engraftment (162). Clinical outcome deteriorated for patients transplanted with more advanced disease: median survival was 36 months for patients in accelerated phase, and all patients at the blast crisis stage died within 3 years after transplantation. In vitro purging was used at only two centers, where either gamma-interferon (148) or long-term culture (150) was used to deplete Ph+ progenitors. Relapse rates were not improved in patients receiving purged versus unpurged grafts, but eligibility criteria and stem-cell sources varied between centers, and the small number of patients in each center prevents statistical comparisons of adequate power.

Following autologous transplantation, most patients show persistence of *bcr-abl*+ cells detectable by PCR. While interferon has proven capable of enhanced control over residual CML cells, it is likely that if the host immune system could be recruited at this time, when the leukemic load is at its lowest, similar and potentially better responses could be observed. One strategy to enhance host reactivity against CML cells is the administration of antigen-presenting cells. Dendritic cells are highly efficient antigen-presenting cells and are probably the most effective stimulators of T-cell responses, both in vitro and in vivo (163–165). In addition, dendritic cells generate not only class II (166,167) but also class I MHC-restricted cytotoxic T-lymphocytes against murine tumor cells (168–170). Moreover, the scarce CD1a+ dendritic cells can now be induced to proliferate and mature from CD34+ precursors in BM (171,172). Dendritic cells are not the only cells capable of inducing host reactivity, and several strategies could be devised to take advantage of the specificity of mAbs to isolate and administer cells with potential for immunization. Thus, cellular manipulation has the potential to go beyond the processing of stem-cell grafts and to serve as a crucial intermediate for active immunotherapy.

C. Acute Lymphoblastic Leukemia

Acute lymphoblastic leukemia (ALL) is a heterogeneous disease affected by numerous parameters, including patient age, clinical presentation, cytogenetics, and immunophenotype. Thus, a standardized therapeutic approach for this disease has been difficult to establish. The treatment of children with ALL usually consists of conventional-dose chemotherapy regimens and leads to high complete remission (CR) rates reaching approximately 95% and long-term DFS rates of over 60% (173,174). Unfortunately, conventional chemotherapy regimens yield less impressive results in adult patients. Despite high CR rates, long-term DFS rates in adults treated with combination chemotherapy range only between 20% and 35% (175–177).

Such results leave considerable room for improvement, and the lack of HLA-compatible donors in a majority of patients has prompted the development of autologous PCT strategies to try to improve the outcome of adults with ALL and pediatric patients with poor prognostic features. Preparative regimens include high doses of cyclophosphamide, etoposide, or melphalan in combination with total-body irradiation, and, as shown in Table 3, most trials take advantage of progenitor-cell purging (178–180). Chemotherapy has been used for purging of autologous ALL progenitor-cell grafts, with mafosfamide and 4-HC being the agents most widely used for such purposes (181,182). Immunologic approaches remain the cornerstone of stem-cell purging. Indeed, antigens on the surface of lymphoblasts, both normal and malignant, are well characterized; mAbs can specifically target these antigens, and third-party (toxins, beads) molecules can induce high levels of elimination of target cells.

1. Antigens on the Surface of ALL Cells

Acute lymphoblastic leukemia cells are subdivided by immunologic criteria based on the B- or T-cell origin of leukemic lymphoblasts. The majority are B-lineage cells, the rest deriving primarily from T-cells. The maturation stages of B-lineage leukemia cells, hence their classification and also their prognosis, are defined by specific combinations of surface antigens and by their antigen receptor gene rearrangements (183–185). The cell-surface molecules HLA-DR, CD19, CD10, CD9, and CD24 are expressed on both proliferating and nonproliferating ALL cells and become appealing targets, allowing not only for the detection but also the elimination of clonogenic ALL cells (184,186,187). Monoclonal antibodies with potential for antileukemia therapy may not all identify B-cell maturational stages, for a mAb directed at *bcr-abl*+ ALL cells also recognizes a 90-kDa antigen also present on neutrophils and AML-M2 cells but not normal CD19+ cells (188). However, this mAb, KOR-SA3544, awaits further characterization.

An immunophenotypic classification can also be applied to T-lineage ALL cells where three groups have been identified: CD7+CD2−CD5− leukemic prothymocytes, CD7+(CD2 or CD5)+CD3− leukemic immature thymocytes, and CD7+CD2+CD5+CD3+ leukemic mature thymocytes. These leukemic maturational stages were useful in identifying a worse 4-year event-free survival in pro-thymocytic leukemia patients treated under treatment protocols of the Children's Cancer Group (189). Immunophenotyping can therefore be used as a prognostic indicator, helping define which ALL patients are best suited for more aggressive approaches, as is the case for patients with poorly differentiated T-lineage ALL, and which antigen to target in stem-cell purging.

2. Purging Strategies

Immunological purging methods are based primarily upon the binding of mAbs to specific antigen markers on the surface of target cells. As previously discussed, such mAbs are not usually cytotoxic and depend on an effector component such as rabbit complement, immunomagnetic beads, or toxins. Interestingly, bispecific CD3/CD19 mAbs alone were used in vitro to activate PB mononuclear cells, namely, CD3+ T-cells, of ALL patients in remission (190). The anti-CD19 fraction of the bispecific antibody then binds to one of the numerous adjacent malignant B-cells. The new proximity created between CD19+ cells and activated T-cells leads to the destruction of malignant B-cells.

Complement (C)-mediated lysis of ALL cells has been achieved in preclinical and clinical settings using either a single mAb, J5 (CD10) (80), or combinations of several mAbs characterizing the ALL cells, J2 (CD9) + J5 (CD10) (180,191), BA-1 (CD24) + BA-2 (CD9) + BA-3 (CD10) (192), or FMC-8 (CD9) + WM-21 (CD10) (193). Monoclonal antibody cocktails have been found to deplete up to 5 logs of tumor cells, whereas 2–3 logs of clonogenic tumor cells were depleted by single mAbs (194,195). Other factors important for efficient depletion include antibody and target-cell concentrations, type (human or rabbit), and dilution of complement, as well as the number of mAb and complement treatments (196,197).

Naturally occurring toxins, such as native ricin, ricin A-chain, deglycosylated ricin A-chain, and blocked whole ricin form, have been conjugated to mAbs specific for ALL cells. These immunotoxins are directed at B- (CD19) or T- (CD5 and CD7) antigens, which are preponderant on most ALL cells and their clonogenic subsets (91,198). Efforts to increase the biologic half-life of immunotoxins have resulted in the development of several linker molecules with potential for increasingly stable attachment of toxins to mAbs. However, linkers designed to hinder the in vivo breakdown of the toxin/antibody disulfide bond do not necessarily increase immunotoxin efficacy. In fact, anti-CD7 immunotoxins made with the ''standard'' heterobifunctional cross-linker *N*-succinimidyl-3(2-pyridyl-dithiolproprionate) (SPDP) demonstrate pharmacokinetics and biodistribution similar to those of more complex linkers (199). In this case, production factors and cytotoxicity profile against CD7+ leukemia cells favor the development of the more conventional former conjugate for both in vitro and in vivo use. Also, intracellular signaling by immunotoxins may differ from signaling from mAb alone, and this may actually affect the activity of the immunotoxin. Indeed, CD19 modulation induced by Anti-B4-bR was higher than that induced by Anti-B4 mAb

Table 3 Autologous Bone Marrow Transplantation for Patients with ALL

Authors	Purging	N	Age range	Remission status	Preparative regimen	Relapse	DFS (3–4 y)
Carey et al. (178)	No purging	15	18–51	CR1+	Mel + TBI	52%	48%
Rizzoli et al. (210)	Maf or no purging	82	2–57	CR1-2+	CY + TBI		38% CR1 27% CR2
Schroeder et al. (294)	Campath-1 or no purging	24	0–16	CR2-3+	Mel + TBI		45%
Powles R et al. (295)	Campath-1 or no purging	38	15–52	CR1+		31%	56% CR1+
Gorin et al. (211)	mAb + C or Maf or no purging	438	1–55	CR1-2+	Multiple CT ± TBI		41% CR1 29% CR2
Cahn et al. (214)	mAbs + C ± Maf	26	2–38	CR1-3+ Rel	TBI + Ara C + Mel	62%	28%
Kersey et al. (212)	B: Anti-CD9 + CD10 + CD24 + C T: Anti-CD3 ± CD5 ± CD18 + Ricin	45	0–50	CR1-3+	CY + TBI ± 6MP ± MTX	79%	20%
Janossy et al. (196)	Anti-CD10 ± CD19 ± CD7 + C	36	6–42	CR1-3+	Multiple CT + TBI		90% CR1 57% CR2+
Simonsson et al. (207)	B: Anti-CD10 ± CD19 + C T: Anti-CD7 + C	54	3–55	CR1-3+	TBI + multiple CT		65% CR1 31% CR2+
Sallan et al. (213)	Anti-CD9 + CD10 + C	44	1–14	CR1-3+ Rel	CY + Ara C + VM26 + TBI		29%
Gilmore et al. (296)	B: Anti-CD10 ± CD19 + C T: Anti-CD7 + C	27	11–45	CR1+	CY + TBI + Ara C	65%	32%

Antibodies for Graft Processing and Purging

Study	Purging	N	Status	Conditioning	Survival	Relapse
Schmid et al. (179)	B: Anti-CD10 + CD19 + CD24 + IB T: Anti-CD2 + CD3 + CD5 + CD7 + IB	22	1–16	CR2-3+ Rel	VP16 + TBI	80%	18%
Uckun et al. (122)	B: Anti-CD9 + CD10 + CD24 + C + 4HC or Anti-CD19 – PAP + 4HC T: Anti-CD5 + CD7 – Ricin + 4HC	83	1–48	CR1-3+	TBI ± AraC ± VP-16 ± CTX	85%	15%
Soiffer et al. (297)	Anti-CD9 + CD10 + C	22	18–54	CR1-3+ Rel	CY ± AraC ± VM26 + TBI	75%	20%
Doney et al. (208)	mAb + C or 4HC	89	2–47	CR1-3+ Rel	CY ± VP16 + TBI	27% 69% 90%	50% CR1 21% CR2+ 0% Rel
Morishima et al. (209)	Anti-CD10 + C	17	4–51	CR1-3+ Rel	Multiple CT + TBI		75% CR1 20% CR2 0% CR3
Fiere et al. (41)	B: Anti-CD10 + CD19 + C ± Maf T: Anti-CD2 + CD5 + CD7 ± Maf	63	15–50	CR1+	CY ± TBI	51%	
Garcia et al. (298)	mAbs + C	32	4–40	CR1+	CY + TBI	41%	50%

Abbreviations—N: number of patients; Rel: relapse; 6MP: 6-mercaptopurine; MTX: methotrexate; TBI: total-body irradiation; CY: cyclophosphamide; B: B-cells; T: T-cells; C: complement; IB: immunomagnetic beads; Maf: mafosfamide; Mel: Melphalan, CT: chemotherapy, 4HC: 4-hydroperoxycyclophosphamide.

alone, and was associated with increased internalization of the immunotoxin (200). These findings suggest that the residual binding activity of the blocked ricin B-chain to cell-surface molecules plays an important role in the greater calcium fluxes and greater internalization rate of Anti-B4-bR, and may modify the functional mechanism of cellular intoxication by the immunotoxin.

Immunomagnetic bead–mediated purging is another alternative to rabbit complement–mediated purging. Magnetic beads coated with mAbs against either B-cells (Anti-CD10, -CD19, -CD24) or T-cells (anti-CD2, -CD3, -CD5, -CD7) were shown to sequester more than 4 logs of malignant cells in preclinical studies. As described for mAb and C purging, a double incubation with ABL2 (CD9) and Bg4 (CD10) mAbs, in a two-step immunomagnetic bead procedure, was sufficient to achieve a 3-log reduction of B-lineage tumor cells (201). Moreover, the high levels of depletion achieved with immunomagnetic beads still lead to good preservation of normal hematopoietic progenitors (202,203) and to complete and stable engraftment even in patients with high-risk disease and exposure to previously intense chemotherapy protocols (179,204). Similar 2–4-log depletions of Ph+ ALL cells and adequate engraftment were reported for purging cells with AB4 (HLA-DR), Anti-CD19 and -CD10 bead combinations (205,206). This remained true for both bone marrow and mobilized peripheral blood grafts. However, the capacity to mobilize progenitor cells decreased with the number of intensive chemotherapy courses (205).

3. Clinical Trials of Autologous Progenitor-Cell Transplantation

Several clinical trials of autologous progenitor-cell transplantation (PCT) for the treatment of patients with ALL who do not have a histocompatible donor have been reported. As shown in Table 3, most studies used mAbs and C as the preferred purging option. Although mAb selection varied between centers, targeted antigens were mainly CD9, CD10, and CD19 for B-lineage ALL, and CD5 and CD7 for T-ALL. Immunological purging used for patients in CR1 induces DFS rates higher than 50% at 3–4 years in the majority of studies (41,196,207–209). However, when autologous harvests are unpurged or treated with mafosfamide, poorer DFS rates are observed (178,210,211). For high-risk patients (CR2+), DFS rates at 3–4 years posttransplant average 25% (122,179,180,196,207–209,212–214). The latter group of patients is also characterized by high relapse rates regardless of purging (122,179,180,208,214). Autologous PCT with multiple-mAb-purged marrow grafts was compared to unrelated transplantation in a nonrandomized study (215). Autologous PCT led to significantly lower transplant-related mortality, while unrelated PCT offered greater protection against relapse. Older patients and those with more advanced disease had increased treatment-related mortality. Nevertheless, both strategies resulted in long-term survival for high-risk patients and with comparable results, particularly in the younger population.

Randomized studies are definitely needed to define the application of these different treatment strategies, but ALL patient populations are so heterogeneous that the number of patients to enroll remains formidable. A potential answer may be a better classification of patients and their diseases. In this context, a quantitative minimal residual disease detection assay, combining fluorescence-activated multiparameter flow cytometry and cell sorting with a leukemic progenitor colony assay, was devised to try to identify the contribution of residual leukemia cells in the graft to relapse (43). Not surprisingly, grafts with a higher leukemic content were associated with a higher probability of relapse. However, definitive conclusions cannot be drawn, since such tools also measure the endogenous tumor mass that may evade toxicity by the preparative regimen. Thus, it would be important to evaluate the leukemogenic potential of autologous grafts before and after purging, and in the patient before and after conditioning. Interestingly, new strategies are being developed to measure the self-renewal potential of B-lineage ALL cells from high-risk cases (216). Such stroma-based culture methods, which yield high levels of leukemic cell growth, represent appealing tools to measure leukemic cell loads accurately and present significant potential, not only for clarifying purging issues, but also for identifying high-risk candidates for aggressive therapy.

D. Non-Hodgkin's Lymphoma

1. In Vitro Negative-Selection Purging Methods

The majority of non-Hodgkin's lymphoma cells are of B-cell origin and display cell-surface antigens characteristic of a mature immunophenotype. However, the nature of the clonogenic lymphoma cells remains obscure. To bypass the problem of identifying target antigens present on clonogenic cells, several groups have relied on chemotherapeutic agents, primarily 4-hydroperoxycyclophosphamide or mafosfamide (217,218), to purge malignant cells from stem-cell grafts. Nevertheless, the identification of conditions to culture non-Hodgkin's lymphoma cells of both high and low-grade has provided important insights into the nature of such cells, and substantiates indirect evidence that NHL cells, which harbor a more mature immunophenotype than ALL cells, also have clonogenic precursors of a more mature antigenic profile (184). Moreover, several in vitro approaches are able to eliminate more than 3 and sometimes up to 6 logs of malignant lymphoma cells by targeting antigens present on the majority of these cells, but with a pattern of expression spanning early pre-B-cells. Indeed, when mAbs directed at the B-lineage antigens, such as CD10, CD20, and B5, are used individually with complement, they can eliminate 2–3 logs of lymphoma cells, and when used in combination these mAbs eliminate clonogenic lymphoma cell lines below the level of detection of limiting dilution assay (more than 4.5 logs) (61,83). Importantly, these experiments performed on cell lines are corroborated by studies evaluating the efficacy of purging on patient lymphoma cells. These studies demonstrate that purging can eliminate all cells harboring the 14;18 translocation using a highly sensitive PCR assay (53,61). In addition, after purging with CD20 or a combination of Anti-CD10, Anti-CD20, and B5 mAbs, the bcl-2-IgH rearrangement is detectable in only half of patients where rearranged cells are present before purging (61). Similarly, after mAb- and rabbit-C-mediated purging with anti-CD9, -CD10, -CD19, and -CD20, the PCR-amplified signal is reduced, with no reduction of CFU-GM with purging (53,61). In both previous studies, the probability of eliminating malignant cells from BM grafts with morphologic involvement by lymphoma cells is much lower than from those without microscopically detectable cells, confirming the limitations of the purging methodologies. However, other factors, such as specific histology, are involved, since mantle-cell lymphoma cells seem particularly difficult to eradicate (219).

Purging methods relying on the capacity of immunomagnetic beads to select negatively for lymphoma cells are able to purge 3–5 logs of lymphoma cells when multiple mAbs are combined and the selection process is repeated (86,220). Immunoglobulin-G and/or IgM mAbs have the capacity to bind to even weakly expressed cell-surface antigens (86,220). Another alternative to purging, technically simpler than rabbit complement or immunomagnetic microspheres, is the use of immunotoxins. These molecules are able to eliminate similar numbers of clonogenic lymphoma cells (91,124,221). Most ITs developed to date target CD19, a pan-B-cell antigen expressed on all B-lineage cells and disappearing only when B-cells transform into plasma cells (184). Monoclonal antibodies of interest are linked to toxin moieties such as whole blocked ricin (Anti-B4-bR), deglycosylated ricin A-chain, or PAP (B43-PAP) (91,221,222). The possibility of administering residual agents in vivo even represents an important advantage over previously described purging strategies, and several ITs were tested in vivo in clinical Phase I–II trials (221,223–225). In vitro, their increased potency, because high IT concentrations can be attained, and minimum manipulation requirements represent important advantages over other methodologies.

Patients with non-Hodgkin's lymphoma of intermediate- or high-grade histologies who relapse following conventional chemotherapy usually have a poor prognosis when treated by salvage chemotherapy only (226). Autologous PCT in these high-risk patients results in prolonged DFS rates ranging from 30% to 59% (218,227–231). These impressive results were confirmed in a randomized study of autologous PCT versus salvage chemotherapy (229). Patients undergoing transplantation had a 46% DFS at 5 years in comparison to a 12% DFS for patients in the chemotherapy group ($p = 0.001$), and results were also significantly better in terms of survival. Unpurged marrow grafts were used, but these patients had no marrow involvement at the time of harvest and preferentially at any time since diagnosis (229,230,232). Nevertheless, a large proportion of patients with diffuse NHL demonstrate histologic documentation of bone marrow infiltration at the time of diagnosis or relapse. In addition, several groups have cultured lymphoma cells from histologically uninvolved bone marrows (45,233). Moreover, molecular rearrangements found in lymphoma cells are detectable by polymerase chain reaction (PCR) in all relapsed patients, whether or not they attain complete remission (49).

Autologous transplantation with immunologically purged grafts was performed in 114 patients presenting a bcl-2-IgH rearrangement (61) and 25 patients with a clonal rearrangement of the third-complementarity-determining region of the immunoglobulin heavy-chain gene (234) detectable by PCR in their marrow grafts before purging. Disease-free survival was significantly poorer in patients receiving a marrow with detectable residual lymphoma cells. The ability to purge residual lymphoma cells was not associated with the degree of bone marrow involvement or previous response to therapy. Since the inability to purge residual lymphoma cells was the most important prognostic indicator of relapse, these results provide further evidence of the clinical utility of ex vivo purging of bone marrow prior to autologous transplantation. Moreover, data from institutions using unpurged progenitor-cell grafts corroborate the higher likelihood of relapse observed in patients receiving grafts contaminated by detectable clonogenic lymphoma cells (52).

Autologous transplantation in patients with follicular lymphoma, where bone marrow and peripheral blood infiltration is particularly prominent, is usually performed with purged grafts. In this setting, at least two groups have reported a 3–5-year DFS of approximately 45% after autologous BM transplantation for patients with relapsed low-grade NHL (235,236). Treatment with a single anti-CD20 mAb and C resulted in only 14% of marrow samples becoming negative for the bcl-2-IgH rearrangement by PCR (236). This study questions the validity of single mAb purging and indicates that further steps must be taken to ensure effective purging, particularly in this patient population, where circulating lymphoma cells are common and where complete remission rates are low. The intensity of purging is further underlined by studies in patients without prior therapy who were initially cytoreduced with CHOP chemotherapy and immediately underwent autologous purged transplantation (237). Again patients in which lymphoma cells were eradicated by the purging procedure had a better DFS than those with PCR-detectable lymphoma cells after purging. Similarly, the detection of bcl-2-IgH–rearranged cells posttransplant was indicative of subsequent relapse (237).

The immunotoxin Anti-B4-bR was used for marrow purging in a phase I/II clinical trial of autologous PCT in patients with refractory or relapsed NHL (238). Preliminary results on 41 patients show that all evaluable patients demonstrated engraftment with purged marrow, without signs of delayed neutrophil or platelet engraftment. Immunotoxin purging eliminated approximately 3 logs of NHL cells in preclinical experiments (91), but its clinical efficacy could not be measured because of the delay required for this family of compounds to eliminate targeted cells. At 62%, the 4-year DFS for these relapsed patients is encouraging, but patients will have to be followed for longer periods before definitive conclusions can be drawn.

The increased popularity of peripheral blood progenitor cell transplantation is attributable primarily to the high efficiency and nontraumatic acquisition of hematopoietic progenitors as well as the shortened engraftment period. Some studies also suggest that PB might show significant advantages in terms of infiltration by lymphoma cells, and may thus be a better source of progenitor cells than BM (51,52). This finding was not shared by several groups who, rather, found similar frequencies of infiltration by bcl-2/IgH–rearranged cells in PB and BM (53–55,239,240). Other investigators also reported that mobilization regimens could promote the release of tumor cells from BM into PB (56,57,58).

We developed a quantitative competitive PCR assay (QC-PCR) to measure the number of bcl-2/IgH–rearranged cells and monitor the infiltration by lymphoma cells in BM, PB, and mobilized PB (59). This QC-PCR approach showed numbers of BM and PB lymphoma cells varying from 1 to 107,245 per million mononuclear cells evaluated in patients in complete or partial remission. A comparison of lymphoma cell content in BM and PB sampled from the same patient and at the same time revealed that BM was infiltrated by more lymphoma cells than was PB. However, the difference in NHL cell number was extremely small, in the order of 1 log or less in most (88%) patients. We also analyzed levels of NHL cells before and after chemotherapy and growth factor mobilization, and found that lymphoma cell content in PB also increased with mobilization in a majority of patients. In fact, no difference in the proportion of bcl-2/IgH–rearranged cells present in BM and mobilized PB could be identified. Thus, the slight advantage of steady-state PB in terms of tumor-cell contamination is completely abolished following mobilization with growth factor and chemotherapy. Moreover, the increased number of cells infused with mobilized PB progenitor-cell grafts suggests instead that such grafts contain higher numbers of malignant cells than with BM.

These results indicate that in vivo progenitor-cell mobilization is not an efficient purging strategy. They are also in line with a semiquantitative study demonstrating that purged BM is less contaminated with t(14;18)-positive cells than are unpurged PB mononuclear cells, which are frequently contaminated with tumor cells (53). Therefore, strategies implemented for the purging of marrow grafts should also apply to PB stem-cell collections. A few patients have undergone PCT with peripheral blood progenitor-cell grafts purged with immunomagnetic beads: These patients had adequate engraftment, suggesting that PB grafts have the same capacity to tolerate the trauma associated with purging as do BM grafts (95,242).

2. Positive Selection of Normal Hematopoietic Progenitors

CD34 Selection Procedures

Rather than purging progenitor-cell grafts of their lymphoma cells, refinements in our comprehension of the nature of hematopoietic cells and in the identification of crucial cell-surface antigens have promoted the development of strategies to try selectively to administer normal stem and progenitor cells in the context of autologous transplantation (243,244). As previously discussed, the CD34 antigen is present on hematopoietic progenitor cells. Several lines of evidence also suggest that few (possibly even a single) CD34+ hematopoietic stem cells may be sufficient for both short-term and long-term engraftment, not only of myeloid but also of lymphoid cells (245,246). These findings generated much enthusiasm and prompted the design of immunologic approaches to identify and isolate these cells for transplant purposes. Indeed, positive selection has the potential to eliminate the need for negative purging approaches, either of malignant cells for autologous transplants or T-cells for allogeneic transplants, while the limited numbers of cells necessary for engraftment would reduce both patient (dimethylsulfoxide-related) toxicity and freezing space requirements.

Principal methodologies for the selection of CD34+ cells include: (a) flow cytometry, (b) chromatography with an avidin-biotin column, (c) immunomagnetic bead isolation, and (d) panning. Results in terms of cell yield, purity, and T-cell elimination, as well as clinical characteristics, are shown in Table 4.

Cell sorting with a (a) high-speed flow cytometer is a particularly precise and flexible approach enabling the isolation of extremely well-defined cell populations through the use of several mAb combinations and scatter characteristics (156,247). The availability of such an approach is still limited by the sophisticated equipment required, but commercial interests may change the situation in the future by providing broad accessibility through centralized facilities. (b) Avidin-biotin chromatography uses instead very large spheres with avidin on their surface, providing a substrate for the attachment and retention of CD34+ cells coated with biotinylated CD34 mAbs (248,249). The nature of the avidin matrix and the tight avidin-biotin bond prevent the release of both antibody and substrate into the graft (250). This approach has now been evaluated in numerous studies, demonstrating both the efficiency and feasibility of this approach for autologous and also T-cell depletion prior to allogeneic transplantation (247,251–253).

CD34+ cells can also be isolated with (c) immunomagnetic microspheres made of ferric oxide–treated polystyrene and coated with sheep antimouse IgG that recognizes murine mAbs attached to the surface of CD34+ cells (254). CD34+ cells are then magnetically recovered and subsequently released from the antibody-bead complex after exposure to an epitope (PR-34) that competes with the CD34 antigen on the surface of progenitor cells for binding to the Fab

Table 4 CD34 Positive Selection Methodologies

Method	Yield median (range)	Purity median (range)	T-cell depletion	Neutrophil engraftment ($>0.5 \times 10^9/L$)	Platelet engraftment ($20-50 \times 10^9/L$)
Avidin-biotin chromatography (58,244,247,251,252,274,275,299–304)	45% (27–92)	71.5% (42–92)	3 logs	13.5 days[a] (10–34)	22 days[a] (9–156)
Immunomagnetic separation (251,258,300,302,305–307)	8% (3–79)	36.5% (13–94)	3.5 logs	10 days[a] (8–15)	10 days[a] (10–20)
Panning (251,262,263,308)	44% (4–66)	56.5% (31–94)			

Abbreviations: [a]: infusion of unexpanded ± ex vivo expanded CD34+ selected cells

fragment of the Anti-CD34 mAb (255). The biologic as well as clinical characteristics of this selection procedure are very similar to those of the avidin-biotin column (256–259).

CD34+ cells can also be obtained following incubation in polysterene flasks coated with Anti-CD34 mAbs. Such a panning technique is commonly used for laboratory experiments, but its clinical application raises concerns about sterility. In addition, the large number of cells to be treated usually involve prior enrichment steps, consisting of (a) mononuclear cell isolation and (b) T-cell depletion with soybean agglutinin, which complicate the selection process, explaining its limited clinical applications (260,261). The small number of cells obtained from umbilical cord harvest is particularly well suited to this approach (251,262,263).

Clinical Applications of CD34-Positive Selection

CD34 is expressed on early normal progenitor cells and not surprisingly in a large number of neoplastic counterparts (7), including acute myeloid leukemia (AML) (40%) (264–266), chronic myelogenous leukemia (CML) (267,268), blast crisis following myelodysplasia (269), B-lineage ALL (70%), and a minority of T-lineage ALL (270). Thus, CD34 selection is not usually favored in these patients.

Lymphoma cells in patients with non-Hodgkin's disease usually harbor a mature immunophenotype and do not express CD34. Thus, CD34 selection is particularly popular for the treatment of these patients. However, the finding of CD34+CD19+ precursors positive for the bcl-2-IgH rearrangement in some patients with follicular lymphoma warrants caution with CD34 selection as a purging strategy in these patients (271). To date, chronic lymphocytic leukemia, multiple myeloma, and most solid tumor cells do not seem to express CD34 (7,272). Thus, most clinical studies using CD34+-selected cells are performed in patients with these diseases (7,273).

The infusion of CD34+ progenitor grafts does not usually impair neutrophil or platelet engraftment (Table 4). Also, mobilized PB- or CD34+-selected cells engraft within the same time if they harbor the same CD34+ cell content, and engraftment remains shorter than with unmanipulated or CD34-selected BM grafts (244,274). The avidin-biotin or immunomagnetic selection process recovers less than 1% of the nucleated BM cell count but approximately 50% of CD34+ cells in patients with non-Hodgkin's lymphoma (275,276). In this study, the percentage of CD34+/CD33− cells correlated with the cloning efficiency of early CFU-GM and the percentage of CD34+/CD33+ cells with the cloning efficiency of late CFU-GM. Although these patients received a relatively small graft (median dose of 1×10^6 CD34+ cells/kg), the median time to neutrophil engraftment was 15 days and to platelet engraftment was 23 days. It is also important to note that high-efficiency CD34 selection can even be performed upon thawing of unselected peripheral blood cells without delaying engraftment (252). More recently, when CD34 selection was performed on a larger patient population and assessed for both bone marrow and peripheral blood grafts, it was found to eliminate bcl-2/IgH+ cells or IgH rearrangements to below detectable levels in 10 of 27 harvests (277). Nevertheless, the majority of stem-cell grafts retained PCR-detectable rearrangements, confirming the persistence of malignant cells and the difficulty of their eradication with CD34 positive selection alone. This is not entirely surprising, since the CD34+ fraction can contain a high proportion of CD34+CD19+ B-lymphoid progenitors, which may not only falsely elevate the CD34+ cell count but also contain lymphoma progenitor cells (275). Although purity levels remain far from optimum after CD34 selection, the presence of CD34+ B-cell lymphoma precursors indicates that improvements in the purity of the CD34 product will not solve the problem completely. In this context, additional efforts are warranted to eliminate residual malignant cells, either by the isolation of earlier progenitors, through additional positive selection of CD34+Thy1+ cells or sorting of CD34+CD38− cells or by combining negative selection with Anti-CD19 and other mAbs (17,245).

Another option to improve the efficacy of purging and potentially of engraftment characteristics is the ex vivo culture of stem cells (278,279). Culture conditions are such that normal hematopoietic progenitor growth is favored, at the expense of a loss in malignant cells. This has been demonstrated clearly in patients with CML (150,280), and the same may be true for patients with non-Hodgkin's lymphoma (281). Indeed, CD34-selected BM or -mobilized PB cells from patients with NHL and presenting a t(14;18) were expanded in suspension culture in the presence of stem-cell factor, IL-1 beta, IL-3, and IL-6. After 7–14 days in culture, the rearrangement was not PCR-detectable in six of the seven patients evaluated. In addition to this purging effect, stem-cell expansion eliminates the need for cryopreservation and could decrease the number of cells required for engraftment. Studies in mice (282) and humans (283,284) support the thesis of enhanced hematopoietic reconstitution following infusion of higher numbers of mature progenitor cells (285).

Patients receiving BM grafts contaminated by lymphoma cells seem to have a poorer DFS than patients receiving grafts without PCR detectable malignant cells. One would like to conclude that purging of lymphoma cells is the sole explanation for the better results observed in these patients, yet it is difficult to subscribe definitely to such a thesis. Indeed, complete elimination of lymphoma cells by purging may reflect lower tumor burdens in these patients and also a higher likelihood of eliminating lymphoma cells in the host with the chemo- and/or radiation therapy preparative regimen. Although several laboratory and clinical findings do not support these assertions, there is a dire need for clearly defining not only the presence but more importantly the number of lymphoma cells present in peripheral blood and bone marrow to determine the endogenous tumor burden in these patients, and also of measuring lymphoma cells before and after purging to assess the contribution of purging to the success of progenitor-cell transplantation. Fortunately, methodologies to measure lymphoma cell content accurately are now available, and they should help clarify these roles by assessing the efficacy of each different treatment strategy.

IV. CONCLUSION

Thirty years ago, autologous bone marrow transplantation was a true revelation. Most of the energy was focused on protecting the hematopoietic reconstituting ability of the graft through freezing. Monoclonal antibody purging was among the first practical approaches to eliminate malignant cells from progenitor-cell grafts. Today, monoclonal antibodies remain at the center of these issues, and they are now leading us through a novel and exciting path: the identification and isolation of the normal hematopoietic stem cell. This journey is educating us on the biology of normal and malignant cell proliferation and differentiation. Minimal disease measurements are providing important clues on the biology of the disease and its treatments. Ex vivo culture of normal progenitors is helping us to explore the requirements for normal and malignant cell growth, engraftment, and dissemination while opening the door to genetic engineering. Selective expansion of cell populations such as B-cells and dendritic cells is gradually leading to effective and reliable cellular immunotherapy. Tomorrow, monoclonal antibody–derived targeting molecules will enable the precise manipulation of defined cellular subsets to devise therapeutic approaches tailored to the physiology of each malignant cell population. In the meantime, we need to take advantage of the full potential of monoclonal antibodies to provide patients with the highest possible quality of hematopoietic grafts.

REFERENCES

1. Goldman JM, Th'ng KH, Park DS. Collection, cryopreservation and subsequent viability of haemopoietic stem cells intended for treatment of chronic granulocytic leukaemia in transformation. Br J Haematol 1978; 40:185–195.
2. Korbling M, Burke P, Braine H, Elfenbein G, Santos BW, Kaizer H. Successful engraftment of blood derived normal hemopoietic stem cells in chronic myelogenous leukemia. Exp Hematol 1981; 9:684–690.
3. Pettengell R, Luft T, Henschler R, Hows JM, Dexter TM, Ryder D, et al. Direct comparison by limiting dilution analysis of long-term culture-initiating cells in hu-

man bone marrow, umbilical cord blood, and blood stem cells. Blood 1994; 84: 3653–3659.
4. Hirao A, Kawano Y, Takaue Y, Suzue T, Abe T, Sato J, et al. Engraftment potential of peripheral and cord blood stem cells evaluated by a long-term culture system. Exp Hematol 1994; 22:521–526.
5. Civin CI, Strauss LC, Brovall C, Fackler MJ, Schwartz JF, Shaper JH. Antigenic analysis of hematopoiesis. III. A hematopoietic progenitor cell surface antigen defined by a monoclonal antibody raised against KG-1a cells. J Immunol 1984; 133: 157–165.
6. Young PE, Baumhueter S, Lasky LA. The sialomucin CD34 is expressed on hematopoietic cells and blood vessels during murine development. Blood 1995; 85:96–105.
7. Krause DS, Fackler MJ, Civin CI, May WS. CD34—structure, biology, and clinical utility. Blood 1996; 87:1–13.
8. Andrews RG, Singer JW, Bernstein ID. Monoclonal antibody 12-8 recognizes a 115-kd molecule present on both unipotent and multipotent hematopoietic colony-forming cells and their precursors. Blood 1986; 67:842–845.
9. Watt SM, Karhi K, Gatter K, Furley AJ, Katz FE, Healy LE, et al. Distribution and epitope analysis of the cell membrane glycoprotein (HPCA-1) associated with human hemopoietic progenitor cells. Leukemia 1987; 1:417–426.
10. Berenson RJ, Andrews RG, Bensinger WI, Kalamasz D, Knitter G, Buckner CD, et al. Antigen CD34+ marrow cells engraft lethally irradiated baboons. J Clin Invest 1988; 81:951–955.
11. Fina L, Molgaard HV, Robertson D, Bradley NJ, Monaghan P, Delia D, et al. Expression of the CD34 gene in vascular endothelial cells. Blood 1990; 75:2417–2426.
12. Brown J, Greaves MF, Molgaard HV. The gene encoding the stem cell antigen, CD34, is conserved in mouse and expressed in haemopoietic progenitor cell lines, brain, and embryonic fibroblasts. Int Immunol 1991; 3:175–184.
13. Strauss LC, Rowley SD, La Russa VF, Sharkis SJ, Stuart RK, Civin CI. Antigenic analysis of hematopoiesis. V. Characterization of My-10 antigen expression by normal lymphohematopoietic progenitor cells. Exp Hematol 1986; 14:878–886.
14. Bernstein ID, Leary AG, Andrews RG, Ogawa M. Blast colony-forming cells and precursors of colony-forming cells detectable in long-term marrow culture express the same phenotype (CD33− CD34+). Exp Hematol 1991; 19:680–682.
15. Krause DS, Ito T, Fackler MJ, Smith OM, Collector MI, Sharkis SJ, et al. Characterization of murine CD34, a marker for hematopoietic progenitor and stem cells. Blood 1994; 84:691–701.
16. Andrews RG, Singer JW, Bernstein ID. Precursors of colony-forming cells in humans can be distinguished from colony-forming cells by expression of the CD33 and CD34 antigens and light scatter properties. J Exp Med 1989; 169:1721–1731.
17. Huang S, Terstappen LW. Lymphoid and myeloid differentiation of single human CD34+, HLA-DR+, CD38− hematopoietic stem cells. Blood 1994; 83:1515–1526.
18. Lapointe C, Forest L, Lussier P, Busque L, Lagace F, Perreault C, et al. Sequential analysis of early hematopoietic reconstitution following allogeneic bone marrow

transplantation with fluorescence in situ hybridization (FISH). Bone Marrow Transplant. 1996; 17:1143–1148.
19. Larochelle A, Vormoor J, Hanenberg H, Wang JCY, Bhatia M, Lapidot T, et al. Identification of primitive human hematopoietic cells capable of repopulating nod/scid mouse bone marrow—implications for gene therapy. Nature Med 1996; 2: 1329–1337.
20. Bertolini F, Battaglia M, Lanza A, Gibelli N, Palermo B, Pavesi L, et al. Multilineage long-term engraftment potential of drug-resistant hematopoietic progenitors. Blood 1997; 90:3027–3036.
21. Kessinger A, Armitage JO, Landmark JD, Weisenburger DD. Reconstitution of human hematopoietic function with autologous cryopreserved circulating stem cells. Exp Hematol 1986; 14:192–196.
22. Bender JG, Unverzagt KL, Walker DE, Lee W, Van Epps DE, Smith DH, et al. Identification and comparison of CD34-positive cells and their subpopulations from normal peripheral blood and bone marrow using multicolor flow cytometry. Blood 1991; 77:2591–2596.
23. To LB, Shepperd KM, Haylock DN, Dyson PG, Charles P, Thorp DL, et al. Single high doses of cyclophosphamide enable the collection of high numbers of hemopoietic stem cells from the peripheral blood. Exp Hematol 1990; 18:442–447.
24. Kotasek D, Shepherd KM, Sage RE, Dale BM, Norman JE, Charles P, et al. Factors affecting blood stem cell collections following high-dose cyclophosphamide mobilization in lymphoma, myeloma and solid tumors. Bone Marrow Transplant. 1992; 9:11–17.
25. Gianni AM, Siena S, Bregni M, Tarella C, Stern AC, Pileri A, et al. Granulocyte-macrophage colony-stimulating factor to harvest circulating haemopoietic stem cells for autotransplantation. Lancet 1989; 2:580–585.
26. Sheridan WP, Begley CG, Juttner CA, Szer J, To LB, Maher D, et al. Effect of peripheral-blood progenitor cells mobilised by filgrastim (G-CSF) on platelet recovery after high-dose chemotherapy. Lancet 1992; 339:640–644.
27. Gheilmini M, Pettengell R, Coutinho LH, Testa N, Crowther D. The effect of the GM-CSF/IL-3 fusion protein PIXY321 on bone marrow and circulating haemopoietic cells of previously untreated patients with cancer. Br J Hematol 1996; 93: 6–12.
28. Siena S, Bregni M, Brando B, Belli N, Ravagnani F, Gandola L, et al. Flow cytometry for clinical estimation of circulating hematopoietic progenitors for autologous transplantation in cancer patients. Blood 1991; 77:400–409.
29. Pettengell R, Morgenstern GR, Woll PJ, Chang J, Rowlands M, Young R, et al. Peripheral blood progenitor cell transplantation in lymphoma and leukemia using a single apheresis. Blood 1993; 82:3770–3777.
30. Copelan EA, Ceselski SK, Ezzone SA, Lasky LC, Penza SL, Bechtel TP, et al. Mobilization of peripheral-blood progenitor cells with high-dose etoposide and granulocyte colony-stimulating factor in patients with breast cancer, non-Hodgkin's lymphoma, and Hodgkin's disease. J Clin Oncol 1997; 15:759–765.
31. Watts MJ, Sullivan AM, Jamieson E, Pearce R, Fielding A, Devereux S, et al. Progenitor-cell mobilization after low-dose cyclophosphamide and granulocyte colony-stimulating factor: an analysis of progenitor-cell quantity and quality and

factors predicting for these parameters in 101 pretreated patients with malignant lymphoma. J Clin Oncol 1997; 15:535–546.
32. Sutherland DR, Keating A, Nayar R, Anania S, Stewart AK. Sensitive detection and enumeration of CD34+ cells in peripheral and cord blood by flow cytometry. Exp Hematol 1994; 22:1003–1010.
33. Elliott C, Samson DM, Armitage S, Lyttelton MP, McGuigan D, Hargreaves R, et al. When to harvest peripheral-blood stem cells after mobilization therapy: prediction of CD34-positive cell yield by preceding day CD34-positive concentration in peripheral blood. J Clin Oncol. 1996; 14:970–973.
34. Bensinger W, Appelbaum F, Rowley S, Storb R, Sanders J, Lilleby K, et al. Factors that influence collection and engraftment of autologous peripheral-blood stem cells. J Clin Oncol 1995; 13:2547–2555.
35. Haas R, Witt B, Mohle R, Goldschmidt H, Hohaus S, Freuhauf S, et al. Sustained long-term hematopoiesis after myeloablative therapy with peripheral blood progenitor cell support. Blood 1995; 85:3754–3761.
36. Haynes A, Hunter A, McQuaker G, Anderson S, Bienz N, Russell NH. Engraftment characteristics of peripheral blood stem cells mobilised with cyclophosphamide and the delayed addition of G-CSF. Bone Marrow Transplant 1995; 16:359–363.
37. Civin CI, Almeida-Porada G, Lee MJ, Olweus J, Terstappen LW, Zanjani ED. Sustained, retransplantable, multilineage engraftment of highly purified adult human bone marrow stem cells in vivo. Blood 1996; 88:4102–4109.
38. Brenner MK, Rill DR, Moen RC, Krance RA, Mirro JJ, Anderson WF, et al. Gene marking to trace origin of relapse after autologous bone marrow transplantation. Lancet 1993; 341:85–86.
39. Deisseroth AB, Zu Z, Claxton D, Hanania EG, Fu S, Ellerson D, et al. Genetic marking shows that Ph+ cells present in autologous transplants of chronic myelogenous leukemia (CML) contribute to relapse after autologous bone marrow in CML. Blood 1994; 83:3068–3076.
40. Gorin NC, Aegerter P, Auvert B, Meloni G, Goldstone AH, Burnett A, et al. Autologous bone marrow transplantation for acute myelocytic leukemia in first remission: a European survey of the role of marrow purging. Blood 1990; 75:1606–1614.
41. Fiere D, Lepage E, Sebban C, Boucheix C, Gisselbrecht C, Vernant JP, et al. Adult acute lymphoblastic leukemia: a multicentric randomized trial testing bone marrow transplantation as postremission therapy. J Clin Oncol 1993; 11:1990–2001.
42. Stahel RA, Mabry M, Skarin AT, Speak J, Bernal SD. Detection of bone marrow metastasis in small-cell lung cancer by monoclonal antibody. J Clin Oncol 1985; 3:455–461.
43. Uckun FM, Kersey JH, Haake R, Weisdorf D, Ramsay NK. Autologous bone marrow transplantation in high-risk remission B-lineage acute lymphoblastic leukemia using a cocktail of three monoclonal antibodies (BA-1/CD24, BA-2/CD9, and BA-3/CD10) plus complement and 4-hydroperoxycyclophosphamide for ex vivo bone marrow purging. Blood 1992; 79:1094–1104.
44. Estrov Z, Grunberger T, Dube ID, Wang YP, Freedman MH. Detection of residual acute lymphoblastic leukemia cells in cultures of bone marrow obtained during remission. N Engl J Med 1986; 315:538–542.
45. Sharp JG, Joshi SS, Armitage JO, Bierman P, Coccia PF, Harrington DS, et al.

Significance of detection of occult non-Hodgkin's lymphoma in histologically uninvolved bone marrow by a culture technique. Blood 1992; 79:1074–1080.

46. Yamada M, Wasserman R, Lange B, Reichard BA, Womer RB, Rovera G. Minimal residual disease in childhood B-lineage lymphoblastic leukemia. Persistence of leukemic cells during the first 18 months of treatment. N Engl J Med 1990; 323:448–455.

47. Jonsson OG, Kitchens RL, Scott FC, Smith RG. Detection of minimal residual disease in acute lymphoblastic leukemia using immunoglobulin hypervariable region specific oligonucleotide probes. Blood 1990; 76:2072–2079.

48. Ngan BY, Nourse J, Cleary ML. Detection of chromosomal translocation t(14;18) within the minor cluster region of bcl-2 by polymerase chain reaction and direct genomic sequencing of the enzymatically amplified DNA in follicular lymphomas. Blood 1989; 73:1759–1762.

49. Gribben JG, Freedman As, Woo SD, Blake K, Shu RS, Freeman G, et al. All advanced-stage non-Hodgkin's lymphomas with a polymerase chain reaction amplifiable breakpoint of bcl-2 have residual cells containing the bcl-2 rearrangement at evaluation and after treatment. Blood 1991; 78:3275–3280.

50. Hetu F, Coutlee F, Roy DC. A non-isotopic nested polymerase chain reaction method to quantitate minimal residual disease in patients with non-Hodgkin's lymphoma. Mol Cell Probes 1994; 8:449–457.

51. Gribben JG, Neuberg D, Barber M, Moore J, Pesek KW, Freedman AS, et al. Detection of residual lymphoma cells by polymerase chain reaction in peripheral blood is significantly less predictive for relapse than detection in bone marrow. Blood 1994; 83:3800–3807.

52. Sharp JG, Kessinger A, Mann S, Crouse DA, Armitage JO, Bierman P, et al. Outcome of high-dose therapy and autologous transplantation in non-Hodgkin's lymphoma based on the presence of tumor in the marrow or infused hematopoietic harvest. J Clin Oncol 1996; 14:214–219.

53. Negrin RS, Pesando J. Detection of tumor cells in purged bone marrow and peripheral-blood mononuclear cells by polymerase chain reaction amplification of bcl-2 translocations. J Clin Oncol 1994; 12:1021–1027.

54. Berinstein NL, Reis MD, Ngan BY, Sawka CA, Jamal HH, Kuzniar B. Detection of occult lymphoma in the peripheral blood and bone marrow of patients with untreated early-stage and advanced-stage follicular lymphoma. J Clin Oncol 1993; 11:1344–1352.

55. Yuan R, Dowling P, Zucca E, Diggelmann H, Cavalli F. Detection of bcl-2/JH rearrangement in follicular and diffuse lymphoma: concordant results of peripheral blood and bone marrow analysis at diagnosis. Br J Cancer 1993; 67:922–925.

56. Ross AA, Cooper BW, Lazarus HM, Mackay W, Moss TJ. Detection and viability of tumor cells in peripheral blood stem cell collections from breast cancer patients using immunocytochemical and clonogenic assay techniques. Blood 1992; 10:936–941.

57. Brugger W, Bross KJ, Glatt M, Weber F, Mertelsmann R, Kanz L. Mobilization of tumor cells and hematopoietic progenitor cells into peripheral blood of patients with solid tumors. Blood 1994; 83:636–640.

58. Lemoli RM, Fortuna A, Motta MR, Rizzi S, Giudice V, Nannetti A, et al. Concomi-

tant mobilization of plasma cells and hematopoietic progenitors into peripheral blood of multiple myeloma patients-positive selection and transplantation of enriched CD34(+) cells to remove circulating tumor cells. Blood 1996; 87:1625–1634.
59. Leonard BM, Hetu F, Busque L, Gyger M, Belanger R, Perreault C, et al. Lymphoma cell burden in progenitor cell grafts measured by competitive polymerase chain reaction: Less than one log difference between bone marrow and peripheral blood sources. Blood 1998; 91:331–339.
60. Rowley SD, Jones RJ, Piantadosi S, Braine HG, Colvin OM, Davis J, et al. Efficacy of ex vivo purging for autologous bone marrow transplantation in the treatment of acute nonlymphoblastic leukemia. Blood 1989; 74:501–506.
61. Gribben JG, Freedman AS, Neuberg D, Roy DC, Blake KW, Woo SD, et al. Immunologic purging of marrow assessed by PCR before autologous bone marrow transplantation for B-cell lymphoma. N Engl J Med 1991; 325:1525–1533.
62. Dicke KA, Zander A, Spitzer G, Verma DS, Peters L, Vellekoop L, et al. Autologous bone-marrow transplantation in relapsed adult acute leukaemia. Lancet 1979; 1:514–517.
63. Wagner JE, Santos GW, Noga SJ, Rowley SD, Davis J, Vogelsang GB, et al. Bone marrow graft engineering by counterflow centrifugal elutriation: results of a Phase I–II clinical trial. Blood 1990; 75:1370–1377.
64. Preijers F, Ruijs P, Schattenberg A, de Witte T. T-cell depletion from allogeneic bone marrow by counterflow centrifugation is not associated with a substantial loss of CD34-positive cells. Prog Clin Biol Res 1994; 389:339–344.
65. Young JW, Papadopoulos EB, Cunningham I, Castro-Malaspina H, Flomenberg N, Carabasi MH, et al. T-cell-depleted allogeneic bone marrow transplantation in adults with acute nonlymphocytic leukemia in first remission. Blood 1992; 79: 3380–3387.
66. Lazzaro GE, Meyer BF, Willis JI, Erber WN, Herrmann RP, Davies JM. The synthesis of a peanut agglutinin-ricin A chain conjugate—potential as an in vitro purging agent for autologous bone marrow in multiple myeloma. Exp Hematol 1995; 23:1347–1352.
67. Min W, Kim D, Lee J, Park J, Kim C. Autologous bone marrow rescue for patients with acute myelogenous leukemia: purging with hyperthermia and ether lipid in vitro. Prog Clin Biol Res 1994; 389:197–203.
68. Yeager AM, Kaizer H, Santos GW, Saral R, Colvin OM, Stuart RK, et al. Autologous bone marrow transplantation in patients with acute nonlymphocytic leukemia, using ex vivo marrow treatment with 4-hydroperoxycyclophosphamide. N Engl J Med 1986; 315:141–147.
69. Douay L, Mary JY, Giarratana MC, Najman A, Gorin NC. Establishment of a reliable experimental procedure for bone marrow purging with mafosfamide (ASTA Z 7557). Exp Hematol 1989; 17:429–432.
70. Uckun FM, Gajl-Peczalska K, Meyers DE, Ramsay NC, Kersey JH, Colvin M, et al. Marrow purging in autologous bone marrow transplantation for T-lineage acute lymphoblastic leukemia: efficacy of ex vivo treatment with immunotoxins and 4-hydroperoxycyclophosphamide against fresh leukemic marrow progenitor cells. Blood 1987; 69:361–366.

71. Rowley SD, Miller CB, Piantadosi S, Davis JM, Santos GW, Jones RJ. Phase I study of combination drug purging for autologous bone marrow transplantation. J Clin Oncol 1991; 9:2210–2218.
72. Juneja HS, Harvey WH, Brasher WK, Thompson EB. Successful in vitro purging of leukemic blasts from marrow by cortivazol, a pyrazolosteroid: a preclinical study for autologous transplantation in acute lymphoblastic leukemia and non-Hodgkin's lymphoma. Leukemia 1995; 9:1771–1778.
73. Traul DL, Anderson GS, Bilitz JM, Krieg M, Sieber F. Potentiation of merocyanine-540-mediated photodynamic therapy by salicylate and related drugs. Photochem Photobiol 1995; 62:790–799.
74. Jamieson C, Richter A, Levy JG. Efficacy of benzoporphyrin derivative, a photosensitizer, in selective destruction of leukemia cells using a murine tumor model. Exp Hematol 1993; 21:629–634.
75. Pal P, Zeng HL, Durocher G, Girard D, Li TC, Gupta AK, et al. Phototoxicity of some bromine-substituted rhodamine dyes—synthesis, photophysical properties and application as photosensitizers. Photochem Photobiol 1996; 63:161–168.
76. Scheffold C, Brandt K, Johnston V, Lefterova P, Degen B, Schontube M, et al. Potential of autologous immunologic effector cells for bone marrow purging in patients with chronic myeloid leukemia. Bone Marrow Transplant 1995; 15:33–39.
77. Cesano A, Pierson G, Visonneau S, Migliaccio AR, Santoli D. Use of a lethally irradiated major histocompatibility complex nonrestricted cytotoxic T-cell line for effective purging of marrows containing lysis-sensitive or -resistant leukemic targets. Blood 1996; 87:393–403.
78. Arbour S, Toupin S, Belanger R, Gyger M, Halle JP, Perreault C, et al. Phenotypic and functional characterization of peripheral blood and bone marrow natural killer cells prior to autologous transplantation. Bone Marrow Transplant 1996; 17:315–322.
79. Bishop MR, Warkentin PI, Jackson JD, Bayever E, Iversen PL, Whalen VI, et al. Antisense oligonucleotide OL (1) p53 for in vitro purging of autologous bone marrow in acute myelogenous leukemia. Prog Clin Biol Res 1994; 389:183–187.
80. Ritz J, Sallan SE, Bast RC, Jr., Lipton JM, Clavell LA, Feeney M, et al. Autologous bone-marrow transplantation in CALLA-positive acute lymphoblastic leukemia after in-vitro treatment with J5 monoclonal antibody and complement. Lancet 1982; 2:60–63.
81. Stepan DE, Bartholomew RM, LeBien TW. In vitro cytodestruction of human leukemic cells using murine monoclonal antibodies and human complement. Blood 1984; 63:1120–1124.
82. Zola H, Potter A, Neoh SH, Juttner CA, Haylock DN, Rice AM, et al. Evaluation of a monoclonal IgM antibody for purging of bone marrow for autologous transplantation. Bone Marrow Transplant 1987; 1:297–301.
83. Roy DC, Felix M, Cannady WG, Cannistra S, Ritz J. Comparative activities of rabbit complements of different ages using an in-vitro marrow purging model. Leukemia Res 1990; 14:407–416.
84. Casellas P, Canat X, Fauser AA, Gros O, Laurent G, Poncelet P, et al. Optimal

elimination of leukemic T cells from human bone marrow with T101-ricin A-chain immunotoxin. Blood 1985; 65:289–297.
85. Stong RC, Uckun F, Youle RJ, Kersey JH, Vallera DA. Use of multiple T-cell-directed intact ricin immunotoxins for autologous bone marrow transplantation. Blood 1985; 66:627–635.
86. Kvalheim G, Sorensen O, Fodstad O, Funderud S, Kiesel S, Dorken B, et al. Immunomagnetic removal of B-lymphoma cells from human bone marrow: a procedure for clinical use. Bone Marrow Transplant 1988; 3:31–41.
87. Reading CL, Thomas MW, Hickey CM, Chandran M, Tindle S, Ball ED, et al. Magnetic affinity colloid (MAC) cell separation of leukemia cells from autologous bone marrow aspirates. Leukemia Res 1987; 11:1067–1077.
88. Negrin RS, Kiem HP, Schmidt-Wolf IG, Blurne KG, Cleary ML. Use of the polymerase chain reaction to monitor the effectiveness of ex vivo tumor cell purging. Blood 1991; 77:654–660.
89. Gribben JG, Saporito L, Barber M, Blake KW, Edwards RM, Griffin JD, et al. Bone marrows of non-Hodgkin's lymphoma patients with a bcl-2 translocation can be purged of polymerase chain reaction-detectable lymphoma cells using monoclonal antibodies and immunomagnetic bead depletion. Blood 1992; 80:1083–1089.
90. Roy DC, Ouellet S, Le Houillier C, Ariniello PD, Perreault C, Lambert JM. Elimination of neuroblastoma and small cell lung cancer cells with an anti-neural cell adhesion molecule immunotoxin. J Natl Cancer Inst 1996; 88:1136–1145.
91. Roy DC, Perreault C, Bélanger R, Gyger M, Le Houillier C, Blättler WA, et al. Elimination of B-lineage leukemia and lymphoma cells from bone marrow grafts using anti-B4-blocked-ricin immunotoxin. J Clin Immunol 1995; 15:51–57.
92. Lemoli RM, Gasparetto C, Scheinberg DA, Moore MA, Clarkson BD, Gulati SC. Autologous bone marrow transplantation in acute myelogenous leukemia: in vitro treatment with myeloid-specific monoclonal antibodies and drugs in combination. Blood 1991; 77:1829–1836.
93. Yokota S, Hara H, Luo Y, Seon BK. Synergistic potentiation of in vivo antitumor activity of anti-human T-leukemia immunotoxins by recombinant alpha-interferon and daunorubicin. Cancer Res 1990; 50:32–37.
94. Deggerdal AH, Pettersen F, Kvalheim G, Hornes E, Smeland E, Fodstad O, et al. Semiquantitative polymerase chain reaction for t(14;18) in follicular lymphomas: a colorimetric approach. Laboratory Investigation 1995; 72:411–418.
95. Straka C, Drexler E, Mitterer M, Langenmayer I, Pfefferkorn L, Stade B, et al. Autotransplantation of B-cell purged peripheral blood progenitor cells in B-cell lymphoma. Lancet 1995; 345:797–798.
96. Zittoun RA, Mandelli F, Willemze R, de Witte T, Labar B, Resegotti L, et al. Autologous or allogeneic bone marrow transplantation compared with intensive chemotherapy in acute myelogenous leukemia. N Engl J Med 1995; 332:217–223.
97. Imrie K, Dicke KA, Keating A. Autologous bone marrow transplantation for acute myeloid leukemia. Stem Cells 1996; 14:69–78.
98. Korbling M, Hunstein W, Fliedner TM, Cayeux S, Dorken B, Fehrentz D, et al.

Disease-free survival after autologous bone marrow transplantation in patients with acute myelogenous leukemia. Blood 1989; 74:1898–1904.
99. Giarratana MC, Gorin NC, Douay L. Plasma interacts with mafosfamide toxicity to normal haematopoietic progenitor cells: impact on in vitro marrow purging. Nouvelle Revue Francaise d'Hematologie 1995; 37:125–130.
100. Douay L, Hu C, Giarratana MC, Bouchet S, Conlon J, Capizzi RL, et al. Amifostine improves the antileukemic therapeutic index of mafosfamide: implications for bone marrow purging. Blood 1995; 86:2849–2855.
101. Ball ED, Mills LE, Coughlin CT, Beck JR, Cornwell GG. Autologous bone marrow transplantation in acute myelogenous leukemia: in vitro treatment with myeloid cell-specific monoclonal antibodies. Blood 1986; 68:1311–1315.
102. Griffin JD, Lowenberg B. Clonogenic cells in acute myeloblastic leukemia. Blood 1986; 68:1185–1195.
103. Ball ED, Schwarz LM, Bloomfield CD. Expression of the CD15 antigen on normal and leukemic myeloid cells: effects of neuraminidase and variable detection with a panel of monoclonal antibodies. Mol Immunol 1991; 28:951–958.
104. Ball ED, Vredenburgh JJ, Mills LE, Cornwell GG, Schwarz L, Howell AL, et al. Autologous bone marrow transplantation for acute myeloid leukemia following in vitro treatment with neuraminidase and monoclonal antibodies. Bone Marrow Transplant 1990; 6:277–280.
105. De Fabritiis P, Ferrero D, Sandrelli A, Tarella C, Meloni G, Pulsoni A, et al. Monoclonal antibody purging and autologous bone marrow transplantation in acute myelogenous leukemia in complete remission. Bone Marrow Transplant 1989; 4:669–674.
106. Selvaggi KJ, Wilson JW, Mills LE, Cornwell GG, Hurd D, Dodge W, et al. Improved outcome for high-risk acute myeloid leukemia patients using autologous bone marrow transplantation and monoclonal antibody-purged bone marrow. Blood 1994; 83:1698–1705.
107. Ball ED, Phelps V, Wilson JW. Acute bone marrow transplantation for acute myeloid leukemia in remission or first relapse using monoclonal antibody-purged marrow (abstr). Blood 1997; 88(suppl 1): 485a.
108. Freeman SD, Kelm S, Barber EK, Crocker PR. Characterization of CD33 as a new member of the sialoadhesin family of cellular interaction molecules. Blood 1995; 85:2005–2012.
109. Griffin JD, Linch D, Sabbath K, Larcom P, Schlossman SF. A monoclonal antibody reactive with normal and leukemic human myeloid progenitor cells. Leukemia Res 1984; 8:521–534.
110. Takahashi M, Maruyama S, Moriyama Y, Shibata A. Applicability of antimyeloid monoclonal antibodies (L4F3, 1G10) to autologous bone marrow transplantation for patients with acute myelogenous leukemia. Transplantation Proc 1992; 24:416–418.
111. Roy DC, Griffin JD, Belvin M, Blattler WA, Lambert JM, Ritz J. Anti-MY9-blocked-ricin: an immunotoxin for selective targeting of acute myeloid leukemia cells. Blood 1991; 77:2404–2412.
112. Robertson MJ, Soiffer RJ, Freedman AS, Rabinowe SL, Anderson KC, Ervin TJ,

et al. Human bone marrow depleted of CD33-positive cells mediates delayed but durable reconstitution of hematopoiesis: clinical trial of MY9 monoclonal antibody-purged autografts for the treatment of acute myeloid leukemia. Blood 1992; 79: 2229–2236.
113. Robertson MJ, Roy DC, Stone RM, Ritz J. Use of CD33 monoclonal antibodies in bone marrow transplantation for acute myeloid leukemia. Prog Clin Biol Res 1994; 389:47–63.
114. Stiff PJ, Schulz WC, Bishop M, Marks L. Anti-CD33 monoclonal antibody and etoposide/cytosine arabinoside combinations for the ex vivo purification of bone marrow in acute nonlymphocytic leukemia. Blood 1991; 77:355–362.
115. Zhong RK, Kozii R, Ball ED. Homologous restriction of complement-mediated cell lysis can be markedly enhanced by blocking decay-accelerating factor. Br J Haematol 1995; 91:269–274.
116. Gee AP, Boyle MD. Purging tumor cells from bone marrow by use of antibody and complement: a critical appraisal. J Natl Cancer Inst 1988; 80:154–159.
117. Schwartz MA, Lovett DR, Redner A, Finn RD, Graham MC, Divgi CR, et al. Dose-escalation trial of M195 labeled with iodine-131 for cytoreduction and marrow ablation in relapsed or refractory myeloid leukemias. J Clin Oncol 1993; 11:294–303.
118. Myers DE, Uckun FM, Ball ED, Vallera DA. Immunotoxins for ex vivo marrow purging in autologous bone marrow transplantation for acute nonlymphocytic leukemia. Transplantation 1988; 46:240–245.
119. Vitetta ES, Fulton RJ, May RD, Till M, Uhr JW. Redesigning nature's poisons to create anti-tumor reagents. Science 1987; 238:1098–1104.
120. Blakey DC, Thorpe PE. An overview of therapy with immunotoxins containing ricin or its A chain. Antibody Immunoconjugates Radiopharmaceuticals 1988; 1: 1–16.
121. Tecce R, Fraioli R, De Fabritiis P, Sandrelli A, Savarese A, Santoro L, et al. Production and characterization of two immunotoxins specific for M5b ANLL leukaemia. Int J Cancer 1991; 49:310–316.
122. Uckun FM, Kersey JH, Haake R, Weisdorf D, Nesbit ME, Ramsay NK. Pretransplantation burden of leukemic progenitor cells as a predictor of relapse after bone marrow transplantation for acute lymphoblastic leukemia. N Engl J Med 1993; 329: 1296–1301.
123. Lambert JM, McIntyre G, Gauthier MN, Zullo D, Rao V, Steeves RM, et al. The galactose-binding sites of the cytotoxic lectin ricin can be chemically blocked in high yield with reactive ligands prepared by chemical modification of glycopeptides containing triantennary N-linked oligosaccharides. Biochemistry 1991; 30:3234–3247.
124. Lambert JM, Goldmacher VS, Collinson AR, Nadler LM, Blattler WA. An immunotoxin prepared with blocked ricin: a natural plant toxin adapted for therapeutic use. Cancer Res 1991; 51:6236–6242.
125. Harousseau JL, Cahn JY, Pignon B, Witz F, Milpied N, Delain M, et al. Comparison of autologous bone marrow transplantation and intensive chemotherapy as postremission therapy in adult acute myeloid leukemia. The Groupe Ouest Est Leucemies Aigues Myeloblastiques (GOELAM). Blood 1997; 90:2978–2986.

126. Griffin JD, Davis R, Nelson DA, Davey FR, Mayer RJ, Schiffer C, et al. Use of surface marker analysis to predict outcome of adult acute myeloblastic leukemia. Blood 1986; 68:1232–1241.
127. Wang JC, Beauregard P, Soamboonsrup P, Neame PB. Monoclonal antibodies in the management of acute leukemia. Am J Hematol 1995; 50:188–199.
128. Griffin JD, Ritz J, Nadler LM, Schlossman SF. Expression of myeloid differentiation antigens on normal and malignant myeloid cells. J Clin Invest 1981; 68:932–941.
129. Griffin JD, Mayer RJ, Weinstein HJ, Rosenthal DS, Coral FS, Beveridge RP, et al. Surface marker analysis of acute myeloblastic leukemia: identification of differentiation-associated phenotypes. Blood 1983; 62:557–563.
130. Neame PB, Soamboonsrup P, Browman GP, Meyer RM, Benger A, Wilson WE, et al. Classifying acute leukemia by immunophenotyping: a combined FAB-immunologic classification of AML. Blood 1986; 68:1355–1362.
131. Sabbath KD, Ball ED, Larcom P, Davis RB, Griffin JD. Heterogeneity of clonogenic cells in acute myeloblastic leukemia. J Clin Invest 1985; 75:746–753.
132. Sirard C, Lapidot T, Vormoor J, Cashman JD, Doedens M, Murdoch B, et al. Normal and leukemic SCID-repopulating cells (SRC) coexist in the bone marrow and peripheral blood from CML patients in chronic phase, whereas leukemic SRC are detected in blast crisis. Blood 1996; 87:1539–1548.
133. Bonnet D, Dick JE. Human acute myeloid leukemia is organized as a hierarchy that originates from a primitive hematopoietic cell. Nat Med 1997; 3:730–737.
134. Lapidot T, Sirard C, Vormoor J, Murdoch B, Hoang T, Caceres-Cortes J, et al. A cell initiating human acute myeloid leukaemia after transplantation into SCID mice. Nature 1994; 367:645–648.
135. Lowenberg B, Verdonck LJ, Dekker AW, Willemze R, Zwaan FE, de Planque M, et al. Autologous bone marrow transplantation in acute myeloid leukemia in first remission: results of a Dutch prospective study. J Clin Oncol 1990; 8:287–294.
136. Wognum AW, Krystal G, Eaves CJ, Eaves AC, Lansdorp PM. Increased erythropoietin-receptor expression on CD34-positive bone marrow cells from patients with chronic myeloid leukemia. Blood 1992; 79:642–649.
137. Dube ID, Kalousek DK, Coulombel L, Gupta CM, Eaves CJ, Eaves AC. Cytogenetic studies of early myeloid progenitor compartments in Ph1-positive chronic myeloid leukemia. II. Long-term culture reveals the persistence of Ph1-negative progenitors in treated as well as newly diagnosed patients. Blood 1984; 63:1172–1177.
138. Leemhuis T, Leibowitz D, Cox G, Silver R, Srour EF, Tricot G, et al. Identification of BCR/ABL-negative primitive hematopoietic progenitor cells within chronic myeloid leukemia marrow. Blood 1993; 81:801–807.
139. Kantarjian HM, Talpaz M, Hester J, Feldman E, Korbling M, Liang J, et al. Collection of peripheral-blood diploid cells from chronic myelogenous leukemia patients early in the recovery phase from myelosuppression induced by intensive-dose chemotherapy. J Clin Oncol 1995; 13:553–559.
140. Simonsson B, Oberg G, Bjoreman M, Bjorkholm M, Carneskog J, Gahrton G, et al. Intensive treatment in order to minimize the Ph-positive clone in CML. Bone Marrow Transplant 1996; 17(suppl 3): S63–S64

141. De Fabritiis P, Sandrelli A, Meloni G, Alimena G, Montefusco E, Lo Coco F, et al. Prolonged suppression of myeloid progenitor cell numbers after stopping interferon treatment for CML may necessitate delay in harvesting marrow cells for autografting. Bone Marrow Transplant 1990; 6:247–251.
142. Boque C, Petit J, Sarra J, Cancelas JA, Munoz J, Espanol JI, et al. Mobilization of peripheral stem cells with intensive chemotherapy (ICE regimen) and G-CSF in chronic myeloid leukemia. Bone Marrow Transplant 1996; 18:879–884.
143. Carella AM, Cunningham I, Lerma E, Dejana A, Benvenuto F, Podesta M, et al. Mobilization and transplantation of Philadelphia-negative peripheral-blood progenitor cells early in chronic myelogenous leukemia. J Clin Oncol 1997; 15:1575–1582.
144. Carella AM, Chimirri F, Podesta M, Pitto A, Piaggio G, Dejana A, et al. High-dose chemoradiotherapy followed by autologous Philadelphia chromosome-negative blood progenitor cell transplantation in patients with chronic myelogenous leukemia. Bone Marrow Transplant 1996; 17:201–205.
145. Carlo-Stella C, Mangoni L, Almici C, Caramatti C, Cottafavi L, Dotti GP, et al. Autologous transplant for chronic myelogenous leukemia using marrow treated ex vivo with mafosfamide. Bone Marrow Transplant 1994; 14:425–432.
146. Jazwiec B, Mahon FX, Pigneux A, Pigeonnier V, Reiffers J. 5-Fluorouracil-resistant CD34(+) cell population from peripheral blood of CML patients contains BCR-ABL-negative progenitor cells. Exp. Hematol. 1995; 23:1509–1514.
147. Einat M, Lishner M, Amiel A, Nagler A, Yarkorli S, Rudi A, et al. Eilatin—a novel marine alkaloid inhibits in vitro proliferation of progenitor cells in chronic myeloid leukemia patients. Exp Hematol 1995; 23:1439–1444.
148. McGlave PB, Arthur D, Miller WJ, Lasky L, Kersey J. Autologous transplantation for CML using marrow treated ex vivo with recombinant human interferon gamma. Bone Marrow Transplant 1990; 6:115–120.
149. Tari AM, Tucker SD, Deisseroth A, Lopez-Berestein G. Liposomal delivery of methylphosphonate antisense oligodeoxynucleotides in chronic myelogenous leukemias. Blood 1994; 84:601–607.
150. Barnett MJ, Eaves CJ, Phillips GL, Gascoyne RD, Hogge DE, Horsman DE, et al. Autografting with cultured marrow in chronic myeloid leukemia: results of a pilot study. Blood 1994; 84:724–732.
151. Petzer AL, Eaves CJ, Barnett MJ, Eaves AC. Selective expansion of primitive normal hematopoietic cells in cytokine-supplemented cultures of purified cells from patients with chronic myeloid leukemia. Blood 1997; 90:64–69.
152. Coutinho LH, Chang J, Brereton ML, Morgenstern GR, Scarffe JH, Harrison CJ, et al. Autografting in Philadelphia (Ph)+ chronic myeloid leukaemia using cultured marrow: an update of a pilot study. Bone Marrow Transplant 1997; 19:969–976.
153. Podesta M, Piaggio G, Sessarego M, Pitto A, Benvenuto F, Vassallo F, et al. Spontaneous exodus of high numbers of normal early progenitor cells (Ph-negative LTC-IC) in the peripheral blood of patients with chronic myeloid leukaemia at the beginning of the disease. Br J Haematol 1997; 97:94–98.
154. Petzer AL, Eaves CJ, Lansdorp PM, Ponchio L, Barnett MJ, Eaves AC. Characterization of primitive subpopulations of normal and leukemic cells present in the

blood of patients with newly diagnosed as well as established chronic myeloid leukemia. Blood 1996; 88:2162–2171.
155. Sauvageau G, Lansdorp PM, Eaves CJ, Hogge DE, Dragowska WH, Reid DS, et al. Differential expression of homeobox genes in functionally distinct CD34+ subpopulations of human bone marrow cells. Proc Natl Acad Sci USA 1994; 91: 12,223–12,227.
156. Verfaillie CM, Bhatia R, Miller W, Mortari F, Roy V, Burger S, et al. BCR/ABL-negative primitive progenitors suitable for transplantation can be selected from the marrow of most early-chronic phase but not accelerated-phase chronic myelogenous leukemia patients. Blood 1996; 87:4770–4779.
157. Eaves CJ, Cashman JD, Wolpe SD, Eaves AC. Unresponsiveness of primitive chronic myeloid leukemia cells to macrophage inflammatory protein 1 alpha, an inhibitor of primitive normal hematopoietic cells. Proc Natl Acad Sci USA 1993; 90:12,015–12,019.
158. Chasty RC, Lucas GS, Owen-Lynch PJ, Pierce A, Whetton AD. Macrophage inflammatory protein-1 alpha receptors are present on cells enriched for CD34 expression from patients with chronic myeloid leukemia. Blood 1995; 86:4270–4277.
159. Traycoff CM, Kosak ST, Grigsby S, Srour EF. Evaluation of ex vivo expansion potential of cord blood and bone marrow hematopoietic progenitor cells using cell tracking and limiting dilution analysis. Blood 1995; 85:2059–2068.
160. Veena P, Cornetta K, Davidson A, Aguero B, McMahel J, Traycoff CM, et al. Preferential sequestration in vitro of BCR/ABL negative hematopoietic progenitor cells among cytokine nonresponsive CML marrow CD34+ cells. Bone Marrow Transplant 1997; 19:1213–1221.
161. Bhatia R, McGlave PB, Miller JS, Wissink S, Lin WN, Verfaillie CM. A clinically suitable ex vivo expansion culture system for LTC-IC and CFC using stroma-conditioned medium. Exp Hematol 1997; 25:980–991.
162. McGlave PB, De Fabritiis P, Deisseroth A, Goldman J, Barnett M, Reiffers J, et al. Autologous transplants for chronic myelogenous leukaemia: results from eight transplant groups. Lancet 1994; 343:1486–1488.
163. Steinman RM. The dendritic cell system and its role in immunogenicity. Ann Rev Immunol 1991; 9:271–296.
164. Grabbe S, Beissert S, Schwarz T, Granstein RD. Dendritic cells as initiators of tumor immune responses: a possible strategy for tumor immunotherapy? Immunol Today 1995; 16:117–121.
165. Paglia P, Girolomoni G, Robbiati F, Granucci F, Ricciardi-Castagnoli P. Immortalized dendritic cell line fully competent in antigen presentation initiates primary T cell responses in vivo. J Exp Med 1993; 178:1893–1901.
166. Cohen PJ, Cohen PA, Rosenberg SA, Katz SI, Mule JJ. Murine epidermal Langerhans cells and splenic dendritic cells present tumor-associated antigens to primed T cells. Eur J Immunol 1994; 24:315–319.
167. Flamand V, Sornasse T, Thielemans K, Demanet C, Bakkus M, Bazin H, et al. Murine dendritic cells pulsed in vitro with tumor antigen induce tumor resistance in vivo. Eur J Immunol 1994; 24:605–610.
168. Zitvogel L, Mayordomo JI, Tjandrawan T, DeLeo AB, Clarke MR, Lotze MT, et al. Therapy of murine tumors with tumor peptide-pulsed dendritic cells: dependence

on T cells, B7 costimulation, and T helper cell 1–associated cytokines. J Exp Med 1996; 183:87–97.
169. Celluzzi CM, Mayordomo JI, Storkus WJ, Lotze MT, Falo LD, Jr. Peptide-pulsed dendritic cells induce antigen-specific CTL-mediated protective tumor immunity. J Exp Med 1996; 183: 283–287.
170. Paglia P, Chiodoni C, Rodolfo M, Colombo MP. Murine dendritic cells loaded in vitro with soluble protein prime cytotoxic T lymphocytes against tumor antigen in vivo. J Exp Med 1996; 183:317–322.
171. Romani N, Gruner S, Brang D, Kampgen E, Lenz A, Trockenbacher B, et al. Proliferating dendritic cell progenitors in human blood. J Exp Med 1994; 180:83–93.
172. Szabolcs P, Avigan D, Gezelter S, Ciocon DH, Moore MA, Steinman RM, et al. Dendritic cells and macrophages can mature independently from a human bone marrow-derived, post-colony-forming unit intermediate. Blood 1996; 87:4520–4530.
173. Rivera GK, Pinkel D, Simone JV, Hancock ML, Crist WM. Treatment of acute lymphoblastic leukemia. 30 years' experience at St. Jude Children's Research Hospital [see comments]. N Engl J Med 1993; 329:1289–1295.
174. Steinherz PG, Gaynon P, Miller DR, Reaman G, Bleyer A, Finklestein J, et al. Improved disease-free survival of children with acute lymphoblastic leukemia at high risk for early relapse with the New York regimen—a new intensive therapy protocol: a report from the Children's Cancer Study Group. J Clin Oncol 1986; 4: 744–752.
175. Linker CA, Levitt LJ, O'Donnell M, Forman SJ, Ries CA. Treatment of adult acute lymphoblastic leukemia with intensive cyclical chemotherapy: a follow-up report. Blood 1991; 78:2814–2822.
176. Hussein KK, Dahlberg S, Head D, Waddell CC, Dabich L, Weick JK, et al. Treatment of acute lymphoblastic leukemia in adults with intensive induction, consolidation, and maintenance chemotherapy. Blood 1989; 73:57–63.
177. Ritz J, Ramsay NK, Kersey JH. Autologous bone marrow transplantation for acute lymphoblastic leukemia. In: Forman SJ, Blume KG, Thomas ED, eds. Bone Marrow Transplantation. Boston: Blackwell Scientific Publications, 1994:731–742.
178. Carey PJ, Proctor SJ, Taylor P, Hamilton PJ. Autologous bone marrow transplantation for high-grade lymphoid malignancy using melphalan/irradiation conditioning without marrow purging or cryopreservation. The Northern Regional Bone Marrow Transplant Group. Blood 1991; 77:1593–1598.
179. Schmid H, Henze G, Schwerdtfeger R, Baumgarten E, Besserer A, Scheffler A, et al. Fractionated total body irradiation and high-dose VP-16 with purged autologous bone marrow rescue for children with high-risk relapsed acute lymphoblastic leukemia. Bone Marrow Transplant 1993; 12:597–602.
180. Soiffer RJ, Roy DC, Gonin R, Murray C, Anderson KC, Freedman AS, et al. Monoclonal antibody-purged autologous bone marrow transplantation in adults with acute lymphoblastic leukemia at high risk of relapse. Bone Marrow Transplant 1993; 12:243–251.
181. Almici C, Manoni L, Carlo-Stella C, Garau D, Cottafavi L, Rizzoli V. Natural killer cell regeneration after transplantation with mafosfamide purged autologous bone marrow. Bone Marrow Transplant 1995; 16:95–101.

182. Nagler A, Peacock M, Tantoco M, Lamons D, Okarma TB, Okrongly DA. Separation of hematopoietic progenitor cells from human umbilical cord blood. J Hematother 1993; 2:243–245.
183. Anderson KC, Bates MP, Slaughenhoupt BL, Pinkus GS, Schlossman SF, Nadler LM. Expression of human B-cell–associated antigens on leukemias and lymphomas: a model of human B-cell differentiation. Blood 1984; 63:1424–1433.
184. Freedman AS. Cell surface antigens in leukemias and lymphomas. Cancer Invest 1996; 14:252–276.
185. Jennings CD, Foon KA. Recent advances in flow cytometry: application to the diagnosis of hematologic malignancy. Blood 1997; 90:2863–2892.
186. Hudson AM, Makrynikola V, Kabral A, Bradstock KF. Immunophenotypic analysis of clonogenic cells in acute lymphoblastic leukemia using an in vitro colony assay. Blood 1989; 74:2112–2120.
187. Uckun FM, Ledbetter JA. Immunobiologic differences between normal and leukemic human B-cell precursors. Proc Natl Acad Sci USA 1988; 85:8603–8607.
188. Mori T, Sugita K, Suzuki T, Okazaki T, Manabe A, Hosoya R, et al. A novel monoclonal antibody, KOR-SA3544 which reacts to Philadelphia chromosome-positive acute lymphoblastic leukemia cells with high sensitivity. Leukemia 1995; 9:1233–1239.
189. Uckun FM, Gaynon PS, Sensel MG, Nachman J, Trigg ME, Steinherz PG, et al. Clinical features and treatment outcome of childhood T-lineage acute lymphoblastic leukemia according to the apparent maturational stage of T-lineage leukemic blasts: a Children's Cancer Group study. J Clin Oncol 1997; 15:2214–2221.
190. Csoka M, Strauss G, Debatin KM, Moldenhauer G. Activation of T cell cytotoxicity against autologous common acute lymphoblastic leukemia (cALL) blasts by CD3×CD19 bispecific antibody. Leukemia 1996; 10:1765–1772.
191. Billett AL, Kornmehl E, Tarbell NJ, Weinstein HJ, Gelber RD, Ritz J, et al. Autologous bone marrow transplantation after a long first remission for children with recurrent acute lymphoblastic leukemia. Blood 1993; 81:1651–1657.
192. LeBien TW, Stepan DE, Bartholomew RM, Stong RC, Anderson JM. Utilization of a colony assay to assess the variables influencing elimination of leukemic cells from human bone marrow with monoclonal antibodies and complement. Blood 1985; 65:945–950.
193. Hudson AM, Makrynikola V, Kalral A, Bradstock KF. Immunophenotypic analysis of clonogenic cells in acute lymphoblastic leukemia using an in vitro colony assay. Blood 1989; 74:2112–2120.
194. Bast RC, Jr., De Fabritiis P, Lipton J, Gelber R, Maver C, Nadler L, et al. Elimination of malignant clonogenic cells from human bone marrow using multiple monoclonal antibodies and complement. Cancer Res 1985; 45:499–503.
195. Racadot E, Herve P, Lamy B, Peters A. Preclinical studies of a panel of 12 monoclonal antibodies in view of bone marrow purging in acute lymphoblastic leukemia. Leuk Res 1987; 11:987–994.
196. Janossy G, Campana D, Burnett A, Coustan-Smith E, Timms A, Bekassy AN, et al. Autologous bone marrow transplantation in acute lymphoblastic leukemia—preclinical immunologic studies. Leukemia 1988; 2:485–495.
197. Howell AL, Fogg-Leach M, Davis BH, Ball ED. Continuous infusion of comple-

ment by an automated cell processor enhances cytotoxicity of monoclonal antibody sensitized leukemia cells. Bone Marrow Transplant. 1989; 4:317–322.
198. Preijers FW, De WT, Wessels JM, De GG, Van LE, Capel PJ, et al. Autologous transplantation of bone marrow purged in vitro with anti-CD7-(WT1-) ricin A immunotoxin in T-cell lymphoblastic leukemia and lymphoma. Blood 1989; 74:1152–1158.
199. Vallera DA, Burns LJ, Frankel AE, Sicheneder AR, Gunther R, Gajl-Peczalska K, et al. Laboratory preparation of a deglycosylated ricin toxin A chain containing immunotoxin directed against a CD7 T lineage differentiation antigen for Phase I human clinical studies involving T cell malignancies. J Immunol Methods 1996; 197:69–83.
200. Goulet AC, Goldmacher VS, Lambert JM, Baron C, Roy DC, Kouassi E. Conjugation of blocked ricin to an anti-CD19 monoclonal antibody increases antibody-induced cell calcium mobilization and CD19 internalization. Blood 1997; 90:2364–2375.
201. Stoppa AM, Hirn J, Blaise D, Delaage M, Novakovitch G, Viens P, et al. Autologous bone marrow transplantation for B cell malignancies after in vitro purging with floating immunobeads. Bone Marrow Transplant 1990; 6:301–307.
202. Kiesel S, Haas R, Moldenhauer G, Kvalheim G, Pezzutto A, Dorken B. Removal of cells from a malignant B-cell line from bone marrow with immunomagnetic beads and with complement and immunoglobulin switch variant mediated cytolysis. Leuk Res 1987; 11:1119–1125.
203. Trickett AE, Ford DJ, Lam PTP, Vowels MR. Immunomagnetic bone marrow purging of common acute lymphoblastic leukemia cells: suitability of BioMag particles. Bone Marrow Transplant 1991; 7:199–203.
204. Korbling M, Knauf W, Funderud S, Kvalheim G, Hunstein W. Autologous transplantation of an immunomagnetic bead purged marrow in patients with relapsed acute lymphoblastic leukemia. Haematologica 1991; 76(suppl 1):29–36.
205. Martin H, Atta J, Zumpe P, Eder M, Elsner S, Rode C, et al. Purging of peripheral blood stem cells yields BCR-ABL-negative autografts in patients with BCR-ABL-positive acute lymphoblastic leukemia. Exp Hematol 1995; 23:1612–1618.
206. Atta J, Martin H, Bruecher J, Elsner S, Wassmann B, Rode C, et al. Residual leukemia and immunomagnetic bead purging in patients with BCR-ABL-positive acute lymphoblastic leukemia. Bone Marrow Transplant 1996; 18:541–548.
207. Simonsson B, Burnett AK, Prentice HG, Hann IH, Brenner MK, Gibson B, et al. Autologous bone marrow transplantation with monoclonal antibody purged marrow for high-risk acute lymphoblastic leukemia. Leukemia 1989; 3:631–636.
208. Doney K, Buckner CD, Fisher L, Petersen FB, Sanders J, Appelbaum FR, et al. Autologous bone marrow transplantation for acute lymphoblastic leukemia. Bone Marrow Transplant 1993; 12:315–321.
209. Morishima Y, Miyamura K, Kojima S, Ueda R, Morishita Y, Sao H, et al. Autologous BMT in high-risk patients with CALLA-positive ALL: possible efficacy of ex vivo marrow leukemia cell purging with monoclonal antibodies and complement. Bone Marrow Transplant 1993; 11:255–259.
210. Rizzoli V, Mangoni L, Carella AM, Aglietta M, Porcellini A, Coleselli P, et al.

Drug-mediated marrow purging: mafosfamide in adult acute leukemia in remission. The experience of the Italian study group. Bone Marrow Transplant 1989; 4(suppl 1):190–194.

211. Gorin NC, Aegerter P, Auvert B. Autologous bone marrow transplantation for acute leukemia in remission: an analysis of 1322 cases. Bone Marrow Transplant 1989; 4(suppl 2):3–5.

212. Kersey JH, Weisdorf D, Nesbit ME, LeBien TW, Woods WG, McGlave PB, et al. Comparison of autologous and allogeneic bone marrow transplantation for treatment of high-risk refractory acute lymphoblastic leukemia. N Engl J Med 1987; 317:461–467.

213. Sallan SE, Niemeyer CM, Billett AL, Lipton JM, Tarbell NJ, Gelber RD, et al. Autologous bone marrow transplantation for acute lymphoblastic leukemia. J Clin Oncol 1989; 7:1594–1601.

214. Cahn JY, Bordigoni P, Souillet G, Pico JL, Plouvier E, Reiffers J, et al. The TAM regimen prior to allogeneic and autologous bone marrow transplantation for high-risk acute lymphoblastic leukemias: a cooperative study of 62 patients. Bone Marrow Transplant 1991; 7:1–4.

215. Weisdorf DJ, Billett AL, Hannan P, Ritz J, Sallan SE, Steinbuch M, et al. Autologous versus unrelated donor allogeneic marrow transplantation for acute lymphoblastic leukemia. Blood 1997; 90:2962–2968.

216. Nishigaki H, Ito C, Manabe A, Kumagai M, Coustan-Smith E, Yanishevski Y, et al. Prevalence and growth characteristics of malignant stem cells in B-lineage acute lymphoblastic leukemia. Blood 1997; 89:3735–3744.

217. Gulati S, Yahalom J, Acaba L, Reich L, Motzer R, Crown J, et al. Treatment of patients with relapsed and resistant non-Hodgkin's lymphoma using total body irradiation, etoposide, and cyclophosphamide and autologous bone marrow transplantation. J Clin Oncol 1992; 10:936–941.

218. Colombat P, Gorin NC, Lemonnier MP, Binet C, Laporte JP, Douay L, et al. The role of autologous bone marrow transplantation in 46 adult patients with non-Hodgkin's lymphomas. J Clin Oncol 1990; 8:630–637.

219. Andersen NS, Donovan JW, Borus JS, Poor CM, Neuberg D, Aster JC, et al. Failure of immunologic purging in mantle cell lymphoma assessed by polymerase chain reaction detection of minimal residual disease. Blood 1997; 90:4212–4221.

220. Kvalheim G, Fjeld JG, Pihl A, Funderud S, Ugelstad J, Fodstad O, et al. Immunomagnetic removal of B-lymphoma cells using a novel mono- sized magnetizable polymer bead, M-280, in conjunction with primary IgM and IgG antibodies. Bone Marrow Transplant 1989; 4:567–574.

221. Uckun FM, Reaman GH. Immunotoxins for treatment of leukemia and lymphoma (review). Leuk Lymphoma 1995; 18:195–201.

222. Ghetie V, Engert A, Schnell R, Vitetta ES. The in vivo anti-tumor activity of immunotoxins containing two versus one deglycosylated ricin A chains. Cancer Lett 1995; 98:97–101.

223. Sausville EA, Headlee D, Stetler-Stevenson M, Jaffe ES, Solomon D, Figg WD, et al. Continuous infusion of the anti-CD22 immunotoxin IgG-RFB4-SMPT-dgA in patients with B-cell lymphoma: a Phase I study. Blood 1995; 85:3457–3465.

224. Grossbard ML, Lambert JM, Goldmacher VS, Spector NL, Kinsella J, Eliseo L, et al. Anti-B4-blocked ricin: a Phase I trial of 7-day continuous infusion in patients with B-cell neoplasms. J Clin Oncol 1993; 11:726–737.
225. Grossbard ML, Gribben JG, Freedman AS, Lambert JM, Kinsella J, Rabinowe SN, et al. Adjuvant immunotoxin therapy with anti-B4-blocked ricin after autologous bone marrow transplantation for patients with B-cell non-Hodgkin's lymphoma. Blood 1993; 81:2263–2271.
226. Philip T, Armitage JO, Spitzer G, Chauvin F, Jagannath S, Cahn JY, et al. High-dose therapy and autologous bone marrow transplantation after failure of conventional chemotherapy in adults with intermediate-grade or high-grade non-Hodgkin's lymphoma. N Engl J Med 1987; 316:1493–1498.
227. Freedman AS, Takvorian T, Anderson KC, Mauch P, Rabinowe SN, Blake K, et al. Autologous bone marrow transplantation in B-cell non-Hodgkin's lymphoma: very low treatment-related mortality in 100 patients in sensitive relapse. J Clin Oncol 1990; 8:784–791.
228. Petersen FB, Appelbaum FR, Hill R, Fisher LD, Bigelow CL, Sanders JE, et al. Autologous marrow transplantation for malignant lymphoma: a report of 101 cases from Seattle. J Clin Oncol 1990; 8:638–647.
229. Philip T, Guglielmi C, Hagenbeek A, Somers R, Van der Lelie H, Bron D, et al. Autologous bone marrow transplantation as compared with salvage chemotherapy in relapses of chemotherapy-sensitive non-Hodgkin's lymphoma. N Engl J Med 1995; 333:1540–1545.
230. Stahel RA, Jost LM, Pichert G, Widmer L. High-dose chemotherapy and autologous bone marrow transplantation for malignant lymphomas. Cancer Treat Rev 1995; 21:3–32.
231. Haioun C, Lepage E, Gisselbrecht C, Bastion Y, Coiffier B, Brice P, et al. Benefit of autologous bone marrow transplantation over sequential chemotherapy in poor-risk aggressive non-Hodgkin's lymphoma: updated results of the prospective study LNH87-2. Groupe d'Etude des Lymphomes de l'Adulte. J Clin Oncol 1997; 15:1131–1137.
232. Williams CD, Goldstone AH, Pearce RM, Philip T, Hartmann O, Colombat P, et al. Purging of bone marrow in autologous bone marrow transplantation for non-Hodgkin's lymphoma: a case-matched comparison with unpurged cases by the European Blood and Marrow Transplant Lymphoma Registry. J Clin Oncol 1996; 14:2454–2464.
233. Philip I, Favrot M. [Cell cultures in Burkitt's lymphoma. Detection of residual disease and application to autologous graft purging]. [French]. Pathologie Biologie 1988; 36:79–82.
234. Zwicky CS, Maddocks AB, Andersen N, Gribben JG. Eradication of polymerase chain reaction detectable immunoglobulin gene rearrangement in non-Hodgkin's lymphoma is associated with decreased relapse after autologous bone marrow transplantation. Blood 1996; 88:3314–3322.
235. Freedman AS, Ritz J, Neuberg D, Anderson KC, Rabinowe SN, Mauch P, et al. Autologous bone marrow transplantation in 69 patients with a history of low-grade B-cell non-Hodgkin's lymphoma. Blood 1991; 77:2524–2529.
236. Johnson PW, Price CG, Smith T, Cotter FE, Meerabux J, Rohatiner AZ, et al.

Detection of cells bearing the t(14;18) translocation following myeloablative treatment and autologous bone marrow transplantation for follicular lymphoma. J Clin Oncol 1994; 12:798–805.
237. Freedman AS, Gribben JG, Neuberg D, Mauch P, Soiffer RJ, Anderson KC, et al. High-dose therapy and autologous bone marrow transplantation in patients with follicular lymphoma during first remission. Blood 1996; 88:2780–2786.
238. Roy DC, Bélanger R, Perreault C, Bonny Y, Busque L, Kassis J, et al. Autologous bone marrow transplantation for patients with non-Hodgkin's lymphoma using anti-B4-bR immunotoxin purging. Proc Fourth Int Symp Immunotoxins 1995; 158–150.
239. Meijerink JP, Smetsers TF, Raemaekers JM, Bogman MJ, de Witte T, Mensink EJ. Quantitation of follicular non-Hodgkin's lymphoma cells carrying t(14;18) by competitive polymerase chain reaction. Br J Haematol 1993; 84:250–256.
240. McCann JC, Kanteti R, Shilepsky B, Miller KB, Sweet M, Schenkein DP. High degree of occult tumor contamination in bone marrow and peripheral blood stem cells of patients undergoing autologous transplantation for non-Hodgkin's lymphoma. Biol Blood Marrow Transplant 1996; 2:37–43.
241. Roy DC, Robertson MJ, Bélanger R, Gyger M, Perreault C, Bonny Y, et al. Engraftment following anti-my9-bR depleted autologous marrow transplantation for patients with acute myeloid leukemia. Blood 1992; 80(suppl 1):376a.
242. Dreger P, Vonneuhoff N, Suttorp M, Loffler H, Schmitz N. Rapid engraftment of peripheral blood progenitor cell grafts purged with B-cell-specific monoclonal antibodies and immunomagnetic beads. Bone Marrow Transplant 1995; 16:627–629.
243. Spangrude GJ. Hematopoietic stem-cell differentiation. Curr Opin Immunol 1991; 3:171–178.
244. Shpall EJ, Jones RB, Bearman SI, Franklin WA, Archer PG, Curiel T, et al. Transplantation of enriched CD34-positive autologous marrow into breast cancer patients following high-dose chemotherapy: influence of CD34-positive peripheral-blood progenitors and growth factors on engraftment. J Clin Oncol 1994; 12:28–36.
245. Baum CM, Weissman IL, Tsukamoto AS, Buckle AM, Peault B. Isolation of a candidate human hematopoietic stem-cell population. Proc Natl Acad Sci USA 1992; 89:2804–2808.
246. Huang S, Terstappen LW. Formation of haematopoietic microenvironment and haematopoietic stem cells from single human bone marrow stem cells. Nature 1992; 360:745–749.
247. Korbling M, Drach J, Champlin RE, Engel H, Huynh L, Kleine HD, et al. Large-scale preparation of highly purified, frozen/thawed CD34+, HLA-DR− hematopoietic progenitor cells by sequential immunoadsorption (CEPRATE SC) and fluorescence-activated cell sorting: implications for gene transduction and/or transplantation. Bone Marrow Transplant 1994; 13:649–654.
248. Berenson RJ, Bensinger WI, Kalamasz D. Positive selection of viable cell populations using avidin-biotin immunoadsorption. J Imm Meth 1986; 91:11–19.
249. Lemoli RM, Gobbi M, Tazzari PL, Tassi TC, Dinota A, Visani G, et al. Bone marrow purging for multiple myeloma by avidin-biotin immunoadsorption. Transplantation 1989; 47:385–387.

250. Auditore-Hargreaves K, Heimfeld S, Berenson RJ. Selection and transplantation of hematopoietic stem and progenitor cells. Bioconjugate Chem 1994; 5:287–300.
251. Dewynter EA, Coutinho LH, Pei X, Marsh JCW, Hows J, Luft T, et al. Comparison of purity and enrichment of CD34(+) cells from bone marrow, umbilical cord and peripheral blood (primed for apheresis) using five separation systems. Stem Cells 1995; 13:524–532.
252. Bohbot A, Lioure B, Faradji A, Schmitt M, Cuillerot JM, Laplace A, et al. Positive selection of CD34(+) cells from cryopreserved peripheral blood stem cells after thawing—technical aspects and clinical use. Bone Marrow Transplant 1996; 17:259–264.
253. McQuaker IG, Haynes AP, Anderson S, Stainer C, Owen RG, Morgan GJ, et al. Engraftment and molecular monitoring of CD34+ peripheral-blood stem-cell transplants for follicular lymphoma: a pilot study. J Clin Oncol 1997; 15:2288–2295.
254. Hardwick RA, Kulcinski D, Mansour V, Ishizawa L, Law P, Gee AP. Design of large-scale separation systems for positive and negative immunomagnetic selection of cells using superparamagnetic microspheres. J Hematother 1992; 1:379–386.
255. Hansen M, Yacob D, Schaeffer A, Jain R, Guha M, Deans R. A comparison of expansion potential and phenotype of cultured CD34+ cells released from immunomagnetic beads by chymopapain or a peptide epitope release reagent. Blood 1995; 86(suppl 1):666a.
256. Paulus U, Dreger P, Viehmann K, von NN, Schmitz N. Purging peripheral blood progenitor cell grafts from lymphoma cells: quantitative comparison of immunomagnetic CD34+ selection systems. Stem Cells 1997; 15:297–304.
257. Roots-Weiss A, Papadimitriou C, Serve H, Hoppe B, Koenigsmann M, Reufi B, et al. The efficiency of tumor cell purging using immunomagnetic CD34+ cell separation systems. Bone Marrow Transplant 1997; 19:1239–1246.
258. Williams SF, Lee WJ, Bender JG, Zimmerman T, Swinney P, Blake M, et al. Selection and expansion of peripheral blood CD34(+) cells in autologous stem cell transplantation for breast cancer. Blood 1996; 87:1687–1691.
259. Kemshead JT. The immunomagnetic manipulation of bone marrow. In: Gee AP, ed. Bone Marrow Processing and Purging. Boca Raton, Fl.: CRC Press, 1991:293–305.
260. Okarma TB. Stem cell selection for autologous bone marrow transplantation. Sem Hematol 1992; 29:9–20.
261. Lebkowski JS, Schain LR, Okrongly D, Levinsky R, Harvey MJ, Okarma TB. Rapid isolation of human CD34 hematopoietic stem cells-purging of human tumor cells. Transplantation 1992; 53:1011–1019.
262. Cardoso AA, Watt SM, Batard P, Li ML, Hatzfeld A, Genevier H, et al. An improved panning technique for the selection of CD34+ human bone marrow hematopoietic cells with high recovery of early progenitors. Exp Hematol 1995; 23:407–412.
263. Cardoso AA, Li ML, Batard P, Sansilvestri P, Hatzfeld A, Levesque JP, et al. Human umbilical cord blood CD34+ cell purification with high yield of early progenitors. J Hematother 1993; 2:275–279.
264. Borowitz MJ, Gockerman JP, Moore JO, Civin CI, Page SO, Robertson J, et al.

Clinicopathologic and cytogenic features of CD34(My 10)-positive acute non-lymphocytic leukemia. Am J Clin Pathol 1989; 91:265–270.
265. Soligo D, Delia D, Oriani A, Cattoretti G, Orazi A, Bertolli V, et al. Identification of CD34+ cells in normal and pathological bone marrow biopsies by QBEND10 monoclonal antibody. Leukemia 1991; 5:1026–1030.
266. Geller RB, Zahurak M, Hurwitz CA, Burke PJ, Karp JE, Piantadosi S, et al. Prognostic importance of immunophenotyping in adults with acute myelocytic leukaemia: the significance of the stem-cell glycoprotein CD34 (My 10). Br J Haematol 1990; 76:340–347.
267. Silvestri F, Banavali S, Baccarani M, Preisler HD. The CD34 hemopoietic progenitor cell associated antigen: biology and clinical applications. Haematologica 1992; 77:265–273.
268. Katz FE, Watt SM, Martin H, Lam G, Capellaro D, Goldman JM, et al. Coordinate expression of BI.3C5 and HLA-DR antigens on haemopoietic progenitors from chronic myeloid leukaemia. Leuk Res 1986; 10:961–971.
269. Guyotat D, Campos L, Thomas X, Vila L, Shi ZH, Charrin C, et al. Myelodysplastic syndromes: a study of surface markers and in vitro growth patterns. Am J Hematol 1990; 34:26–31.
270. Gore SD, Kastan MB, Civin CI. Normal human bone marrow precursors that express terminal deoxynucleotidyl transferase include T-cell precursors and possible lymphoid stem cells. Blood 1991; 77:1681–1690.
271. Macintyre EA, Belanger C, Debert C, Canioni D, Turhan AG, Azagury M, et al. Detection of clonal CD34(+)19(+) progenitors in bone marrow of bcl-2-IgH-positive follicular lymphoma patients. Blood 1995; 86:4691–4698.
272. Vescio RA, Hong CH, Cao J, Kim A, Schiller GJ, Lichtenstein AK, et al. The hematopoietic stem cell antigen, CD34, is not expressed on the malignant cells in multiple myeloma. Blood 1994; 84:3283–3290.
273. Sankey EA, More L, Dhillon AP. QBEnd/10: a new immunostain for the routine diagnosis of Kaposi's sarcoma. J Pathol 1990; 161:267–271.
274. Brugger W, Henschler R, Heimfeld S, Berenson RJ, Mertelsmann R, Kanz L. Positively selected autologous blood CD34+ cells and unseparated peripheral blood progenitor cells mediate identical hematopoietic engraftment after high-dose VP16, ifosfamide, carboplatin, and epirubicin. Blood 1994; 84:1421–1426.
275. Gorin NC, Lopez M, Laporte JP, Quittet P, Lesage S, Lemoine F, et al. Preparation and successful engraftment of purified CD34+ bone marrow progenitor cells in patients with non-Hodgkin's lymphoma. Blood 1995; 85:1647–1654.
276. Hohaus S, Pforsich M, Murea S, Abdallah A, Lin YS, Funk L, et al. Immunomagnetic selection of CD34+ peripheral blood stem cells for autografting in patients with breast cancer. Br J Haematol 1997; 97:881–888.
277. Lopez M, Lemoine FM, Firat H, Fouillard L, Laporte JP, Lesage S, et al. Bone marrow versus peripheral blood progenitor cells CD34 selection in patients with non-Hodgkin's lymphomas: different levels of tumor cell reduction. Implications for autografting. Blood 1997; 90:2830–2838.
278. To LB, Haylock DN, Simmons PJ, Juttner CA. The biology and clinical uses of blood stem cells. Blood 1997; 89:2233–2258.
279. Roy DC, Beauger N, Gyger M. Progenitor cell preparation and purging. In: Matzku

S, Stahel RA, eds. Antibodies in Diagnosis and Therapy: Technologies, Mechanisms and Clinical Data. Frankfort: Merck, 1997. In press.
280. Coutinho LH, Brereton ML, Santos AM, Ryder WD, Chang J, Harrison CJ, et al. Evaluation of cytogenetic conversion to Ph-haemopoiesis in long-term bone marrow culture for patients with chronic myeloid leukaemia on conventional hydroxyurea therapy, on pulse high-dose hydroxyurea and on interferon-alpha. Br J Hematol 1996; 93:869–877.
281. Widmer L, Pichert G, Jost LM, Stahel RA. Fate of contaminating t(14; 18)+ lymphoma cells during ex vivo expansion of CD34-selected hematopoietic progenitor cells. Blood 1996; 88:3166–3175.
282. Muench MO, Moore MA. Accelerated recovery of peripheral blood cell counts in mice transplanted with in vitro cytokine-expanded hematopoietic progenitors. Exp Hematol 1992; 20:611–618.
283. To LB, Roberts MM, Haylock DN, Dyson PG, Branford AL, Thorp D, et al. Comparison of haematological recovery times and supportive care requirements of autologous recovery phase peripheral blood stem cell transplants, autologous bone marrow transplants and allogeneic bone marrow transplants. Bone Marrow Transplant 1992; 9:277–284.
284. Haylock DN, To LB, Dowse TL, Juttner CA, Simmons PJ. Ex vivo expansion and maturation of peripheral blood CD34+ cells into the myeloid lineage. Blood 1992; 80:1405–1412.
285. Korbling M. Blood stem cell transplantation and gene therapy of cancer. Stem Cells 1995; 13:106–113.
286. Sierra J, Granena A, Garcia J, Valls A, Carreras E, Rovira M, et al. Autologous bone marrow transplantation for acute leukemia: results and prognostic factors in 90 consecutive patients. Bone Marrow Transplant 1993; 12:517–523.
287. Mitus AJ, Miller KB, Schenkein DP, Ryan HF, Parsons SK, Wheeler C, et al. Improved survival for patients with acute myelogenous leukemia. J Clin Oncol 1995; 13:560–569.
288. de la Rubia J, Sanz GF, Martin G, Sempere A, Picon I, Carral A, et al. Autologous bone marrow transplantation for patients with acute myeloblastic leukemia in relapse after autologous blood stem cell transplantation. Bone Marrow Transplant 1996; 18:1167–1173.
289. Tomas F, Gomez-Garcia dS, Lopez-Lorenzo JL, Arranz R, Figuera A, Camara R, et al. Autologous or allogeneic bone marrow transplantation for acute myeloblastic leukemia in second complete remission. Importance of duration of first complete remission in final outcome. Bone Marrow Transplant 1996; 17:979–984.
290. Stein AS, O'Donnell MR, Chai A, Schmidt GM, Nademanee A, Parker PM, et al. In vivo purging with high-dose cytarabine followed by high-dose chemoradiotherapy and reinfusion of unpurged bone marrow for adult acute myelogenous leukemia in first complete remission. J Clin Oncol 1996; 14:2206–2216.
291. Petersen FB, Lynch MH, Clift RA, Appelbaum FR, Sanders JE, Bensinger WI, et al. Autologous marrow transplantation for patients with acute myeloid leukemia in untreated first relapse or in second complete remission. J Clin Oncol 1993; 11:1353–1360.
292. Linker CA, Damon LE, Ries CA, Rugo HS, Wolf JL. Busulfan plus etoposide as

a preparative regimen for autologous bone marrow transplantation for acute myelogenous leukemia: an update. Semin Oncol 1993; 20:40–48.
293. Laporte JP, Douay L, Lopez M, Labopin M, Jouet JP, Lesage S, et al. One hundred twenty-five adult patients with primary acute leukemia autografted with marrow purged by mafosfamide: a 10-year single-institution experience. Blood 1994; 84: 3810–3818.
294. Schroeder H, Pinkerton CR, Powles RL, Meller ST, Tait D, Milan S, et al. High-dose melphalan and total-body irradiation with autologous marrow rescue in childhood acute lymphoblastic leukaemia after relapse. Bone Marrow Transplant 1991; 7:11–15.
295. Powles R, Mehta J, Singhal S, Horton C, Tait D, Milan S, et al. Autologous bone marrow or peripheral blood stem cell transplantation followed by maintenance chemotherapy for adult acute lymphoblastic leukemia in first remission: 50 cases from a single center. Bone Marrow Transplant 1995; 16:241–247.
296. Gilmore MJ, Hamon MD, Prentice HG, Katz F, Slaper-Cortenbach IC, Hunter AE, et al. Failure of purged autologous bone marrow transplantation in high-risk acute lymphoblastic leukaemia in first complete remission. Bone Marrow Transplant 1991; 8:19–26.
297. Soiffer RJ, Roy DC, Gonin R, Murray C, Anderson KC, Freedman AS, et al. Monoclonal antibody-purged autologous bone marrow transplantation in adults with acute lymphoblastic leukemia at high risk of relapse. Bone Marrow Transplant 1993; 12:243–251.
298. Garcia J, Punti C, Picon M, Tigues D, Amill B, Canals C, et al. Bone marrow purging in acute lymphoblastic leukemia: biological and clinical features. J Hematother 1994; 3:203–211.
299. De Bruyn C, Delforge A, Bron D, Bernier M, Massy M, Ley P, et al. Comparison of the coexpression of CD38, CD33 and HLA-DR antigens on CD34+ purified cells from human cord blood and bone marrow. Stem Cells 1995; 13:281–288.
300. Dreger P, Viehmann K, Steinmann J, Eckstein V, Muller-Ruchholtz W, Loffler H, et al. G-CSF-mobilized peripheral blood progenitor cells for allogeneic transplantation: comparison of T cell depletion strategies using different CD34+ selection systems or CAMPATH-1. Exp Hematol. 1995; 23:147–154.
301. Mahe B, Menard A, Accard F, Pineau D, Robillard N, Hermouet S. In vitro expansion of CD34+ cells from peripheral blood of myeloma and lymphoma patients. Nouvelle Revue Francaise d'Hematologie 1995; 37:335–341.
302. David S, Rice A, Vianes I, Duperray V, Dupouy M, Reiffers J. Expansion of blood CD34 positive cells—committed precursors expansion does not affect immature hematopoietic progenitors. Nouvelle Revue Francaise d'Hematologie 1995; 37: 343–349.
303. Link H, Arseniev L, Bahre O, Berenson RJ, Battmer K, Kadar JG, et al. Combined transplantation of allogeneic bone marrow and CD34+ blood cells. Blood 1995; 86:2500–2508.
304. Brugger W, Heimfeld S, Berenson RJ, Mertelsmann R, Kanz L. Reconstitution of hematopoiesis after high-dose chemotherapy by autologous progenitor cells generated ex vivo. N Engl J Med 1995; 333:283–287.
305. Bensinger WI, Buckner CD, Shannon-Dorcy K, Rowley S, Appelbaum FR, Beny-

unes M, et al. Transplantation of allogeneic CD34+ peripheral blood stem cells in patients with advanced hematologic malignancy. Blood 1996; 88:4132–4138.
306. Cornetta K, Gharpure V, Mills B, Hromas R, Abonour R, Broun ER, et al. Rapid engraftment after allogeneic transplantation using CD34-enriched marrow cells. Bone Marrow Transplant 1998; 21:65–71.
307. Lane TA, Law P, Maruyama M, Young D, Burgess J, Mullen M, et al. Harvesting and enrichment of hematopoietic progenitor cells mobilized into the peripheral blood of normal donors by granulocyte-macrophage colony-stimulating factor (GM-CSF) or G-CSF: potential role in allogeneic marrow transplantation. Blood 1995; 85:275–282.
308. Holyoake TL, Alcorn MJ, Richmond LJ, Freshney MG, Pearson C, Fitzsimons E, et al. Efficient isolation of human CD34 positive hemopoietic progenitor cells by immune panning. Stem Cells 1994; 12:114–124.

12
Monoclonal Antibody Therapy for Solid Tumors: An Overview

Panos Fidias*
Harvard Medical School and Massachusetts General Hospital, Boston, Massachusetts

I. INTRODUCTION

The use of traditional cytotoxic therapy for malignant tumors has met with significant successes but also has demonstrated several important limitations. Both chemotherapy and radiation therapy are toxic to normal as well as malignant cells, a fact that prohibits dose escalation of these agents without unacceptable side effects. Additionally, even with aggressive approaches, the majority of advanced solid tumors remain incurable, reflecting the intrinsic insensitivity of the malignant clone to currently employed therapies. It would be optimal if antitumor agents could be delivered specifically to the tumor cell, thus allowing for highly toxic modalities to be utilized without dose-limiting systemic toxicity.

The discovery by Kohler and Milstein of extremely specific antibodies produced by immortalized mouse myeloma cells opened the stage for such an approach (1), and for the past 20 years monoclonal antibody (mAb) therapy has attempted to make this expectation a reality (2). The first clinical trial with serotherapy was performed in 1980, involving the use of a monoclonal antibody in a patient with lymphoma (3). The initial enthusiasm, however, was blunted by the practical difficulties observed during the course of the clinical development of antibody therapy (2).

Monoclonal antibodies can be administered in either an unconjugated or a conjugated form. "Naked" antibodies target a specific determinant on tumor

---

* *Current affiliation:* Hematology-Oncology Associates of South Texas, San Antonio, Texas.

cells but are usually not directly toxic. Instead, they rely on the body's effector systems for the eradication of the tumor. The Fc fragment of the intact immunoglobulin can activate the complement cascade, with potency depending on its isotype (4). Moreover, cellular components of the immune system, especially monocytes, lymphocytes, and natural killer (NK) cells, can be recruited on site through their Fc receptors. Therefore, mAb therapy can activate both complement-dependent cytotoxicity (CDC) and antibody-dependent cellular cytotoxicity (ADCC) specific for the tumor (5). Alternatively, antibodies can act as carriers of potent agents, such as chemotherapy drugs, radioisotopes, or toxins. This approach can allow for the delivery of highly cytotoxic therapy without systemic nonspecific side effects. All subsequent modifications in the area of monoclonal antibody therapy still are based on these basic approaches, and have attempted mainly to overcome the obstacles encountered in clinical trials through technical refinement of the constructs or the more rational use of mAbs, based on the biology of solid tumors.

II. OBSTACLES TO EFFECTIVE IMMUNOTHERAPY

Adequate access of any therapeutic substance to its target tissue is central to the success of the treatment. This is especially important in solid tumors, in which poor blood flow and areas of necrosis and fibrosis are common. Solid tumors demonstrate variations in their vascularity, and therefore only well-perfused areas can be reached by monoclonal antibodies. Experiments using video micrography and direct visualization of human tumors grown in immunodeficient mice demonstrate that the vascular network of solid tumors is quite complex and provides little help to the optimal delivery of drugs. Blood flow is inadequate and often intermittent; the vessels are tortuous, they have bends and loops, and they frequently exhibit arteriovenous shunts (6). Additional barriers are raised by the high interstitial pressures within solid tumors. Usually, the hydrostatic pressure in the circulation exceeds the interstitial pressures, promoting the diffusion of molecules into the interstitium. However, tumors have been shown to have high interstitial pressures opposing the influx of monoclonal antibodies (7). Even if they do diffuse across the vessel wall, mAbs are large molecules that can encounter significant limitations in diffusion in areas of low interstitial volume and high tumor cell volume. In vitro studies have shown greater penetration of antibody fragments into tumors, compared with the full-length molecule (8). However, the exclusion of molecules from cells is independent of molecular weight, which means that even smaller molecules might encounter the same obstacles (9).

In addition to physical limitations to drug diffusion, antibodies can be trapped outside their target area, due to the formation of antigen–antibody complexes. Such immune complex formation can occur either within the tumor or at the periphery. Studies have shown that in the presence of high antigen density, mAbs are attached to perivascular tumor cells, limiting their access to the bulk of the disease (10). Even more important is the well-characterized rapid clearance of antibodies from the circulation in the presence of significant antigenic load. This was shown in studies with hematologic malignancies, where large numbers of circulating cells carrying the targeted antigen would lead to a shortened half-life of the monoclonal antibody (11). Circulating tumor cells obviously are less prominent in the case of solid tumors; however, antigenic shedding can lead to similar results. Almost all antigens can be shed into the circulation to some degree (5), leading to the formation of immune complexes and trapping the antibody in the periphery. The same effect occurs when patients develop high titers of antibodies against the infused foreign proteins (12).

The actual binding of mAbs to tumor cells is influenced not only by the ability of antibodies to penetrate into tissues but also by the properties of the targeted antigen. Solid tumors are known to exhibit marked heterogeneity in the expression of cell-surface antigens (13). Moreover, antigen-negative clones can emerge during the course of therapy, as has been clearly established in the case of non-Hodgkin's lymphomas (14). This process of immunoselection is different from a similar process that can impair antibody binding, called *antigenic modulation*. The mechanism behind antigenic modulation involves downregulation of surface molecules when they engage a ligand, due to capping and internalization, which is not compensated for by a higher rate of antigen cycling and expression (15). Even when the targeted antigen is present constantly, there is a certain threshold of antigen density and antibody concentration below which binding is not effective.

In several trials, the ability of mAbs to bind to target tissue was evaluated with biopsies of tumor sites following the administration of antibodies. These biopsies have yielded conflicting results, an unsurprising finding considering all the different factors that can influence antibody penetration and binding to tumor. The immunotoxin 260F9-ricin A was given to five patients with metastatic breast cancer, and two underwent biopsies of chest wall lesions: no mAb binding was appreciated (16). In another study with the same antibody, a patient with metastatic breast cancer was biopsied at the end of an 8-day treatment cycle, and again no antibody binding was seen (17). Weiner et al. used the monoclonal CO17-A (with interferon-γ) in the treatment of 19 patients with metastatic colorectal cancer. Out of nine biopsies of antigen-positive tumors, three stained positive by immunohistochemistry (IHC) for the presence of antibody (18). Other studies have suggested that binding of antibody is related to the total dose administered. Two out of fifteen patients treated with the bispecific antibody MDX-210 had positive IHC on repeat biopsies. Both were treated at the higher dose of 10 mg/m^2 (19). Elias et al. saw binding of KS1/4 in nearly all lung cancer patients treated with a total dose of 500–1000 mg of antibody (20). Similarly, binding of L6 mAb was appreciated in patients with a variety of malignancies who received a dose above 35 mg/m^2 (21).

Once the mAbs have attached to their target, they should exert their cytotoxicity as potently as possible. Unconjugated, whole antibodies rely predominantly on the activation of the host's immune system, especially complement proteins and cellular effectors. Laboratory studies have shown that murine IgG2a antibodies are superior to other subclasses in exerting ADCC, possibly because of stronger Fc receptor interactions (4). Murine IgG3 is the second most favorable subclass. However, murine proteins are less potent than human antibodies in eliciting an immune response, due to species differences. Evidence suggesting activation of human effectors is sporadic. The murine mAb KS1/4 (IgG2a) was used to treat eleven patients with non-small-cell lung cancer; on posttherapy biopsies, complement deposition was noted in the presence of antibody binding (20). Similar complement deposition was seen with the use of R24, an anti-GD3 ganglioside antibody used in the treatment of malignant melanoma (22). In another study, the bispecific murine antibody MDX-210 was identified in posttreatment biopsies of patients with breast cancer; in one case, a mononuclear cell infiltrate also was appreciated (19). The true significance of these findings is unclear, for they have been inconsistent and only rarely associated with tumor response.

Immunoconjugates were designed in an effort to overcome these limitations. The intrinsic sensitivity of the tumor to the specific modality employed is of great importance, since the targeting of ineffective agents will not improve on the clinical results. The question still remains whether adequately tumoricidal doses of chemotherapy drugs, radiation, or toxins can be delivered to the tumor site by antibodies without prohibitive toxicity. In general, clinical responses have been too limited to draw any firm conclusions (Tables 1–3).

Another important factor limiting the usefulness of mAbs is the occurrence of nonspecific toxicity against normal tissues. In contrast to hematologic malignancies, solid tumors do not express unique tumor-specific antigens; therefore, monoclonal antibodies cross-react to a certain degree with nonmalignant tissue (5). Insight into such interactions often is provided by preclinical studies on animal models (23). However, occasionally unexpected toxicities are encountered as a result of unsuspected binding of mAbs to vital structures (16,24). This is especially worrisome in the case of immunoconjugates, which carry a higher cytotoxic potential than "naked" antibodies.

Lastly, the efficacy of passive immunotherapy with mAbs can be blunted by the development of human antimouse antibodies (HAMA) or human antitoxin antibodies. In theory, allergic reactions are possible, due to the formation of immune complexes, which can be deposited in tissues and lead to serum sickness (25,26). This is especially true with the large quantities of antibody required for therapy with unconjugated mAbs. Moreover, high titers of these antibodies can rapidly clear the infused antibody from the circulation, limiting its access to the

Table 1 Clinical Studies of Monoclonal Antibodies in Colorectal Cancer

Reference	Antibody	Responses	Immune responses[a]
28	B72.3-^{131}I	0/12	9/12
12	B72.3-^{131}I	NR	7/12
27	CC49-^{131}I	0/24	24/24
29	B72.3-^{131}I	0/12	7/12
71	17-1A	2/20	NR
76	17-1A	1/4	3/4
39	17-1A	Improved OS	80%
66	28A32-^{131}I	0/28	None
21	L6	0/2	NR
73	791T/36-RTA	2/17	16/17
79	CC49-^{131}I	0/13	12/13
65	16.88-^{131}I	NR	0/20
81	MAb 33-^{131}I	0/23	23/23
69	17-1A	1/25	21/25
78	17-1A	1/20	10/20
18	17-1A	0/19	NR
48	D612	0/?	NR
37	I-1-bR	0/8	3/8
83	A7-NCS	2/8	NR
82	ch17-1A-^{125}I	0/28	1/15

[a] Includes the formation of human antimouse and human antitoxin antibodies.
NR: not reported; OS: overall survival; bR: blocked ricin; NCS: neocarsinostatin; ch17-1A: chimeric 17-1A; RTA: ricin toxin A.

Table 2 Clinical Studies of Monoclonal Antibodies in Ovarian Cancer

Reference	Antibody	Responses	Immune responses[a]
35	NR-LU-10-186Re	4/17	17/17
34	CC49-177Lu	1/12	12/12
21	L6	0/9	NR
38	HMFG1-90Y	NA	52/52
19	MDX-210	1/6[b]	NR
26	HMFG1-90Y	NR	12/12
24	OVB3-PE	0/23	23/23

[a] Includes the formation of human antimouse and human antitoxin antibodies.
[b] Mixed response.
PE: pseudomonas exotoxin; NA: not applicable; NR: not reported.

Table 3 Clinical Studies with Monoclonal Antibodies in Breast Cancer

Reference	Antibody	Responses	Immune responses[a]
52	rhuMAb HER-2/neu	8/36[b]	NR
64	rhuMAb HER-2/neu	5/43	0/43
16	260F9-RTA	0/5	3/5
21	L6	1/5	NR
17	260F9-RTA	1/4	4/4
19	MDX-210	1/9	NR
84	BR 55-2	1/9	NR

[a] Includes the formation of human antimouse and human antitoxin antibodies.
[b] With cisplatin.
NR: not reported.

tumor (12). Many trials have restricted therapeutic infusions to only one course or to a limited number of courses until the development of measurable antimouse/antitoxin response. Clinical experience has shown that rapid clearance and peripheral trapping are more frequent events than the development of significant allergic reactions (27–29).

III. STRATEGIES FOR EFFECTIVE IMMUNOTHERAPY

Whole immunoglobulin (Ig) molecules have high molecular weight and large size, which can impede their diffusion into bulky tumors. Moreover, they are very immunogenic and their Fc portion contributes to poor pharmacokinetics and nonspecific uptake by Fc receptors (30). Antibody access to tumor sites can be improved with the development of mAb fragments lacking the Fc portion of the Ig molecule. Through biochemical digestion techniques, bivalent antigen-binding fragments F(ab')$_2$ or monovalent fragments Fab' can be produced. Genetic engineering techniques can be used to join only the variable regions of the heavy (V_H) and light (V_L) chains with a unique peptide linker, giving rise to single-chain antigen-binding proteins (sFvs) (31). Generally, these constructs have retained their capacity to bind to target antigens, have demonstrated potent cytotoxicity, and have shown more rapid clearance with less immunogenicity (32). Moreover, they were found to exhibit a greater degree of tumor penetration compared to whole Igs. Yokota et al. treated athymic mice xenografted with LS-174T human colon carcinoma with intravenous injections of either radiolabeled mAb CC49 (murine IgG1), its respective F(ab')$_2$ and Fab', or CC49 sFv(8). The animals were sacrificed at different time points and the tumors examined with microautoradiographic analysis for the presence of antibody. Most of the IgG was concentrated adjacent to vessels, the sFv was present throughout the tumor mass, and the F(ab')$_2$ and Fab' fragments showed intermediate penetration. Moreover, the sFv demonstrated its peak penetration very early, at 0.5 hours postinjection, compared to the IgG, which had equivalent tumor penetration at 48–96 hours posttherapy. This study suggested that the actual degree of tumor uptake for sFvs may be higher than expected based on their rapid clearance.

At a more practical level, improvement in antibody access can be achieved by direct delivery to the tumor site. Malignancies that tend to remain localized in a specific anatomic location lend themselves to such an approach. The most common clinical scenario is the intraperitoneal injection of radioimmunoconjugates for the treatment of ovarian cancer (33–35). Typically, patients who have demonstrated free flow of peritoneal fluid are given the antibody through a peritoneal dialysis catheter, mixed with 1–2 liters of normal saline or Hartman's solution. The patients then change positions frequently to allow even distribution of the drug throughout the peritoneal cavity. Hospitalization lasts less than a week, until radioactivity levels fall within a safe range.

Similarly, intralesional therapy can be applied to other tumors. Riva et al. treated 24 patients with recurrent malignant gliomas with the mAbs BC-2 and BC-4 conjugated to iodine-131 (36). Following surgical resection, an indwelling catheter was introduced into the cavity and subsequently connected to a subcutaneous reservoir. A series of injections could be performed without local untoward effects. Zalceberg et al. utilized the intralesional route to treat patients with hepatic metastases of gastrointestinal origin with the Anti-CEA antibody I-1 conjugated to the toxin blocked–ricin (37). Toxicity generally was mild, with the most common side effect being hepatic capsular pain 24–48 hours following each injection.

Bulky tumors frequently are associated with areas of necrosis and fibrosis, making antibody access problematic. Several investigators have attempted to overcome this limitation by treating patients in the adjuvant setting. This approach has many theoretical advantages: accessibility should be much enhanced, tumor volume is considerably smaller, and circulating tumor antigen should be limited. Based on their previous experience with HMFG1 mAb conjugated to yttrium-90, Hird et al. treated women with ovarian cancer following cytoreductive surgery and chemotherapy with intraperitoneal administration of the radioimmunoconjugate (38). Survival was improved compared to a historical control group from a previous clinical trial, but the limitations of such an analysis are obvious. In another study, patients with lymph-node-positive colon cancer were randomized following potentially curative surgery to receive a placebo or unconjugated antibody 17-1A (39). Survival was improved for the group of patients receiving the antibody. Lynch et al. reported on the toxicity and efficacy of the N-901 mAb linked to the toxin-blocked ricin in patients with either limited- or extensive-stage small-cell lung cancer, administered in the setting of a complete response or near complete response following traditional chemotherapy (40). Twelve patients were treated, and one patient with limited-stage disease remains free of disease more than 2 years after the start of therapy (personal communication, T.J. Lynch).

Unmodified murine antibodies have limited potential to activate human immune pathways. Constructing antibodies with specificity both for the target tumor antigen and molecules on effector cells could theoretically lead to recruitment of large numbers of cytotoxic cells into the neoplastic tissue. Such bispecific constructs can enhance in vitro tumor lysis by effector cells, and also have demonstrated these effects in murine models of human tumor xenografts.

The therapeutic effect of the bispecific mAb 2B1, which targets the human Fcγ receptor III (CD16) and the extracellular domain of the c-erbB-2 oncogene product, was examined in SCID mice xenografted with human SK-OV-3 ovarian carcinoma (41). Cytokines, lymphocytes, and lymphokine-activated killer cells had minimal effect on tumor growth, but the addition of 2B1 led to significantly improved survival. This antibody was administered in a Phase I study to patients with c-erbB-2-expressing tumors. Peak serum levels of tumor necrosis factor (TNF), IL-6, IL-8, and elastase were found 1–4 hours following the start of the infusion, and tumor localization of ^{111}In-labeled autologous leukocytes also was noted, suggesting effective activation and targeting of host immune response.

A similar antibody, MDX-210, targets the same oncogene product but binds to FcγRI (CD64), present on monocytes and macrophages. Preclinical studies demonstrated that monocytes, macrophages, and interferon-γ- (IFN-γ)-treated neutrophils could phagocytose tumor cells expressing c-erbB-2 in the presence of MDX-210 (42). Valone et al. used this antibody in a Phase I study in patients with advanced breast or ovarian cancer overexpressing c-erbB-2 and found evidence of monocyte activation. Doses of MDX-210 greater than 3.5 mg/m^2 saturated at least 80% of monocyte FcγRI and were associated with elevated levels of TNFα, IL-6, and granulocyte colony-stimulating factor (CSF) (19).

Alternatively, cytokines can be administered directly to patients during therapy with monoclonal antibodies, in an effort to upregulate expression of tumor antigens or more effectively activate human immune response. The administration of IFN-γ to athymic mice harboring human colon carcinoma HT-29 led to a time- and dose-dependent increase in expression of both CEA and the tumor-associated antigen TAG-72 (43). Furthermore, Anti-TAG and Anti-CEA antibodies showed enhanced localization to the HT-29 tumors. More importantly, experiments using the combination of interferon with ^{131}I-CC49, an Anti-TAG mAb, resulted in a statistically significant improvement in therapeutic efficacy, compared with ^{131}I-CC49 alone (43). Similar results have been obtained in humans (44). Johnson et al. (44) administered IFN-2α at a dose 1 × 10^6 units intramuscularly for 4 days to five patients with a variety of adenocarcinomas. The expression of the TAG-72 antigen was evaluated on tumor specimens prior to and 1 day following therapy with interferon. Three of the five patients exhibited increases in both the percentage of cells expressing TAG-72 and the intensity of the staining. Weiner et al. used a low-dose interferon schedule in an attempt to enhance the efficacy of the unmodified mAb CO17-1A for patients with metastatic colorectal cancer. Enhancement of monocyte ADCC was seen by 24 hours; lymphocyte ADCC and natural killer activity directed against K562 cells was enhanced to a lesser degree (18).

Polymorphonuclear cells (PMN) are capable of lysing a variety of tumor cell lines and freshly obtained tumor cells (45,46). Compared with PMN cells from healthy donors, PMN cells stimulated by G-CSF demonstrate augmented cytotoxicity in ADCC assays against human glioma and squamous cell carcinoma cell lines, sensitized with mAb 425 to the EGF receptor (47). Based on these preclinical results, Repp et al. conducted a Phase I trial of MDX-210 combined with G-CSF in patients with advanced breast cancer. Even at the lower dose levels, patients showed elevated plasma levels of IL-6 and TNF-α 4 hours postinfusion and a delayed increase in G-CSF plasma levels and soluble IL-2 receptor, suggesting effective activation of the immune system. Moreover, in vitro cytotoxicity assays against SK-BR3 breast cancer cells with isolated neutrophils showed enhanced cytotoxicity in the presence of MDX-210 during, but not before or after, G-CSF administration (47).

In another study, patients with metastatic adenocarcinomas of gastrointestinal origin were treated with the mAb D612, directed at a membrane glycoprotein expressed on gastrointestinal tumors, in combination with recombinant monocyte colony-stimulating factor (rhM-CSF) (48). The majority of the patients demonstrated a greater than two-fold increase in peripheral monocyte counts. Although no specific trend was seen for IL-1b, IL-1ra, IL-6, TNF-α, or TNF-β, serum neopterin levels showed a definite increase in five of the six patients studied. Therefore, it is conceivable that coadministration of cytokines can mobilize human immune responses and enhance the cytotoxicity of mAb therapy. Clinical experience is too limited at this point to confirm or exclude such an effect.

Preclinical studies have evaluated the addition of traditional chemotherapy to mAb treatment. The effect of combining doxorubicin with mAbs 528 and 225 against the epidermal growth factor receptor (EGFR) was evaluated in squamous cell carcinoma and breast carcinoma cell lines, as well as in xenografted BALB/c nude mice (49). Whereas treatment with either mAbs or doxorubicin alone temporarily inhibited growth of established tumor xenografts, the combination of both agents substantially enhanced antitumor activity. Similar results were obtained with the use of these antibodies and cisplatin against epidermoid carcinoma xenografts (50).

In another experiment, nude mice bearing human breast adenocarcinoma were treated with combinations of chemotherapy with mAb 4D5, which targets HER-2/neu, a receptor closely related to EGFR (51). Treatment with antibody therapy alone produced 35% growth inhibition compared with control mAb; therapy with paclitaxel and doxorubicin led to a 35% and 27% growth inhibition, respectively. Combined treatment with either mAb/paclitaxel or mAb/doxorubicin combinations was associated with 70–93% tumor inhibition, without increasing overall toxicity. Based on these observations, a Phase II trial was initiated in patients with advanced breast cancer overexpressing HER-2/neu, in which mAb Anti-p185 HER-2 was administered together with cisplatin (52). Therapy was tolerated well, with a toxicity profile similar to that expected with cisplatin alone. No randomized trials are available yet to determine the superiority, if any, of such a combination over standard chemotherapy.

Even without the addition of cytotoxic drugs, mAbs targeting biologically important molecules can have direct toxicity for tumors. As just noted, mAbs against growth factor receptors, when given alone, can be toxic to cell lines overexpressing these receptors. Epidermal growth factor receptor is present at high levels in many human epithelial tumors, and antibodies that block the interaction of the receptor with its ligands, EGF and TGF-α, have been shown to inhibit growth of tumors in vitro (53). Unconjugated murine mAbs ICR16, ICR62, and ICR64, which target the extracellular domain of EGFR, were given to athymic mice bearing a variety of human tumors (squamous cell carcinoma, breast adenocarcinoma, and vulvar carcinoma). Complete regression of tumors was seen, even when therapy was delayed until the tumors already were established. In vitro studies with a humanized version of an Anti-HER-2/neu monoclonal antibody showed antiproliferative effect against HER-2/neu overexpressing tumors (54).

Another potential target for mAb therapy is the P-glycoprotein, responsible for the multiple-drug-resistant (MDR) phenotype of many human neoplasms. Anti-P-gp mAb, MRK16, and its $F(ab')_2$ fragment were evaluated for their therapeutic effect on P-gp-mediated MDR human colorectal carcinoma cell lines in a nude mouse model (55). MRK16 alone showed significant inhibition of tumor growth of P-gp positive cell lines. This inhibition was enhanced when the mAb was given in combination with doxorubicin. In contrast, doxorubicin alone had no effect on tumor growth.

Several other novel targets can be identified. Ferrara et al. attempted to block the signal inducing new vessel formation in human tumors. An antibody that blocks vascular endothelium growth factor (VEGF), a substance that is overexpressed in almost all tumors, produced dramatic suppression of tumor growth in animals xenografted with human rhabdomyosarcoma (56). Rettig et al. discovered that the mAb F19 interacts with the highly specific antigen fibroblast activation protein (FAP) on the surface of reactive fibroblasts present in tumor stroma, which are capable of producing a variety of potentially important cytokines (57). In a pilot clinical trial, mAb ^{131}I-F19 was administered intravenously to patients with hepatic metastases from colorectal carcinomas scheduled to undergo resection or insertion of hepatic artery catheters (58). Immunohistochemical studies of biopsy tissues showed expression of FAP in tumor stroma but not in normal liver, and confirmed that the FAP-positive stromal cells were interposed between the tumor capillaries and the malignant colon epithelial cells. At the time of surgery, tumor-to-liver drug ratio was up to 21:1 and tumor-to-serum ratio was up to 9:1, suggesting the possible therapeutic application of such an antibody.

There are two important limitations in the use of murine proteins for immunotherapy: they are weaker than their human counterparts in inducing immune responses, and they are themselves immunogenic to the host, even in patients inherently immunosuppressed due to their disease (59). Smaller molecules, such as Fab' or sFvs, may be less immunogenic but lose any ability to activate immune effectors through the Fc portion. An alternative approach is to add human sequences to the mouse variable regions, in order to limit immunogenicity and enhance activity. Chimeric antibodies combine the variable regions of a murine antibody with the constant region of a human Fc, which determines effector functions (60). Both preclinical and clinical studies have established that chimeric antibodies retain their specificity for their targets and may be more active than their murine counterparts (61). Immune responses to murine proteins are seen with chimeric constructs; however, they frequently are reported as delayed and less severe than those seen with pure murine monoclonals. LoBuglio et al. treated ten patients with colon cancer with a chimeric 17-1A mAb and noted that only one patient receiving three doses of the chimeric monoclonal developed modest antibody reactivity against the murine variable region (62). However, even with chimeric constructs, repeated dosing can lead to anamnestic response and rapid disappearance of the mAb from the circulation, along with the formation of immune complexes (12). In clinical trials, HAMA formation can be seen in up to 75% of patients treated with chimeric antibodies (12,28).

Antibody variable regions have loop areas of high variability in amino acid sequences, referred to as *complementarity-determining regions* (CDRs), which are central in antigen binding. Humanized antibodies take primarily the CDRs from rodents, whereas the variable region frameworks and the constant regions are human (30). Tokuda et al. compared the cytotoxicity of a murine and a humanized 4D5 antibody against a human gastric carcinoma xenograft. Antibody-dependent cellular cytotoxicity assays using peripheral blood mononuclear cells showed that the humanized antibody augmented cytotoxicity, whereas the murine antibody did not (54). In clinical trials with humanized antibodies, no significant immune responses were noted (63,64).

A more fundamental solution would be to produce human antibodies; however, there are several problems with this approach. There is difficulty in finding a cell that would yield hybridomas with a stable production of human mAbs. Also, there is an ethical problem of obtaining suitably immunized B-cells from human donors. Nevertheless, trials with human antibodies have been performed. Haisma et al. used the IgM mAb ^{131}I-16.88 derived from peripheral blood B-cells of a patient immunized with irradiated autologous colon cancer cells admixed with BCG to treat twenty colorectal cancer patients. Immunogenicity was assessed with enzyme-linked immunosorbent assay (ELISA), radioimmunoassay, and dot-blot assay, none of which showed any evidence of antihuman antibody response (65). In a similar study, patients with metastatic colon cancer were treated with either mAb 16.88 or mAb 28A32, which is derived from a human–mouse heterohybridoma (66). No patient developed an antibody response to 16.88, but two patients developed localized urticarial reactions following injection with 28A32. More work remains to define better the properties and clinical usefulness of such constructs.

IV. MONOCLONAL ANTIBODIES IN SOLID TUMORS: CLINICAL EXPERIENCE

A. Toxicities

Table 4 lists the most common toxicities associated with a variety of mAbs used for the treatment of solid tumors. One of the major concerns in antibody therapy is the possibility of developing life-threatening allergic reactions; this concern is heightened for patients who form antimouse/antitoxin antibodies during the course of therapy.

Clinical experience has shown that although true allergic reactions are possible, they are relatively rare. In a large overview evaluating the toxicity profile of unconjugated mAbs in 177 patients with twenty different malignancies receiving 291 infusions of twenty-two different mAbs, the incidence of possible allergic reactions ranged from less than 1% to 18% of all infusions (5). Relatively benign manifestations, such as urticaria and pruritus, occurring in 18% and 6% of infusions, respectively, were more common than severe reactions, such as bronchospasm and anaphylaxis, which were present in almost 1% of infusions. Similar findings are reported in other large trials. Riethmueller et al. administered 371 infusions of the mAb 17-1A to 90 patients with colon cancer, and reported that the incidence of allergic or anaphylactic reactions was 1.6% of all infusions (39). Similarly, Mellstedt et al., using the same antibody, encountered anaphylactic reactions in 1% of infusions (67). These authors also noted that infusions of mAbs in patients who had developed a HAMA response led to a reduction of antimouse antibody titers without detection of immune complexes or development of clinical sequelae. They suggested that in the presence of excess antigen, immune complexes are small and are cleared rapidly by the reticuloendothelial system. In the latter study, the pharmacokinetics of the infused antibody were not altered in patients with HAMA. The same conclusion was reached in a study by Khazaeli et al. using the same antibody (68).

However, most trials with conjugated or unconjugated antibodies have

Table 4 Toxicities Associated with Monoclonal Antibody Therapy

Antibody	Allergic/fever[a]	Hematologic	Hepatic	Neuro	GI	CLS	Cardiac	Respiratory	Other
3F8	+++	—	—	—	—	—	—	—	++++ severe pain
17-1A	+	—	+	+	+-++	—	—	—	—
rhu mAb HER-2/neu	+	—	—	—	+	—	—	—	+ pain
L6	++	—	—	+	—	—	—	—	—
MDX-210	+++-++++	—	++	—	++	—	—	+	—
BR 55-2	+	—	—	—	+	—	—	—	++ hematuria
KS1/4 (MTX)	++-+++	—	++	—	++	—	—	—	—
A7-NCS	++	—	—	—	++	—	—	—	—
NR LU10-^{186}Re	++	++	+++	—	+	—	—	—	—
B 72.3-^{131}I	++	+++	—	—	+	—	—	—	—
CC 49-^{131}I	+	++	—	+	+	—	—	+	—
CC 49-^{177}Lu	+	+++	—	—	+	—	—	—	—
HMFG1-^{90}Y	++	++++	—	—	—	—	—	—	—
mAb 33-^{131}I	—	++	++	+++	++	—	—	—	++ fatigue
260F9-RTA	++++	—	++++	+	—	+++	—	++	—
N901-bR	+++	++	—	++	—	++-+++	+	—	++ myalgia
79IT/36-RTA	++	—	+	—	—	++-+++	—	—	—
I-1 bR[b]	+	—	—	—	++	—	—	—	++ liver pain

[a] Includes all cases with fever, rash, arthralgias, bronchospasm, or anaphylaxis. However, not all cases of fever represent true allergic reactions.
[b] Intralesional therapy of hepatic metastases.

shown a clear change in the pharmacokinetic profile of mAbs when given to patients with antimouse or antitoxin response. The half-life of the infused antibody and the severity of nonallergic toxicities are dramatically reduced (12, 28,29). In contrast, allergic reactions appear to be more frequent, presumably due to the formation of antibody–antigen complexes (69,70). Such immune complexes were detected during rechallenge in patients who had a high antibody response to the initial infusion of the chimeric antibody chB72.3 (12). In a study by Dillman et al., three out of eighty-two patients receiving 186 infusions developed bronchospasm or anaphylaxis (70). All patients were treated more than once, at least 2 weeks after a previous treatment. Ragnhammar et al. noted that the incidence of immediate-type allergic reactions increased from 5% of patients in the initial cycle of therapy with mAb 17-1A in combination with GM-CSF, to as high as 78% during the third cycle (71). Thus, it appears that repeated infusions of mAbs should be given with extreme caution, especially in patients known to have antimouse or antitoxin antibodies.

Fever is seen in approximately one-fourth of patients during infusion (5). Although the fever can be associated with chills, rigors, diaphoresis, or even blood pressure changes, it is not always related to allergic reactions. Dillman et al. noted toxicity in twenty out of eighty-two first infusions with antibodies reacting with antigens on circulating cells, compared to zero of fifty-five first infusions with antibodies that did not demonstrate such reactivity (70). Although clearance of circulating cells is more common with antibodies against hematologic malignancies, cross-reactivity with antigens on blood cells can be seen with mAb therapy targeting solid tumors as well. Patients receiving an Anti-CEA mAb developed fevers, rigors, nausea, and vomiting associated with a rapid decrease in the number of PMN cells (72).

Cross-reactivity with antigens expressed on normal tissues can be a source of significant side effects. Occasionally, such toxicities are anticipated, based on preclinical studies on animal models (23); however, they also can be unpredictable. Severe, dose-limiting encephalopathy was seen in patients treated with the immunotoxin OVB3-PE administered intraperitoneally to patients with ovarian cancer, although such interaction with brain tissue was not appreciated during preclinical testing (24). Similarly, Gould et al. administered the mAb 260F9 conjugated to ricin A-chain to five patients with metastatic breast cancer (16). Three patients suffered debilitating neuropathy/plexopathy, which led to inability for self-care lasting for 6 months. It subsequently was established that human nerves express the 260F9 antigen on Schwann cells or myelin.

With immunoconjugates, the toxicity of the conjugated molecule needs to be considered as well. Studies with radioisotopes have frequently shown significant myelosuppression, for both the white cells and platelets (27–29,34,35). The degree of this toxicity depends on the total radiation dose, fractionation, and extent of pretreatment with conventional cytototoxic medications (27,28). The toxin ricin has been associated with capillary leak syndrome, manifested predominantly by weight gain, hypoalbuminemia, and hyponatremia, progressing to peripheral edema, dyspnea, and noncardiogenic pulmonary edema (17,23,73). Careful monitoring of drug levels, albumin, and body weight is important, since neither diuretics nor steroids consistently are helpful in severe cases of capillary leak syndrome.

Other toxicities, such as nausea, vomiting, liver function test abnormalities, and diarrhea, are reported inconsistently for a variety of mAbs and are rarely clinically significant. Tumor pain also has been associated with mAb therapy (64). Severe pain involving the abdomen and lower back and spreading peripherally to the ankles and feet was seen in all patients treated with the antiganglioside antibody 3F8 (74). The exact cause of this syndrome is unclear. The same antibody was also associated with significant hypertension, infrequently requiring antihypertensive therapy. Another antiganglioside antibody, R24, caused fatal hemorrhagic tumor necrosis in a patient with widespread melanoma (75).

B. Clinical Trials with mAbs in Solid Tumors

Table 5 lists the mAbs used in immunotherapy of solid tumors, their target antigen, and the clinical setting in which they are more commonly employed. This

Table 5 Monoclonal Antibodies and Targeted Antigens in Solid Tumors

Antibody	Antigen	Disease
B72.3	TAG-72	Colorectal cancer
3F8	GD2	Neuroblastoma
CC49	TAG-72	Colorectal cancer, ovarian cancer
17-1A	CO 17-1A	Colorectal cancer
4D5	HER-2/neu	Breast cancer
N-901	CD56	Small cell lung cancer
HMFG1	PEM	Ovarian cancer
MoAb 255	EGFR	SCCA lung
MoAb 33	A33	Colorectal cancer
MDX-210[a]	HER-2/neu FcγRI	Breast cancer, ovarian cancer
BC-2/BC-4	Tenascin	Glioma
BR 55-2	Le^y	Breast cancer
I-1	CEA	Adenocarcinomas

[a] Bispecific antibody.
TAG: tumor-associated glycoprotein; GD: ganglioside; PEM: polymorphic epithelial mucin; EGFR: epidermal growth factor receptor; Le^y: Lewis^y antigen; HMFG1: human milk fat globulin 1.

section will provide an overview of the clinical results of mAb therapy in solid tumors.

1. Colorectal Cancer

Gastrointestinal (GI) malignancies have been the focus of clinical trials since the early days of immunotherapy. In 1982, four patients with advanced GI tumors, three of whom had colorectal cancer, were given a single infusion of the mAb 17-1A, in an attempt to define the safety profile and pharmacokinetics of this antibody (76). The 17-1A antibody recognizes a 47-40 Kd glycoprotein on the surface on many malignant and normal cells, which may be involved in cellular adhesion to the extracellular matrix. Subsequently, Sears et al. treated forty patients with this antibody in two sequential trials. In the first study, patients received a single dose of 15–1000 mg of protein (77). Three of twenty patients entered complete remission (CR), and two remained in remission 2 years after the therapy (77,78). However, some patients in that trial received standard therapy concurrently with the immunotherapy. In the second study, twenty patients with advanced colorectal cancer and no therapy for at least 1 month prior to mAb therapy were given 200–850 mg of 17-1A, with one patient having a partial response (PR) (78). Another patient had stable disease, and a third one had partial regression of a liver metastasis while he developed progression of his abdominal wall disease. Of note, radioimaging with iodinated $F(ab')_2$ fragment of 17-1A in this particular patient was positive in the liver but negative in the abdominal wall. Using the mAb L6, Goodman et al. treated two patients with colon cancer without any objective clinical benefit (21).

The value of repeated doses of mAb was examined in a study by LoBuglio et al., who treated 25 patients with minimally pretreated metastatic GI cancers, twenty of whom had colon primaries (69). No patient received concurrent chemotherapy. The number of infusions varied from a single dose of 400 mg up to four doses administered at weekly intervals. One patient with liver metastases who received two infusions entered a CR within 6 weeks, which lasted for 56 weeks. Of the twenty patients receiving more than one infusion, one developed facial flushing and two had an anaphylactic reaction; all three of these patients developed HAMA.

Based on promising preclinical data showing enhanced activity of mAbs given together with cytokines, Ragnhammar et al. administered four monthly cycles of GM-CSF at a dose of 250 $\mu g/m^2$ daily for 10 days to twenty patients with metastatic colorectal carcinoma expressing the antigen CO17-1A (71). On day 3 of each cycle, 400 mg of mAb 17-1A were infused. Two patients with predominantly lymph node metastases (one also had lung metastasis) remained in CR 23 and 29 months after the start of therapy. Due to the development of hypersensitivity reactions, the number of patients able to receive full doses of the mAb decreased significantly during the course of therapy: all patients received 400 mg at the first cycle, fourteen patients had full dose on cycle two, three out of eighteen patients had full dose on cycle three, and only one of eleven patients without disease progression had 400 mg at the last cycle.

In an effort to upregulate antigen expression on tumor cells, interferon gamma was given to nineteen patients with metastatic colorectal cancer as an intravenous infusion for 4 days (18). On days 2, 3, and 4, 150 mg of 17-1A was infused over 2 hours. A single patient had stable disease, but no objective responses were seen.

The combination of D612, which targets a 48 Kd glycoprotein expressed on GI tumors, and recombinant M-CSF has shown potent ADCC in vitro. In a Phase II study, fourteen patients with metastatic GI adenocarcinoma were treated. Although some degree of monocyte activation was seen, no patient responded (48).

More recently, investigators have evaluated the toxicity and activity of immunoconjugates in patients with colorectal cancer. The majority of these trials involve the use of radioisotopes, with iodine-131 used most commonly. The chimeric antibody chB72.3 is directed against the tumor-associated glycoprotein TAG-72, expressed on many adenocarcinomas. In a Phase I study, patients were given chB72.3-^{131}I at doses ranging from 18 mCi/m^2 to 36 mCi/m^2 (29). The maximum tolerated dose was reached at 36 mCi/m^2 and was defined by myelosuppression. Although the tumor areas were estimated to have been exposed to 2.3–5.9 cGy/mCi, no responses were seen in the twelve patients treated. An additional twelve patients received the same immunoconjugate at a dose of 28–36 mCi/m^2 in either two or three fractions administered 1 week apart (28). There was a trend toward less myelosuppression for the group of patients receiving fractionated mAb therapy compared to the previous group receiving a single dose of chB72.3-^{131}I. Out of twelve patients, one minor response was observed.

A second-generation Anti-TAG-72 antibody, CC49, also has been utilized in radioimmunotherapy. Divgi et al. used an ^{131}I-CC49 mAb to treat twenty-four patients with measurable metastatic colorectal cancer with radiation doses ranging from 15 mCi/m^2 to 90 mCi/m^2 (27). As in other radioimmunotherapy trials, the major toxicity was transient myelosuppression. Although imaging studies showed satisfactory tumor targeting, no responses were seen. The same mAb was administered to fifteen patients by Murray et al. at a dose of 75 mCi/m^2 as a 1-hour infusion (79). Once again, despite favorable imaging of known disease sites, no patient responded to treatment. CC49 was conjugated to lutetium-177 (177-Lu), which poses less radiation risks than ^{131}I, and was given to six patients with advanced adenocarcinomas, but no responses were seen (80).

The mAb A33 targets an antigenic epitope on a high-molecular-weight glycoprotein expressed on malignant, as well as normal, intestinal tissue. The conjugate A33-iodine-131 was infused in twenty-three patients with metastatic colon cancer at doses ranging from 30 mCi/m^2 to 90 mCi/m^2 (81). The maximum tolerated dose was reached at 75 mCi/m^2, due to hematologic toxicity. No significant toxicity attributable to binding of the mAb to normal tissues was appreciated, and no patient responded. Iodine-131 also has been conjugated to human monoclonal antibodies 16.88 and 28A32 and given to patients with advanced colorectal cancers (65,66). Host immunologic response was minimal, but no patient had objective clinical benefit. Meredith et al. treated patients with metastatic colorectal cancer with the chimeric antibody 17-1A linked to iodine-125, which is a low-energy Auger electron emitter that can spare neighboring tissues (82). Indeed, myelosuppression was minimal up to a dose of 250 mCi, but no responses were evident.

Immunotoxin therapy has been used less frequently. Byers et al. undertook a trial of the immunotoxin XomaZyme-791, which combines the mAb 791T/36 with the A-chain of the plant toxin ricin, in patients with metastatic colon cancer (73). The immunotoxin was infused over 1 hour daily for 5 days. Two out of seventeen patients showed evidence of response, with decreasing size of large liver metastases and disappearance of smaller ones. Another modified version of the ricin toxin, blocked ricin, was linked to the anti-CEA antibody I-1 and administered intralesionally to twenty-seven patients with hepatic metastases from colorectal primaries (37). Therapy generally was well tolerated, with liver pain being the most common toxicity. Although seven patients showed minor responses, such as decreases in liver function tests, CEA levels, or pain, no objective responses were observed.

A single trial from Japan has evaluated the benefit of antibody targeted chemotherapy for colorectal cancer (83). The mAb A7 and the chemotherapeutic agent neocarsinostatin (NCS) were bound covalently to form the conjugate A7-NCS. This conjugate was given through the hepatic artery to eight patients with liver metastases, two of whom entered a PR while two others showed a minor response.

2. Ovarian Cancer

Table 2 lists the clinical trials of mAb therapy in ovarian cancer. The majority involve the intraperitoneal instillation of conjugates, although unconjugated antibodies also have been used. Goodman et al. treated nine patients with ovarian cancer with seven daily intravenous infusions of mAb L6, which binds to a variety of carcinomas, including ovary, breast, colon, and non-small cell lung cancer. Treatment was tolerated well, but no responses were seen (21). Another unconjugated mAb, MDX-210, has specificity for both the high-affinity type I Fc receptor and the cell-surface protein c-erbB-2, which can be overexpressed in breast and ovarian cancer. It can be used in these tumor types to recruit effector cells to the tumor site. Valone et al. administered this construct to six patients with stage III or IV platinum-refractory ovarian cancer shown to overexpress c-erbB-2 (19). A single patient had a mixed response, with a more than 50% reduction in the size of her cervical adenopathy but also with evidence of worsening bowel obstruction.

A number of studies have evaluated the role of radioimmunotherapy delivered directly into the peritoneum through a peritoneal dialysis catheter in women with ovarian cancer. The murine IgG1 mAb HMFG1 recognizes an epitope on the polymorphic epithelial mucin (PEM), present in almost all cases of ovarian cancer. Maraveyas et al. administered the HMFG1 mAb conjugated to yttrium-90 to nineteen patients following second-look laparoscopy, nine of whom had no evidence of disease (26). Hematologic toxicity was seen in all patients, lasting as long as 56 days posttherapy, and five patients showed evidence of hypersensitivity reactions. The maximum tolerated dose was established at 18.5 mCi/m^2. Based on their preliminary results, the same group of investigators treated women with ovarian cancer in an adjuvant setting, following cytoreductive surgery and chemotherapy (38). The survival of a subgroup of fifteen patients with stages IIb and III was compared to a historical control of a similar group of patients treated at the same center. Despite the relatively small numbers, a large difference in survival was noted, suggesting that adjuvant radioimmunotherapy for ovarian cancer possibly should be evaluated in a randomized fashion.

In contrast, results of radioimmunotherapy remain poor in studies where patients with macroscopic disease are treated. Meredith et al. treated twelve women with relapsed or refractory ovarian cancer with the immunoconjugate ^{177}Lu-CC49. Despite successful localization of tumor on imaging studies in eleven of twelve patients, only one of eight patients with gross disease achieved a PR (34). In another study in relapsed/refractory ovarian cancer patients treated with the mAb NR-LU-10 bound to rhenium-186, responses were seen only in four of seven patients with pretreatment tumor size of less than 1 cm (35).

The single study with intraperitoneally delivered immunotoxin therapy with *Pseudomonas* exototin linked to the mAb OVB3 was associated with dose-limiting encephalopathy and no responses (24).

3. Breast Cancer

Patients with metastatic breast cancer were treated with the immunotoxin 260F9-RTA (ricin A-chain), which targets a 55 Kd antigen expressed in almost half of breast cancer specimens. Four women received this immunotoxin as a 1-hour infusion daily for 8 consecutive days (17). One patient with a solitary lung nodule entered CR, which lasted for 3.5 months. However, therapy was associated with capillary leak syndrome, manifested as weight gain, hypoalbuminemia, edema, and dyspnea, at doses insufficient to saturate antigen-expressing tumor tissue. Moreover, in a similar study of continuous infusion 260F9-RTA, three out of five patients experienced severe neuropathy, and no patient responded (16).

More recently, unconjugated antibodies have entered into clinical trials in patients with advanced breast cancer. The mAb L6 was given to five patients as a daily infusion for 7 days (21). One patient who received 400 mg/m^2/d achieved complete resolution of a chest wall soft tissue mass at 14 weeks following therapy. Of note, at 6 weeks posttreatment, biopsies revealed a marked inflammatory response, consisting of a population of plasma cells, lymphocytes, and other mononuclear cells. Breast cancer patients whose tumors expressed the Lewis antigen Le^y were given the Anti-Le^y antibody BR55-2 on 5 consecutive days at a total dose of 50–400 mg/m^2 (84). Out of the first nine evaluable patients, one minor response of an anterior mediastinal soft tissue mass was noted.

Approximately one-third of breast cancers have high levels of HER-2/neu, which may also carry prognostic significance. A humanized Anti-HER-2/neu antibody, 4D5, directed against the extracellular domain of the HER-2/neu protein (p185^{HER2}) was used to treat patients with metastatic breast cancer (64). After a loading dose of 250 mg, ten weekly infusions at a dose of 100 mg each were given to forty-six eligible patients. Out of forty-three evaluable patients, five showed an objective response: a patient with chest wall disease entered a CR, and four other patients achieved a partial response lasting for 1–7.7 months. The same antibody was administered for a total of 8 weeks to thirty-six evaluable patients with advanced breast cancer in combination with 75 mg/m^2 of cisplatin on days 1, 29, and 57 (52). One CR and seven PRs were recorded. The toxicity was similar to that anticipated with cisplatin alone. The bispecific antibody MDX-210 (against HER-2/neu and FcγRI) was evaluated in a Phase I study in nine patients with breast cancer, one of whom had a tumor inflammatory response during therapy and eventually entered a PR (19).

4. Other Solid Tumors

Experience with mAb therapy in other solid tumors is limited, despite encouraging in vitro studies in a variety of histologies (85–88). Divgi et al. targeted the EGF receptor in nineteen patients with unresectable or metastatic squamous cell lung cancer with the mAb 225 linked to indium-111 (89). No patient responded to therapy. Elias et al. used the mAb KS1/4 conjugated to methotrexate in a study of eleven patients with stage IIIB or IV nonsmall-cell lung cancer (25). A single patient treated with the immunoconjugate achieved a minimal response but subsequently progressed. The immunotoxin N901-bR was administered in a Phase I study to patients with refractory or relapsed small-cell lung cancer (SCLC) (23). Dose escalation was limited by capillary leak syndrome, but one patient achieved a PR.

Thirty-three patients with metastatic renal cell cancer were treated with the mAb G250 conjugated to iodine-131, but no responses were seen (90). Patients with hormone-refractory metastatic prostate cancer received the mAb CC49-^{131}I as a single intravenous infusion (91). Out of fifteen patients, no responses in PSA or tumor bulk were seen, but six out of ten evaluable patients had improvement in their pain level. Riva et al. studied the value of intralesional radioimmunotherapy in patients with recurrent malignant gliomas (36). Following placement of a catheter at the tumor site, patients received BC-2 or BC-4 antitenascin antibodies linked to iodine-131 for a total of 2–4 injections. Of the seventeen evaluable patients, three entered a PR and three more achieved CR with a median duration of 15 months. Juweid et al. treated patients with advanced medullary carcinoma of the thyroid with Anti-CEA mAbs linked to iodine-131 (including one patient receiving high-dose radiatioimmunotherapy with autologous bone marrow transplantation) (92). Out of ten evaluable patients, six had evidence of response lasting up to 26 months. Patients with neuroblastoma, two of whom had undergone allogeneic bone marrow transplant, were treated with the antiganglioside GD2 mAb 3F8 (74). One of these patients achieved a PR lasting for 17 weeks, whereas the other patient was not assessable for response but remained progression free 63 weeks following therapy with 3F8 (93).

V. CONCLUSION

Monoclonal antibody therapy of solid tumors is an elegant and powerful modality, which has produced many promising results in animal models and in vitro studies but only sporadic clinical successes. The many requirements for effective immunotherapy, especially access to tumor, lack of nonspecific toxicity, and low immunogenicity, have raised many obstacles in the efforts to achieve more consistent results. Newer constructs are being developed that aim to address these issues. Encouraging clinical results suggested that mAb therapy may be most useful in the setting of minimal residual disease. More importantly, the identification of biologically important molecules that can serve as antigenic targets will be central to the development of more powerful immunotherapeutic tools.

REFERENCES

1. Kohler G, Milstein C. Continuous cultures of fused cells secreting antibody of predefined specificity. Nature 1975; 256:495–497.
2. Hall SS. Monoclonal antibodies at age 20: promise at last? Science 1995; 270:915–916.
3. Nadler LM, Stashenko P, Hardy R, et al. Serotherapy of a patient with a monoclonal antibody directed against a human lymphoma-associated antigen. Cancer Res 1980; 40:3147–3154.
4. Imai K, Pellegrino MA, Wilson BS, Ferrone S. Higher cytolytic efficiency of an

IgG2 alpha than of an IgG1 monoclonal antibody reacting with the same (or spatially close) determinant on a human high-molecular-weight melanoma-associated antigen. Cell Immunol 1982; 72:239–247.
5. Dillman RO. Antibodies as cytotoxic therapy. J Clin Oncol 1994; 12:1497–1515.
6. Jain RK. Hemodynamic and transport barriers to the treatment of solid tumors. Int J Radiat Biol 1991; 60:85–100.
7. Jain RK, Baxter LT. Mechanisms of heterogeneous distribution of monoclonal antibodies and other macromolecules in tumors: significance of elevated interstitial pressure. Cancer Res 1988; 48:7022–7032.
8. Yokota T, Milenic DE, Whitlow M, Schlom J. Rapid tumor penetration of a single-chain Fv and comparison with other immunoglobulin forms. Cancer Res 1992; 52: 3402–3408.
9. El-Kareh AW, Braunstein SL, Secomb TW. Effect of cell arrangement and interstitial volume fraction on the diffusivity of monoclonal antibodies in tissue. Biophys J 1993; 64:1638–1646.
10. Juweid M, Neumann R, Paik C, et al. Micropharmacology of monoclonal antibodies in solid tumors: direct experimental evidence for a binding site barrier. Cancer Res 1992; 52:5144–5153.
11. Laurent G, Frankel AE, Hertler AA, Schlossman DM, Casellas P, Jansen FK. Treatment of leukemia patients with T101 ricin A chain immunotoxins. Cancer Treat Res 1988; 37:483–491.
12. Khazaeli MB, Saleh MN, Liu TP, et al. Pharmacokinetics and immune response of 131I-chimeric mouse/human B72.3 (human gamma 4) monoclonal antibody in humans. Cancer Res 1991; 51:5461–5466.
13. Heppner GH. Tumor heterogeneity. Cancer Res 1984; 44:2259–2265.
14. Meeker T, Lowder J, Cleary ML, et al. Emergence of idiotype variants during treatment of B-cell lymphoma with anti-idiotype antibodies. N Engl J Med 1985; 312: 1658–1665.
15. Shawler DL, Miceli MC, Wormsley SB, Royston I, Dillman RO. Induction of in vitro and in vivo antigenic modulation by the anti-human T-cell monoclonal antibody T101. Cancer Res 1984; 44:5921–5927.
16. Gould BJ, Borowitz MJ, Groves ES, et al. Phase I study of an anti–breast cancer immunotoxin by continuous infusion: report of a targeted toxic effect not predicted by animal studies. J Natl Cancer Inst 1989; 81:775–781.
17. Weiner LM, O'Dwyer J, Kitson J, et al. Phase I evaluation of an anti–breast carcinoma monoclonal antibody 260F9-recombinant ricin A-chain immunoconjugate. Cancer Res 1989; 49:4062–4067.
18. Weiner LM, Moldofsky PJ, Gatenby RA, et al. Antibody delivery and effector cell activation in a Phase II trial of recombinant gamma-interferon and the murine monoclonal antibody CO17-1A in advanced colorectal carcinoma. Cancer Res 1988; 48: 2568–2573.
19. Valone FH, Kaufman PA, Guyre PM, et al. Phase Ia/Ib trial of bispecific antibody MDX-210 in patients with advanced breast or ovarian cancer that overexpresses the proto-oncogene HER-2/neu. J Clin Oncol 1995; 13:2281–2292.
20. Elias DJ, Hirschowitz L, Kline LE, et al. Phase I clinical comparative study of mono-

clonal antibody KS1/4 and KS1/4-methotrexate immunconjugate in patients with non-small-cell lung carcinoma. Cancer Res 1990; 50:4154–4159.
21. Goodman GE, Hellstrom I, Brodzinsky L, et al. Phase I trial of murine monoclonal antibody L6 in breast, colon, ovarian, and lung cancer. J Clin Oncol 1990; 8:1083–1092.
22. Vadhan-Raj S, Cordon-Cardo C, Carswell E, et al. Phase I trial of a mouse monoclonal antibody against GD3 ganglioside in patients with melanoma: induction of inflammatory responses at tumor sites. J Clin Oncol 1988; 6:1636–6148.
23. Lynch TJ, Jr., Lambert JM, Coral F, et al. Immunotoxin therapy of small-cell lung cancer: a phase I study of N901-blocked ricin. J Clin Oncol 1997; 15:723–734.
24. Pai LH, Bookman MA, Ozols RF, et al. Clinical evaluation of intraperitoneal Pseudomonas exotoxin immunoconjugate OVB3-PE in patients with ovarian cancer. J Clin Oncol 1991; 9:2095–2103.
25. Elias DJ, Kline LE, Robbins BA, et al. Monoclonal antibody KS1/4-methotrexate immunoconjugate studies in non-small cell lung carcinoma. Am J Resp Crit Care Med 1994; 150:1114–1122.
26. Maraveyas A, Snook D, Hird V, et al. Pharmacokinetics and toxicity of an yttrium-90-CITC-DTPA-HMFG1 radioimmunoconjugate for intraperitoneal radioimmunotherapy of ovarian cancer. Cancer 1994; 73:1067–1075.
27. Divgi CR, Scott AM, Dantis L, et al. Phase I radioimmunotherapy trial with iodine-131-CC49 in metastatic colon carcinoma. J Nucl Med 1995; 36:586–592.
28. Meredith RF, Khazaeli MB, Liu T, et al. Dose fractionation of radiolabeled antibodies in patients with metastatic colon cancer. J Nucl Med 1992; 33:1648–1653.
29. Meredith RF, Khazaeli MB, Plott WE, et al. Phase I trial of iodine-131-chimeric B72.3 (human IgG4) in metastatic colorectal cancer. J Nucl Med 1992; 33:23–29.
30. Boleti E, George AJ, Epenetos AA. Therapeutic monoclonals. Biochem Soc Trans 1995; 23:1044–1047.
31. Huston JS, Mudgett-Hunter M, Tai MS, et al. Protein engineering of single-chain Fv analogs and fusion proteins. Methods Enzymol 1991; 203:46–88.
32. Bird RE, Hardman KD, Jacobson JW, et al. Single-chain antigen-binding proteins [published erratum appears in Science 1989 (Apr 28); 244(4903):409]. Science 1988; 242:423–426.
33. Maraveyas A, Epenetos AA. Targeted immunotherapy. An update with special emphasis on ovarian cancer. Acta Oncol 1993; 32:741–746.
34. Meredith RF, Partridge EE, Alvarez RD, et al. Intraperitoneal radioimmunotherapy of ovarian cancer with lutetium-177-CC49. J Nucl Med 1996; 37:1491–1496.
35. Jacobs AJ, Fer M, Su FM, et al. A phase I trial of a rhenium 186-labeled monoclonal antibody administered intraperitoneally in ovarian carcinoma: toxicity and clinical response. Obstet Gynecol 1993; 82:586–593.
36. Riva P, Arista A, Tison V, et al. Intralesional radioimmunotherapy of malignant gliomas. An effective treatment in recurrent tumors. Cancer 1994; 73:1076–1082.
37. Zalcberg JR, Pietersz G, Toohey B, et al. A Phase I/II study of the intralesional injection of ricin-monoclonal antibody conjugates in patients with hepatic metastases. Eur J Cancer 1994; 30A:1227–1231.

38. Hird V, Maraveyas A, Snook D, et al. Adjuvant therapy of ovarian cancer with radioactive monoclonal antibody. Br J Cancer 1993; 68:403–406.
39. Riethmuller G, Schneider-Gadicke E, Schlimok G, et al. Randomized trial of monoclonal antibody for adjuvant therapy of resected Dukes' C colorectal carcinoma. German Cancer Aid 17-1A Study Group. Lancet 1994; 343:1177–1183.
40. Lynch TJ, Grossbard M, Fidias P, et al. Immunotoxin therapy of small cell lung cancer (SCLC): clinical trials of N901-blocked ricin (N901-bR). Proc Annu Meet Am Soc Clin Oncol 1995; 14:A1350.
41. Weiner LM, Holmes M, Adams GP, LaCreta F, Watts P, Garcia de Palazzo I. A human tumor xenograft model of therapy with a bispecific monoclonal antibody targeting c-erbB-2 and CD16. Cancer Res 1993; 53:94–100.
42. Valone FH, Kaufman PA, Guyre PM, et al. Clinical trials of bispecific antibody MDX-210 in women with advanced breast or ovarian cancer that overexpresses HER-2/neu. J Hematother 1995; 4:471–475.
43. Greiner JW, Ullmann CD, Nieroda C, et al. Improved radioimmunotherapeutic efficacy of an anticarcinoma monoclonal antibody (131I-CC49) when given in combination with gamma-interferon. Cancer Res 1993; 53:600–608.
44. Johnson E, Byrne B, Pestka S, Schlom J, Alwan D, Goldberg J. In vivo upregulation of TAG 72 by systemic interferon alpha 2a (IFN). Proc Annu Meet Am Soc Clin Oncol 1994; 13:A953.
45. Cemerlic D, Dadey B, Han T, Vaickus L. Cytokine influence on killing of fresh chronic lymphocytic leukemia cells by human leukocytes. Blood 1991; 77:2707–2715.
46. Valerius T, Repp R, de Wit TP, et al. Involvement of the high-affinity receptor for IgG (Fc gamma RI; CD64) in enhanced tumor cell cytotoxicity of neutrophils during granulocyte colony-stimulating factor therapy. Blood 1993; 82:931–939.
47. Repp R, Valerius T, Wieland G, et al. G-CSF-stimulated PMN in immunotherapy of breast cancer with a bispecific antibody to Fc gamma RI and to HER-2/neu (MDX-210). J Hematother 1995; 4:415–421.
48. Saleh MN, Khazaeli MB, Wheeler RH, Bucy RP, Schlom J, LoBuglio AF. A Phase II trial of murine MoAb D612 combined with recombinant human M-CSF (rhM-CSF) in patients with metastatic gastrointestinal (GI) cancer. Proc Annu Meet Am Assoc Cancer Res 1994; 35:A1505.
49. Baselga J, Norton L, Masui H, et al. Antitumor effects of doxorubicin in combination with anti-epidermal growth factor receptor monoclonal antibodies. J Natl Cancer Inst 1993; 85:1327–1333.
50. Fan Z, Baselga J, Masui H, Mendelsohn J. Antitumor effect of anti-epidermal growth factor receptor monoclonal antibodies plus *cis*-diamminedichloroplatinum on well-established A431 cell xenografts. Cancer Res 1993; 53:4637–4642.
51. Baselga J, Norton L, Shalaby R, Mendelsohn J. Anti-HER2 humanized monoclonal antibody (MAb) alone and in combination with chemotherapy against human breast carcinoma xenografts. Proc Annu Meet Am Soc Clin Oncol 1994; 13:A53.
52. Pegram M, Lipton A, Pietras R, et al. Phase II study of intravenous recombinant humanized anti-p185 HER-2 monoclonal antibody (rhuMAb HER-2) plus cisplatin in patients with HER-2/neu overexpressing metastatic breast cancer. Proc Annu Meet Am Soc Clin Oncol 1995; 14:A124.

53. Modjtahedi H, Eccles S, Box G, Styles J, Dean C. Immunotherapy of human tumour xenografts overexpressing the EGF receptor with rat antibodies that block growth factor–receptor interaction. Br J Cancer 1993; 67:254–261.
54. Tokuda Y, Ohnishi Y, Shimamura K, et al. In vitro and in vivo anti-tumor effects of a humanised monoclonal antibody against c-erbB-2 product. Br J Cancer 1996; 73:1362–1365.
55. Iwahashi T, Okochi E, Ariyoshi K, et al. Specific targeting and killing activities of anti-P-glycoprotein monoclonal antibody MRK16 directed against intrinsically multidrug-resistant human colorectal carcinoma cell lines in the nude mouse model. Cancer Res 1993; 53:5475–5482.
56. Borgstrom P, Hillan KJ, Sriramarao P, Ferrara N. Complete inhibition of angiogenesis and growth of microtumors by anti-vascular endothelial growth factor neutralizing antibody: novel concepts of angiostatic therapy from intravital videomicroscopy. Cancer Res 1996; 56:4032–4039.
57. Garin-Chesa P, Old LJ, Rettig WJ. Cell surface glycoprotein of reactive stromal fibroblasts as a potential antibody target in human epithelial cancers. Proc Natl Acad Sci USA 1990; 87:7235–7239.
58. Welt S, Divgi CR, Scott AM, et al. Antibody targeting in metastatic colon cancer: a Phase I study of monoclonal antibody F19 against a cell-surface protein of reactive tumor stromal fibroblasts. J Clin Oncol 1994; 12:1193–1203.
59. Grossbard ML, Press OW, Appelbaum FR, Bernstein ID, Nadler LM. Monoclonal antibody-based therapies of leukemia and lymphoma. Blood 1992; 80:863–878.
60. Owens RJ, Young RJ. The genetic engineering of monoclonal antibodies. J Immunol Methods 1994; 168:149–165.
61. Shitara K, Kuwana Y, Nakamura K, et al. A mouse/human chimeric anti-(ganglioside GD3) antibody with enhanced antitumor activities. Cancer Immunol Immunother 1993; 36:373–380.
62. LoBuglio AF, Wheeler RH, Trang J, et al. Mouse/human chimeric monoclonal antibody in man: kinetics and immune response. Proc Natl Acad Sci USA 1989; 86:4220–4224.
63. Jones PT, Dear PH, Foote J, Neuberger MS, Winter G. Replacing the complementarity-determining regions in a human antibody with those from a mouse. Nature 1986; 321:522–525.
64. Baselga J, Tripathy D, Mendelsohn J, et al. Phase II study of weekly intravenous recombinant humanized anti-p185HER2 monoclonal antibody in patients with HER2/neu-overexpressing metastatic breast cancer. J Clin Oncol 1996; 14:737–744.
65. Haisma HJ, Pinedo HM, Kessel MA, et al. Human IgM monoclonal antibody 16.88: pharmacokinetics and immunogenicity in colorectal cancer patients. J Natl Cancer Inst 1991; 83:1813–1819.
66. Steis RG, Carrasquillo JA, McCabe R, et al. Toxicity, immunogenicity, and tumor radioimmunodetecting ability of two human monoclonal antibodies in patients with metastatic colorectal carcinoma. J Clin Oncol 1990; 8:476–490.
67. Mellstedt H, Frodin JE, Masucci G, et al. The therapeutic use of monoclonal antibodies in colorectal carcinoma. Semin Oncol 1991; 18:462–477.
68. Khazaeli MB, Saleh MN, Wheeler RH, et al. Phase I trial of multiple large doses

of murine monoclonal antibody CO17-1A. II. Pharmacokinetics and immune response. J Natl Cancer Inst 1988; 80:937–942.
69. LoBuglio AF, Saleh MN, Lee J, et al. Phase I trial of multiple large doses of murine monoclonal antibody CO17-1A. I. Clinical aspects. J Natl Cancer Inst 1988; 80: 932–936.
70. Dillman RO, Beauregard JC, Halpern SE, Clutter M. Toxicities and side effects associated with intravenous infusions of murine monoclonal antibodies. J Biol Response Mod 1986; 5:73–84.
71. Ragnhammar P, Fagerberg J, Frodin JE, et al. Effect of monoclonal antibody 17-1A and GM-CSF in patients with advanced colorectal carcinoma—long-lasting, complete remissions can be induced. Int J Cancer 1993; 53:751–758.
72. Dillman RO, Beauregard JC, Sobol RE, et al. Lack of radioimmunodetection and complications associated with monoclonal anticarcinoembryonic antigen antibody cross-reactivity with an antigen on circulating cells. Cancer Res 1984; 44:2213–2218.
73. Byers VS, Rodvien R, Grant K, et al. Phase I study of monoclonal antibody-ricin A chain immunotoxin Xomazyme-791 in patients with metastatic colon cancer. Cancer Res 1989; 49:6153–6160.
74. Cheung NK, Lazarus H, Miraldi FD, et al. Ganglioside GD2 specific monoclonal antibody 3F8: a Phase I study in patients with neuroblastoma and malignant melanoma. J Clin Oncol 1987; 5:1430–1440.
75. Minasian LM, Szatrowski TP, Rosenblum M, et al. Hemorrhagic tumor necrosis during a pilot trial of tumor necrosis factor-alpha and anti-GD3 ganglioside monoclonal antibody in patients with metastatic melanoma. Blood 1994; 83:56–64.
76. Sears HF, Atkinson B, Mattis J, et al. Phase I clinical trial of monoclonal antibody in treatment of gastrointestinal tumors. Lancet 1982; 1:762–765.
77. Sears HF, Herlyn D, Steplewski Z, Koprowski H. Effects of monoclonal antibody immunotherapy on patients with gastrointestinal adenocarcinoma. J Biol Response Mod 1984; 3:138–150.
78. Sears HF, Herlyn D, Steplewski Z, Koprowski H. Phase II clinical trial of a murine monoclonal antibody cytotoxic for gastrointestinal adenocarcinoma. Cancer Res 1985; 45:5910–5913.
79. Murray JL, Macey DJ, Kasi LP, et al. Phase II radioimmunotherapy trial with 131I-CC49 in colorectal cancer. Cancer 1994; 73:1057–1066.
80. Mulligan T, Carrasquillo J, Chung Y, et al. Phase I study of intravenous lutetium-177 (177Lu)-labeled CC49 monoclonal antibody (MAb) in patients with advanced adenocarcinoma. Proc Annu Meet Am Soc Clin Oncol 1993; 12:A956.
81. Welt S, Divgi CR, Kemeny N, et al. Phase I/II study of iodine-131-labeled monoclonal antibody A33 in patients with advanced colon cancer. J Clin Oncol 1994; 12: 1561–1571.
82. Meredith RF, Khazaeli MB, Plott WE, et al. Initial clinical evaluation of iodine-125-labeled chimeric 17-1A for metastatic colon cancer. J Nucl Med 1995; 36:2229–2233.
83. Takahashi T, Yamaguchi T, Kitamura K, et al. Clinical application of monoclonal antibody–drug conjugates for immunotargeting chemotherapy of colorectal carcinoma. Cancer 1988; 61:881–888.

84. Theodoulou M, Gilewski TA, Welt S, et al. Anti-Lewis Y (LeY) monoclonal antibody (mAb) BR55-2 (IgG2a) in patients with advanced breast cancer. Proc Annu Meet Am Soc Clin Oncol 1994; 13:A974.
85. Anderson PM, Meyers DE, Hasz DE, et al. In vitro and in vivo cytotoxicity of an anti-osteosarcoma immunotoxin containing pokeweed antiviral protein. Cancer Res 1995; 55:1321–1327.
86. Stastny JJ, Das Gupta TK. The use of daunomycin-antibody immunoconjugates in managing soft tissue sarcomas: nude mouse xenograft model. Cancer Res 1993; 53:5740–5744.
87. Snider JM, Bushnell LJ, Chen LC, Lanza LA. c-erbB-2/p185-directed therapy in human lung adenocarcinoma. Ann Thorac Surg 1996; 62:1454–1459.
88. Zangemeister-Wittke U, Lehmann HP, Waibel R, Wawrzynczak EJ, Stahel RA. Action of a CD24-specific deglycosylated ricin-A-chain immunotoxin in conventional and novel models of small-cell-lung-cancer xenograft. Int J Cancer 1993; 53:521–528.
89. Divgi CR, Welt S, Kris M, et al. Phase I and imaging trial of indium 111-labeled anti-epidermal growth factor receptor monoclonal antibody 225 in patients with squamous cell lung carcinoma. J Natl Cancer Inst 1991; 83:97–104.
90. Divgi CR, Bander NH, Welt S, et al. Phase I/II trial with I-131-labeled monoclonal antibody (MA) G250 in metastatic renal cell cancer (RCC). Proc Annu Meet Am Soc Clin Oncol 1995; 14:A1345.
91. Meredith RF, Bueschen AJ, Khazaeli MB, et al. Treatment of metastatic prostate carcinoma with radiolabeled antibody CC49. J Nucl Med 1994; 35:1017–1022.
92. Juweid M, Sharkey RM, Behr T, et al. Targeting and treatment of medullary thyroid cancer (MTC) with radiolabeled monoclonal antibodies (MAbs) against carcinoembryonic antigen (CEA). Proc Annu Meet Am Soc Clin Oncol 1995; 14:A1342.
93. Cheung NV, Lazarus H, Miraldi FD, et al. Reassessment of patient response to monoclonal antibody 3F8. J Clin Oncol 1992; 10:671–672.

13
Monoclonal Antibody-Based Therapy of Breast Cancer

Francisco J. Esteva* and Daniel F. Hayes
Georgetown University Medical Center, Washington, D.C.

I. INTRODUCTION

Currently, the mainstays of treatment for metastatic human cancers are radiation and chemotherapy. The efficacy of these crude modalities is based on exploiting the differential growth rates of cancer cells versus normal cells. Since these differences are small, the toxicity of these therapies is substantial. Such considerations have engendered an enthusiastic search for therapies directed toward biological processes that might be more specific for cancer cells than for normal tissues. For many reasons, breast cancer is a particularly appealing disease to approach with such biologic therapies. The disease is common and it causes great suffering. More importantly, specific treatment targeted toward a single overexpressed molecule (e.g., the estrogen receptor) has been applied successfully to breast cancer patients in the form of hormonal therapy for over 100 years (1).

In this regard, investigators have, for nearly this entire century, studied a variety of methods designed to manipulate the immune system to stimulate a host-versus-tumor response. In 1896, Dr. William Coley (2) reported regressions of inoperable soft tissue sarcomas using a combination of bacterial toxins. In the 1960s and 1970s, *Bacillus Calmette-Guerin* (BCG) and levamisole were tested in patients with breast cancer in hopes of providing nonspecific immunostimulatory effects. These studies were performed in the adjuvant and metastatic settings and, although Phase II studies indicated beneficial effects (3,4), randomized trials

---

* *Current affiliation:* The University of Texas M. D. Anderson Cancer Center, Houston, Texas.

showed no impact on survival (5). Indeed, if anything, patients treated with BCG had a worse outcome than controls. In the 1970s, the availability of polyclonal antisera raised hopes of passive immunotherapy (6,7). Unfortunately, this approach also was unsuccessful in producing major clinical effects. In 1975, Kohler and Milstein (8) described the generation of monoclonal antibodies (MAbs) by hybridoma technology. The availability of highly specific murine antibodies led to the discovery of several previously unrecognized human tumor-associated proteins that, in turn, became targets for therapy. The discovery of proto-oncogenes in the 1980s (9), together with the availability of monoclonal antibodies, generated great excitement about the possibility of targeted anticancer therapy.

Breast cancer cells often express antigens that normally are not expressed on breast tissue, and/or they overexpress antigens that normally are expressed but at low levels. These antigens are often immunostimulants and are defined as tumor-associated antigens (TAAs). Few if any TAA are truly "tumor specific," and most if not all can be detected at some point in the development of the normal cell. Breast cancer-associated antigens include proteins normally expressed on fetal cells (e.g., carcinoembryonic antigen), proteins involved in mammary cell differentiation (e.g., MUC-1), and products of activated oncogenes (e.g., *erb*B2) or mutated tumor suppressor genes (e.g., p53) (Table 1). Several of these TAAs are undergoing preclinical and clinical testing as novel treatment targets for patients with breast cancer (10). Monoclonal antibody-based therapies are particularly appealing because of antibody selectivity for specific antigens both in vitro

Table 1 Breast Cancer–Associated Antigens

TAA	Abnormality in breast cancer	Percentage of positive breast cancers
EGFR	Protein overexpression	20–30
*erb*B2	Gene amplification	20–30
	Protein overexpression	
CEA	Protein overexpression	50
TAG-72	Protein overexpression	80–90
Le^y antigen	Protein overexpression	90
MUC-1	Protein overexpression	80 (fully glycosylated)
		20 (underglycosylated)
TN antigen	Protein expression (cryptic antigen in normal cells)	80–90
L6 antigen	Protein overexpression	80–90
p53	Mutation	50

TAA: tumor-associated antigen; CEA: carcinoembryonic antigen; EGFR: epidermal growth factor receptor.

and in animal models of breast cancer. Unfortunately, clinical development of monoclonal antibody-based therapy has proved more complex than originally expected. In this review we will discuss the most important limitations to the clinical development of antibody-based therapy of breast cancer. Potential strategies to overcome these barriers will be presented, with an emphasis on present clinical trials.

II. IMMUNOTHERAPY FOR BREAST CANCER

Directing a potent immune response to cancers without damaging normal tissues is the "holy grail" of tumor immunology. However, as just discussed, nonspecific stimulation of the immune system generally has been unsuccessful. If immunotherapy is to succeed, most investigations have demonstrated that it must be antigen directed and not just nonspecific stimulation of undirected immune effector cells.

Monoclonal antibody therapy may lead to cancer cell death in one of many ways (Table 2). Historically, therapies involving modulation of the immune system were defined as "passive" or "active." Passive immunotherapy relates to the intravenous administration of antibodies directed against specific tumor-associated antigens. Extensive preclinical testing indicates that this approach has potential value in the treatment of breast cancer. Monoclonal antibodies directed against breast cancer-associated growth factor receptors have been shown to induce cytotoxicity in vitro and in animal models (11,12). The mechanisms of action of passively administered antibodies include complement activation and enhancement of antibody-dependent cellular cytotoxicity (ADCC) (13).

Table 2 Mechanisms of MAb-Induced Cell Death

1. Induction of immune response
   - Passive
   - Active
2. Delivery of cytotoxic agents
   - Radioactive moiety
   - Bacterial or plant toxin
   - Chemotherapy
3. Induction of biological response
   - Apoptosis
   - Differentiation
   - Growth inhibition
   - Modulation of chemotherapy resistance

Active immunotherapy involves the generation of a long-lasting, vaccinelike T-cell-mediated immune response. This can be achieved by administering whole cancer cell extracts or small antigenic peptides isolated from tumors to experimental animals or cancer patients. In addition to T-cell activation, MAbs mimicking breast cancer antigens (anti-idiotype MAbs) can result in a humoral autoantibody-like immune response (14).

Because of their specificity, MAbs have also been used to deliver covalently coupled toxic agents to cancer sites. These include radioactive isotopes (15), bacterial or plant toxins (16,17), cytokines (18), or conventional chemotherapy (19). Monoclonal antibodies also may directly induce a biological response that leads to cell growth inhibition or death, such as stimulating a signal for apoptosis by mimicking a natural ligand (20). Moreover, MAbs also might regulate cellular mechanisms of resistance to other drugs and therefore enhance sensitivity (21,22), even if the MAb itself has little or no detectable effect on cell growth or viability.

In addition, MAbs can induce biological responses that lead to growth inhibition (23), cell differentiation (24), programmed cell death (apoptosis) (25), and modulation of chemotherapy sensitivity (26). Recently, passive Anti-*erb*B2 MAb therapy has been associated with tumor responses in patients with chemotherapy-resistant metastatic breast cancer (27).

Although most MAbs have been directed to cell membrane proteins, intracellular antibodies (also called *intrabodies*) have been developed (28). Potential targets include molecules involved in the intracellular processing of growth factor receptors, proteins involved in the signal transduction pathways, and some cyclins. For example, a single-chain Fv antibody fragment has been generated that binds *erb*B2 in the endoplasmic reticulum, resulting in downregulation of the receptor and reversal of the malignant phenotype (29). However, intracellular targeting will require adequate delivery systems to be clinically effective.

III. MECHANISMS INHERENT IN HOST IMMUNE RESPONSE THAT RESULT IN LIMITED EFFICACY OF IMMUNOTHERAPY FOR BREAST CANCER

Perhaps the most desired effect of immunotherapy, including antibody-based therapy, is the generation of a long-lasting, cellular-based, ''vaccine''-like immune response. However, given the complexity of antitumor immune responses, if immunotherapy is to be successful it must encompass several strategies simultaneously. For purposes of this review we will broadly define immune resistance (or ''tolerance'') as a failure successfully to eliminate TAA-expressing breast cancer cells from the host. It is probable that resistance is multifactorial and occurs anywhere along the immune pathway. Immunologic barriers that contribute to resistance of breast cancer cells to immune surveillance and immunotherapy, as well as technical and pharmacodynamic barriers associated with MAb-based therapy of breast cancer, will be discussed.

A. Immunologic Barriers

Several mechanisms can account for the ability of tumors to escape immunosurveillance and to resist immunotherapy (Table 3). The first step in mounting a potent antitumor immune response involves effective presentation of tumor-associated antigens to T-lymphocytes, either by "professional" antigen-presenting cells (APC) (e.g., macrophages) or by the cancer cells themselves. Antigen presentation requires appropriate expression of MHC class II proteins, adhesion molecules, and costimulatory molecules by the APC. Downregulation of any of these important molecules in macrophages may lead to inefficient APC function. Breast cancer cells are known to be poor antigen-presenting cells, despite MHC class II expression (30). Another mechanism of T-cell recognition is by direct binding of malignant cells to helper lymphocytes in an MHC class I-restricted fashion. However, MHC class I molecules often are downregulated in patients with breast cancer (31). Patients with large tumor burdens also may develop a state of systemic T-cell unresponsiveness due to abnormalities in T-cell receptor signal transduction pathways. Even if tumor antigen-specific T-cells exist in patients and circulate to the tumor, lack of expression of costimulatory molecules, or insufficient antigen/MHC complexes, may not lead to cytotoxic T-lymphocyte (CTL) activation (32,33).

It is possible that tumor cells actively produce agents that may alter effector cell recognition or function. Secretion of transforming growth factor-beta by breast cancer cells can inhibit several lymphocyte and macrophage functions (34). One study showed that the placental isoferritin-associated p43 protein can inhibit

Table 3 Mechanisms of Resistance to Immunotherapy for Breast Cancer

1. Downregulation of MHC class I and class II antigens in cancer cells
2. Development of altered T-cell function
    - Loss of costimulatory molecules (e.g., B7) by cancer cells
    - Loss of z-chain (T-cell receptor)
3. Production of immunosuppressant molecules by cancer cells
    - Production of TGFβ
    - Production of p43 placental isoferritin
    - Induction of T-cell apoptosis by MUC-1 gene product
4. Antigen modulation
5. Antigen masking

activation of T-lymphocytes in patients with breast cancer but not in women with benign pathology (35). Experimental and clinical data indicate that the MUC-1 gene product may function as an immunosuppressant molecule in patients with breast cancer. Overexpression of the MUC-1 protein by breast cancer cells has been associated with impaired cell–cell interaction and T-cell recognition (36), and inhibition of eosinophil adhesion to antibody-coated cells (37). In one study, the serum level of MUC-1 antigen was detected by MAb CA27.29 in breast cancer patients undergoing Anti-Tn antigen vaccination. Patients with high levels of circulating MUC-1 before vaccination mounted a lower number of CD69+ peripheral blood lymphocytes and had lower overall survival compared to patients with low levels of serum MUC-1 before treatment (38). This result supports the hypothesis that MUC-1 is associated with resistance (''tolerance'') to immunotherapy.

Binding of endogenous antibodies to tumor-associated antigens may lead to immune resistance because of loss of antigen expression. In this case, the antigen–antibody complexes may undergo endocytosis or may be shed into the circulation. If the complex is released into the systemic circulation and the antibody does not fix complement, the presence of antibody–antigen complexes would protect cancer cells from other complement-activating antibodies (39). This mechanism of resistance, known as *antigen modulation,* may complicate delivery of passive immunotherapy in the form of antitumor antibodies.

In summary, antibodies directed against tumor-associated antigens are unlikely to produce substantial antibreast cancer effects when administered alone. Likewise, although antitumor responses are attributed mostly to the cellular arm of the immune system, cumulative data suggest that nonspecific T-cell therapy alone is also insufficient (40). Indeed, cancer patients often develop antibodies and T-cell responses directed against specific TAAs (41) and yet their tumors progress to lethal metastatic disease. These data suggest that if immune therapy of breast cancer is to be successful, multiple strategies will need to be combined to overcome inherent resistance (or ''tolerance'').

Several investigators have considered strategies that might overcome some of these immunologic barriers. One such strategy involves the use of bispecific monoclonal antibodies (Bi-MAbs) (42). These are antibody constructs designed to link tumor cells expressing TAA directly with effector immune cells. Originally, Bi-MAbs were developed to identify triggering molecules of cytotoxicity. Triggering of the CD3 molecule, for example, was found to induce T-cell-mediated cytotoxicity. In vitro studies showed that Bi-MAb with specificity to one of the different classes of Fc receptors could be triggered by antibody binding outside the binding site for IgG, indicating that Bi-MAb-mediated cytotoxicity may not be inhibited by the presence of natural IgG. This is a potential advantage compared to conventional monoclonal antibodies. Bispecific antibodies have been shown to be as effective as their parental antibodies in inducing antibody-dependent cellular cytotoxicity (ADCC) both in vitro and in vivo (43,44). Perhaps more importantly, certain BiMAbs mediate antibody-dependent cell-mediated phagocytosis (ADCP), (45) which may translate into a long-lasting vaccinelike response.

B. Technical and Pharmacodynamic Barriers

In addition to the biologic concerns already discussed, technical and pharmacodynamic barriers must be minimized before MAb-based therapy can be widely applied to patients with breast cancer. These include the development of human antimouse antibodies (HAMA), difficulties associated with the delivery of large molecules to solid tumors, heterogeneous antigen expression in tumors, and expression of tumor-associated antigens in normal tissues (Table 4).

1. Development of Human AntiMouse Antibodies (HAMA)

Development of HAMA results in rapid clearance of the antibody from the circulation upon reinfusion. Recently, genetic engineering technology has allowed production of completely humanized antibodies that do not elicit host antihuman antibodies (HAHA), allowing for multiple repeated doses with adequately maintained circulating MAb levels. At least one such antibody, rhuMAbHER2, directed against HER2/neu, has undergone extensive Phase I, II, and III clinical testing, and HAHA production has not been a problem in these clinical trials (27).

Table 4 Barriers Associated with Clinical Development of MAb-Based Therapy

A. Development of HAMA
   Strategy: Antibody humanization
B. Limited tumor penetration
   Strategies: Antibody fragment (Fab)
                Liposomal formulation
C. Heterogeneous antigen expression in the tumor
   Strategies: Induction of "innocent bystander" effect by radiolabeled MAb
                Upregulation of antigen expression by interferon
                Combination of several antibodies ("cocktail")
D. TAA expression on normal cells
   Strategies: Accept limited toxicity
                Use growth factors (e.g., G-CSF)

2. Delivery of Monoclonal Antibodies to Solid Tumors

Theoretical and experimental evidence suggest that tumor penetration may limit efficacy of monoclonal antibodies in solid tumors (46). Delivery of MAb to metastatic cancers is compromised by intratumoral barriers, such as increased interstitial fluid pressure in the tumor compared to normal tissues and poor perfusion of tumor vasculature. Antibody-related factors include pharmacokinetics, capillary permeability, and binding to target antigens (47).

In order to improve delivery of MAb to solid tumors, small antibody fragments that contain the specific combining region (sFv) have been developed (48). These fragments are as specific as the parental antibodies and have been shown to induce objective responses in patients with breast cancer. Another strategy associated with improved tumor penetration and increased biological activity involves the use of liposomal formulations. For example, liposomes conjugated to an Anti-HER/neu antibody fragment results in higher uptake by breast cancer cells in vitro (49) and in vivo (50). In one study, combination of monoclonal antibody MAbp120 with liposomes (Lipo) and hyperthermia (HT) resulted in enhanced antitumor effects in a human breast cancer cell line (MCF-7) when compared to MAb alone. In this experiment, cell growth inhibition by the combination of MAbp120 + Lipo + HT was 65%, whereas irrelevant control antibodies produced only slight cytotoxicity (51).

3. Heterogeneous Antigen Expression in Tumors and Expression of Tumor-Associated Antigens in Normal Tissues

One distinct feature of human breast cancers is the heterogeneity of TAAs between different tumors and among different cells within the same tumor. For example, one study showed high heterogeneity in the level of *erb*B2 gene amplification and mRNA expression in 61 samples of primary breast cancer (52). This difference in TAA expression may lead to a decreased efficacy of MAb-based therapy.

Interferon can upregulate antigen expression in human breast cancer in vitro and in vivo. A clinical trial using interferon in combination with an Anti-TAG-72 monoclonal antibody showed a significant increase in expression of the target antigen (53). This approach is currently under active investigation.

Another strategy to enhance killing of cells with heterogeneous antigen expression is the use of radioimmunotherapy. In this case, although radiopharmaceutical agents linked to antibodies are delivered to high-antigen-expressing cells, an "innocent bystander" effect may result from the emission of radioactivity to surrounding cancer cells that do not bind the immunoconjugate (54). Radioimmunotherapy has been associated with complete erradication of solid tumors in animal models (55). Clinical trials are currently testing the feasibility and safety of this approach in patients with breast cancer (Table 5).

Finally, combination of several MAbs may be more effective than single therapy. One study showed that antibody "cocktails" were significantly more sensitive in differentiating cancer cells from normal cells in primary human breast tumors (56). A combination of two ricin-based immunotoxins directed against two different epitopes of the transferrin receptor has been shown to induce synergistic cytotoxicity in breast cancer cell lines (57). Of course, one loses relative specificity with such an approach and toxicity may be higher. This promising strategy has not been tested in clinical trials and awaits completion of toxicity studies using single-immunotoxin therapy.

4. Expression of Tumor-Associated Antigen in Normal Cells

One of the most important barriers to the clinical development of MAbs as therapeutic agents is the potential damage to normal cells. Since TAAs are not truly tumor-specific and are expressed at some level by normal tissues, MAb specificity is critical. For a MAb-based therapy to enter clinical trial, the agent must be as specific as possible and cause the least toxicity to normal tissues in appropriate animal models (usually involving nonhuman primates). However, unanticipated toxicity may occur. For example, Gould et al. (58) reported the development of unexpected neurological toxicity in breast cancer patients receiving an immunotoxin that had been generated against a carcinoma antigen. In this study, the antibody recognized a myelin antigenic epitope, and many patients developed a demyelinating syndrome.

IV. CLINICAL DEVELOPMENT OF MONOCLONAL ANTIBODY-BASED THERAPY FOR BREAST CANCER

Clinical trials of monoclonal antibodies are currently under way in patients with breast cancer. At the time of this review, thirteen clinical trials are accruing patients with different stages of breast cancer in the United States (Table 5). Available data according to the target tumor-associated antigen will be presented.

A. The Epidermal Growth Factor Receptor Family

Several oncogenes have been implicated in the pathogenesis of breast cancer. One of the most extensively studied groups of oncogenes encodes growth factor receptors that, upon activation, initiate signal transduction pathways that result in altered gene expression and mitogenesis (59). The type 1 growth factor receptor family consists of four transmembrane glycoproteins with tyrosine kinase activity. These include the epidermal growth factor receptor (EGFR) (60), *erb*B2 (61), *erb*B3 (62), and *erb*B4 (63). Ligands known to bind and activate these

Table 5 Active Clinical Trials Using MAb-Based Therapy for Patients with Metastatic Breast Cancer

Phase	Target	Monoclonal antibody	Trial objectives	Lead organization(s) and trial ID
I	EGFR	MDX447 (BsAb) ± G-CSF	• Safety and tolerability of BsAb with and without G-CSF • OBD and/or MTD of BsAb with and without G-CSF • Biochemical and immunological marker response • Pharmacokinetics • Binding of Bi-MAb to breast tumor tissue after treatment with antibody alone and in combination with G-CSF • Preliminary assessment of antitumor effects	Medarex (Annandale, NJ) MDX-95-062 Memorial Sloan Kettering Cancer Ctr (New York, NY) NCI-V95-0771 MSKCC-95062
I	EGFR	C225 (Chimeric Ab) + Paclitaxel	• Safety profile • Efficacy • Estimate the optimal biologic dose (OBD) or the MTD • Pharmacokinetics and immunokinetics	Memorial Sloan Kettering Cancer Ctr (New York, NY) NCI-V96-0832
I	erbB2	520C9xH22 [MDX-H210] (BsAb)	• Safety and toxicity • MTD and OBD • Pharmacokinetics and immunologic effects • Effects on tumor regression • Assess binding of 520C9xH22 Ab to cancer tissue	National Cancer Institute (Bethesda, MD) NCI-95-C-0023K
I	erbB2	MDX 520xH22 (BsAb) + G-CSF	• MTD • Pharmacokinetics • Immunologic effects of Bi-MAb alone and in combination with G-CSF • Binding of Bi-MAb to breast tumor tissue after treatment with antibody alone and in combination with G-CSF • Preliminary assessment of antitumor effects	Medarex (Annandale, NJ) MDX-1B-95-2 University of Southern California (Los Angeles, CA) NCI-V95-0658 LAC-USC-1B952

Phase	Target	Agent	Objectives	Institution
IA/AB	erbB2	520C9xH22 (MDX-H210) (BsAb) + Interferon gamma	• Toxicity of 520C9xH22 in combination with interferon gamma MTD and OBD • Degree of activation of effector cell populations (monocytes, neutrophils, T- and B-lymphocytes, and NK cells) • Localization of antibody to tumor masses • Extent and localization of infiltrating macrophages, granulocytes, and lymphocytes in tumors • Assess capacity of IFNg to increase monocyte and neutrophil expression of the human Ig receptor Fcg RI	Medarex (Annandale, NJ) Dartmouth Medical School (Lebanon, NH) NCI-V94-0450 DMS-9318
III	erbB2	RhuMAb HER2 (recombinant human antibody)	• Determine overall response rate (CR and PR) • Characterize further the MAb safety profile • Determine the duration of response, 1-year survival, and the time to disease progression • Evaluate the quality of life of these patients (EORTC model)	University of California at Los Angeles UCLA-HSPC-9510492
I	CEA	^{131}I-MN-14 • Intact Ig • F(ab)	• MTD and appropriate dose of antibody for Phase II studies • Pharmacokinetics of intact Ig and Ab fragment • Tumor and organ dosimetry of intact Ig and Ab fragment • Magnitude and significance of HAMA on the biodistribution of intact Ig and Ab fragment	Garden State Cancer Ctr (Belleville, NJ) NCI-V93-0306
I	TAG	^{131}I-CC49	• Assess feasibility and side effects of radioimmunotherapy with ^{131}I-CC49 followed by TBI and Thiotepa with autologous PBSCR MTD • Determine impact of TBI/thiotepa on the frequency and magnitude of HAMA • Determine objective clinical responses	University of Alabama at Birmingham UAB-9505

Table 5 Continued

Phase	Target	Monoclonal antibody	Trial objectives	Lead organization(s) and trial ID
I	B3	LMB-1 immunotoxin (Anti-B3-PE)	• Toxicity profile • Clinical responses • Pharmacokinetics • Development of HAMA, both to the murine MAb and to PE	National Cancer Institute (Bethesda, MD) NCI-T92-0223N NCI-MB-313
I	B3	• ^{90}Y-B3 • ^{111}In-B3	• Ability of ^{111}In-B3 to image known metastases • MTD of ^{90}Y-B3 • Toxicity profiles of ^{90}Y-B3 and ^{111}In-B3 • Pharmacokinetics, in vivo stability and antibody biodistribution • Dosimetry for ^{111}In-B3 • HAMA development • Antitumor effects	National Cancer Institute (Bethesda, MD) NCI-94-C-0075B NCI-T93-0046N NCI-NMOB-9304
I	B3	LMB-7 immunotoxin (Anti-B3-PE recombinant single-chain immunotoxin)	• Toxicity profile • Clinical responses • Pharmacokinetics • Development of HAMA, both to the murine MAb and to PE	National Cancer Institute (Bethesda, MD) NCI-94-C-0172H NCI-T94-0037N
I	BR55	BR55-2 (IgG2a)	• Toxicity profile • Pharmacokinetics • Development of HAMA • Determine whether MAb BR55-2 mediates in vitro ADCC or complement-dependent cell lysis, complement activation in blood or tumor tissue, induction of an inflammatory infiltrate in tumor tissue, or binding to and reduction of tumor cells in bone marrow	Memorial Sloan Kettering Cancer Ctr (New York, NY)

I/II	NR-LU-10	NR-LU-10 conjugated to streptavidin → ^{90}Y linked to Biotin	• MTD of ^{90}Y-Biotin following administration of MAb NR-LU-10 conjugated to streptavidin as part of a pretargeting approach • Evaluate the safety of the pretargeting approach • Evaluate the ability of ^{90}Y-Biotin to localize to known and occult tumor sites via the pretargeting approach using indium-111-biotin • Estimate the radiation dose achieved by ^{90}Y-Biotin at tumor sites and in normal organs based on measurements of ^{111}In-Biotin uptake • Evaluate objective tumor responses • Assess immunogenicity of the pretargeting components given i.v.	Virginia Mason Medical Ctr (Seattle, WA) VMRC-6366 Stanford University Medical Ctr (Stanford, CA)

MAb: monoclonal antibody; PE: *Pseudomonas* exotoxin; ^{90}Y: yttrium-90; ^{111}In: indium-111; MTD: maximum tolerated dose; OBD: optimal biologic dose; HAMA: human antimouse antibodies; EGFR: epidermal growth factor receptor; IFNg: interferon gamma; G-CSF: granulocyte-colony stimulation factor; NK: natural killer; TBI: total-body irradiation; PBSCR: peripheral blood stem-cell rescue; CR: complete response; PR: partial response; EORTC: European Organization for Research and Treatment of Cancer; i.v.: intravenously; CEA: carcinoembryonic antigen; Ig: immunoglobulin.

receptors include the epidermal growth factor (EGF) (64), the transforming growth factor alpha (65), amphiregulin (66), and heregulin (67).

1. Epidermal Growth Factor Receptor

The epidermal growth factor receptor is a 170-Kd transmembrane glycoprotein that is overexpressed in 20–30% of human breast cancers (68). Activation of the EGFR by ligand binding induces malignant transformation in mammalian cells, indicating that this receptor/ligand system plays a role in cellular transformation (64,69). Patients whose tumors overexpress the EGFR have a poor prognosis compared to patients with no EGFR overexpression (70,71). Overexpression of the EGFR has been associated with downregulation of the estrogen receptor and resistance to tamoxifen therapy in breast cancer patients (72).

Monoclonal antibodies that block signal transduction pathways activated by epidermal growth factor receptor can inhibit the growth of EGFR-overexpressing cells in vitro and in animal models (73). The MAbs 225 IgG1 and 528 IgG2A bind to the EGF receptor with affinity comparable to the natural ligands. This leads to competition for receptor binding between the antibody and the endogenous ligands and inhibition of ligand-induced activation of the EGFR tyrosine kinase (74–77).

In preclinical studies, Anti-EGFR antibodies appear to act synergistically to cause tumor cell death when combined with conventional chemotherapy. Combination of MAb with cisplatin or doxorubicin leads to long-lasting complete responses in most animals (21,22).

In a Phase I clinical trial, multiple doses of chimeric (human:murine) Anti-EGFR MAb C225 were administered to breast cancer patients whose tumors overexpressed EGFR. Preliminary data suggest adequate pharmacokinetics with receptor-blocking serum levels and low toxicity (78).

Anti-EGFR bispecific antibodies have been developed, in attempts to direct a potent immune response to EGFR-expressing tumors. The MDX447 bispecific monoclonal antibody combines a fragment of MAb H425 (Anti-EGFR) and a fragment of MAb H22 (to Fc-γ RI). A Phase I clinical trial using MDX447 in combination with G-CSF showed minimal toxicity and evidence of G-CSF-induced upregulation of Fc-γ RI on neutrophils. Furthermore, in vivo binding of MDX447 to polymorphonuclear cells was increased in patients receiving G-CSF. No responses have been seen at 3.5 mg/m^2 dose level. However, fifteen out of twenty-two patients had stable disease beyond the first month of therapy, and dose escalation continues (79).

In summary, EGFR-blocking antibodies can be administered safely to breast cancer patients, and further development of this approach is warranted. However, the specific ''niche'' of interrupting this important receptor/ligand system has not been established yet.

2. *erb*B2

One of the first genetic abnormalities identified in human breast cancer was amplification of the *erb*B-2 gene (also called HER-2, or *neu*) (80). This amplification results in overexpression of a 185-Kd transmembrane protein with tyrosine kinase activity (81) that shares high homology with EGFR (82). The *erb*B-2 protein is amplified and/or overexpressed in 60% of patients with ductal carcinoma in situ (83) and in 20–30% of patients with invasive breast cancer (84). Amplification of the *erb*B-2 proto-oncogene and/or overexpression of the *erb*B-2 protein are associated with a worse prognosis in patients with breast cancer who have involvement of the axillary lymph nodes (85).

The *erb*B2 gene product is an excellent therapeutic target for the following reasons: (a) it is localized to the cell membrane; (b) it is present in a very high proportion of cancer cells in tumors that overexpress *erb*B2, and (c) it is usually overexpressed both in the primary tumor and at metastatic sites, indicating that patients whose primary tumors overexpress *erb*B2 could be effectively treated in the metastatic setting with Anti-*erb*B2 directed therapy (86). Monoclonal anti-*erb*B2 antibodies have been shown to reduce the growth rate of human breast cancer cells in vitro and in vivo (87).

In 1996, Baselga et al. (27) reported a Phase II clinical trial using a humanized version of the Anti-*erb*B2 murine monoclonal antibody 4D5 (RhuMAb HER2). In this study, 45 patients with metastatic breast cancer refractory to multiple chemotherapies and hormone manipulations received weekly rhuMAb HER2 antibody therapy. The response rate in this heavily pretreated group was 11%. In addition, 37% of patients had stable disease after multiple doses. The results of this study showed that binding a tumor-associated antigen (*erb*B2) with a specific monoclonal antibody may result in objective clinical responses in patients with breast cancer.

Extensive preclinical and clinical data suggest that *erb*B2 may be associated with modulation of response to certain therapeutic agents. These include cisplatin (21,88), paclitaxel (89), doxorubicin (90), and hormone therapies (91). In one study, patients with breast cancer whose tumors overexpressed *erb*B2 had lower survival after adjuvant cyclophosphamide, methotrexate, and 5-fluorouracil (CMF) chemotherapy (92). Interestingly, *erb*B2 overexpression recently has been associated with a high response rate to taxol chemotherapy in patients with metastatic breast cancer (89). These observations led to clinical trials evaluating the combination of Anti-*erb*B2 monoclonal antibodies with other therapeutic agents. Multicenter Phase III trials are currently in progress in the United States and Europe using rhuMAb HER2 alone and in combination with conventional chemotherapy, in both the adjuvant and the metastatic settings (Table 5).

Ideally, the *erb*B2 protein might serve as a cancer "vaccine." For example, *erb*B2 overexpression has been associated with the presence of dense lymphocyte infiltration in the primary tumors of patients with breast cancer (93). Specific cytotoxic T-lymphocytes have been identified in the peripheral blood of patients whose tumors overexpress *erb*B2 (94). Bispecific MAbs that recognize *erb*B2 and CD3 can induce tumor regressions in nude mice bearing *erb*B2 overexpressing human xenografts (95). Also, Anti-*erb*B2 Bi-MAbs have been generated that recognize the Fc gamma receptors present on macrophages and monocytes. These include the Fc-γ RI (CD64), Fc-γ RII (CDw32), and Fc-γ RIII receptors (96,97). Phase I clinical trials have shown minimal toxicity, evidence of biological activity, and even objective clinical responses (98,99). Several studies indicate that the biological activity of Bi-MAb can be enhanced by combination with G-CSF, GM-CSF, and interferon. The mechanism of action of these cytokines may be related to an increase in the number of immune effector cells to tumor sites (by colony-stimulating factors) and upregulation of antigen expression (by interferon) (100). Phase I/II trials addressing the feasibility and toxicity profile of Anti-*erb*B2 bispecific antibodies in combination with cytokines are ongoing (Table 5).

In order to increase their antitumor activity, Anti-*erb*B2 monoclonal antibodies have been combined with bacterial or plant toxins. This initially was achieved by chemically linking an antibody fragment to a toxin, resulting in large, highly immunogenic proteins. More recently, smaller immunotoxins have been generated by genetic engineering techniques. For example, 23(Fv)PE is a recombinant toxin that shows strong selectivity for *erb*B2 binding and can induce tumor regressions in animal models with low toxicity (101). A Phase I clinical trial using e23(Fv)PE anti-*erb*B2 recombinant toxin has been initiated at the National Cancer Institute. In an attempt to improve delivery of these immunotoxins, Chen et al. (102) transfected the genetic sequence encoding the e23(Fv)PE Anti-*erb*B2 immunotoxin into tumor infiltrating lymphocytes (TILs). Administration of these modified TILs resulted in tumor responses in an animal xenograft model.

A novel therapeutic approach using Anti-*erb*B2 MAb involves intracellular targeting. A single-chain Fv antibody fragment has been generated that binds *erb*B2 in the endoplasmic reticulum, resulting in downregulation of the receptor and reversal of the malignant phenotype (29,103). This approach has not reached clinical testing yet.

B. Carcinoembryonic Antigen

Oncofetal TAAs are expressed during embryonic development and downregulated in adult tissues. The best characterized in breast cancer is the human carcinoembryonic antigen (CEA). Indeed, CEA was the first TAA identified (104). Although initial studies suggested CEA was a gastrointestinal-related tumor marker, subsequent studies demonstrated that CEA overexpression occurs in nearly all epithelial malignancies (105). Carcinoembryonic antigen is overexpressed in 50% of patients with invasive breast cancer as disclosed by immunohistochemical methods (106) and can be detected in the serum of patients with all stages of breast cancer (107).

Because CEA is overexpressed in many types of carcinomas, it has been extensively evaluated as a target for immunotherapy (108,109). Monoclonal antibodies against CEA can eradicate CEA-overexpressing cancer cells in vitro and human tumors growing in mice. A Phase I study of the chimeric T84.66 anti-CEA antibody in patients with metastatic CEA-producing malignancies reported no toxicity from the antibody administration and good localization of the antibody to metastatic sites (110). However, to date, no studies have reported impressive clinical results with Anti-CEA-directed therapy.

C. Mucin Antigens

A number of proteins expressed by normal mammary cells can be altered or produced at high levels by breast cancer cells. This differential expression in neoplastic versus normal cells may provide novel targets for immunotherapy of breast cancer. The most extensively studied antigens involved in mammary cell differentiation belong to the family of mucin glycoproteins.

1. Tumor-Associated Glycoprotein 72

The tumor-associated glycoprotein 72 (TAG-72) is a high-molecular-weight mucin that is overexpressed in a wide range of human adenocarcinomas. These include breast, ovary, endometrial, prostate, gastrointestinal, and non-small-cell lung cancer (111).

Monoclonal antibodies that react with the TAG-72 antigen include B72.3 (112) and CC49 (113). These antibodies can eliminate TAG-72 overexpressing human xenografts growing in athymic mice. Clinical trials have shown that CC49 antibody localizes well to metastatic sites. A Phase I study using ^{131}I-CC49 in combination with total-body irradiation and high-dose thiotepa is in progress (Table 5).

2. Lewis^y Antigen

The Lewis^y (Le^y) antigen is a complex carbohydrate that belongs to the Lewis blood group, although it is rarely detected in normal erythrocytes. Interestingly, Le^y is expressed in many human carcinomas (pancarcinoma antigen), including breast cancer. Although the normal function of this molecule is unclear, its glycosylation pattern has been found to be altered in cancer cells (114).

Monoclonal antibody B3 is a murine antibody (IgG1k) that recognizes the Le^y antigen. A series of B3-based immunotoxins are undergoing clinical testing at the National Cancer Institute (NCI). LMB-1 was constructed by chemically linking B3 to a truncated *Pseudomonas* exotoxin that lacks its binding domain

(PE38). Preclinical data showed excellent antitumor activity and low toxicity in nonhuman primates (115). Although Phase I clinical testing has not been completed, preliminary data indicate that the major toxicity is capillary leak syndrome. Of note, one patient with metastatic breast cancer had a complete response to LMB-1 therapy (116).

Monoclonal antibody BR96 binds Le^y antigen with high affinity in cancer cells (117). Upon recognition of the antigenic carbohydrate, BR96 is internalized rapidly by cancer cells but not by normal cells. This makes BR96 an excellent vehicle to transport toxic agents to cancer cells. For example, conjugation of BR96 with doxorubicin resulted in cures of human breast cancer xenografts growing in nude mice (118). Phase I clinical trials have been initiated using this approach, and the main toxicity observed has been gastrointestinal (severe vomiting) (119). A BR96(sFv)PE recombinant immunotoxin combining BR96 with a truncated *Pseudomonas* exotoxin has been shown to be active in vitro (120) and in animal models (121). Clinical testing is under way.

3. MUC-1 Protein

The polymorphic epithelial mucin (PEM), also known as human milk fat globule (HMFG), MAM6 and DF3-antigen, is a transmembrane protein encoded by the MUC-1 gene (122). The MUC-1 protein extracellular domain is highly glycosylated, resulting in an extended mucinlike structure. Although glycosylated MUC-1 is expressed on most normal epithelial cells, it is overexpressed on the cell surface of 80% of human breast cancers (123). Furthermore, the cancer-associated glycosylation pattern of MUC-1 appears to be different from the glycosylated protein found in normal cells. Cancer-associated MUC-1 may be underglycosylated compared to the normal gene product (124,125). The underglycosylated protein, which may be more tumor-specific, is detected less often, perhaps in only 20% of patients with breast cancer. The MUC-1 protein is shed by tumor cells to the circulation, and serial serum levels can be used to monitor patients with breast cancer (107).

Specific MAbs have been developed that recognize the fully glycosylated MUC-1 protein, such as HMFG-1, HMFG-2 (126), and DF3 (127). Antibodies that react only with the underglycosylated MUC-1 species include SM3 (128) and DF3-P (129).

Of note, preclinical and clinical studies suggest MUC-1 protein may be a good target for immunotherapy (130,131). In cancer cells the MUC-1 antigen is expressed throughout the cell membrane, whereas it is located almost exclusively on the ductal luminal surface in normal cells (127). Cytotoxic T-lymphocytes (CTL) that attack MUC-1-overexpressing cells have been reported in vitro (132). Human dendritic cells overexpressing the MUC-1 gene have been generated as a vaccine approach for the treatment of patients whose tumors overexpress

MUC-1 (133). A Phase I clinical trial of an MUC-1 peptide vaccine showed induction of a specific immune response in breast cancer patients (134).

4. Tn Antigen

The syalin Tn is a glycoprotein expressed in a subset of human primary breast tumors. Tn is not expressed in normal mammary cells, where it behaves as a "cryptic" antigen, hidden from immune effector cells by complex carbohydrates (135).

The differential expression pattern of the Tn antigen makes it an interesting target for immunotherapy. Clinical trials indicate that Tn-based vaccines can be administered with minimal toxicity to patients with breast cancer and that specific humoral immune responses can be generated. In two studies, the levels of Anti-Tn antibodies detected using this approach were enhanced by pretreatment with cyclophosphamide (136,137). However, thus far, it is not clear that these studies have resulted in measurable beneficial effects in breast cancer patients.

5. L6 Antigen

The L6 monoclonal antibody recognizes a protein epitope expressed on most breast cancers. Although the normal L6 protein structure is not known, it requires the presence of membranes, and it is unaffected by the removal of carbohydrate side chains (138).

Phase I clinical trials using murine and chimeric (human:mouse) Anti-L6 monoclonal antibodies have demonstrated good tumor localization at tolerable doses (139,140). In one study, one patient had a complete response, and serial tumor biopsies revealed infiltration by helper and suppressor T-cells but no evidence of NK cells (139). Radioimmunotherapy using a humanized murine monoclonal antibody (chimeric L6) resulted in objective tumor responses in 50% of chemotherapy-refractory patients with metastatic breast cancer (141). Although the number of patients was small, a greater response was observed in patients with elevated levels of interleukin-2 receptor in the serum. One of the main toxicities was myelosupression. The same investigators have shown that bone marrow toxicity can be minimized if the antibody is administered in combination with G-CSF or autologous peripheral blood stem-cell support (142).

V. CONCLUSION

In summary, the field of MAb-based therapy of breast cancer is moving forward in both the experimental and the clinical arenas. A significant number of antibodies are undergoing clinical trials and preliminary reports indicate promising biological effects and objective clinical responses. Unfortunately, except for the promising Phase II results reported for the Anti-HER2 MAb 4D5, few real clinical benefits have been observed. To date, the activity of MAbs or strategies discussed are insufficient to be used in noninvestigational settings. Biologic, technical, and pharmacodynamic problems remain unsolved, and potential strategies to overcome these barriers are actively being investigated. In the future, monoclonal antibodies will most likely be used in combination with chemotherapy, cytokines, and other biological therapies in patients with minimal disease. Antibody-based therapy may also contribute to the development of anti-breast cancer vaccines. Thus, a better understanding of the immune system, coupled with laboratory molecular biology techniques offer promise of successful immunotherapy in the future.

REFERENCES

1. Beatson GT. On the treatment of inoperable cases of carcinoma of the mamma: suggestions for a new method of treatment, with illustrative cases (abstr). Lancet 1896; ii:104–107.
2. Coley WB. Recurrent sarcoma of the palm of the hand successfully treated with the toxines of Erysipelas and Bacillus Prodigiosus (abstr). Ann Surg 1896; 24:501–502.
3. Hortobagyi GN, Yap HY, Blumenschein GR, Gutterman JU, Buzdar AU, Tashima CK, Hersh EM. Response of disseminated breast cancer to combined modality treatment with chemotherapy and levamisole with or without Bacillus Calmette-Guerin. Cancer Treat Rep 1978; 62:1685–1692.
4. Gutterman JU, Mavligit GM, Blumenshein G, Burgess MA, McBride CM, Hersh EM. Immunotherapy of human solid tumors with Bacillus Calmette-Guerin: prolongation of disease-free interval and survival in malignant melanoma, breast, and colorectal cancer. Ann N Y Acad Sci 1976; 277:135–159.
5. Buzdar AU, Blumenschein GR, Smith TL, Powell KC, Hortobagyi GN, Yap HY, Schell FC, Barnes BC, Ames FC, Martin RG, et al. Adjuvant chemotherapy with fluorouracil, doxorubicin, and cyclophosphamide, with or without *Bacillus Calmette-Guerin* and with or without irradiation in operable breast cancer. A prospective randomized trial. Cancer 1984; 53:384–389.
6. Anderson JM, Kelly F, Wood SE, Halnan KE. Stimulatory immunotherapy in mammary cancer. Br J Surg 1974; 61:778–784.
7. Oettgen HF, Old LJ, Farrow JH, Valentine FT, Lawrence HS, Thomas L. Effects of dialyzable transfer factor in patients with breast cancer. Proc Natl Acad Sci USA 1974; 71:2319–2323.
8. Kohler G, Milstein C. Continuous cultures of fused cells secreting antibody of predefined specificity. Nature 1975; 256:495–497.
9. Bishop JM. Molecular themes in oncogenesis. Cell 1991; 64:235–248.
10. Schlom J, Greiner J, Hand PH, Colcher D, Inghirami G, Weeks M, Pestka S, Fisher PB, Noguchi P, Kufe D. Monoclonal antibodies to breast cancer-associated antigens

as potential reagents in the management of breast cancer. Cancer 1984; 54:2777–2794.
11. Schnurch HG, Stegmuller M, Vering A, Beckmann MW, Bender HG. Growth inhibition of xenotransplanted human carcinomas by a monoclonal antibody directed against the epidermal growth factor receptor. Eur J Cancer 1994; 30A:491–496.
12. Masui H, Kawamoto T, Sato JD, Wolf B, Sato G, Mendelsohn J. Growth inhibition of human tumor cells in athymic mice by anti-epidermal growth factor receptor monoclonal antibodies. Cancer Res 1984; 44:1002–1007.
13. Pegram MD, Baly D, Wirth C, Gilkerson E, Slamon DJ, Sliwkowski MX, Bauer K, Fox JA. Antibody dependent cell-mediated cytotoxicity in breast cancer patients in Phase III clinical trials of a humanized anti-HER2 antibody (abstr). Proc Am Assoc Cancer Res 1997; 38:602.
14. Chakraborty M, Mukerjee S, Foon KA, Kohler H, Ceriani RL, Bhattacharya-Chatterjee M. Induction of human breast cancer-specific antibody responses in cynomolgus monkeys by a murine monoclonal anti-idiotype antibody. Cancer Res 1995; 55:1525–1530.
15. Goldenberg DM, Larson SM, Reisfeld RA, Schlom J. Targeting cancer with radio-labeled antibodies. Immunol Today 1995; 16:261–264.
16. Batra JK, Kasprzyk PG, Bird RE, Pastan I, King CR. Recombinant anti-*erb*B2 immunotoxins containing *Pseudomonas* exotoxin. Proc Natl Acad Sci USA 1992; 89:5867–5871.
17. Weiner LM, O'Dwyer J, Kitson J, Comis RL, Frankel AE, Bauer RJ, Konrad MS, Groves ES. Phase I evaluation of an anti-breast carcinoma monoclonal antibody 260F9-recombinant ricin a chain immunoconjugate. Cancer Res 1989; 49:4062–4067.
18. Kopreski MS, Lipton A, Harvey HA, Kumar R. Growth inhibition of breast cancer cell lines by combinations of anti-P185HER2 monoclonal antibody and cytokines. Anticancer Res 1996; 16:433–436.
19. Aboud-Pirak E, Hurwitz E, Bellot F, Schlessinger J, Sela M. Inhibition of human tumor growth in nude mice by a conjugate of doxorubicin with monoclonal antibodies to epidermal growth factor receptor. Proc Natl Acad Sci USA 1989; 86:3778–3781.
20. Ennis BW, Valverius EM, Bates SE, Lippman ME, Bellot F, Kris R, Schlessinger J, Masui H, Goldenberg A, Mendelsohn J, et al. Anti-epidermal growth factor receptor antibodies inhibit the autocrine-stimulated growth of MDA-468 human breast cancer cells. Mol Endocrinol 1989; 3:1830–1838.
21. Fan Z, Baselga J, Masui H, Mendelsohn J. Antitumor effect of anti-epidermal growth factor receptor monoclonal antibodies plus cis-diamminedichloroplatinum on well established A431 cell xenografts. Cancer Res 1993; 53:4637–4642.
22. Baselga J, Norton L, Masui H, Pandiella A, Coplan K, Miller WH Jr, Mendelsohn J. Antitumor effects of doxorubicin in combination with anti-epidermal growth factor receptor monoclonal antibodies. J Natl Cancer Inst 1993; 85:1327–1333.
23. Sarup JC, Johnson RM, King KL, Fendly BM, Lipari MT, Napier MA, Ullrich A, Shepard HM. Characterization of an anti-p185her2 monoclonal antibody that stimulates receptor function and inhibits tumor cell growth. Growth Regul 1991; 1:72–82.

24. Bacus SS, Stancovski I, Huberman E, Chin D, Hurwitz E, Mills GB, Ullrich A, Sela M, Yarden Y. Tumor-inhibitory monoclonal antibodies to the HER-2/Neu receptor induce differentiation of human breast cancer cells. Cancer Res 1992; 52: 2580–2589.
25. Deshane J, Grim J, Loechel S, Siegal GP, Alvarez RD, Curiel DT: Intracellular antibody against *erb*B-2 mediates targeted tumor cell eradication by apoptosis. Cancer Gene Ther 1996; 3:89–98.
26. Pegram MD, Finn RS, Arzoo K, Beryt M, Pietras RJ, Slamon DJ. The effect of her-2/neu overexpression on chemotherapeutic drug sensitivity in human breast and ovarian cancer cells. Oncogene 1997; 15:537–472.
27. Baselga J, Tripathy D, Mendelsohn J, Baughman S, Benz CC, Dantis L, Sklarin NT, Seidman AD, Hudis CA, Moore J, Rosen PP, Twaddell T, Henderson IC, Norton L. Phase II study of weekly intravenous recombinant humanized anti-p185HER2 monoclonal antibody in patients with HER2/neu-overexpressing metastatic breast cancer. J Clin Oncol 1996; 14:737–744.
28. Richardson JH, Marasco WA. Intracellular antibodies: development and therapeutic potential. Trends Biotechnol 1995; 13:306–310.
29. Deshane J, Siegal GP, Alvarez RD, Wang MH, Feng M, Cabrera G, Liu T, Kay M, Curiel DT. Targeted tumor killing via an intracellular antibody against *erb*B-2. J Clin Invest 1995; 96:2980–2989.
30. Gimmi CD, Morrison BW, Mainprice BA, Gribben JG, Boussiotis VA, Freeman GJ, Park SY, Watanabe M, Gong J, Hayes DF, Kufe DW, Nadler LM. Breast cancer-associated antigen, DF3/MUC1, induces apoptosis of activated human T cells. Nat Med 1996; 2:1367–1370.
31. Cabrera T, Angustias Fernandez M, Sierra A, Garrido A, Herruzo A, Escobedo A, Fabra A, Garrido F. High frequency of altered HLA Class I phenotypes in invasive breast carcinomas. Hum Immunol 1996; 50:127–134.
32. Boussiotis VA, Freeman GJ, Gray G, Gribben J, Nadler LM. B7 but not intercellular adhesion molecule-1 costimulation prevents the induction of human alloantigen-specific tolerance. J Exp Med 1993; 178:1753–1763.
33. Ochoa AC, Longo DL. Alteration of signal transduction in T cells from cancer patients. Important Adv Oncol 1995; 43–54.
34. Kehrl JH, Taylor A, Kim SJ, Fauci AS. Transforming growth factor-beta is a potent negative regulator of human lymphocytes. Ann N Y Acad Sci 1991; 628:345–353.
35. Rosen HR, Ausch C, Reiner G, Reinerova M, Svec J, Tuchler H, Schiessel R, Moroz C. Immunosuppression by breast cancer associated p43-effect of immunomodulators. Breast Cancer Res Treat 1996; 41:171–176.
36. van de Wiel-van Kemenade E, Ligtenberg MJ, de Boer AJ, Buijs F, Vos HL, Melief CJ, Hilkens J, Figdor CG. Episialin (MUC1) inhibits cytotoxic lymphocyte-target cell interaction. J Immunol 1993; 151:767–776.
37. Hayes DF, Silberstein DS, Rodrique SW, Kufe DW. DF3 antigen, a human epithelial cell mucin, inhibits adhesion of eosinophils to antibody-coated targets. J Immunol 1990; 145:962–970.
38. Reddish MA, MacLean GD, Poppema S, Berg A, Longenecker BM. Pre-immunotherapy serum CA27.29 (MUC-1) mucin level and CD69+ lymphocytes

correlate with effects of theratope sialyl-Tn-KLH cancer vaccine in active specific immunotherapy. Cancer Immunol Immunother 1996; 42:303–309.
39. Ting CC, Tsai SC, Rogers MJ. Host control of tumor growth. Science 1977; 197: 571–573.
40. Rosenberg SA, Lotze MT, Muul LM, Chang AE, Avis FP, Leitman S, Linehan WM, Robertson CN, Lee RE, Rubin JT, et al. A progress report on the treatment of 157 patients with advanced cancer using lymphokine-activated killer cells and interleukin-2 or high-dose interleukin-2 alone. N Engl J Med 1987; 316:889–897.
41. Disis ML, Smith JW, Murphy AE, Chen W, Cheever MA. In vitro generation of human cytolytic T-cells specific for peptides derived from the HER-2/neu proto-oncogene protein. Cancer Res 1994; 54:1071–1076.
42. Fanger MW, Morganelli PM, Guyre PM. Bispecific antibodies. Crit Rev Immunol 1992; 12:101–124.
43. Weiner LM, Holmes M, Richeson A, Godwin A, Adams GP, Hsieh-Ma ST, Ring DB, Alpaugh RK. Binding and cytotoxicity characteristics of the bispecific murine monoclonal antibody 2B1. J Immunol 1993; 151:2877–2886.
44. Mezzanzanica D, Garrido MA, Neblock DS, Daddona PE, Andrew SM, Zurawski VR Jr, Segal DM, Wunderlich JR. Human T-lymphocytes targeted against an established human ovarian carcinoma with a bispecific F(ab′)2 antibody prolong host survival in a murine xenograft model. Cancer Res 1991; 51:5716–5721.
45. Watanabe M, Wallace P, Graziano R, Deo Y, Kufe DW, Hayes DF. Antibody dependent cellular phagocytosis (ADCP) against HER-2/*neu* positive human breast cancer cells mediated by bispecific monoclonal antibody (BsAb) MDX-210 (abstr). Breast Cancer Res Treat 1996; 41:247.
46. Jain RK. Barriers to drug delivery in solid tumors. Sci Am 1994; 271:58–65.
47. Sung C, Youle RJ, Dedrick RI. Pharmacokinetic analysis of immunotoxin uptake in solid tumors: role of plasma kinetics, capillary permeability, and binding. Cancer Res 1990; 50:7382–7392.
48. Raag R, Whitlow M: Single-chain Fvs. FASEB J 1995; 9:73–80.
49. Kirpotin D, Park JW, Hong K, Zalipsky S, Li WL, Carter P, Benz CC, Papahadjopoulos D. Sterically stabilized anti-HER2 immunoliposomes: design and targeting to human breast cancer cells in vitro. Biochemistry 1997; 36:66–75.
50. Park JW, Colbern GT, Hong K, Kirpotin D, Shao Y, Baselga J, Papahadjopoulos D, Benz CC. Targeted intracellular drug delivery via anti-HER2 immunoliposomes yields superior antitumor efficacy (abstr). Proc Am Soc Clin Oncol 1997; 16:430a.
51. Perlaky L, Busch RK, Busch H. Combinatorial effects of monoclonal anti-p120 antibody (Mabp120), liposomes and hyperthermia on MCF-7 and LOX tumor cell lines. Oncol Res 1996; 8:363–369.
52. King CR, Swain SM, Porter L, Steinberg SM, Lippman ME, Gelmann EP. Heterogeneous expression of *erb*B-2 messenger rna in human breast cancer. Cancer Res 1989; 49:4185–4191.
53. Murray JL, Macey DJ, Grant EJ, Rosenblum MG, Kasi LP, Zhang HZ, Katz RL, Riger PT, Le Bherz D, Bhadkamkar V, et al. Enhanced TAG-72 expression and tumor uptake of radiolabeled monoclonal antibody CC49 in metastatic breast cancer patients following alpha-interferon treatment. Cancer Res 1995; 55:5925s–5928s.

54. Maraveyas A, Epenetos AA. An overview of radioimmunotherapy. Cancer Immunol Immunother 1991; 34:71–73.
55. Wahl RL. Experimental radioimmunotherapy: a brief overview. Cancer 1994; 73: 989–992.
56. Boyer CM, Borowitz MJ, McCarty KS Jr, Kinney RB, Everitt L, Dawson DV, Ring D, Bast RC Jr. Heterogeneity of antigen expression in benign and malignant breast and ovarian epithelial cells. Int J Cancer 1989; 43:55–60.
57. Crews JR, Maier LA, Yu YH, Hester S, O'Briant K, Leslie DS, De Sombre K, George SL, Boyer CM, Argon Y, et al. A combination of two immunotoxins exerts synergistic cytotoxic activity against human breast-cancer cell lines. Int J Cancer 1992; 51:772–779.
58. Gould BJ, Borowitz MJ, Groves ES, Carter PW, Anthony D, Weiner LM, Frankel AE. Phase I study of an anti-breast cancer immunotoxin by continuous infusion: report of a targeted toxic effect not predicted by animal studies. J Natl Cancer Inst 1989; 81:775–781.
59. Dickson RB, Lippman ME. Growth factors in breast cancer. Endocr Rev 1995; 16: 559–589.
60. Schlessinger J. Regulation of cell growth and transformation by the epidermal growth factor receptor. Adv Exp Med Biol 1988; 234:65–73.
61. Bargmann CI, Hung MC, Weinberg RA. The neu oncogene encodes an epidermal growth factor receptor-related protein. Nature 1986; 319:226–230.
62. Prigent SA, Lemoine NR, Hughes CM, Plowman GD, Selden C, Gullick WJ. Expression of the c-*erb*B-3 protein in normal human adult and fetal tissues. Oncogene 1992; 7:1273–1278.
63. Plowman GD, Culouscou JM, Whitney GS, Green JM, Carlton GW, Foy L, Neubauer MG, Shoyab M. Ligand-specific activation of HER4/p180*erb*B4, a fourth member of the epidermal growth factor receptor family. Proc Natl Acad Sci USA 1993; 90:1746–1750.
64. Di Fiore PP, Pierce JH, Fleming TP, Hazan R, Ullrich A, King CR, Schlessinger J, Aaronson SA. Overexpression of the human EGF receptor confers an EGF-dependent transformed phenotype to NIH 3T3 cells. Cell 1987; 51:1063–1070.
65. Wong ST, Winchell LF, McCune BK, Earp HS, Teixido J, Massague J, Herman B, Lee DC. The tgf-alpha precursor expressed on the cell surface binds to the egf receptor on adjacent cells, leading to signal transduction. Cell 1989; 56:495–506.
66. Shoyab M, Plowman GD, McDonald VL, Bradley JG, Todaro GJ. Structure and function of human amphiregulin: a member of the epidermal growth factor family. Science 1989; 243:1074–1076.
67. Plowman GD, Green JM, Culouscou JM, Carlton GW, Rothwell VM, Buckley S. Heregulin induces tyrosine phosphorylation of HER4/p180*erb*B4. Nature 1993; 366:473–475.
68. Real FX, Rettig WJ, Chesa PG, Melamed MR, Old LJ, Mendelsohn J. Expression of epidermal growth factor receptor in human cultured cells and tissues: relationship to cell lineage and stage of differentiation. Cancer Res 1986; 46:4726–4731.
69. Velu TJ, Beguinot L, Vass WC, Willingham MC, Merlino GT, Pastan I, Lowy DR. Epidermal-growth-factor-dependent transformation by a human EGF receptor proto-oncogene. Science 1987; 238:1408–1410.

70. Klijn JG, Berns PM, Schmitz PI, Foekens JA. The clinical significance of epidermal growth factor receptor (EGF-R) in human breast cancer: a review on 5232 patients. Endocr Rev 1992; 13:3–17.
71. Klijn JG, Look MP, Portengen H, Alexieva-Figusch J, van Putten WL, Foekens JA. The prognostic value of epidermal growth factor receptor (EGF-R) in primary breast cancer: results of a 10-year follow-up study. Breast Cancer Res Treat 1994; 29:73–83.
72. Toi M, Tominaga T, Osaki A, Toge T. Role of epidermal growth factor receptor expression in primary breast cancer: results of a biochemical study and an immunocytochemical study. Breast Cancer Res Treat 1994; 29:51–58.
73. Mendelsohn J. Epidermal growth factor receptor as a target for therapy with antireceptor monoclonal antibodies. Monogr Natl Cancer Inst 1992; 13:125–131.
74. Kawamoto T, Sato JD, Le A, Polikoff J, Sato GH, Mendelsohn J. Growth stimulation of A431 cells by epidermal growth factor: identification of high-affinity receptors for epidermal growth factor by an anti-receptor monoclonal antibody. Proc Natl Acad Sci USA 1983; 80:1337–1341.
75. Sato JD, Kawamoto T, Le AD, Mendelsohn J, Polikoff J, Sato GH. Biological effects in vitro of monoclonal antibodies to human epidermal growth factor receptors. Mol Biol Med 1983; 1:511–529.
76. Rodeck U, Williams N, Murthy U, Herlyn M. Monoclonal antibody 425 inhibits growth stimulation of carcinoma cells by exogenous egf and tumor-derived egf/tgf-alpha. J Cell Biochem 1990; 44:69–79.
77. Aboud-Pirak E, Hurwitz E, Pirak ME, Bellot F, Schlessinger J, Sela M. Efficacy of antibodies to epidermal growth factor receptor against KB carcinoma in vitro and in nude mice. J Natl Cancer Inst 1988; 80:1605–1611.
78. Bos M, Mendelsohn J, Bowden C, Pfister D, Cooper MR, Cohen R, Burtness B, D'Andrea G, Waksal H, Norton L, Baselga J. Phase I studies of anti-epidermal growth factor receptor (EGFR) chimeric monoclonal antibody C225 in patients with EGFR overexpressing tumors (abstr). Proc Am Soc Clin Oncol 1996; 15:443.
79. Curnow RT, Keeperman KL, Malone T. A Phase I trial of bispecific antibody (BsAb) MDX447 without and with granulocyte colony-stimulating factor (G-CSF) in patients with adult solid tumors (abstr). Proc Am Soc Clin Oncol 1997; 16:438a.
80. King CR, Kraus MH, Aaronson SA. Amplification of a novel v-*erb*B-related gene in a human mammary carcinoma. Science 1985; 229:974–976.
81. Akiyama T, Tong T, Ogawara H, Toyoshima K, Yamamoto T. The product of the human c-*erb*B-2 gene: a 185-kilodalton glycoprotein with tyrosine kinase activity. Science 1986; 232:1644–1646.
82. Kruh GD, King CR, Kraus MH, Popescu NC, Amsbaugh SC, McBride WO, Aaronson SA. A novel human gene closely related to the *abl* proto-oncogene. Science 1986; 234:1545–1548.
83. Allred DC, Clark GM, Molina R, Tandon AK, Schnitt SJ, Gilchrist KW, Osborne CK, Tormey DC, McGuire WL. Overexpression of HER-2/neu and its relationship with other prognostic factors change during the progression of in situ to invasive breast cancer. Hum Pathol 1992; 23:974–979.
84. Paik S, Hazan R, Fisher ER, Sass RE, Fisher B, Redmond C, Schlessinger J, Lippman ME, King CR. Pathologic findings from the National Surgical Adjuvant Breast

and Bowel Project: prognostic significance of *erb*B-2 protein overexpression in primary breast cancer. J Clin Oncol 1990; 8:103–112.
85. Slamon DJ, Clark GM, Wong SG, Levin WJ, Ullrich A, McGuire WL. Human breast cancer: correlation of relapse and survival with amplification of the HER-2/neu oncogene. Science 1987; 235:177–182.
86. King CR, Kraus MH, Di Fiore PP, Paik S, Kasprzyk PG. Implications of *erb*B-2 overexpression for basic science and clinical medicine. Semin Cancer Biol 1990; 1:329–337.
87. Harwerth IM, Wels W, Schlegel J, Muller M, Hynes NE. Monoclonal antibodies directed to the *erb*B-2 receptor inhibit in vivo tumour cell growth. Br J Cancer 1993; 68:1140–1145.
88. Hancock MC, Langton BC, Chan T, Toy P, Monahan JJ, Mischak RP, Shawver LK. A monoclonal antibody against the c-*erb*B-2 protein enhances the cytotoxicity of *cis*-diamminedichloroplatinum against human breast and ovarian tumor cell lines. Cancer Res 1991; 51:4575–4580.
89. Baselga J, Seidman AD, Rosen PP, Norton L. Her2 overexpression and paclitaxel sensitivity in breast cancer: therapeutic implications. Oncology (Huntingt) 1997; 11:43–48.
90. Harris LN, Trock B, Berris M, Esteva-Lorenzo F, Paik S. The role of *erb*B-2 extracellular domain in predicting response to chemotherapy in breast cancer patients (abstr). Proc Am Soc Clin Oncol 1996; 15:108.
91. Yamauchi H, O'Neill A, Gelman R, Carney W, Tenney DY, Hosch S, Hayes DF. Prediction of response to antiestrogen therapy in advanced breast cancer patients by pretreatment circulating levels of extracellular domain of the her-2/c-neu protein. J Clin Oncol 1997; 15:2518–2525.
92. Gusterson BA, Gelber RD, Goldhirsch A, Price KN, Save-Sod*erb*orgh J, Anbazhagan R, Styles J, Rudenstam CM, Golouh R, Reed R, et al. Prognostic importance of c-*erb*B-2 expression in breast cancer. International (Ludwig) breast cancer study group. J Clin Oncol 1992; 10:1049–1056.
93. Tang RP, Kacinski B, Validire P, Beuvon F, Sastre X, Benoit P, dela Rochefordiere A, Mosseri V, Pouillart P, Scholl S. Oncogene amplification correlates with dense lymphocyte infiltration in human breast cancers: a role for hematopoietic growth factor release by tumor cells? J Cell Biochem 1990; 44:189–198.
94. Disis ML, Calenoff E, McLaughlin G, Murphy AE, Chen W, Groner B, Jeschke M, Lydon N, McGlynn E, Livingston RB, et al. Existent T-cell and antibody immunity to HER-2/neu protein in patients with breast cancer. Cancer Res 1994; 54: 16–20.
95. Shalaby MR, Carter P, Maneval D, Giltinan D, Kotts C. Bispecific HER2 $\times$ CD3 antibodies enhance T-cell cytotoxicity in vitro and localize to HER2-overexpressing xenografts in nude mice. Clin Immunol Immunopathol 1995; 74:185–192.
96. Weiner LM, Holmes M, Adams GP, La Creta F, Watts P, Garcia de Palazzo I. A human tumor xenograft model of therapy with a bispecific monoclonal antibody targeting c-*erb*B-2 and CD16. Cancer Res 1993; 53:94–100.
97. Weiner LM, Alpaugh RK, Amoroso AR, Adams GP, Ring DB, Barth MW. Human neutrophil interactions of a bispecific monoclonal antibody targeting tumor and human Fc gamma RIII. Cancer Immunol Immunother 1996; 42:141–150.

98. Valone FH, Kaufman PA, Guyre PM, Lewis LD, Memoli V, Ernstoff MS, Wells W, Barth R, Deo Y, Fisher J, et al. Clinical trials of bispecific antibody MDX-210 in women with advanced breast or ovarian cancer that overexpresses HER-2/neu. J Hematother 1995; 4:471–475.
99. Valone FH, Kaufman PA, Guyre PM, Lewis LD, Memoli V, Deo Y, Graziano R, Fisher JL, Meyer L, Mrozek-Orlowski M, et al. Phase IA/IB trial of bispecific antibody MDX-210 in patients with advanced breast or ovarian cancer that overexpresses the proto-oncogene HER-2/neu. J Clin Oncol 1995; 13:2281–2292.
100. Guadagni F, Roselli M, Nieroda C, Dansky-Ullmann G, Schlom J, Greiner JW. Biological response modifiers as adjuvants in monoclonal antibody-based treatment (review). In Vivo 1993; 7:591–599.
101. King CR, Fischer PH, Rando RF, Pastan I. The performance of e23(Fv)PE, recombinant toxins targeting the erbB-2 protein. Sem Cancer Biol 1996; 7:79–86.
102. Chen SY, Yang AG, Chen JD, Kute T, King CR, Collier J, Cong Y, Yao C, Huang XF. Potent antitumor activity of a new class of tumor-specific killer cells. Nature 1997; 385:78–80.
103. Deshane J, Loechel F, Conry RM, Siegal GP, King CR, Curiel DT. Intracellular single-chain antibody directed against erbB2 down-regulates cell surface erbB2 and exhibits a selective anti-proliferative effect in erbB2 overexpressing cancer cell lines. Gene Ther 1994; 1:332–337.
104. Gold P, Freedman SO. Demonstration of tumor-specific antigens in human colonic carcinomata by immunological tolerance and absorption techniques (abstr). J Exp Med 1965; 121:439–462.
105. Fletcher RH. Carcinoembryonic antigen. Ann Intern Med 1986; 104:66–73.
106. Robbins PF, Eggensperger D, Qi CF, Schlom J. Definition of the expression of the human carcinoembryonic antigen and non-specific cross-reacting antigen in human breast and lung carcinomas. Int J Cancer 1993; 53:892–897.
107. Hayes DF, Zurawski VR Jr, Kufe DW. Comparison of circulating CA15-3 and carcinoembryonic antigen levels in patients with breast cancer. J Clin Oncol 1986; 4:1542–1550.
108. Schlom J, Weeks MO. Potential clinical utility of monoclonal antibodies in the management of human carcinomas. Important Adv Oncol 1985; 170–192.
109. Schlom J, Kantor J, Abrams S, Tsang KY, Panicali D, Hamilton JM. Strategies for the development of recombinant vaccines for the immunotherapy of breast cancer. Breast Cancer Res Treat 1996; 38:27–39.
110. Wong JY, Williams LE, Yamauchi DM, Odom-Maryon T, Esteban JM, Neumaier M, Wu AM, Johnson DK, Primus FJ, Shively JE, et al. Initial experience evaluating 90ytitrium-radiolabeled anti-carcinoembryonic antigen chimeric T84.66 in a Phase I radioimmunotherapy trial. Cancer Res 1995; 55:5929s–5934s.
111. Guadagni F, Roselli M, Ferroni P, Amato T, Colcher D, Greiner JW, Schlom J. Clinical evaluation of the new tumor marker TAG-72. Anticancer Res 1991; 11:1389–1394.
112. Roselli M, Hitchcock CL, Molinolo A, Milenic DE, Colcher D, Martin EW Jr, Hinkle GH, Schlom J. Autoradiographic evaluation of radiolabeled monoclonal antibody B72.3 distribution in tumor and lymph nodes of adenocarcinoma patients. Anticancer Res 1995; 15:975–984.

113. Kashmiri SV, Shu L, Padlan EA, Milenic DE, Schlom J, Hand PH. Generation, characterization, and in vivo studies of humanized anticarcinoma antibody CC49. Hybridoma 1995; 14:461–473.
114. Leoni F, Colnaghi MI, Canevari S, Menard S, Colzani E, Facheris P, Figini M, Miotti S, Magnani JL. Glycolipids carrying Le(y) are preferentially expressed on small-cell lung cancer cells as detected by the monoclonal antibody MLUC1. Int J Cancer 1992; 51:225–231.
115. Pai LH, Batra JK, Fitz Gerald DJ, Willingham MC, Pastan I. Antitumor effects of B3-PE and B3-LysPE40 in a nude mouse model of human breast cancer and the evaluation of B3-PE toxicity in monkeys. Cancer Res 1992; 52:3189–3193.
116. Pai LH, Wittes RE, Setser A, Willingham MC, Pastan I. Phase I study of the immunotoxin LMB-1, an anti-cancer murine MAb B3, coupled to a recombinant form of *Pseudomonas* Exotoxin, PE38 (abstr). Proc Am Soc Clin Oncol 1996; 15:481.
117. Sheriff S, Chang CY, Jeffrey PD, Bajorath J. X-ray structure of the uncomplexed anti-tumor antibody BR96 and comparison with its antigen-bound form. J Mol Biol 1996; 259:938–946.
118. Trail PA, Willner D, Lasch SJ, Henderson AJ, Hofstead S, Casazza AM, Firestone RA, Hellstrom I, Hellstrom KE. Cure of xenografted human carcinomas by BR96-doxorubicin immunoconjugates. Science 1993; 261:212–215.
119. Giantonio BJ, Gilewski TA, Bookman MA, Norton L, Kilpatrick D, Dougan MA, Slichenmyer WJ, Onetto NM, Canetta RM. A Phase I study of weekly BR96-doxorubicin (BR-96-DOX) in patients with advanced carcinoma expressing the Lewis^y (Le^y) antigen (abstr). Proc Am Soc Clin Oncol 1996; 15:443.
120. Friedman PN, McAndrew SJ, Gawlak SL, Chace D, Trail PA, Brown JP, Siegall CB. Br96 sFv-PE40, a potent single-chain immunotoxin that selectively kills carcinoma cells. Cancer Res 1993; 53:334–339.
121. Siegall CB, Chace D, Mixan B, Garrigues U, Wan H, Paul L, Wolff E, Hellstrom I, Hellstrom KE. In vitro and in vivo characterization of BR96 sFv-PE40. A single-chain immunotoxin fusion protein that cures human breast carcinoma xenografts in athymic mice and rats. J Immunol 1994; 152:2377–2384.
122. Hilkens J. CA 15-3 assay for the detection of episialin, a serum marker for breast cancer. In: S Sell, ed. Serological Cancer Markers. City: Totowa, NJ: Humana Press, 1992: 261–280.
123. Hayes DF, Mesa-Tejada R, Papsidero LD, Croghan GA, Korzun AH, Norton L, Wood W, Strauchen JA, Grimes M, Weiss RB, et al. Prediction of prognosis in primary breast cancer by detection of a high molecular weight mucin-like antigen using monoclonal antibodies DF3, F36/22, and CU18: a Cancer and Leukemia Group B study. J Clin Oncol 1991; 9:1113–1123.
124. Lloyd KO, Burchell J, Kudryashov V, Yin BWT, Taylor-Papadimitriou J. Comparison of *O*-linked carbohydrate chains in MUC-1 mucin from normal breast epithelial cell lines and breast carcinoma cell lines. Demonstration of simpler and fewer glycan chains in tumor cells. J Biol Chem 1996; 271:33,325–33,334.
125. Hull SR, Bright A, Carraway KL, Abe M, Hayes DF, Kufe DW. Oligosaccharide differences in the DF3 sialomucin antigen from normal human milk and the BT-20 human breast carcinoma cell line. Cancer Commun 1989; 1:261–267.
126. Taylor-Papadimitriou J, Burchell J, Moss F, Beverley P. Monoclonal antibodies to

epithelial membrane antigen and human milk fat globule mucin define epitopes expressed on other molecules. Lancet 1985; 1:458.
127. Kufe D, Inghirami G, Abe M, Hayes D, Justi-Wheeler H, Schlom J. Differential reactivity of a novel monoclonal antibody (DF3) with human malignant versus benign breast tumors. Hybridoma 1984; 3:223–232.
128. Girling A, Bartkova J, Burchell J, Gendler S, Gillett C, Taylor-Papadimitriou J. A core protein epitope of the polymorphic epithelial mucin detected by the monoclonal antibody SM-3 is selectively exposed in a range of primary carcinomas. Int J Cancer 1989; 43:1072–1076.
129. Perey L, Hayes DF, Maimonis P, Abe M, O'Hara C, Kufe DW. Tumor selective reactivity of a monoclonal antibody prepared against a recombinant peptide derived from the DF3 human breast carcinoma-associated antigen. Cancer Res 1992; 52:2563–2568.
130. Finn OJ, Jerome KR, Henderson RA, Pecher G, Domenech N, Magarian-Blander J, Barratt-Boyes SM. Muc-1 epithelial tumor mucin-based immunity and cancer vaccines. Immunol Rev 1995; 145:61–89.
131. Taylor-Papadimitriou J, Stewart L, Burchell J, Beverley P. The polymorphic epithelial mucin as a target for immunotherapy. Ann N Y Acad Sci 1993; 690:69–79.
132. Jerome KR, Barnd DL, Bendt KM, Boyer CM, Taylor-Papadimitriou J, McKenzie IF, Bast RC Jr, Finn OJ. Cytotoxic T-lymphocytes derived from patients with breast adenocarcinoma recognize an epitope present on the protein core of a mucin molecule preferentially expressed by malignant cells. Cancer Res 1991; 51:2908–2916.
133. Henderson RA, Nimgaonkar MT, Watkins SC, Robbins PD, Ball ED, Finn OJ. Human dendritic cells genetically engineered to express high levels of the human epithelial tumor antigen mucin (MUC-1). Cancer Res 1996; 56:3763–3770.
134. Goydos JS, Elder E, Whiteside TL, Finn OJ, Lotze MT. A Phase I trial of a synthetic mucin peptide vaccine. Induction of specific immune reactivity in patients with adenocarcinoma. J Surg Res 1996; 63:298–304.
135. Longenecker BM, Rahman AF, Leigh JB, Purser RA, Greenberg AH, Willans DJ, Keller O, Petrik PK, Thay TY, Suresh MR, et al. Monoclonal antibody against a cryptic carbohydrate antigen of murine and human lymphocytes. I. Antigen expression in non-cryptic or unsubstituted form on certain murine lymphomas, on a spontaneous murine mammary carcinoma, and on several human adenocarcinomas. Int J Cancer 1984; 33:123–129.
136. Miles DW, Towlson KE, Graham R, Reddish M, Longenecker BM, Taylor-Papadimitriou J, Rubens RD: A randomized Phase II study of sialyl-Tn and DETOX-B adjuvant with or without cyclophosphamide pretreatment for the active specific immunotherapy of breast cancer. Br J Cancer 1996; 74:1292–1296.
137. MacLean GD, Miles DW, Rubens RD, Reddish MA, Longenecker BM. Enhancing the effect of theratope sTn-KLH cancer vaccine in patients with metastatic breast cancer by pretreatment with low-dose intravenous cyclophosphamide. J Immunother Emphasis Tumor Immunol 1996; 19:309–316.
138. Fell HP, Gayle MA, Yelton D, Lipsich L, Schieven GL, Marken JS, Aruffo A, Hellstrom KE, Hellstrom I, Bajorath J. Chimeric L6 anti-tumor antibody. Genomic construction, expression, and characterization of the antigen binding site. J Biol Chem 1992; 267:15,552–15,558.

139. Goodman GE, Hellstrom I, Brodzinsky L, Nicaise C, Kulander B, Hummel D, Hellstrom KE. Phase I trial of murine monoclonal antibody L6 in breast, colon, ovarian, and lung cancer. J Clin Oncol 1990; 8:1083–1092.
140. Goodman GE, Hellstrom I, Yelton DE, Murray JL, O'Hara S, Meaker E, Zeigler L, Palazollo P, Nicaise C, Usakewicz J, et al. Phase I trial of chimeric (human-mouse) monoclonal antibody L6 in patients with non-small-cell lung, colon, and breast cancer. Cancer Immunol Immunother 1993; 36:267–273.
141. De Nardo SJ, Mirick GR, Kroger LA, O'Grady LF, Erickson KL, Yuan A, Lamborn KR, Hellstrom I, Hellstrom KE, De Nardo GL. The biologic window for chimeric L6 radioimmunotherapy. Cancer 1994; 73:1023–1032.
142. Richman CM, De Nardo SJ, O'Grady LF, De Nardo GL. Radioimmunotherapy for breast cancer using escalating fractionated doses of ^{131}I-labeled chimeric L6 antibody with peripheral blood progenitor cell transfusions. Cancer Res 1995; 55: 5916s–5920s.

14
Monoclonal Antibody-Based Therapy of Melanoma

Marcus O. Butler
Harvard Medical School and Dana-Farber/Partners CancerCare, Boston, Massachusetts

Frank G. Haluska
Harvard Medical School, Massachusetts General Hospital, and Dana-Farber/Partners CancerCare, Boston, Massachusetts

I. INTRODUCTION

The incidence of malignant melanoma in the United States is rising faster than that of any other cancer. It appears that the number of new cases is doubling each decade (1). In 1997, an estimated 40,300 new cases of melanoma were diagnosed, and though many patients will be cured by surgical excision, 7,300 deaths are expected, due mainly to metastatic disease (2). Unfortunately, therapeutic options for metastatic melanoma are limited. Melanoma is a relatively chemotherapy-resistant disease. Dacarbazine, the most active agent, induces response rates in 19–25% of patients. Combination chemotherapy regimens have been developed, some with moderately high response rates. However, in randomized multicenter trials, results are much more modest, with response rates similar to those obtained with dacarbazine alone (3).

II. MELANOMA AND TUMOR IMMUNITY

Though the prognosis for patients with metastatic melanoma is generally poor, occasional patients will exhibit clinical and histologic evidence of spontaneous tumor regression. Many investigators postulate that host immunity may be responsible for this phenomenon (4,5). In support of this, an autoimmune response directed against shared melanocyte and melanoma antigens has been suggested to explain the better course of melanoma patients who develop vitiligo (6). Furthermore, both cellular and humoral immune responses against malignant melanoma have been observed. In melanoma, the presence of tumor-infiltrating lymphocytes (TILs) has been associated with a favorable prognosis. Many of these cells, which are predominantly CD3+ T-lymphocytes, appear to bind autologous melanoma cells and acquire cytotoxic T-cell activity after incubation with interleukin-2 (IL-2) (7). A role for cellular immunity in the treatment of melanoma has been supported by the tumor regressions seen in 10–20% of patients given high-dose IL-2 or IL-2 plus lymphokine-activated killer cells (8–10). Furthermore, adoptive transfer of TILs along with IL-2 therapy has been shown to induce tumor responses (11,12). T-cells present in tumor or obtained from peripheral blood appear to recognize specific antigens on melanoma cells and may be cytotoxic in the context of class I MHC restriction (13). With respect to a humoral response, patients with melanoma have been shown to produce antibodies against melanoma antigens, though a correlation with survival is not clear (14,15). Additionally, patients can be induced to produce antibodies after immunization with melanoma cells or purified antigen (16,17).

Recent work has shown that melanoma-specific T-cells recognize three general categories of melanoma antigens, which include the melanocyte lineage proteins (tryosinase, gp100, MART-1/Melan-A, TRP1, and TRP2); the MAGE gene family, which are expressed developmentally in a variety of nonmelanocyte tissues; and tumor-mutated antigens (β-catenin, MUM-1, and CDK4) (18). Like T-cell immunity, some antibodies produced by melanoma patients appear to bind to unique antigens that are found only on autologous and not allogeneic tumor (19). Presumably, these antibodies recognize mutated antigens that are unique to the cancer and not shared with other tumors or normal cells. Patients also produce antibodies that recognize tumor antigens expressed on different tumors. Interestingly, the best-characterized antibodies recognize different antigens than those recognized by T-cells. These antigens are classified as differentiation antigens, which are expressed in normal cells and regulated during normal differentiation. In particular, host autoantibodies have been identified that recognize gangliosides, which are glycolipids found in tissues of neurectodermal origin (20).

Since host cellular and humoral tumor immunity are active in patients with melanoma, immunotherapeutic strategies directed against melanoma have been studied. As discussed, cytokine therapy (i.e., IL-2) appears to have activity in the treatment of melanoma. Also, efforts have focused on therapies aimed at directing host defenses against tumor antigens. Currently, several ongoing trials are investigating vaccines derived from the antigens recognized by T-cells, although the results are not yet available. However, efforts to use monoclonal antibodies directed against melanoma antigens began in the 1980s, and this experience has been instructive. In this review, we shall discuss trials that have utilized monoclonal antibody technology in the treatment of malignant melanoma.

III. MONOCLONAL ANTIBODIES AS THERAPY

Use of monoclonal antibody technology has provided a wealth of experience in attempting to direct host immune responses against tumor. Investigators have produced monoclonal antibodies to melanoma antigens by using the hybridoma technology originally reported by Kohler (21). Clinical trials are ongoing, and several strategies have been published. These include antibody alone, antibody in combination with cytokines, antibody linked to a toxin or radioactive isotope, and monoclonal idiotypic antibody used as a vaccine. In this review, we shall discuss examples of each of these strategies applied to patients with melanoma.

The search for melanoma antigens has identified molecular epitopes recognized by several monoclonal antibodies. These antibodies were usually produced by injecting human melanoma material into mice and producing mouse antihuman monoclonal antibodies, using hybridoma technology. None of these surface antigens are entirely melanoma specific. However, some of these antigens have characteristics of differentiation antigens that mark cells of neuroectodermal origin, including melanoma (22). Abnormally high expression of these antigens sometimes occurs, with transformation of the cell to a malignant state. Table 1 identifies these antigens and the corresponding monoclonal antibodies used in humans.

Use of monoclonal antibody alone can theoretically induce tumor regression via several mechanisms. Antibodies may bind tumor receptors and act to inhibit vital cellular functions or trigger the induction of apoptosis (23). Additionally, therapeutic action of monoclonal antibodies can occur through recruitment of cytotoxic components of the immune system (24,25). Single molecules of IgM and dimers of IgG can fix and activate complement. This complement-dependent

Table 1 Melanoma Antigens and the Monoclonal Antibodies Developed and Used in Clinical Studies

Melanoma antigen	Monoclonal antibody
GD2	14G2a, ME36.1, ch14.18, 3F8
GD3	R24, ME36.1, MG-22
GM2	L72, L55
Melanotransferrin (p97)	8.2, 96.5
HMW-MAA (p240 or mCSP)	9.2.27, 225.28S, 48.7, ZME-018, XOMAZYME-MEL
Idiotype antibodies generated with p240	IMe1-1, IMe1-2, MF11-30, MK2-23

Table 2 Melanoma Monoclonal Antibodies Administered to Patients with Additional Agents Systemically or Conjugated to Antibody

Monoclonal antibody	Second agent
R24	WR-2721/Cisplatin, GM-CSF, M-CSF, IL-2, TNF-α
ch14.18	GM-CSF, IL-2
14.G2a	IL-2
96.5	Interferon-α
XOMAZYME-MEL	Ricin-A (conjugated to antibody)
MG-22	IL-2

cytotoxicity (CDC) has been demonstrated in vitro by some of the monoclonal antibodies discussed in this review. Antibody-dependent cellular cytotoxicity (ADCC) also has been demonstrated to occur. Here, target cells are coated by antibody, which then is recognized by the Fc receptors of effector cells such as lymphocytes, monocytes, tissue macrophages, granulocytes, and eosinophils. In conducive situations, effector cells can then release cytolysins and induce cell killing.

Investigators also have attempted to enhance the antitumor activity of antimelanoma monoclonal antibodies. Monoclonal antibodies have been administered with cytokines, toxins, and radioisotopes (see Table 2). Some trials involved administration of drug systemically, with the intent that local antitumor effects might be enhanced by the specific binding of MAbs, while limiting unwanted toxicity. Other trials have utilized antibodies manipulated so that the coadministered drug or radioisotope is covalently bound to the MAb, resulting in improved delivery to specific tumor sites.

IV. OBSTACLES TO MONOCLONAL ANTIBODY-BASED THERAPY

Mechanisms of MAb efficacy may be hindered by: (a) heterogeneous expression of antigen among tumor cells; (b) downregulation of antigen expression; (c) poor tumor vascularity; (d) decreased vascular permeability of vessels feeding tumor; and (e) creation of a binding site barrier of antigen/antibody complexes, thereby preventing additional antibody binding (26,27). Additionally, the host immune response to foreign monoclonal protein can nullify any possible response. This human antimurine antibody (HAMA) response produces antibodies directed to foreign epitopes present on the infused monoclonal antibody. Some of these host antibodies can bind to the antigen-binding sites of the MAb. However, in nonhuman-derived monoclonal antibody administration, host responses to the constant domain (Fc) of whole antibodies can be equally significant. By administering the antigen-binding Fab fragment alone, researchers have attempted to decrease this immune response and to improve access of antibody to tumor by decreasing the antibody's size. Additional work to genetically engineer MAbs such that the non-antigen-binding portions are human sequences is ongoing. This potentially would limit the HAMA response, and allow effector cell cytotoxicity through the Fc portion to occur.

Of note, one of the monoclonal antibody strategies under investigation in melanoma tries to harness the HAMA response. In this example, antiidiotype antibodies, which are MAbs containing binding domains that have similar structure to tumor epitopes, are used as a vaccine. The aim is to produce a HAMA response that cross-reacts with melanoma antigens, breaking tolerance and conferring antitumor effects. Antiidiotype antibodies generated with the p240 melanoma antigen will be discussed further in this review.

V. TUMOR ANTIGENS RECOGNIZED BY MONOCLONAL ANTIBODIES

The known melanoma antigens recognized by the humoral immune system are predominantly differentiation antigens. Monoclonal antibodies produced by murine vaccination with human melanoma cells or extracts recognize ganglioside antigens, p97, and high-molecular-weight melanoma-associated antigens. Although these proteins are not unique to melanoma cells, expression on normal tissues is limited, and, importantly, the level of expression on tumor cells is upregulated. In this section, we will discuss the structure, function, and distribution of these melanoma antigens.

The ganglioside antigens, GD2, GD3, GM2, are glycolipid molecules composed of a sialylated oligosaccharide chain linked to a ceramide core. These cell-surface molecules appear to be involved in cell–cell and cell–substrate recognition (28,29). Each ganglioside differs slightly in its oligosaccharide chain and in the arrangement of one or more sialic acid residues. Melanoma cells express gangliosides at high levels, which makes them potential targets for monoclonal antibody therapy (30). GD3 is most highly expressed, followed by GD2 and GM2. Additionally, though these antigens are not restricted to melanoma, they are present in higher number on the surface of melanoma cells. Thus, although antibody therapy may preferentially impact the tumor, toxicity to normal tissues displaying antigen must be considered.

GD3 is one of the most widely expressed gangliosides, present on the surface of normal and malignant cells. Importantly, the concentration of GD3 molecules on tumor cells is five to ten times that of normal melanocytes (31). In the

1980s, Dippold et al. generated the IgG3 mouse monoclonal antibody, R24, which recognizes GD3's trisaccharide structure, NeuAcα2-8NeuAcα2-3Gal (32). This antibody reacts with melanocytes, astrocytes, melanomas, astrocytomas, and a subset of sarcomas (33). Also, R24 has been shown to detect GD3 on fetal thymocytes and a fraction of peripheral T-lymphocytes (34). R24 has been the most extensively studied melanoma MAb in clinical trials.

GD2 differs from GD3 by only a single sugar moiety (GalNAc) and, while upregulated on transformed melanocytes, is also present in normal brain and other neuroectoderm-derived tissues (30,35). Limited clinical use of MAbs against GD2 also will be discussed. Finally, monoclonal antibodies to GM2 have been administered to patients. Though the expression of GM2 in normal tissues may be more limited, it appears to be expressed on only a subset of tumor cells (36).

Melanotransferrin, or p97/gp95, is a 95,000–97,000-dalton phosphorylated sialoglycoprotein that is expressed on most normal adult tissues, including uterus, bladder, muscle, colon, and liver. Expression on melanoma cells, however, is much higher (10–1000-fold higher expression) (30,37–39). Monoclonal antibodies have been developed and employed in radiolocalization.

High-molecular-weight melanoma-associated antigen (HMW-MAA, or mCSP) is a proteoglycan of 240–280 kDa to which are added high-molecular-weight chondroitin sulfate glycosoaminoglycan side chains (30). This antigen is expressed on most melanomas and nevi. It also is seen on cultured melanocytes, though it has not been detected on normal epidermal melanocytes (40). The antigen is expressed on microspikes found on the surface of melanoma cells (41). Its location and the increased concentration on metastatic tumor suggest that it may be involved in the metastatic potential gained by melanoma. Consequently, it has been hypothesized that inhibition of HMW-MAA function may improve the clinical course of patients with melanoma by impeding metastatic spread.

VI. SOLE ADMINISTRATION OF UNCONJUGATED MONOCLONAL ANTIBODIES

R24 is a monoclonal antibody that recognizes the ganglioside GD3. Although this antigen is not truly tumor specific, it is tumor enriched in many melanoma tumors. In vitro studies have shown that R24 may have promising antimelanoma properties, since binding of GD3 by R24 can mediate antibody-dependent cellular cytotoxicity (ADCC), fix complement (CDC), inhibit cell growth, and induce morphologic changes of cells in culture (42,43). Dippold et al. initiated in vivo R24 administration in the early 1980s (44). Their experience showed that R24 antibody infusions in patients with melanoma and other neuroectodermal tumors induced few toxic side effects, despite the presence of GD3 on some normal cells. With doses of 1 mg to 200 mg, serial neurologic and opthalmic examinations failed to demonstrate toxicity. Patients receiving antibody usually complained of pain in bulky tumor masses 3 hours after infusion. Additionally, reactions around cutaneous melanoma nodules included bright inflammatory halos and/or blister formation. In several cases, different metastases in the same patient responded differently, some regressing and some progressing.

Houghton et al. expanded this work by treating a total of twenty-one melanoma patients in a Phase I trial (45). Like Dippold, they observed few toxic drug effects. At the lowest dose level of 8 mg/m^2, no clinical effects were noted. However, with doses greater than 10 mg/m^2, all patients developed urticaria and pruritus, frequently over cutaneous lesions. At higher doses, not only were cutaneous reactions more severe, but patients also had marked gastrointestinal symptoms, including nausea, vomiting, and diarrhea. Of note, these investigators observed four partial responses and two minor responses in the series of twenty-one patients. Interestingly, these responses occurred in patients receiving lower doses of drug. More importantly, this Phase I trial extended its observations through the microscopic analysis of biopsy specimens. R24 was detected in tumors as late as 30 days posttreatment. In twelve of the fourteen patients biopsied after R24 infusion, inflammatory changes included infiltration of CD3+/CD8+/Ia+ T-cells, mast cells with mast cell degranulation, and deposition of complement components C3, C5, and C9. Most patients were shown to develop human IgG antimouse antibodies after 8–40 days. Confirmatory studies were conducted by Raymond et al., who also demonstrated that rare (2/6) responses can occur. Patients experienced tumor pain, edema, erythema, and urticaria. In their study, the drug was administered by continuous infusion, and two patients suffered fluid overload. Chemical pancreatitis was seen in one patient (46).

Recently, Dippold et al. have extended their work with the R24 antibody (47). In a spectacular case of a patient with melanosis of the meninges, complete remission with no evidence of recurrence at 6 years was documented in one patient who received intrathecal injection of R24 monoclonal antibody. Another patient treated with intrathecal R24 had a brief clearing of melanoma from the CSF, but died a few weeks later from relapse. Additionally, fifteen more patients without CNS involvement were treated with intravenous R24. Urticarea, burning, and pruritis were noted, especially at higher doses. Again, drug activity tended to be seen in patients receiving a lower dose. Though only one of six patients experienced a mixed response at the higher dose, possible activity was seen in four of nine patients given the lower dose. In the low-dose group, two patients had partial responses, one had a minor response, and one had a mixed response. In contrast to Kirkwood et al., who reported that CD8- and CD4-positive tumor-infiltrating lymphocytes changed after R24 treatment (48), Dippold did not demonstrate changes in the peripheral lymphocytes of intravenously treated patients (e.g., NK cell activity or ADCC). Lymphocytes cultured from the complete responder to intrathecal R24, however, demonstrated high cytolytic activity against allogeneic melanoma cells in vitro.

Though the action of R24 on melanoma cells is probably mediated by the binding of antibody to GD3 displayed on the melanoma cell surface, Boussiotis et al. have suggested that R24 binding to T-cells may act as a costimulatory signal, preventing anergy and inducing T-cell proliferation (49). Therefore, R24 may not act solely by binding directly to melanoma cells, but may act by stimulating the host immune system to recognize melanoma antigen.

Several other monoclonal antibodies to gangliosides have been developed for melanoma treatment, though fewer trials with each agent have been completed. The murine monoclonal antibody ME-36.1 recognizes both GD2 and GD3, fixes human complement, mediates ADCC, and inhibits human melanoma growth and metastases in nude mice (50). One report notes no significant toxicity, presence of antibody in six of thirteen patient biopsies, and one 16-month complete response (51). In another study, Cheung et al. saw tumor responses using the Anti-GD2 antibody 3F8 to treat melanoma as well as neuroblastoma and osteogenic sarcoma. Again, mild toxicities included focal pain during infusion, urticaria, fever, diaphoresis, nausea, vomiting, and hypertension. Local inflammatory reactions were commonly observed, as were rare responses (52). Phase I trials of 14G2a, an Anti-GD2 IgG2a monoclonal antibody, have shown modest activity with significant toxicity (53,54). After tracer doses of iodine-131-labeled 14G2a to determine tumor uptake, patients underwent prolonged infusions of antibody. They experienced severe generalized pain, hyponatremia, fever, rash, paresthesias, weakness, and chronic refractory postural hypotension. Sixteen of eighteen patients developed human antimouse antibodies to 14G2a. External immunoscintigraphy had a sensitivity of 86% for detection of known lesions. However, microscopic localization of antibody was seen in only two of six biopsies, despite the presence of antigen in each specimen (53).

VII. RADIOISOTOPE-LABELED ANTIBODY

In contrast to the antiganglioside antibodies, infusions with monoclonal antibodies directed against other antigens (p97 and p240) have not resulted in measurable regressions of tumor (55–57). Dillman has suggested that this may relate to the fact that the monoclonal antibodies studied do not affect in vitro ADCC or CDC (58). Conversely, infusion of most antibodies to these antigens results in virtually no symptoms, making infusions of radiolabeled antibody easily tolerated.

Consequently, research has focused on these antibodies as vehicles of specific and sensitive radiation delivery. Such technology could serve in the delivery of radiation to tumor while sparing normal tissue, or provide a sensitive and specific label for radioimmunodetection. In an attempt to improve targeting, reduce immunogenicity, and increase plasma clearance kinetics, radiolabeled F(ab')2 and Fab' fragments have frequently been used. These are antibody components that contain the V region and first constant domain of the heavy chain only. Because they lack the Fc portion, these fragments are smaller, do not interact with Fc receptors, and have an improved target-to-background concentration ratio (23). Unfortunately, reduction in human antimouse antibody (HAMA) production has been minimal (59).

Isotope-labeled 3F8 has been studied in patients suffering from brain tumors (both primary and metastatic to the brain). In one study (60), Arbit was able to detect a melanoma metastasis to the brain with I-131-labeled antibody while inducing few side effects.

Dillman, Halpern, and others studied the antimelanotransferrin monoclonal antibody P96.5 in radioimmunodetection of metastatic melanoma, and they found that approximately 50% of lesions are detectable with indium-111-labeled whole antibody (61). Of note, however, is that they were able to identify a few previously undetected metastases. Larson et al. conducted imaging studies with iodine-131-labeled monoclonals 96.5 and 8.2, which recognize melanotranferrin. No toxic effects were observed, and 88% of lesions larger than 1.5 cm were detected. They also were the first to use an Fab fragment clinically, with one patient receiving 1 mg of labeled Fab derived from 8.2. In this patient they found that Fab fragments were taken up by tumor and that a higher tumor-to-blood ratio was obtained (62). Larson extended this and has reported some encouraging results with Fab fragments against melanotransferrin (63,64). The finding that Fab fragments may have better efficacy in patients is supported by animal studies, which show a greater target-to-nontarget ratio compared to whole IgG (65). Also, whole antibody has a serum half-life measured in hours compared to that of the Fab, which is measured in minutes (66). Preliminary work with I-131- and I-125-labeled Fab fragments of 8.2 and 96.5 antibodies has suggested possible feasibility for clinical radiotherapy (64).

High-molecular-weight melanoma-associated antigen, or p240, also has been the subject of radiolocalization studies using indium-111-labeled mouse monoclonal antibody. Halpern found that only 43% of known lesions labeled with the monoclonal ZME-018 (67). With the same antibody, Murray et al. showed a greater detection rate with soft-tissue and lymph node metastases (76%) than with visceral metastases (19%) (68). No tumor responses to antibody infusion were noted. As with antimelanotransferrin antibodies, Fab fragments have been used in order to improve detection of tumor. Siccardi et al. have published several reports of multicenter trials that use F(ab')2 fragments of the 225.28S antibody. They reported that 250 of 412 known lesions could be seen with their technique, and 127 previously occult lesions were detected as well (69,70). The European Multicentre Study Group published similar results, with an overall sensitivity of

79%. Again, many unsuspected lesions were identified (20% of the total lesions seen). Most of these lesions were thought to represent metastases, with 56% confirmed as metastatic by other modalities (71,72).

Further preliminary efforts to overcome problems with background antibody uptake have included subcutaneous administration of Fab fragments derived from this antibody (73). This work suggests that subcutaneous administration may result in filtering of possible contaminants by the reticuloendothelial and lymphatic system and result in reduced vascular background and decreased nonspecific accumulation in the liver. Of note, Larson did report an antitumor response to the administration of an I-131-labeled Fab fragment derived from the Anti-HMWA antibody 48.7. In this study, correct localization occurred in 74% of documented metastases (74).

Unfortunately, these optimistic results have been qualified by further investigations using the same antibody Fab fragments but demonstrating significant false positive rates or sensitivities of only 26% (75). However, new methods involving the administration of biotinylated forms of 225.28S MAb may significantly decrease background uptake. After biotinylated monoclonal antibody is administered, avidin then is injected, to precipitate circulating antibody. Finally, radioactive biotin is then given. In this study, high-resolution SPECT scans were then obtained and found to detect uveal melanoma more easily due to improved tumor-to-nontumor ratio (76).

In summary, the administration of monoclonal antibodies alone for the treatment and detection of malignant melanoma has yielded some promising results. The rare responses seen with antiganglioside antibodies are encouraging in this chemoresistant disease. Perhaps most hopeful is that side effects are easily tolerated. Use of antibody for detection of metastatic disease also has produced mixed results. Sensitivity and specificity have differed, depending on the group administering the technology. Additionally, the development of an antibody response to mouse antibodies limits its potential readministration. Together, these limitations on the use of MAb directed at melanoma antigens have stimulated investigation in the field to develop additional strategies.

VIII. THE HUMAN ANTIMURINE ANTIBODY RESPONSE

Host development of antibodies that recognize and bind to an administered monoclonal antibody limits the therapeutic and diagnostic use of this product. If therapeutic antibody is removed from the circulation prior to its binding to target, clinical responses will not be seen. Attempts to "humanize" mouse antibody are ongoing (23). Chimeric antibodies are constructions that contain human constant domains with the murine monoclonal antibody's variable domains. Unfortunately, even these antibodies may still incite a host response, so "humanized," or hyperchimeric, versions are being produced. These antibodies are chimeric antibodies with additional modifications of the variable region's murine framework.

Clinical use of these monoclonal antibodies in melanoma has been limited. Saleh et al. have conducted a Phase I trial with the chimeric Anti-GD2 monoclonal antibody ch14.18 (77). This therapy was associated with abdominal and pelvic pain that sometimes required narcotic analgesia. Unfortunately, no responses were seen, and eight of twelve patients developed an Anti-IgG response to the variable region of the chimeric antibody. Adopting another strategy, Irie used a human lymphoblastoid cell line to produce human monoclonal IgM antibodies recognizing the gangliosides GD2 and GM2. Intralesional administration of L72, which recognizes GD2, in six of eight melanoma patients resulted in a 50% tumor regression (78). L55-81, which recognizes GM2, was shown to react with melanoma as well as some colon, ovarian, breast, renal, and prostate cancers (79). This antibody appears to induce tumor regressions with intralesional administration (80).

IX. ENHANCING AGENTS ADMINISTERED WITH MONOCLONAL ANTIBODIES

In order to improve the marginal response rates seen with monoclonal antibodies (especially those binding to ganglioside antigens), several trials combining the administration of MAbs with other agents have been conducted. These agents include some cytotoxic chemotherapeutic agents as well as biologic agents aimed at enhancing the presumed immunologic mechanisms responsible for clinical responses.

A. Chemotherapy

Given that the antiganglioside antibodies induced CDC and ADCC of melanoma cells in vitro, many of the cytokine/monoclonal antibody trials utilize this class of MAb. In 1994, Bukowski et al. reported results of a Phase I trial combining the Anti-GD3 monoclonal R24 with cisplatin (81). WR-2721, a radioprotective agent, was added as well, due to published response rates of 53% in treating melanoma with cisplatin and WR-2721 (82). In this study, toxicity was moderate, with fever and urticaria attributed to R24 and severe but reversible renal failure attributed to cisplatin. The patients studied were preselected for excellent performance status and for binding of R24 to biopsy specimens. Unfortunately, responses were few, with two out of nineteen patients responding after receiving all three agents, and one out of four responding after receiving only cisplatin and WR-2721. A series of immunologic studies did not show an enhancement of

CD8+ subsets as previously reported (83). Additionally, cisplatin did not prevent development of the HAMA response, limiting the future use of R24 in most patients.

B. Growth Factors

Some investigators have shown that colony-stimulation factors may augment monocyte and granulocyte antibody-dependent cellular cytotoxicity (ADCC) through an increase in Fc receptor number or affinity (84–88). Chachoua et al. administered granulocyte-macrophage colony-stimulating factor (GM-CSF) with R24 (89). Toxicity was similar to that seen with R24 alone, though hypotension was dose limiting and allergic reactions appeared to be more severe. Only two of twenty patients experienced brief responses. Since these patients received the highest dose level of R24 in this study and R24 as a single agent is associated with a few clinical responses, it is difficult to assess whether GM-CSF improves the efficacy of R24. To address this question in vitro, the investigators were able to show increased in vitro monocyte and granulocyte direct-cytotoxicity and ADCC, consistent with GM-CSF effect. GM-CSF also has been studied in combination with the Anti-GD2 chimeric monoclonal antibody ch14.18 (90). In this study, the significant neurologic and painful side effects of ch14.18 administration were seen, but no antitumor effects were documented. However, the investigators were able to demonstrate enhancement of monocyte and neutrophil tumoricidal activity.

Evidence has been published that human macrophage colony-stimulating factor (M-CSF) may enhance cytotoxicity toward melanoma targets better than GM-CSF (91): eighteen patients receiving R24 were randomly assigned also to receive either GM-CSF or M-CSF. Peripheral blood monocytes derived from M-CSF-treated patients exhibited enhanced levels of cytotoxicity toward melanoma target cells as compared to healthy controls and to those treated with GM-CSF. Minasian et al. have administered M-CSF in conjunction with R24 (92). Their earlier work indicated that M-CSF may augment ADCC in melanoma patients (93). Though transient grade III thrombocytopenia due to M-CSF administration was observed, other expected toxicities from R24 and M-CSF were mild and not dose-limiting. ADCC was not measured, though a significant monocytosis with increased expression of HLA-DR on monocytes was consistent with monocyte activation. Mixed responses were documented and this therapy warrants further investigation.

C. Interleukin-2

In vitro, preincubation with IL-2 has been shown to increase ADCC using the murine monoclonal antibody 3F8 as well as other IgG3 MAb (94–97). Goodman et al. have reported on the coadministration of the Anti-GD3 murine monoclonal antibody MG-22 and IL-2 in seven patients. They saw tolerable side effects, though no responses, as they increased IL-2 administration to 18×10^6 IU/m²/day. They did, however, see an augmentation of natural killer and ADCC activity in peripheral blood mononuclear cells with increasing doses of IL-2 (98). Creekmore et al. also have reported the administration of R24 with IL-2 (99). In this study, high doses of IL-2 were administered, with resulting toxicity. Although five of thirty-two patients never received R24 due to the early toxicity of IL-2, ten of twenty-three evaluable patients did obtain partial responses. Consequently, the investigators suggested that R24 may augment the antitumor activity of IL-2. Bajorin et al. administered R24 with IL-2. IL-2 was administered at a dose of 1×10^6 units/m² over 6 hours per day for 5 days in an attempt to expand potential effector cell populations (100). Toxicity was tolerable, and three of the 20 patients treated had responses (one partial and two minor). Interleukin-2 appeared to accelerate the HAMA response, for several patients developed antimouse antibodies on only the fifth day of treatment. Fifteen of the patients treated had increases in LAK activity, though there was no observed correlation with antitumor responses.

The schedule of IL-2 and MAb dosing may be important in the production of HAMA. Based on the observation that IL-2 may modulate HAMA as well as have intrinsic antitumor activity, Albertini et al. have published results of combining IL-2 with the murine Anti-GD2 antibody 14.G2a and its chimeric derivative, ch14.18. These investigators found that all patients given mouse monoclonal antibody prior to IL-2 developed HAMA responses. However, patients receiving IL-2 before, during, and after ch14.18 infusions were much less likely to develop HAMA (3/14). This result is encouraging for the future use of antibodies such as ch14.18, as demonstrated by the blocking of in vitro binding activity of ch14.18 to GD2-expressing cells by serum containing Anti-Id antibody (101).

D. Tumor Necrosis Factor

Recombinant tumor necrosis factor-α (TNF-α) has been shown to have antitumor effects (102). Unfortunately, safe, tolerable systemic doses have little antitumor effect (103–108). As a strategy for focusing TNF-induced inflammation at tumor sites, Minasian et al. have used R24 to induce a local inflammatory response in patients with metastatic melanoma, with deposition of complement and infiltration of neutrophils as discussed earlier. Six hours later, they infused TNF. Seven of the eight study patients had mild toxicity (fever and chills), but no responses were noted. One patient, however, developed a tumor lysis syndrome shortly after treatment. The patient died of respiratory decompensation, and an autopsy revealed selective necrosis of metastatic disease. It is not clear why this patient had such an exaggerated response to treatment whereas others in the trial did not respond at all. The investigators suggested that the patient's polymorphonuclear cells may have been in a stimulated state prior to treatment, as indicated by in vitro white blood cell studies obtained. Potentially, this observation may help in devising new strategies for augmenting tumor necrosis (109).

E. Interferon

Alpha interferon increases the expression of some melanoma-associated antigens on cultured melanoma cells in vitro (110–112). Some animal studies have extended these findings of increased antigen expression (113). Such an effect may be useful in dealing with variable antigen expression, resulting in enhanced antibody binding. As a way to upregulate antigen expression, interferon treatment has been attempted in the setting of monoclonal antibody administration. Whereas some clinical studies failed to demonstrate this effect of interferon administration in patients (114), others have shown enhanced expression (115). Rosenblum et al. performed a pilot study comparing 111-In-labeled antimelanoma antibody 96.5 uptake in patients pretreated with interferon versus controls (116). Five patients with malignant melanoma received interferon 24 hours before the administration of monoclonal antibody. Compared to controls, there was a statistically significant increase in the plasma half-life of the 111-In-label, which, the authors suggested, was due to an increase of extravascular distribution of antibody. Additionally, the apparent volume of distribution increased in the interferon group. Whole-body scans showed a threefold increase in radiolabeled antibody in tumor but no change in liver, spleen, bone, or kidney. Consequently, interferon may improve radiolabeled-antibody targeting to tumor without affecting normal tissues.

In summary, the trials that have combined administration of antimelanoma monoclonal antibodies with systemic chemotherapy or cytokines have been inconclusive. The small numbers of patients treated in these Phase I studies preclude obtaining definitive results. Although we cannot determine whether there is an improved therapeutic effect, there were occasional intriguing responses. With the exception of one case of tumor lysis seen on the TNF trial, therapy was well tolerated, and the addition of monoclonal antibodies did not increase toxicity.

X. MONOCLONAL ANTIBODY CONJUGATES

Some studies have attempted to combine the specificity of the monoclonal antibody with a cytotoxic drug. In an early report, polyclonal antibodies reactive to melanoma cells were linked to chlorambucil. This immunotoxin yielded responses in two of thirteen patients (117). Others have attempted to combine drugs such as adriamycin and mitomycin-C with customized monoclonal antibodies, with variable results (118,119).

Further manipulations of the monoclonal antibody can result in direct target cell toxicity. It is possible to produce hybrid molecules that maintain the specificity of monoclonal antibodies while maintaining the cytotoxic properties of molecules such as the ribosomal-inhibiting protein ricin-A. Ricin is a toxin that contains two polypeptides, an A-chain and a B-chain. The A-chain of ricin causes cell death by inhibiting protein synthesis by the 60S ribosomal subunit; the B-chain facilitates entry of the toxin into cells. By dissociating the A-chain from the B-chain, the toxin does not enter cells easily, and toxicity is at least 1500 times less (120). Thus, by combining ricin A with a monoclonal antibody that may be internalized by the target cell, specificity of toxicity is theoretically possible. In melanoma, the XOMAZYME-MEL immunotoxin, which is a hybrid molecule consisting of a monoclonal antibody and ricin A, has been studied in clinical and preclinical settings. The monoclonal antibody component reacts with melanoma-associated antigens having molecular weights of 220,000 and over 500,000. This immunotoxin has been administered to normal rats at low doses without major toxicity, and higher doses produced only transient weight loss, peripheral edema, leukocytosis, hypoalbuminemia, and mildly elevated liver function tests (121). Engelstad et al. have reported that the monoclonal IgG2a antibody, from which XOMAZME-MEL was made, does localize in metastatic lesions in melanoma patients (122). In 1987, Spitler et al. reported treatment with this ricin-A-linked monoclonal and found mild side effects, including a transient decrease in serum albumin, malaise, myalgia, decreased appetite, and fevers (123). The fall in serum albumin corresponding with edema and weight gain were seen at higher doses and were dose limiting. As with other studies with monoclonal antibodies, most patients did not respond to therapy. However, there were four mixed responses and one complete response noted among the twenty-two patients treated. Finally, localization of immunotoxin to tumor was shown with biopsies performed after infusion of drug. In a second, similar study, six patients were treated with immunotoxin, with comparable results (124). All in all, over 200 patients received the XOMAZME-MEL immunotoxin (125). These patients experienced acceptable toxicity, and some favorable responses were seen. However, therapy was limited by the production of host antibodies to the administered immunotoxin, resulting in rapid clearance of drug after repeated doses. Attempts to inhibit this response with immune suppressants are ongoing (126).

XI. HARNESSING THE ANTI-IDIOTYPIC RESPONSE

The host immune response to infused monoclonal antibody can limit the ability of drug to reach its target. Although inhibiting this immune response may allow repeated administration of antibody, such strategies run counter to attempts to enhance host antitumor immunity. Interestingly, Mittelman, Ferrone, and others have investigated the use of anti-idiotypic antibodies that recognize an antimelanoma monoclonal antibody's antigen binding region. These idiotypic antibodies theoretically have structures that correspond to a melanoma antigen and can serve as material for vaccination. Also, this may serve as a strategy to overcome tolerance. Though an immune response against melanoma antigens recognized as self may be inhibited, patients may produce antibodies in response to administration of foreign monoclonal antibodies. The patient's antibodies may then in turn cross-react with the self antigens (127). In 1990, Mittelman et al. reported two clinical trials in which the mouse anti-idiotypic monoclonal antibody MF11-30 was administered to a total of thirty-seven patients. This monoclonal antibody bears the internal image of the melanoma antigen, human high-molecular-weight melanoma-associated antigen (HMW-MAA). Patients were injected with F(ab')2 fragments in an attempt to eliminate antibody response to the Fc region. Few toxicities were noted, and one complete response and a few minor responses were reported (128). As seen with MF11-30, further studies with a similar anti-idiotypic antibody, MK2-23, showed that humoral Anti-HMW-MAA immunity could be induced and rare responses could be seen (129,130). Another study with the antiidiotype monoclonal antibody, I-Mel-2, showed less specific antibody production but some efficacy and one complete response (131). Additionally, investigators noted a correlation of antibody response with increased survival. This occurred despite the relative low affinity of immune serum for HMW-MAA. Investigators argue that this association is not fortuitous, since there is a temporal relationship between development of Anti-HMW-MAA immunity and response (132,133). Furthermore, increased survival was not markedly affected by prior chemotherapy, tumor burden, or the administration of low-dose cyclophosphamide (134). Since HMW-MAA antigen is not a target of ADCC, binding of anti-anti-idiotype antibodies may interfere with the postulated role that HMW-MAA has with metastatic potential of melanoma cells (135). This might occur through inhibiting the metastatic potential of cells that require HMW-MAA for interaction with the extracellular space (136,137).

XII. CONCLUSION

Monoclonal antibody technology in melanoma has yet to produce a clearly effective therapy or diagnostic tool. Clinical studies to date demonstrate that murine monoclonal antibodies can be administered with minimal toxicity. The several responses reported in this review certainly are provocative. Table 3 summarizes responses seen using the best-studied antibody, R24. Yet, one must be aware of the fact that melanoma can spontaneously regress in the rare patient. Furthermore, most antitumor activity detailed in the monoclonal antibody literature in melanoma is not rigorously defined and includes mixed and partial responses. Though

Table 3 Responses Observed with R24

Drug(s)	Responses/total patients	Ref.
R24	4/21	45
R24	2/6	46
R24	5/15	47
R24/WR-2721/Cisplatin	2/19	81
R24/GM-CSF	2/20	89
R24/M-CSF	3/19	92
R24/IL-2	10/23	99
R24/IL-2	3/20	100
R24/TNF	1 fatal tumor lysis/8	109

this is true, there have been well-documented remissions that must be explained. For example, the intrathecal administration of R24 antibody in a patient with melanosis of the meninges produced a 6-year remission. The rare occurrence of such spectacular responses raises the question of features of tumor biology or host immune responses that set such patients apart. Do the MAb responders share common features with the rare patients who completely respond to IL-2 or to a vaccine mediated by manipulation of T-cell immunity? No data are available to address this question. Thus, understanding the mechanism of such remissions remains one of the goals of tumor immunology and will continue to warrant active investigation.

The tumor antigens recognized by this generation of monoclonal antibodies are limited by a lack of specificity and heterogeneous expression on tumors. Another generation of tumor antigens recognized by T-cells has come under study in the last several years. These antigens may provide more specificity, and attempts to induce a cytotoxic T-cell response against these antigens may obviate the problems caused by HAMA production. The data accumulated from MAb trials ultimately may contribute to an understanding of the host immune response to all of these tumor antigens. Immunotherapy targeted at melanoma antigens will remain an active area of investigation, and it is hoped that the rare response can be made more commonplace for patients suffering from progressive melanoma.

REFERENCES

1. Gin-Jorgensen CM, Rigel DS, Freedman RJ. The worldwide incidence of malignant melanoma. In: Balch CM, et al, eds. Cutaneous Melanoma. Philadelphia: Lippincott, 1992:27–39.

2. Parker SL, et al. Cancer statistics, 1997 [published erratum appears in CA Cancer J Clin 1997 Mar–Apr; 47(2):68]. CA Cancer J Clin 1997; 47(1):5–27.
3. Margolin K, et al. Low antitumor activity of BCNU, DTIC, cisplatin (DDP) and tamoxifen (TAM) in advanced melanoma: a Southwest Oncology Group Study (abstr). Proc Am Soc Clin Oncol 1997; 16:495.
4. Bodurtha AJ, et al. A clinical, histologic, and immunologic study of a case of metastatic malignant melanoma undergoing spontaneous remission. Cancer 1976; 37(2): 735–742.
5. Nathanson L. Spontaneous regression of malignant melanoma: a review of the literature on incidence, clinical features, and possible mechanisms. In: E.F. Lewison EF, ed. Conference on Spontaneous Regression of Cancer. Washington, DC: U.S. Government Printing Office, 1976:67.
6. Nordlund JJ, et al. Vitiligo in patients with metastatic melanoma: a good prognostic sign. J Am Acad Dermatol 1983; 9(5):689–696.
7. Itoh K, Platsoucas CD, Balch CM. Autologous tumor-specific cytotoxic T lymphocytes in the infiltrate of human metastatic melanomas. Activation by interleukin 2 and autologous tumor cells, and involvement of the T cell receptor. J Exp Med 1988; 168(4):1419–1441.
8. Parkinson DR, et al. Interleukin-2 therapy in patients with metastatic malignant melanoma: a Phase II study. J Clin Oncol 1990; 8(10):1650–1656.
9. Rosenberg SA, et al. A progress report on the treatment of 157 patients with advanced cancer using lymphokine-activated killer cells and interleukin-2 or high-dose interleukin-2 alone. N Engl J Med 1987; 316(15):889–897.
10. Rosenberg SA, et al. Treatment of 283 consecutive patients with metastatic melanoma or renal cell cancer using high-dose bolus interleukin 2 [see comments.] JAMA 1994; 271(12):907–913.
11. Rosenberg SA, et al. Use of tumor-infiltrating lymphocytes and interleukin-2 in the immunotherapy of patients with metastatic melanoma. A preliminary report [see comments.] N Engl J Med 1988; 319(25):1676–1680.
12. Rosenberg SA, et al. Treatment of patients with metastatic melanoma with autologous tumor-infiltrating lymphocytes and interleukin 2 [see comments.] J Natl Cancer Inst 1994; 86(15):1159–1166.
13. Wolfel T, et al. Lysis of human melanoma cells by autologous cytolytic T cell clones. Identification of human histocompatibility leukocyte antigen A2 as a restriction element for three different antigens. J Exp Med 1989; 170(3):797–810.
14. Jones PC, et al. Prolonged survival for melanoma patients with elevated IgM antibody to oncofetal antigen. J Natl Cancer Inst 1981; 66(2):249–254.
15. Vlock DR, Kirkwood JM. Serial studies of autologous antibody reactivity to melanoma. Relationship to clinical course and circulating immune complexes. J Clin Invest 1985; 76(2):849–854.
16. Livingston PO, et al. Vaccines containing purified GM2 ganglioside elicit GM2 antibodies in melanoma patients. Proc Natl Acad Sci USA 1987; 84(9):2911–2915.
17. Tai T, et al. Immunogenicity of melanoma-associated gangliosides in cancer patients. Int J Cancer 1985; 35(5):607–612.
18. Kawakami Y, et al. Identification of melanoma antigens recognized by T lympho-

cytes and their use in the immunotherapy of cancer. Updates: Principles and Practice of Oncology, In: DeVita VT, Hellman S, Rosenberg SA, eds. Philadelphia: Lippincott-Raven, 1996:1–20.
19. Old LJ. Cancer immunology: the search for specificity. Natl Cancer Inst Monogr 1982; 60:193–209.
20. Itoh K, Houghton AN, Balch CM. Immune responses to melanoma. In: Balch CM, et al., eds. Cutaneous Melanoma. Philadelphia: Lippincott, 1992:144–162.
21. Kohler G, Milstein C. Continuous cultures of fused cells secreting antibody of predefined specificity. Nature 1975; 256(5517):495–497.
22. Lloyd KO. Human tumor antigens: detection and characterization with monoclonal antibodies. In: Heberman RB, ed. Basic and Clinical Tumor Immunology. Boston: Nijhoff, 1983:159–214.
23. Junghans RP, Sgouros G, Scheinberg DA. Antibody-based immunotherapies for cancer. In: Chabner BA, Longo, DL, eds. Cancer Chemotherapy and Biotherapy. Philadelphia: Lippincott-Raven, 1996:655–689.
24. Frank MM. Complement in the pathophysiology of human disease. N Engl J Med 1987; 316(24):1525–1530.
25. Metzger H, Kinet JP. How antibodies work: focus on Fc receptors. Faseb J 1988; 2(1):3–11.
26. Juweid M, et al. Micropharmacology of monoclonal antibodies in solid tumors: direct experimental evidence for a binding site barrier. Cancer Res 1992; 52(19): 5144–5153.
27. Weinstein JN, van Osdol W. Early intervention in cancer using monoclonal antibodies and other biological ligands: micropharmacology and the ''binding site barrier.'' Cancer Res 1992; 52(9 suppl):2747s–2751s.
28. Cheresh DA, Spiro RC. Biosynthetic and functional properties of an Arg-Gly-Asp-directed receptor involved in human melanoma cell attachment to vitronectin, fibrinogen, and von Willebrand factor. J Biol Chem 1987; 262(36):17,703–17,711.
29. Hakomori S. Aberrant glycosylation in tumors and tumor-associated carbohydrate antigens. Adv Cancer Res 1989; 52: 257–331.
30. Houghton AN, Chapman PB. Melanoma. In: DeVita VT, Hellman S, Rosenberg SA, eds. Biologic Therapy of Cancer. Philadelphia: Lippincott, 1995:567–589.
31. Albino AP, et al. Class II histocompatibility antigen expression in human melanocytes transformed by Harvey murine sarcoma virus (Ha-MSV) and Kirsten MSV retroviruses. J Exp Med 1986; 164(5):1710–1722.
32. Tai T, et al. Monoclonal antibody R24 distinguishes between different N-acetyl- and N-glycolylneuraminic acid derivatives of ganglioside GD3. Arch Biochem Biophys 1988; 260(1):51–55.
33. Dippold WG, et al. Cell surface antigens of human malignant melanoma: definition of six antigenic systems with mouse monoclonal antibodies. Proc Natl Acad Sci US America 1980; 77(10):6114–6118.
34. Kniep B, et al. CDw60 glycolipid antigens of human leukocytes: structural characterization and cellular distribution. Blood 1993; 82(6):1776–1786.
35. Herlyn M, Koprowski H. Melanoma antigens: immunological and biological characterization and clinical significance. Annu Rev Immunol 1988; 6:283–308.

36. Natoli EJ Jr, et al. A murine monoclonal antibody detecting N-acetyl- and N-glycolyl-GM2: characterization of cell surface reactivity. Cancer Res 1986; 46(8): 4116–4120.
37. Brown JP, et al. Quantitative analysis of melanoma-associated antigen p97 in normal and neoplastic tissues. Proc Natl Acad Sci USA 1981; 78(1):539–543.
38. Garrigues HJ, et al. Detection of a human melanoma-associated antigen, p97, in histological sections of primary human melanomas. Int J Cancer 1982; 29(5):511–515.
39. Woodbury RG, et al. Analysis of normal neoplastic human tissues for the tumor-associated protein p97. Int J Cancer 1981; 27(2):145–149.
40. Houghton AN, et al. Surface antigens of melanocytes and melanomas. Markers of melanocyte differentiation and melanoma subsets. J Exp Med 1982; 156(6):1755–1766.
41. Garrigues HJ, et al. The melanoma proteoglycan: restricted expression on microspikes, a specific microdomain of the cell surface. J Cell Biol 1986; 103(5):1699–1710.
42. Hellstrom I, Brankovan V, Hellstrom KE. Strong antitumor activities of IgG3 antibodies to a human melanoma-associated ganglioside. Proc Natl Acad Sci USA 1985; 82(5):1499–1502.
43. Dippold WG, Knuth KRA, Meyer zum Buschenfelde KH. Inhibition of human melanoma cell growth in vitro by monoclonal anti-GD3-ganglioside antibody. Cancer Res 1984; 44(2):806–810.
44. Dippold WG, Knuth KRA, Meyer zum Buschenfelde KH. Inflammatory tumor response to monoclonal antibody infusion. Euro J Cancer Clin Oncol 1985; 21(8): 907–912.
45. Houghton AN, et al. Mouse monoclonal IgG3 antibody detecting GD3 ganglioside: a Phase I trial in patients with malignant melanoma. Proc Natl Acad Sci US America 1985; 82(4):1242–1246.
46. Raymond J, et al. A Phase Ib trial of murine monoclonal antibody R24 (anti-GD3) in metastatic melanoma. Proc ASCO 1991; 10:298.
47. Dippold W, Bernhard H, Meyer zum Buschenfelde KH. Immunological response to intrathecal and systemic treatment with ganglioside antibody R-24 in patients with malignant melanoma. Eur J Cancer 1994; 30A(2):137–144.
48. Kirkwood JM, et al. A Phase Ib trial of murine monoclonal antibody R-24 (anti-GD3) in metastatic melanoma (abstract). Proc Am Assoc Cancer Res 1992; 33: 340.
49. Boussiotis VA, et al. R24 anti-GD3 ganglioside antibody can induce costimulation and prevent the induction of alloantigen-specific T cell clonal anergy. Eur J Immunol 1996; 26(9):2149–2154.
50. Iliopoulos D, et al. Inhibition of metastases of a human melanoma xenograft by monoclonal antibody to the GD2/GD3 gangliosides. J Natl Cancer Inst 1989; 81(6): 440–444.
51. Lichtin A, et al. Therapy of melanoma with an anti-melanoma ganglioside monoclonal antibody: a possible mechanism of a complete response. Proc ASCO 1988; 7:247.
52. Cheung N-K, et al. Murine monoclonal antibody (Mab) specific for GD2 ganglio-

side: a Phase I trial in patients with neuroblastoma, melanoma, and osteogenic sarcoma (abstr). Proc Am Assoc Cancer Res 1986; 27:1260.
53. Murray JL, et al. Phase I trial of murine monoclonal antibody 14G2a administered by prolonged intravenous infusion in patients with neuroectodermal tumors. J Clin Oncol 1994; 12(1):184–193.
54. Saleh MN, et al. Phase I trial of the murine monoclonal anti-GD2 antibody 14G2a in metastatic melanoma. Cancer Res 1992; 52(16):4342–4347.
55. Oldham RK, et al. Monoclonal antibody therapy of malignant melanoma: in vivo localization in cutaneous metastasis after intravenous administration. J Clin Oncol 1984; 2(11):1235–1244.
56. Schroff RW, et al. Monoclonal antibody therapy in malignant melanoma: factors effecting in vivo localization. J Biol Response Mod 1987; 6(4):457–472.
57. Goodman GE, et al. Pilot trial of murine monoclonal antibodies in patients with advanced melanoma. J Clin Oncol 1985; 3(3):340–352.
58. Dillman RO. Antibodies as cytotoxic therapy [see comments.] J Clin Oncol 1994; 12(7):1497–1515.
59. Maher VE, et al. Human antibody response to the intravenous and intraperitoneal administration of the F(ab')2 fragment of the OC125 murine monoclonal antibody. J Immunother 1992; 11(1):56–66.
60. Arbit E, et al. Quantitative studies of monoclonal antibody targeting to disialoganglioside GD2 in human brain tumors. Eur J Nucl Med 1995; 22(5):419–426.
61. Dillman RO, et al. Radioimmunodetection of cancer with the use of indium-111-labeled monoclonal antibodies. NCI Monogr 1987(3):33–36.
62. Larson SM, et al. Imaging of melanoma with L-131-labeled monoclonal antibodies. J Nucl Med 1983; 24(2):123–129.
63. Larson SM, et al. Diagnostic imaging of malignant melanoma with radiolabeled antitumor antibodies. JAMA 1983; 249(6):811–812.
64. Larson SM, et al. Localization of 131I-labeled p97-specific Fab fragments in human melanoma as a basis for radiotherapy. J Clin Invest 1983; 72(6):2101–2114.
65. Houston LL, Nowinski RC, Bernstein ID. Specific in vivo localization of monoclonal antibodies directed against the Thy 1.1 antigen. J Immunol 1980; 125(2): 837–843.
66. Halpern SE, Bartholomew R. Pharmacokinetics of an indium-labeled IgG monoclonal antibody over a prolonged period. Eur J Nucl Med 1995; 22(11):1323–1325.
67. Halpern SE, et al. Scintigraphy with In-111-labeled monoclonal antitumor antibodies: kinetics, biodistribution, and tumor detection. Radiology 1988; 168(2):529–536.
68. Murray JL, et al. Clinical parameters related to optimal tumor localization of indium-111-labeled mouse antimelanoma monoclonal antibody ZME-018. J Nucl Med 1987; 28(1):25–33.
69. Siccardi AG. Immunoscintigraphy of melanoma and of CEA-secreting carcinomas. Multicenter studies of the Italian National Research Council. Int J Rad Appl Instrum B 1989; 16(6):637–639.
70. Siccardi AG, et al. Multicenter study of immunoscintigraphy with radiolabeled monoclonal antibodies in patients with melanoma. Cancer Res 1986; 46(9):4817–4822.

71. Siccardi AG, et al. European multicenter study on melanoma immunoscintigraphy by means of 99mTc-labelled monoclonal antibody fragments. The European Multicenter Study Group. Eur J Nucl Med 1990; 16(4–6):317–323.
72. Siccardi AG. Tumor immunoscintigraphy by means of radiolabeled monoclonal antibodies: multicenter studies of the Italian National Research Council—Special Project ''Biomedical Engineering.'' Cancer Res 1990; 50(3 suppl):899s–903s.
73. Paganelli G, et al. Improved immunoscintigraphy by subcutaneous injection of 99mTc or 111-In labelled F(ab′)2 fragments of an anti-melanoma monoclonal antibody. Int J Rad Appl Instrum B 1986; 13(4):423–428.
74. Larson SM, et al. Use of I-131 labeled, murine Fab against a high molecular weight antigen of human melanoma: preliminary experience. Radiology 1985; 155(2):487–492.
75. Salzillo F, et al. Radioimmunoscintigraphy with 99mTc-225.28S-F(ab′)2 in cutaneous and ocular melanomas: cases of particular clinical interest. J Nucl Biol Med 1993; 37(4):191–197.
76. Magnani P, et al. Quantitative comparison of direct antibody labeling and tumor pretargeting in uveal melanoma. J Nucl Med 1996; 37(6):967–971.
77. Saleh MN, et al. Phase I trial of the chimeric anti-GD2 monoclonal antibody ch14.18 in patients with malignant melanoma. Hum Antibodies Hybridomas 1992; 3(1):19–24.
78. Irie RF, Morton DL. Regression of cutaneous metastatic melanoma by intralesional injection with human monoclonal antibody to ganglioside GD2. Proc Natl Acad Sci USA 1986; 83(22):8694–8698.
79. Nishinaka Y, Ravindranath MH, Irie RF. Development of a human monoclonal antibody to ganglioside G(M2) with potential for cancer treatment. Cancer Res 1996; 56(24):5666–5671.
80. Irie RF, Matsuki T, Morton DL. Human monoclonal antibody to ganglioside GM2 for melanoma treatment [letter.] Lancet 1989; 1(8641):786–787.
81. Bukowski RM, et al. Phase I trial of cisplatin, WR-2721, and the murine monoclonal antibody R24 in patients with metastatic melanoma: clinical and biologic effects. J Immunother Emphasis Tumor Immunol 1994; 15(4):273–282.
82. Glover D, et al. WR-2721 and high-dose cisplatin: an active combination in the treatment of metastatic melanoma. J Clin Oncol 1987; 5(4):574–578.
83. Welte K, et al. Stimulation of T lymphocyte proliferation by monoclonal antibodies against GD3 ganglioside. J Immunol 1987; 139(6):1763–1771.
84. Liesveld JL, et al. Cytokine effects and role of adhesive proteins and Fc receptors in human macrophage-mediated antibody dependent cellular cytotoxicity. J Cell Biochem 1991; 45(4):381–390.
85. Kushner BH, Cheung NK. GM-CSF enhances 3F8 monoclonal antibody-dependent cellular cytotoxicity against human melanoma and neuroblastoma. Blood 1989; 73(7):1936–1941.
86. Chachoua A, et al. Monocyte activation following systemic administration of granulocyte-macrophage colony-stimulating factor. J Immunother Emphasis Tumor Immunol 1994; 15(3):217–224.
87. Liesveld JL, et al. Expression of IgG Fc receptors in myeloid leukemic cell lines.

Effect of colony-stimulating factors and cytokines. J Immunol 1988; 140(5):1527–1533.
88. Munn DH, Cheung NK. Antibody-dependent antitumor cytotoxicity by human monocytes cultured with recombinant macrophage colony-stimulating factor. Induction of efficient antibody-mediated antitumor cytotoxicity not detected by isotope release assays. J Exp Med 1989; 170(2):511–526.
89. Chachoua A, et al. Phase Ib trial of granulocyte-macrophage colony-stimulating factor combined with murine monoclonal antibody R24 in patients with metastatic melanoma. J Immunother Emphasis Tumor Immunol 1994; 16(2):132–41.
90. Murray JL, et al. Phase Ia/Ib trial of anti-GD2 chimeric monoclonal antibody 14.18 (ch14.18) and recombinant human granulocyte-macrophage colony-stimulating factor (rhGM-CSF) in metastatic melanoma. J Immunother Emphasis Tumor Immunol 1996; 19(3):206–217.
91. Schmid I, et al. Alterations in phenotype and cell-surface antigen expression levels of human monocytes: differential response to in vivo administration of rhM-CSF or rhGM-CSF. Cytometry 1995; 22(2):103–110.
92. Minasian LM, et al. A Phase I study of anti-GD3 ganglioside monoclonal antibody R24 and recombinant human macrophage-colony stimulating factor in patients with metastatic melanoma. Cancer 1995; 75(9):2251–2257.
93. Bajorin DF, et al. Recombinant macrophage colony stimulating factor: a Phase 1 trial in patients with metastatic melanoma (abstr). Proc Am Soc Clin Oncol 1990; 9:183.
94. Munn DH, Cheung NK. Interleukin-2 enhancement of monoclonal antibody-mediated cellular cytotoxicity against human melanoma. Cancer Res 1987; 47(24 pt 1):6600–6605.
95. Eisenthal A, et al. Effect of combined therapy with lymphokine-activated killer cells, interleukin 2 and specific monoclonal antibody on established B16 melanoma lung metastases. Cancer Res 1988; 48(24 pt 1):7140–7145.
96. Kawase I, et al. Combined therapy of mice bearing a lymphokine-activated killer-resistant tumor with recombinant interleukin 2 and an antitumor monoclonal antibody capable of inducing antibody-dependent cellular cytotoxicity. Cancer Res 1988; 48(5):1173–1179.
97. Honsik CJ, Jung G, Reisfeld RA. Lymphokine-activated killer cells targeted by monoclonal antibodies to the disialogangliosides GD2 and GD3 specifically lyse human tumor cells of neuroectodermal origin. Proc Natl Acad Sci USA 1986; 83(20):7893–7897.
98. Goodman GE, et al. Phase I trial of murine monoclonal antibody MG-22 and IL-2 in patients with disseminated melanoma (abstr). Proc ASCO 1992; 11:1190.
99. Creekmore S, et al. Phase Ib/II trial of R24 antibody and interleukin-2 (IL2) in melanoma (abstr). Proc ASCO 1992; 11:1186.
100. Bajorin DF, et al. Phase I evaluation of a combination of monoclonal antibody R24 and interleukin 2 in patients with metastatic melanoma. Cancer Res 1990; 50(23):7490–7495.
101. Albertini MR, et al. Systemic interleukin-2 modulates the anti-idiotypic response to chimeric anti-GD2 antibody in patients with melanoma. J Immunother Emphasis Tumor Immunol 1996; 19(4):278–295.

102. Carswell EA, et al. An endotoxin-induced serum factor that causes necrosis of tumors. Proc Natl Acad Sci USA 1975; 72(9):3666–3670.
103. Creaven PJ, et al. A Phase I clinical trial of recombinant human tumor necrosis factor given daily for five days. Cancer Chemother Pharmacol 1989; 23(3):186–191.
104. Creagan ET, et al. A Phase I clinical trial of recombinant human tumor necrosis factor. Cancer 1988; 62(12):2467–2471.
105. Chapman PB, et al. Clinical pharmacology of recombinant human tumor necrosis factor in patients with advanced cancer. J Clin Oncol 1987; 5(12):1942–1951.
106. Creaven PJ, et al. Phase I clinical trial of recombinant human tumor necrosis factor. Cancer Chemother Pharmacol 1987; 20(2):137–144.
107. Feinberg B, et al. A Phase I trial of intravenously administered recombinant tumor necrosis factor-alpha in cancer patients. J Clin Oncol 1988; 6(8):1328–1334.
108. Kimura K, et al. Phase I study of recombinant human tumor necrosis factor. Cancer Chemother Pharmacol 1987; 20(3):223–229.
109. Minasian LM, et al. Hemorrhagic tumor necrosis during a pilot trial of tumor necrosis factor-alpha and anti-GD3 ganglioside monoclonal antibody in patients with metastatic melanoma. Blood 1994; 83(1):56–64.
110. Murray JL, et al. Differential in vitro effects of recombinant alpha-interferon and recombinant gamma-interferon alone or in combination on the expression of melanoma-associated surface antigens. J Biol Response Mod 1988; 7(2):152–161.
111. Giacomini P, et al. Modulation by recombinant DNA leukocyte (alpha) and fibroblast (beta) interferons of the expression and shedding of HLA- and tumor-associated antigens by human melanoma cells. J Immunol 1984; 133(3):1649–1655.
112. Imai K, et al. Differential effect of interferon on the expression of tumor-associated antigens and histocompatibility antigens on human melanoma cells: relationship to susceptibility to immune lysis mediated by monoclonal antibodies. J Immunol 1981; 127(2):505–509.
113. Murray JL, et al. Recombinant alpha-interferon enhances tumor targeting of an antimelanoma monoclonal antibody in vivo. J Biol Response Mod 1990; 9(6):556–363.
114. Cerny T, et al. Immunoscintigraphy with 99mTc labelled F(ab′)2 fragments of an anti melanoma monoclonal antibody (225.28S) in patients with metastatic malignant melanoma. Eur J Nucl Med 1987; 13(3):130–133.
115. Gasparini M, et al. Enhancement of in vivo monoclonal antibody targeting with recombinant interferon and cytokines. Int J Biol Markers 1993; 8(3):160–165.
116. Rosenblum MG, et al. Interferon-induced changes in pharmacokinetics and tumor uptake of ^{111}In-labeled antimelanoma antibody 96.5 in melanoma patients. J Natl Cancer Inst 1988; 80(3):160–165.
117. Ghose T, et al. Immunochemotherapy of malignant melanoma with chlorambucil-bound antimelanoma globulins: preliminary results in patients with disseminated disease. J Natl Cancer Inst 1977; 58(4):845–852.
118. Oldham, RK, et al. Adriamycin custom-tailored immunoconjugates in the treatment of human malignancies. Mol Biother 1988; 1(2):103–113.

119. Orr D, et al. Phase I trial of mitomycin C immunoconjugates cocktails in human malignancies. Mol Biother 1989; 1(4):229–240.
120. Olsnes S, Refsnes K, Pihl A. Mechanism of action of the toxic lectins abrin and ricin. Nature 1974; 249(458):627–631.
121. Harkonen S, et al. Toxicity and immunogenicity of monoclonal antimelanoma antibody-ricin A chain immunotoxin in rats. Cancer Res 1987; 47(5):1377–1382.
122. Engelstad V, et al. Initial clinical experience with intravenous and subcutaneous indium-111 antimelanoma monoclonal radioimmunoimaging (scientific program). Radiology 1985; 157:98.
123. Spitler LE, et al. Therapy of patients with malignant melanoma using a monoclonal antimelanoma antibody-ricin A chain immunotoxin. Cancer Res 1987; 47(6):1717–1723.
124. von Wussow P, et al. Immunotherapy in patients with advanced malignant melanoma using a monoclonal antibody ricin A immunotoxin. Eur J Clin Oncol 1988; 24(supplement 2):S69–S73.
125. Spitler, LE. Monoclonal antibodies in the treatment of malignant melanoma. Front Radiat Ther Oncol 1990; 24:186–93; discussion 202–203.
126. Spitler LE, Mischak R, Scannon P. Therapy of metastatic malignant melanoma using Xomazyme Mel, a murine monoclonal anti-melanoma ricin A chain immunotoxin. Int J Rad Appl Instrum B 1989; 16(6):625–627.
127. Chattopadhyay P, et al. Human high molecular weight-melanoma associated antigen mimicry by an anti-idiotypic antibody: characterization of the immunogenicity and the immune response to the mouse monoclonal antibody IMel-1. Cancer Res 1991; 51(22):6045–6051.
128. Mittelman A, et al. Active specific immunotherapy in patients with melanoma. A clinical trial with mouse antiidiotypic monoclonal antibodies elicited with syngeneic anti-high-molecular-weight-melanoma-associated antigen monoclonal antibodies [published erratum appears in J Clin Invest 1991 Feb; 87(2):757]. J Clin Invest 1990; 86(6):2136–2144.
129. Mittelman A, et al. Humoral antimelanoma immunity: induction by mouse antiidiotypic mAb, MK2-23 and association with survival of patients with advanced melanoma. Mt Sinai J Med 1992; 59(3):234–237.
130. Mittelman A, et al. Human high molecular weight melanoma-associated antigen (HMW-MAA) mimicry by mouse anti-idiotypic monoclonal antibody MK2-23: induction of humoral anti-HMW-MAA immunity and prolongation of survival in patients with stage IV melanoma. Proc Natl Acad Sci USA 1992; 89(2):466–470.
131. Quan WD, Jr, et al. Active specific immunotherapy of metastatic melanoma with an antiidiotype vaccine: a Phase I/II trial of I-Mel-2 plus SAF-m. J Clin Oncol 1997; 15(5):2103–2110.
132. Mittelman A, et al. Kinetics of the immune response and regression of metastatic lesions following development of humoral anti-high molecular weight-melanoma associated antigen immunity in three patients with advanced malignant melanoma immunized with mouse antiidiotypic monoclonal antibody MK2-23. Cancer Res 1994; 54(2):415–421.
133. Ferrone S, et al. Human high molecular weight-melanoma associated antigen mim-

icry by mouse anti-idiotypic monoclonal antibodies MK2-23. Experimental studies and clinical trials in patients with malignant melanoma. Pharmacol Ther 1993; 57(2–3):259–290.
134. Mittelman A, et al. Antiantiidiotypic response and clinical course of the disease in patients with malignant melanoma immunized with mouse antiidiotypic monoclonal antibody MK2-23. Hybridoma 1995; 14(2):175–81.
135. Ferrone S. Anti-idiotypes in melanoma. Hybridoma 1993; 12(5):509–514.
136. Kageshita T, et al. Association of high molecular weight melanoma-associated antigen expression in primary acral lentiginous melanoma lesions with poor prognosis. Cancer Res 1993; 53(12):2830–2833.
137. Bumol TF, Walker LE, Reisfeld RA. Biosynthetic studies of proteoglycans in human melanoma cells with a monoclonal antibody to a core glycoprotein of chondroitin sulfate proteoglycans. J Biol Chem 1984; 259(20):12,733–12,741.

15
Monoclonal Antibodies in the Management of Lung Cancer

Stefan C. Grant
Cornell University Medical College and Memorial Sloan-Kettering Cancer Center, New York, New York

Ellen Early
Memorial Sloan-Kettering Cancer Center, New York, New York

John Mendelsohn
The University of Texas M.D. Anderson Cancer Center, Houston, Texas

I. INTRODUCTION

Lung cancer remains the leading cause of death due to cancer in men and has exceeded breast cancer as a cause of cancer death in women. It is estimated that there were over 180,000 new cases diagnosed in the United States in 1997 (1). Most of these patients will succumb to their disease. Lung cancer is divided into two histologic groups. Roughly 80% of all lung cancers are classified as non-small-cell lung cancer (NSCLC), comprising adenocarcinoma, large-cell carcinoma, and squamous cell (epidermoid) carcinoma. Most of the remaining cases are classified as small-cell lung cancer (SCLC), which has a different biologic behavior, natural history, and treatment. Approximately 10% of lung cancer specimens have mixed histology, with both small-cell and non-small-cell elements.

The various histologic subtypes of NSCLC behave in a similar manner, and standard treatment is identical. Surgery is the mainstay of therapy for early-stage disease, with chemotherapy being employed in more advanced disease. Radiation therapy often is used as a substitute for surgery or in combination with systemic chemotherapy. Over the past several years, the role of systemic chemotherapy in locally advanced disease has been defined. More recently the value of chemotherapy in early-stage disease has been studied. Current therapies have been demonstrated to provided significant improvements in both survival and quality of life. Increasingly, however, it has been recognized that improved staging modalities and treatments are needed to achieve a major impact on this disease.

Small-cell lung cancer, the lung cancer most strongly associated with tobacco use, comprises a number of subtypes, including the classical oat-cell carcinoma. Unlike NSCLC, it metastasizes early and rarely is treated with surgical resection. Instead, the mainstay of treatment is chemotherapy, with the addition of radiation therapy for those patients in whom only locoregional spread is identified. Though systemic chemotherapy is highly effective in SCLC, most patients experience recurrence or progression of the disease and eventually succumb to their cancer. Although median survival time improved after the institution of cisplatin-based chemotherapy regimens, median survival from the time of diagnosis remains poor, ranging from 7 to 14 months. The use of increasing doses of chemotherapy or prolonged treatment has not had a substantial effect on the survival of patients with this disease.

As in other tumor types, biologic agents, including monoclonal antibodies, have been studied in lung cancer. Surface antigens have been identified in both NSCLC and SCLC, and the role of antibodies for both diagnosis and treatment is being evaluated. Monoclonal antibodies or their fragments have the potential to provide improved specificity and sensitivity for staging purposes, with the possibility of greater efficiency if they can be substituted for other, more cumbersome diagnostic tests. In certain cases the antigenic targets identified are growth factor receptors, and monoclonal antibodies are used to block the activation of growth pathways. Other targets have been selected for their relatively high levels of expression on tumor cells and restricted expression on normal tissues. Antibodies directed against these antigens may stimulate an immunologic response by triggering the complement cascade or antibody-dependent cellular cytotoxicity (ADCC) to enhance killing of tumor cells. Antibodies also have been conjugated to toxins, chemotherapeutic molecules, or radionuclides in order to achieve the destruction of viable tumor cells (2).

II. SURFACE MARKERS, GROWTH FACTOR RECEPTORS, AND LIGAND EXPRESSION IN LUNG CANCER

In an attempt to aid in the development of new treatment strategies, there has been a collaborative effort between individual laboratories. The Second and Third International Workshops on Lung Cancer Antigens sought to characterize and define lung cancer cell-surface molecules and the antigenic targets of the monoclonal antibodies directed toward these antigens (3,4). As a result, the nature and function of many of these antigens have been characterized. See Table 1.

Table 1 Cluster Analysis of Lung Cancer Antigens

Cluster	Antigen	Selected Antibodies
1	NCAM extracellular domain	SEN36, SEN 7
1C	NCAM intracellular domain	KD11 MG-5
2	EGP-2/GA-733-2	MOC-31
4	CD24	SWA-11
6	Le^Y hapten	MLuC-1, ABL364
w7	High-molecular-weight mucins	NCC-ST-439
8	Mucins (TAG-72)	B72.3, CC49
9	Mucins (MUC1)	KL-6, KM-432
10	Neurone-specific proteins	RNL-2, RNL-3
11	40-kd membrane	44-3A6, KM195
12	Folic acid receptor	MW207, FBP146
13	EGP-1/GA733-1	RS7, MR54
14	EGF receptor	225, 528, RG83852
w15	Mesothelial membrane antigen	ME-1, ME-2

From the Third International Workshop on Lung Tumors and Differentiation Antigens.
Source: Modified from Ref. 110.

The largest number of antibodies to small-cell lung cancer have been found to react with the cluster-1 antigen, a 145-kDa molecule, later identified as the neural cell adhesion molecule (NCAM) (5). The NCAM is expressed in almost all small-cell lung cancer cells and has been associated with the expression of neuroendocrine markers of differentiation, independent of the histological type of lung cancer (6). Cluster-2 antigen is a 40-kDa surface protein that has a wide distribution on epithelial tissues. This appears to be identical to a transmembrane protein cloned from an adenocarcinoma cell line (7). Cluster-4 antigen is a heavily glycosylated but unusually short protein of only 80 amino acids. It is virtually identical to the leukocyte activation antigen CD24 except for a single valine-alanine substitution, and is reportedly found on virtually all small-cell lung cancer cells (3,8). Cluster-5 and cluster-5A antigens are sialoglycoproteins, expressed on small-cell lung cancer; cluster-6 and cluster-8 antigens are blood-group-related carbohydrate structures; and cluster-W7 antigen is a mucin-related carbohydrate structure. Two other well-defined antigens, CD11B, which binds to ICAM-1, and CD57, originally defined as leukocyte antigens, also have been associated with small-cell lung cancer (9,10). Small-cell lung cancer also expresses beta-1 integrin, and an antibody directed against beta-1 integrin decreases the binding of small-cell lung cancer cells to laminin, suggesting that beta-1 integrin promotes adhesion to extracellular matrix in this system (11).

Compared to normal lung epithelium, NSCLC has been shown to express elevated levels of epidermal growth factor (EGF) receptor as well as its ligand TGFα (transforming growth factor α), and in over one-third of NSCLC specimens, primarily adenocarcinomas, the HER-2/*neu* gene product is overexpressed, providing a potential mechanism to effect tumor growth. Small-cell lung cancer cells have a different pattern of receptor expression. They also secrete bombesin, a peptide commonly produced by neuroendocrine cells.

Nevertheless, despite their specificity, antibodies do have a number of inherent limitations as therapeutic and diagnostic agents that need to be resolved. These include nonuniform distribution and delivery of antibody to tumor sites, antigenic heterogenicity of tumors, short half-lives, cross-reactivity with normal cells, and the immunogenicity of the antibodies themselves, resulting in the production of human antibodies against the xenogeneic proteins. Nonuniform uptake of systemically administered antibody in solid tumor biopsy specimens is due not only to inhomogeneous tumor antigen expression but also to physiological barriers to antibodies, such as a heterogeneous blood supply, elevated interstitial pressures in tumor centers, large transport distances, and inadequate cellular trafficking to tumor cells (12).

Particularly with respect to SCLC, which is highly sensitive to both chemotherapy and radiation, it has been proposed that these modalities be employed as initial therapy. Thereafter, agents such as monoclonal antibodies could be utilized in an attempt to eliminate microscopic residual disease. The effective use of such approaches has the potential to improve the survival of patients with lung cancer and to achieve greater rates of cure.

III. ANTIBODIES AGAINST GROWTH FACTORS IN NON-SMALL-CELL LUNG CANCER

A host of growth factors and receptors have been identified in both normal lung as well as on NSCLC and SCLC tumor cells, with different patterns of growth factor and receptor expression displayed by different histologic subtypes. These factors have been shown to promote or inhibit cellular proliferation, and in many cases both receptor and ligand are coexpressed by the same cell. The mutation of, or alterations in the expression of, growth factors and their receptors may contribute to oncogenic transformation, because an abnormal level of growth factor expression, aberrance in growth factor function, and deviant receptor function appear to play an important role in malignant transformation. In lung cancer, crucial growth factors have been identified and have been targeted for the development of treatment strategies. It has been proposed that blocking the action of growth factors with substances such as antibodies or small peptides could provide a means of inhibiting the in vivo growth of tumors.

A. Antibodies Against the Epidermal Growth Factor Receptor

Compared to normal lung epithelium, NSCLC has been shown to express elevated levels of epidermal growth factor (EGF) receptor as well as its ligand TGFα (transforming growth factor α), providing a potential mechanism for autocrine growth stimulation. The binding of epidermal growth factor (EGF) to the EGF receptor (EGFR), a transmembrane glycoprotein, stimulates tyrosine kinase activity, initiating one of the most critical cellular growth-regulatory signal-transduction cascade systems. Found primarily on cells of epithelial origin (13,14), the overexpression of EGF receptor has been shown to play an important role in the proliferation of several human malignancies and may be a marker of a poor prognosis (15–17). The EGF receptor is activated by a family of growth factors, including EGF, TGFα, amphiregulin, and heparin-binding EGF (18–21). Although there is only 35% homology between TGFα and EGF, the two molecules have identical binding affinity. Overexpression of the EGF receptor has been shown in NSCLC (22–27), the increase in the number of EGF receptors on these cells most often due to increased transcription or postranscription modifications rather than amplification of the EGF receptor gene (28). Previously, EGF receptors were reported to be absent on SCLC cell lines (29). Immune histochemistry studies have detected high levels of EGF receptors on nearly all squamous carcinomas (74–100%), in some adenocarcinomas, but only rarely in SCLC (22,30–32). In a study by Berger et al. 109 serially resected primary lung cancers were analyzed for EGF receptor expression. Seventy-four percent of squamous tumors, 34% of adenocarcinomas, and 33% of large-cell tumors were positive for EGF receptor (33). The prognostic significance of overexpression in lung cancer tissue is unresolved. Overexpression of EGF receptor has been reported to correlate with poor prognosis (24,25,34) or to have no prognostic significance (35). Nevertheless, the high levels of expression in these tumors, with the existence of an autocrine loop, have made it an attractive antigenic target for manipulation by investigators.

1. Preclinical Studies

Although many Anti-EGFR antibodies exist, two that have been studied extensively are the monoclonal mouse antibodies MAb 225, an IgG1, and MAb 523, an IgG2a (36,37). They have been shown to bind to the EGF receptor, compete with EGF for receptor occupancy, bind with an affinity comparable to the natural ligand, and to block receptor activation by EGF or TGFα (37,38). In a series of experiments using the A431 cell line it was shown that only monoclonal antibodies that recognize the EGFR and block ligand binding have an antiproliferative effect (37). Using MAb 528, Reiss et al. demonstrated that blocking ligand binding to EGFR in squamous carcinoma cell lines, including the lung cancer cell line CaLu-1, could inhibit cell growth by approximately 50% (39). Fan et al.

(40) evaluated monovalent 225 Fab′, 225 F(Ab′)$_2$, and intact MAb 225 for their ability to block ligand binding to the receptor and thereby to inhibit activation of tyrosine kinase activity. Though the monovalent 225 Fab′ demonstrated weaker activity when compared to 225 F(Ab′)$_2$ and intact antibody (40,41), the activity of the bivalent F(Ab′)$_2$ and monovalent 225 Fab′ fragments provided strong evidence that the antiproliferative effects were due to pharmacologic blockade of EGF receptors without participation of immune responses mediated by the Fc fragment of the antibody. The same group studied the ability of these antibodies to inhibit tumor growth in athymic mice using a series of human xenografts, including the epidermal lung cancer cell line T222, and reported the ability of MAb 225 and MAb 528 to inhibit tumor formation. In contrast, the use of MAb 455 (which binds the EGFR without blocking ligand binding) lacked this ability (42).

Imanishi et al. evaluated the role of ligand produced by human epithelial tumor cells as an autocrine growth factor in tumors expressing high levels of EGFR (43). They studied the human lung adenocarcinoma cell lines A-549 and PC-9, both of which express high levels of EGFR and produce TGF-α. Using the IgG1 antibodies WA-3 directed against TGFα and KEM-10 directed against the EGFR, they demonstrate that antibodies directed against both ligand and receptor also could inhibit tumor cell growth.

In order to evaluate the ability accurately to target xenografts expressing high levels of EGFR, Goldenberg and co-workers (44) studied the monoclonal antibody 225 radiolabeled with indium-111. In nude mice, they used human tumor xenografts bearing high levels of EGFR to demonstrate that an Anti-EGFR MAb could be delivered to EGFR-bearing tumors, providing additional data supporting clinical trials of Anti-EGFR antibodies.

Following up on the observation of synergy between MAb A108 and cisplatin (45), the efficacy of combining EGF blockade with chemotherapy was examined in xenografts of human squamous carcinoma and adenocarcinoma. The combination of Anti-EGFR MAb 225 or 528 with either doxorubicin or cisplatin eliminated well-established xenografts, which could not be achieved with either therapy alone (46,47). See Figure 1.

2. Clinical Studies

Indium-111-labeled MAb 225 was evaluated in a Phase I and imaging trial at Memorial Sloan-Kettering Cancer Center (48). Patients with stage III and IV inoperable squamous cell carcinoma of the lung were studied. They were divided into groups receiving total doses of MAb 225 ranging from 1 mg to 300 mg. At the first dose level, 1 mg of unlabeled MAb was administered to patients. Thereafter, groups received 4 mg of ^{111}In-labeled MAb 225 mixed with unlabeled MAb to give a total dose of 4, 20, 40, 120, or 300 mg. At a dose of 120 mg and higher

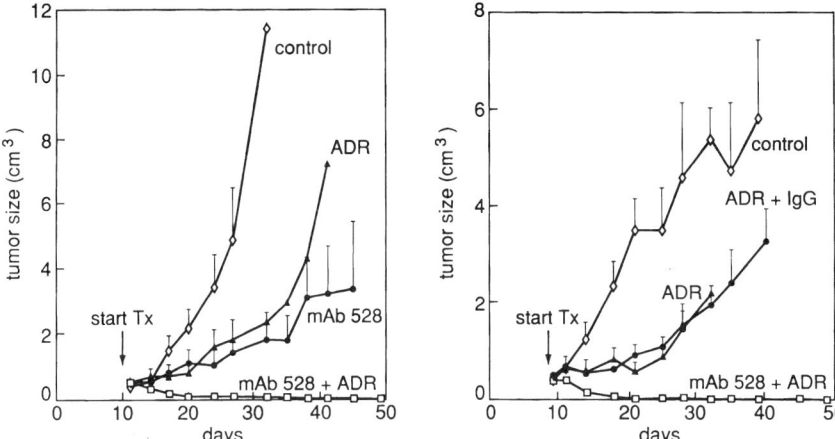

Figure 1 Antitumor effect of chemotherapy in combination with an Anti-EGFR antibody. Results of experiments reported by Baselga et al. Antitumor activity of MAb 528 in combination with doxorubicin (DOXO) on well-established A431 squamous cell carcinoma xenografts in athymic mice. Treatment with either doxorubicin or MAb 528 alone partially inhibited tumor growth. Doxorubicin with a nonspecific mouse IgG did not produce an antitumor effect greater than doxorubicin alone. The combination of MAb 528 with doxorubicin resulted in the disappearance of all tumors in animals surviving on day 30. (From Ref. 46.)

the $t_{1/2}$ was greater than 24 hours, and the serum concentration of MAb 225 was greater than 40 nM at 72 hours postinfusion, more than an order of magnitude greater than the equilibrium dissociation constant for the binding or either 225 or natural ligand to the EGFR. Importantly, no major toxicity was observed, notwithstanding the expression of EGFR on normal tissues such as the liver, and patients tolerated the maximum doses without difficulty. It was estimated that greater than 20 mg of antibody was required to saturate the EGF receptors present in the liver, and this was confirmed by improved imaging of tumors in patients whose dose of 225 exceeded this amount, with eight of eight metastatic tumors exceeding 1 cm in diameter being identified. All patients developed antimouse antibodies (HAMA). This study demonstrated that MAb 225 could be administered safely at the doses studied and that tumor uptake of labeled MAb was dose-dependent.

A second Phase I trial evaluated the Anti-EGF receptor antibody, MAb 528 (49). In this study, the antibody was labeled with ^{131}I in order to compare differences between hepatic uptake of indium and iodine. Squamous cell carcinoma patients of the lung and head and neck were enrolled, and a study design essentially identical to that employed in the trial of 225 was used. Again, in patients receiving an MAb dose of at least 40 mg all primary and metastatic lesions greater than 1 cm in diameter as determined by conventional staging methods were detected. In the liver, ^{131}I-MAb uptake was reduced and liver metastases were identified by radionuclide scanning. Again, toxicity was minimal.

On the basis of the observation of synergy between MAb 225 or MAb 528 with cisplatin or doxorubicin in a nude mouse model (46,47), a Phase I trial is being conducted to evaluate human–mouse chimeric MAb C225 plus cisplatin in patients with advanced lung and head/neck cancer (50).

Another Anti-EGFR antibody that has been studied in clinical trials is RG83852. Also known as A108, it is a mouse IgG2a that has been reported to react with 80% of human NSCLC cell lines tested (51). In a trial conducted at M. D. Anderson Cancer Center (52), fifteen patients with NSCLC or head and neck cancer were treated with escalating doses of RG83852. Cohorts of three patients received a total dose of 50, 100, 200, 400, or 600 mg/m^2 by continuous infusion for 5 days. No significant side effects were reported, and it was estimated that there was greater than 50% EGFR saturation at doses greater than or equal to 200 mg/m^2, with close to 100% saturation at a dose of 600 mg/m^2. Tumor specimens were obtained pretreatment and one day posttreatment in selected patients, and tumor tyrosine kinase activity was shown to be upregulated posttherapy in specimens collected from two of five patients with EGFR-positive tumors. Citing studies that suggest that tumors in which growth is regulated by high levels of EGFR expression may have characteristics that make them more susceptible to chemotherapy or radiotherapy (53–55), the authors proposed that the upregulation of EGFR may be one explanation for the synergistic effects of Anti-EGFR antibodies combined with chemotherapy previously reported (45,56).

In another Phase I trial (57), patients with advanced NSCLC were treated with RG83852 trace labeled with I-131. Thirteen patients received RG83852 at doses ranging from 0.1 mg/kg to 7 mg/kg. Although localization to tumor sites could not be shown by radionuclide scanning, immunohistochemical analysis of tumor biopsies taken from selected patients at the highest dose level demonstrated saturation of EGF receptors on tumor cells after administration of RG83852. Again, minimal side effects were observed, with occasional low-grade fevers postinfusion being the major adverse event.

The rat IgG2b monoclonal antibody ICR62 also has been studied in a Phase I trial in patients with lung cancer (58). Groups of three patients with either lung or head and neck cancer were treated with 2.5, 10, 20, or 40 mg of antibody. An additional eight patients received a dose of 100 mg. In this trial no serious adverse events were reported, and biopsies taken 24 hours postinfusion in four patients who received at least 40 mg MAb demonstrated localization to tumor. The authors report that further trials are planned.

B. HER-2/*neu*/c-*erb*B2

The gene known as c-*erb*B-2, HER-2, and *neu* was independently identified in three different ways. The gene codes for a 185-kDa transmembrane receptorlike phosphoglycoprotein that has 50% amino acid homology to the EGF receptor and has intrinsic tyrosine kinase activity (59–61). Notwithstanding the high degree of homology between the EGF receptor and c-*erb*B-2 (62), EGF does not bind to p185^{HER-2} (63). Studies performed in culture demonstrate that a single-point mutation or the overexpression of c-*erb*B-2/HER-2/*neu* in NIH 313 cells can achieve its transforming potential (62,64,65). Kern et al. demonstrated that p185^{HER-2} is normally expressed in epithelial cells of the respiratory tract, bronchial mucosal glands, and type II pneumocytes (66). Overexpression of HER-2 due to gene amplification occurs frequently in many adenocarcinomas, and increased expression has been implicated in malignant transformation. It has been reported to be present in many cancers, including NSCLC, and has been linked to a poor prognosis (67–72). Although gene amplification has been implicated in many malignancies, in NSCLC overexpression of HER2 may be regulated by transcriptional or posttranscriptional mechanisms (68). Tumor cell resistance to cytotoxicity mediated by activated macrophages or by TNFα also has been correlated with high levels of p185^{HER2} expression (73), as has resistance to cytotoxic agents such as platinum (74).

There is evidence that p185^{HER2} and the EGF receptor may interact. Under certain circumstances, EGF can act through the EGF receptor to stimulate tyrosine phosphorylation on p185^{HER2} (75). It has been postulated that these related receptor proteins may form a heterodimer with growth regulatory activity (76). It can be postulated that the combined use of antibodies directed against each of these receptors could produce an effective antitumor effect.

A number of antibodies directed against the p185^{HER2} protein have been produced (74,77–81) Kern et al. (82) evaluated the Anti-p185^{HER2} monoclonal antibody 4D5, an antibody with known receptor antagonist effects against a series of human lung cancer cell lines. These included adenocarcinoma, large-cell, squamous cell, and adenosquamous cell lines. In a series of experiments it was demonstrated that 4D5 could inhibit the growth of expressing cells in a dose-dependent manner, but this was also dependent on the level of p185^{HER2} expression. The results of their experiments were consistant with the observation that the antibody was cytostatic and not cytotoxic (81). Subsequently it was shown that antibodies that bind the extracellular domain of *erb*B-2 can inhibit the development of xenografts as well as the retardation in the growth of established tumors (83).

A humanized form of 4D5, HumAb 4D5, has been developed (84) and studied in clinical trials. Two Phase I trials have been conducted, weekly doses of antibody being administered in the second without toxicity, as well as a Phase

II trial in breast cancer (85). The Phase II study evaluated the antibody in 46 patients with advanced breast cancer. Forty-three patients were evaluable for response. Patients received weekly doses of antibody until evidence of progression. One complete response was confirmed pathologically and four partial responses were observed. Given the known expression of p185^{HER2} in NSCLC, this would be an appropriate antibody for study in this disease. A Phase II trial of HumAb 4D5 in combination with cisplatin had been conducted in breast cancer based on evidence that the antibody can promote chemotherapy sensitivity (86,87).

IV. GROWTH FACTORS SPECIFIC TO SMALL-CELL LUNG CANCER

Small-cell lung cancer cells express a range of neuropeptides and growth factors (88–91). Several have been evaluated as potential targets for treatment with monoclonal antibodies. These include bombesin (gastrin-releasing polypeptide), neuromedin C, neuromedin B, rantensin, litorin, insulin-like growth factor I (IGF-I) and transferrin (92).

A. Gastrin-Releasing Peptide

1. Preclinical Data

Gastrin-releasing peptide (GRP) is the human homolog of bombesin, a 14-amino-acid peptide (93). Although there is little GRP present in the normal adult lung, it is secreted by a number of human neuroendocrine lung tumors, most notably small-cell lung cancer. Bombesin-like peptides can also be detected throughout the gastrointestinal tract and brain. Gastrin-releasing peptide is encoded by a gene on chromosome 18q (92). Bombesin, GRP, and neuromedin B (NMB) act as mitogenic peptides, and a role in the autocrine growth of certain SCLC tumors has been proposed (94). Bombesin has been shown to be produced by some small-cell carcinoma cell lines, whose proliferation it stimulates (95,96), and GRP antagonists have been reported to inhibit growth in SCLC cell lines studied (97). Most SCLC cell lines show stimulation of formation of colonies in soft agar in the presence of either ligand, and this response can be blocked by a monoclonal antibody directed against a conserved region shared on both molecules (96,98). Classic SCLC cells express high levels of GRP, whereas NMB is present at low concentrations in many lung cancer cell lines (99,100). The usual non-small-cell lung cancers, adenocarcinoma, squamous cell carcinoma, and large-cell carcinoma, do not produce immunoreactive GRP. However, NSCLC tumors with neuroendocrine features, which account for approximately 10–15% of all NSCLC, have been shown to have immunoreactive GRP (101).

In a series of preclinical studies, MAb 2A11, which binds to the carboxyl terminal portion of bombesin-like peptide, was evaluated for its ability to block access of bombesin to its receptor and thereby exert an antitumor effect (96). Studies using an agarose colony assay in serum-free media demonstrated that growth of the SCLC line NCI-N592 was inhibited. A xenograft mouse model also was studied. Mice were treated three times weekly with intraperitoneal 2A11. Tumor suppression was observed in all animals, although after 5 weeks there was subsequent progression in half of the animals. This data supported the hypothesis that the use of MAb 2A11 to prevent bombesin-like peptides from binding to specific receptors could suppress tumor growth.

2. Clinical Studies

A Phase I trial of MAb 2A11 was undertaken in patients with small-cell lung carcinoma (102). Fourteen patients received MAb 2A11 at doses ranging from 10 to 250 mg/m^2/day three times a week for 4 weeks. ^{111}In-labeled MAb localized to the tumor site, and no toxicity was reported.

The results of a subsequent Phase II study were published recently (103). Patients received twelve doses of MAb 2A11, 250 mg/m^2, over a 4-week period. Twelve of thirteen patients were evaluable for response. Of these, one had a complete radiologic response to treatment, shown in Figure 2, four had stable disease, and seven had progression. The responding patient received two cycles of therapy with MAb 2A11 and remained without radiologic evidence of progression for 5 months. When a recurrence was identified, a third cycle was administered, without benefit. Importantly, no patients developed a HAMA response to the administered antibody, permitting readministration of 2A11 to the responding patient. The observed response, seen in a patient with recurrent disease, is encouraging and supports the notion that an autocrine growth loop can be blocked by antibodies directed against either a receptor or its ligand.

B. Insulin-Like Growth Factors

Insulin-like growth factor I is a 70-amino-acid growth factor with approximately 70% homology with EGF-II and 50% sequence homology to insulin (104). Binding sites for IGF-I are present on SCLC tumors and cells (105,106). Small-cell lung cancer cells also secrete IGF-I-like activity, and ligand binding to the receptor protein results in activation of tyrosine kinase. Insulin-like growth factor I can function as an autocrine growth factor in SCLC (92,106,107), but the mitogenic response to IGF-I can be blunted by antibodies to IGF-I receptor or to IGF-I (106–108). More recently, Zia et al. (109) demonstrated that IGF-I may be a regulatory agent in NSCLC as well. The monoclonal antibody αIR-3, which inhibits the specific binding of IGF-I to receptors, was able to inhibit the growth

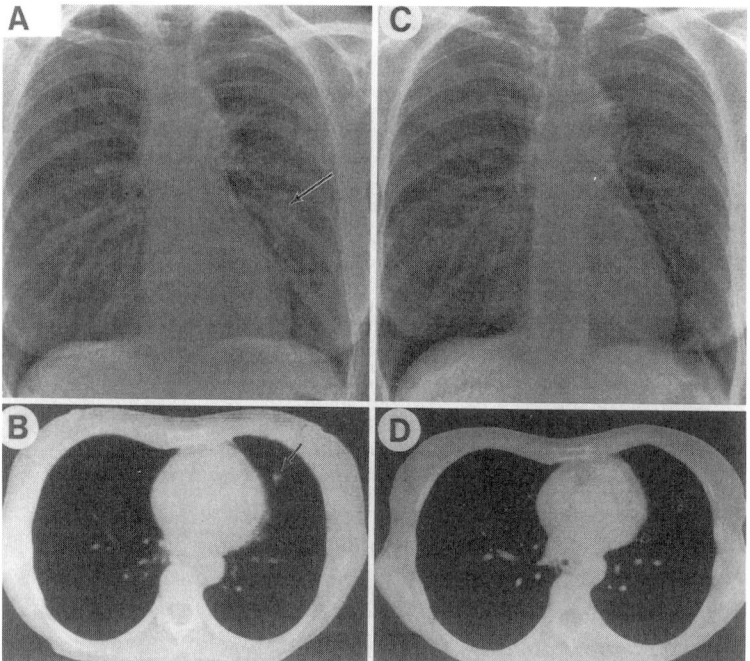

Figure 2 Antitumor effect of MAb 2A11 that binds GRP and inhibits binding of the ligand to receptor. Pretreatment chest X-ray (A) and CT scan (B) showing left midlung and upper lobe masses. Posttreatment chest X-ray (C) and CT scan (D) after one cycle of 2A11. (From Ref. 103.)

of a series of established NSCLC cell lines in vitro and in vivo using a nude mouse model. This represents another possible target in both SCLC and NSCLC.

C. Antibodies Directed Against the Neural Cell Adhesion Molecule

1. Preclinical Data

The neural cell adhesion molecule, or NCAM (CD56, NKH01), designated as a cluster-1 antigen according to the Third International Workshop on Lung Tumor and Differentiation Antigens (110), is expressed by almost all SCLC tumors studied (111–113). The NCAM is expressed on normal tissues such as nerves, endocrine cells, NK cells, and striated and cardiac muscle, but not in major organs such as the liver, kidney, lung, and bowel, (114–116). A number of antibodies have been raised against the NCAM. A mouse Anti-NCAM IgG1 MAb, NE150, was studied in a nude mouse xenograft model (117). Using the SCLC cell line NCI-H69, xenografts were established in athymic mice. The animals were then treated with a single dose of antibody. Six groups of mice were studied. Treatment groups received unlabeled NE150, NE150 radiolabeled with 11.1 or 3.7 Mbq iodine-131, an isotype-matched MAb 59A radiolabeled with 11.1-Mbq ^{131}iodine, or a sham treatment. Each animal received 70 µg of antibody. Therapy with 11.1 Mbq of ^{131}I-Ne150 produced a 60-day mean growth delay. In contrast, treatment with 11.1 Mbq ^{131}I-59A resulted in an 8-day mean growth delay, and no statistically significant growth retardation was seen with either 3.7 Mbq of ^{131}I-NE150 or unlabeled NE150. See Figure 3.

2. Clinical Studies

The use of an immunotoxin targeting the NCAM on SCLC has been reported (118). N901, a mouse IgG1 monoclonal antibody against CD56 antigen, was combined with blocked ricin to form the immunotoxin N901-bR. This had demonstrated a selectivity of greater than 700-fold for antigen-positive cells as com-

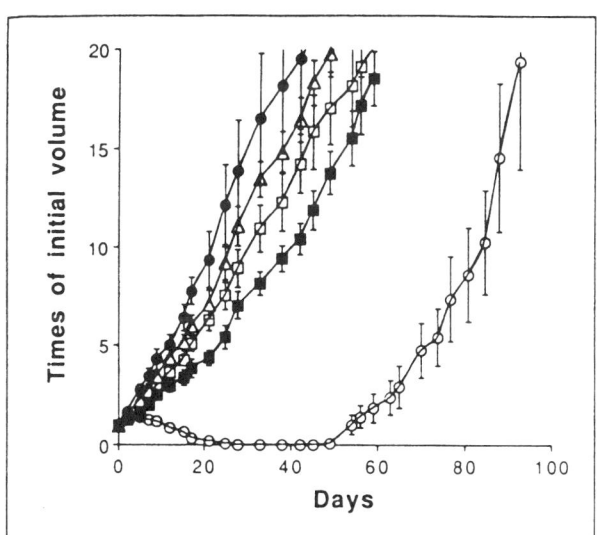

Figure 3 Use of radiolabeled Anti-NCAM MAb in the treatment of established tumors. Changes in the size of NCI-H69 xenografts after radioimmunotherapy. Five groups of mice were treated with 11.1 Mbq (○), 3.7 Mbq of ^{131}I-NE150 (□), unlabeled NE150 (△), ^{131}I-labeled irrelevant MAb (■), or a sham treatment (●). (From Ref. 117.)

pared to antigen-negative cells. In the Phase I trial, twenty-one patients with either relapsed SCLC (eighteen patients) or refractory SCLC (three patients) were studied. Groups of patients were treated with N901-bR daily for 7 days by continuous infusion. Five dose levels were evaluated: 5, 10, 20, 30, and 40 µg/kg/day. Dose-limiting toxicity occurred at a dose of 40 µg/kg/day, when two of three patients developed a capillary leak syndrome. Despite concern about possible cardiac toxicity, this was not observed, and neurotoxicity was limited to the observation that there was a trend toward decreased amplitudes on nerve conduction studies without clinical evidence of neuropathy. Most patients developed either antimouse antibodies (HAMA) or antiricin antibodies (HARA). One patient had a partial response to treatment, which persisted for 3 months without further therapy, and six patients had stable disease. Encouraged by the results of the trial, the authors report that they are conducting a trial evaluating this therapy after completion of initial chemotherapy for patients with SCLC.

V. ANTIBODIES DIRECTED AGAINST CARCINOEMBRYONIC ANTIGEN

Carcinoembryonic antigen (CEA), a tumor-associated glycoprotein first described in patients with colorectal cancer, also has been shown to be present in primary lung cancer (119,120). Said et al. (120) reported that tumors were strongly positive for CEA in six of six patients with adenocarcinoma, six of eight with squamous cell carcinoma, three of three with adenosquamous carcinoma, and eight of ten patients with large-cell carcinoma. Weakly positive or negative CEA was reported in SCLC. These observations have been confirmed by other authors (121). Three studies evaluating the use of CEA as a target for immunoscintigraphy have been published (122–124).

Krishnamurthy et al. studied the Anti-CEA monoclonal antibody ZCE 025, a mouse IgG1 antibody, in twenty men for whom there was a clinical suspicion of a primary lung cancer (122). Patients received 1 mg of antibody labeled with 4–5 mCi of indium-111. Radionuclide scans were performed on days 3 and 6 or 7 postinfusion. Scan results were correlated with chest radiographs, CT scans, bronchoscopic findings, and pathologic analysis of surgical specimens. The scintigraphy was true positive in twelve of sixteen patients with primary lung cancer, eight of nine with squamous cell carcinoma, and four of seven with adenocarcinoma. It was true negative in three of four patients who had benign lung disease. In true positive cases, the ^{111}In Anti-CEA ZCE 025 MAb imaging correlated well with CT and surgical findings.

A second study was reported by Biggi et al. (123). They studied $F(ab')_2$ fragments of the Anti-CEA antibody F023C5 labeled with indium-111 in 66 patients with ciinically suspected lung cancer. An additional eight patients with benign lung diseases also were studied. Sixty-three of 66 patients had pathologically confirmed lung cancer. Of these, 57 patients had positive immunoscintigraphic scans. Five of the six patients with negative scans had tumors less than 2 cm in diameter located in proximity to the mediastinum. Three of the eight control subjects without lung cancer had positive scans. Although SCLC is generally considered to be a non-CEA-expressing tumor, the scans were positive in all SCLC patients studied, despite immunohistochemical analysis of tumors being negative in three of the four specimens evaluated. Similar discrepancies between immunoscintigraphic and immunohistochemical results have previously been reported. Riva reported that whereas 90.7% of SCLC had positive radionuclide scans, only one of 34 specimens stained positive for CEA (125).

The third trial studied twenty-eight patients with lung cancer, twenty-one squamous cell, five adenocarcinoma, one large-cell, and one SCLC. Using unspecified $F(ab')_2$ fragments of an Anti-CEA antibody labeled with indium-111, immunoscintigraphic scans were correlated with conventional staging modalities. In twenty-one patients the primary tumor was imaged using the Anti-CEA MAb, and in seventeen of twenty-one (81%) there was concordance between the conventional preoperative staging and the radionuclide scans. In two patients the Anti-CEA MAb scan overstaged the tumor, and in two others mediastinal disease identified on the antibody scan but not by conventional staging was confirmed at surgery. In all three studies, the presence of the heart and great vessels within the mediastinum limited the utility of the antibody scan as a means of accurately staging mediastinal disease and aiding in the preoperative evaluation of patients with NSCLC.

VI. High-Molecular-Weight Human Milk Fat Globule Antigens

High-molecular-weight human milk fat globule (HMFG) antigens also are expressed on a number of tumors of epithelial origin. A number of monoclonal antibodies that react with HMFG antigens have been reported to react with breast, ovarian, and colorectal tumors (126). Kalofonos and colleagues conducted an imaging trial in fourteen patients with NSCLC (127). They used the $F(ab')_2$ fragments of HMFG1, an IgG1 monoclonal antibody raised against a component of human milk fat globule membranes and shown to react with NSCLC tumors (128). Twelve patients had squamous cell carcinoma and two had adenocarcinoma. Patients received an intravenous infusion of 150–250 µg of MAb with a specific activity of 5 mCi/mg. In addition, seven of the patients were studied using an equal dose of ^{111}In-labeled $F(ab')_2$ fragments of a nonspecific monoclonal antibody 4C4, either 2 weeks prior to or after study with HMFG1 MAb. The primary tumor and four of five known sites of distant metastatic disease were identified by immunoscintigraphy with the specific antibody. However, tumor was identified using the nonspecific MAb 4C4 in five of the seven patients studied, although the specificity index was higher with HMFG1 in three of these patients. Noting the 70% positive scan rate using a nonspecific antibody, compared with the 100% positive scan rate with HMFG1, the authors proposed that imaging with nonspecific antibodies be incorporated into future imaging trials.

In a second trial, the mouse IgG3 monoclonal antibody KC-4G3 that recognizes a human milk fat globule antigen was studied (126). Twenty-four patients with histologically confirmed NSCLC were studied. Twenty-three had been evaluated for the presence of KC-4 antigen on their tumors, and all were positive. Twelve patients had adenocarcinoma, six squamous cell carcinoma, three adenosquamous cell carcinomas, one undifferentiated carcinoma, and one bronchoalveolar carcinoma. In all, 91 sites of disease were identified by conventional staging modalities, including physical examination, chest X-rays, CT scans, and radionuclide scans. One milligram of KC-4G3 antibody was labeled with 5 mCi of indium-111, and patients received a total dose of 1, 10, 50, 100, or 200 mg. Early blood pool activity gradually cleared over 48–72 hours postinfusion. Immunoscintigraphy was most successful in pulmonary lesions (31 of 45) and soft tissue lesions (4 of 5). Successful images were also obtained for four of eleven lymph node metastases, six of nineteen bone lesions, two of four adrenal metastases, two of two liver metastases, and two of two kidney metastases. Overall, 92% of patients had at least one lesion visualized, and 57% of the 91 lesions were identified. The success of imaging correlated with the size of the lesion, and in a few patients areas of antibody localization were seen that did not correlate with known sites of disease and may have represented unidentified metastases. The authors concluded that further study was appropriate, but the sensitivity of the modality needed improvement. Given the findings reported by Kalofonos (127) using a nonspecific MAb, it is apparent that the utility of antibodies directed against HMFG remains to be shown.

VII. NR-LU-10

NR-LU-10 is a mouse IgG2b monoclonal antibody that recognizes a 40-kDa cell-surface glycoprotein antigen expressed by many carcinomas, including those of lung, prostate, colon, breast, and ovary. The antigen has not been well characterized but is present on both SCLC and NSCLC cells. There also is localization to normal thyroid, salivary glands, and anterior pituitary (129). The intact antibody, the F(ab')$_2$ fragments, and the Fab have been studied. Recently, the Fab fragments of the antibody, termed Nofetumomab, radiolabeled with technetium-

99, was approved by the U.S. Food and Drug Administration (FDA) as an imaging modality in SCLC. Currently, clinical trials are ongoing to evaluate it as a therapeutic modality in a number of malignancies, including lung cancer.

The results of a Phase III imaging trail were reported individually by a number of participating investigators. Morris and colleagues reported the results of imaging studies using intact antibody labeled with technetium-99m in patients with small-cell lung cancer (130). Five patients with known SCLC were studied by routine staging modalities, during which fifteen chest lesions, six bone lesions, liver metastases in one patient, adrenal metastases, and one intracranial lesion were identified. Immunoscintigraphy using NR-LU-10 Fab then was performed. Fourteen of the fifteen chest lesions were identified by this means, including one not identified by conventional means. Four of six bone lesions and the liver metastases also were identified by immunoscintigraphy. However, labeled antibody did not concentrate in either the adrenal or the brain lesions. The investigators concluded that NR-LU-10 had potential usefulness as a complementary imaging modality in this disease.

The results in another group of seventeen patients with SCLC was reported by Balaban and colleagues (129). Twenty-two evaluations were performed, five patients being reevaluated after therapy. A total of 73 lesions were identified by conventional staging. Of these, 54 (74%) were detected by the radiolabeled antibody. Seven of eight patients staged as having limited stage disease by conventional imaging modalities were concordantly staged using the labeled NR-LU-10. In the eighth patient, bone marrow involvement was demonstrated by the antibody scan and subsequently confirmed by repeat bone marrow biopsy. Two patients considered to have extensive-stage disease after conventional staging were staged as limited disease by immunoscintigraphy. The overall accuracy of the monoclonal antibody in staging patients was reported to be 88%. Of note, in one patient a brain metastasis seen on CT scan also was identified by the antibody scan. Most lesions not identified by immunoscintigraphy were less than 1 cm in diameter and were located in the liver.

In a second paper, the same group reported their experience with the evaluation of bone marrow involvement in SCLC patients using NR-LU-10 Fab labeled with Tc-99m (131). After fifteen patients underwent antibody scanning, three were diagnosed as having bone marrow involvement, including the one apparently reported in their later paper (129). Although the final results of the Phase III trial have yet to be published, they are reported in the package insert of the FDA-licensed product TC99m Nofetumomab Merpentan (Verluma™). An overall staging accuracy of 82% is reported, superior to any other single test, although conventional imaging studies were individually superior for the evaluation of individual organs or areas, and on the basis of these data the agent was approved by the FDA for the detection of extensive-stage disease in patients with SCLC.

NR-LU-10 also has been evaluated for the staging of patients with NSCLC (132–135). Rusch et al. (132) reported the results in twenty-four previously untreated patients. Fourteen men and ten women with potentially resectable non-small-cell lung cancer were studied. All patients underwent both computerized tomography and immunoscintigraphy. Thereafter patients underwent mediastinoscopy or thoracotomy with complete mediastinal lymph node mapping for pathologic correlation. Patients received 20–30 mCi (5–10 mg) of 99mTc-labeled NR-LU-10 (Fab) intravenously and underwent whole-body and single-photon emission computed tomography (SPECT) 14–17 hours postinfusion. In one patient a prior ventilation perfusion scan precluded adequate imaging. In the remaining twenty-three patients, good-quality images were obtained. Uptake was seen in twenty-two pulmonary lesions later proven to be malignant. In the one patient whose pulmonary lesion was subsequently proven to be benign there was no antibody localization to the lesion. With respect to the evaluation of the mediastinal lymph nodes of the twenty-one patients who underwent a surgical procedure, the NR-LU-10 scans were false positive in five and false negative in one. This was comparable to the results by computerized tomographic (CT) scan, with six false positives and one false negative.

Friedman et al. (135) reported the preliminary results of the imaging trial in NSCLC. Fifty-two patients had been studied at the time of publication. Twenty-six were potential surgical candidates. Staging by means of NR-LU-10 imaging was compared to conventional staging. They calculated the positive predictive value (PPV) of CT scan for (TNM) N2 disease as 100%. However, the negative predictive value (NPV) was only 72–83%; i.e. the correct stage was identified by CT in 72–81% of cases. For antibody scanning, the PPV was 75–100% and the NPV 92%, and the correct stage was identified in 81–90% of patients. In combination, the overall sensitivity was 100%, PPV was 78–100%, and NPV was 100%. Stewart et al. (134) and Vansant et al. (133), who evaluated both SCLC and NSCLC patients, reported similar results.

NR-LU-10 also has been evaluated for immunotherapy of solid tumors and a Phase I/II clinical trial is currently being conducted under the tradename of Avicidin™. In preclinical studies with rhenium-labeled NR-LU-10, responses were seen in nude mice with human lung cancer xenografts (136). Subcutaneous xenografts of the human SCLC cell line SHT-1 were established in nude mice that were then treated with a total dose of 500–600 µCi ^{186}Re-NR-LU-10 in divided doses. Three of sixteen mice had complete remissions, and the remainder showed a mean tumor growth delay of 53 days. This was substantially better than the control arm, in which eight mice were treated with a radiolabeled irrelevant antibody. One of the control mice experienced a treatment-related death, one achieved a complete response, and these mice experienced a mean growth delay of 20 days. The results of a Phase I trial of rhenium-186-labeled NR-LU-10 have been reported in which dose limiting toxicity was seen at a radionuclide dose of 120 mCi/m^2 (137,138). The current clinical trail in solid tumors employs a streptavidin-biotin type of system in which the antibody is administered first followed by the radionuclide.

VII. GANGLIOSIDES IN LUNG CANCER

Gangliosides are glycosphingolipids, composed of a ceramide portion that anchors the ganglioside into the plasma membrane and a carbohydrate moiety oriented to the exterior. They are ubiquitous constituents of mammalian cells. Due to differences in the carbohydrate moiety, a large number of distinct gangliosides exist with differing patterns of distribution. Certain gangliosides have been shown to have high levels of expression in certain tumors, including SCLC, with relatively low levels of expression in normal tissues. These include the gangliosides GD2, GD3, GM2, and fucosyl-GM1 (139–143). Ganglioside function is not well defined but appears to play a role in tumor cell attachment to extracellular matrix in certain malignancies (144). Because of their relatively restricted expression on normal tissues and organs, these three gangliosides represent potential immunologic targets in SCLC. Using the Anti-GD2 antibody 3F8 and the Anti-GD3 antibody R24 we were able to target SCLC xenografts in nude mice (Grant, unpublished data). Studies by Hanibuchi et al. (143) evaluated the ability of KM966, a mouse-human chimeric MAb against GM2, to induce lymphocyte- and monocyte-mediated lysis of SCLC cells in vitro. They also demonstrated lysis of NSCLC cells in the same system.

A. Clinical Trials

1. Imaging of Small-Cell Lung Cancer with Antiganglioside Antibodies

In a pilot study, MAb 3F8 was evaluated for its ability to target tumor sites in patients with SCLC (145). Twelve patients were enrolled in this trial, and ten received intravenous 3F8 labeled with 2 or 10 mCi of I-131. The first five patients had recurrent or progressive disease after chemotherapy, and the remaining seven patients were treated at the time of diagnosis, prior to the initiation of chemotherapy. Radionuclide scanning was performed on days 1, 2, and 3 postinfusion and once between day 5 and day 7. Four patients were imaged with single-photon emission tomography (SPECT). Radionuclide scans demonstrated localization to all known sites of disease, other than small brain metastases in one patient. SPECT/CT fusion images confirmed precise localization. These findings support the role of further studies to evaluate therapeutic application of Anti-GD2 antibodies in SCLC. See Figure 4.

2. Active Immunization Against Gangliosides

Antibodies directed against GD3 have demonstrated antitumor activity against metastic melanoma, another tumor that expresses high levels of GD3 (146). Chapman and co-workers developed a mouse anti-idiotypic IgG2 antibody against GD3 and demonstrated that the antibody, designated BEC2, could induce Anti-GD3 antibodies in rabbits (147). Subsequent trials have evaluated BEC2 in patients with melanoma and small-cell lung cancer (148). BEC2 was combined with BCG as an immune stimulant in an attempt to improve the antibody response to a series of immunizations. Patients with SCLC who had a major response to initial therapy were evaluated for their ability to be immunized against GD3 ganglioside.

Fifteen patients, of whom eight had extensive-stage disease at the time of diagnosis, were evaluated in the trial. BEC-2 was administered intradermally at a dose of 2.5 mg together with BCG, which was used as an immune adjuvant. For each patient, the initial dose of BCG was 3×10^7 CFU. The dose of BCG was reduced for each successive immunization. The BEC-2/BCG mixture was administered on weeks 0, 2, 4, 6, and 10. All patients developed Anti-BEC-2 (HAMA) antibodies. Five of thirteen patients evaluable for a serologic response developed detectable levels of Anti-GD3 IgG antibodies. Adverse effects were limited to local skin toxicity, which necessitated dose attenuation for $\geq 3+$ toxicity in fourteen of fifteen patients. Five patients are alive, without evidence of recurrent or progressive SCLC. Survival from the time of initial diagnosis for these patients ranged from 19.3 to 57.3 months and is superior to historical control groups of patients. Based on the encouraging results of this trial, a Phase III trial

Figure 4 Targeting of SCLC using the Anti-GD2 antibody 3F8. Chest X-ray showing a right lung mass and hilar adenopathy (top left) and radionuclide scan on day 3 postinfusion (top right) of a patient with extensive stage disease. The patient had a primary tumor located in the lower lobe of the right lung. Metastases to mediastinal lymph nodes, as well as three large liver metastases, were present. At the bottom, selected SPECT images are shown. Scan numbers 41–43 show serial cuts through a liver metastasis. Scans 25–27 show coronal sections through the lung primary metastasis and one of the liver metastases. Scans 36–38 are sagittal sections throught the lung primary metastasis and three liver metastases. In the bottom right-hand corner, a volume-averaged SPECT scan demonstrates uptake in the lower lobe of the right lung, mediastinum, and multiple liver metastases. (From Ref. 145.)

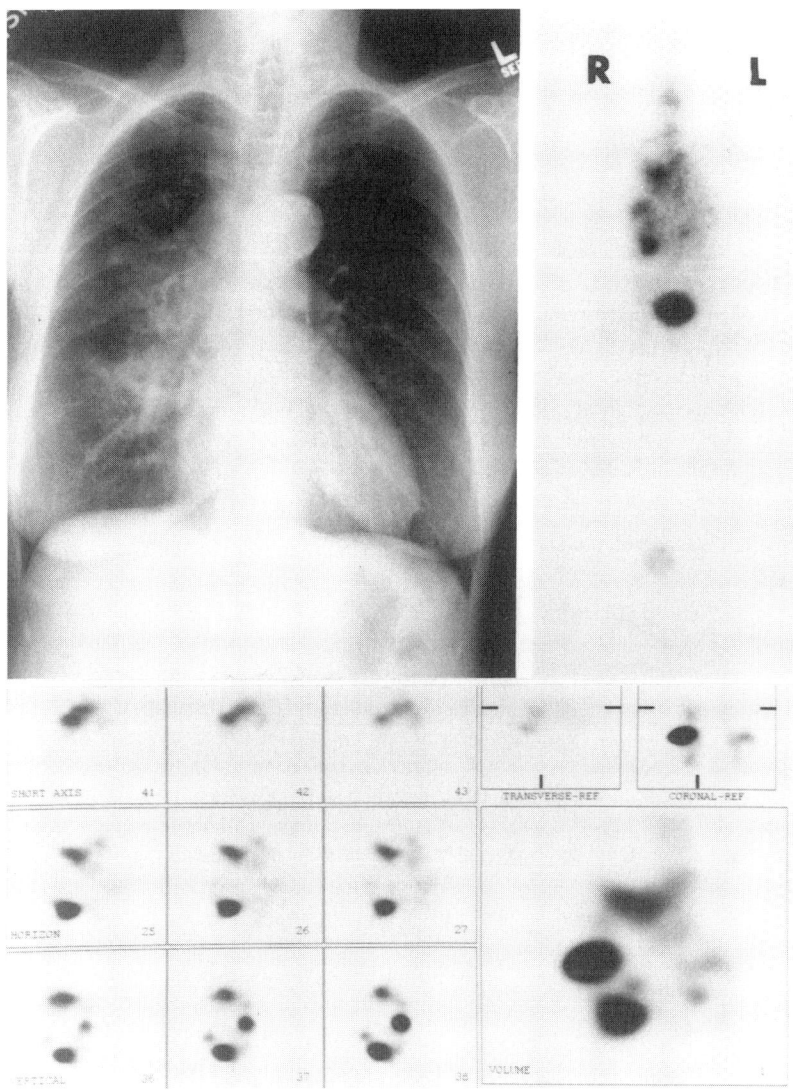

is being initiated. Patients with limited-stage disease will receive standard therapy and then be randomized either to receive BEC2 plus BCG or to observation. Trials evaluating the feasibility of active immunization against other gangliosides are now under way.

IX. CONCLUSION

Lung cancer is an excellent model in which to explore the role of monoclonal antibodies in the diagnosis and treatment of solid tumors. Small-cell lung cancer is highly responsive to therapy, and patients with early-stage NSCLC undergo apparent, complete surgical resections. Despite this, patients in both groups relapse and die from their disease. The experience with monoclonal antibodies suggests that this diagnostic and therapeutic modality has the potential to have a major impact on these diseases. As our knowledge of tumor immunology increases, we can anticipate rapid growth in the study and use of monoclonal antibodies in lung cancer.

REFERENCES

1. Boring CC, Squires TS, Tong T, Montgomery S. Cancer Statistics 1997. CA-A Cancer Journal for Clinicians 1997; 47.
2. Vaikus L, Foon KA. Overview of monoclonal antibodies in the diagnosis and therapy of cancer. Cancer Invest 1991; 9:195–209.
3. Stahel RA, Mabry M, Sabbath K, Speak JA, Bernal SD. Selective cytotoxicity of murine monoclonal antibody LAM2 against human small-cell carcinoma in the presence of human complement: Possible use for in vitro elimination of tumor cells from bone marrow. Int J Cancer 1985; 35:587–592.
4. Souhami RL, Beverly PCL, Bobrow LG, Ledermann JA. Antigens of lung cancer: results of the Second International Workshop on Lung Cancer Antigens. J Natl Cancer Inst 1991; 83:809–812.
5. Patel K, Moore SE, Dickson G, et al. Neural cell adhesion molecule is the antigen recognized by monoclonal antibodies of similar specificity in small cell lung carcinoma and neuroblastoma. Int J Cancer 1989; 44:573–578.
6. Carbone DP, Koros AMC, Linnoila RI, Jewett P, Gazdar AF. Neural cell adhesion molecule expression and messenger RNA splicing patterns in lung cancer cell lines are correlated with neuroendocrine phenotype and growth morphology. Cancer Res 1991; 51:6142–6149.
7. Strnad J, Hamilton AE, Beavers LS, et al. Molecular cloning and characterization of a human adenocarcinoma/epithelial cell surface antigen complementary DNA. Cancer Res 1989; 49:314–317.
8. Jackson D, Waibel R, Weber E, Bell J, Stahel RA. CD24, a signal transduction

molecule expressed on human B cells, is a major surface antigen in small cell lung carcinomas. Cancer Res 1992; 52:5264–5270.
9. Bunn PA, Linnoila I, Minna JD. Small cell lung cancer, endocrine cells of the fetal bronchus, and other neuroendocrine cells express the leu-7 antigenic determinant present on natural killer cells. Blood 1986; 65:764–768.
10. Ruff MR, Pert CB. Small cell carcinoma of the lung: macrophage-specific antigens suggest hemopoietic stem cell origin. Science 1984; 225:1034–1036.
11. Feldman LE, Shink KC, Natale KB, Todd 3d RF. Beta-1 integrin expression on human small cell lung cancer cells. Cancer Res 1991; 51:1065–1070.
12. Schwartz MA, Scheinberg DA, Houghton AN. Monoclonal antibody therapy. Cancer Chemother Biol Response Modif 1992; 13:156–174.
13. Schlessinger J. The epidermal growth factor receptor as a multi-functional allosteric protein. Biochem J 1988; 27:3119–3123.
14. Thompson DM, Gill GN. The EGF receptor: structure, regulation and potential role in malignancy. Cancer Survey 1985; 4:767–788.
15. Neal D, Bennett M, Hall R, et al. Epidermal growth factor receptors in human bladder cancer. Comparison of invasive and superficial tumors. Lancet 1985; 1: 366–368.
16. Sainsbury JRC, Malcolm AJ, Appleton DR, Farndon JR, Harris AL. Presence of epidermal growth factor receptor as an indicator of poor prognosis in patients with breast cancer. Journal of Clinical Pathology 1985; 38.
17. Sainsbury JRC, Farndon JR, Sherbet GV, Harris AL. Epidermal growth-factor receptors and oestrogen receptors in human breast cancer. Lancet 1985; 1:364–366.
18. Carpenter G. Epidermal growth factor. Annu Rev Biochem 1979; 48:193–216.
19. Shoyab M, Plowman GD, McDonald VL, Bradley JG, Todaro GJ. Structure and function of human amphiregulin: a member of the epidermal growth factor family. Science 1989; 243:1074–1076.
20. Massague J. Transforming growth factor-α. J Biol Chem 1990; 265:21,393–21,396.
21. Higashiyama S, Abraham JA, Miller J, Fiddes JC, Klagsbrun M. A heparin-binding growth factor secreted by macrophage-like cells that is related to EGF. Science 1991; 251:936–939.
22. Hendler FJ, Ozanne BW. Human squamous cell lung cancers express increased epidermal growth factor receptors. J Clin Invest 1984; 74.
23. Sobol RE, Astarita RW, Hofeditz C. EGF receptor expression in human lung carcinomas defined by a monclonal antibody. J Natl Cancer Inst 1987; 79:403–407.
24. Veale D, Ashcroft T, Marsh C, Gibson GJ, Harris AL. Epidermal growth factor receptors in non-small cell lung cancer. Br J Cancer 1987; 55:513–516.
25. Hendler F, Shum-Siu A, Nanu L, Yuan D, Ozanne B. Increased EGF receptors and the absence of an alveolar differentiation marker predict a poor survival in lung cancer. Proc Am Soc Clin Oncol 1989; 8.
26. Veale D, Kerr N, Gibson J, Harris A. Characterization of epidermal growth factor receptor in primary human non-small cell lung cancer. Cancer Res 1989; 49:1313–1317.
27. Rusch V, Baselga J, Cordon-Cardo C, et al. Differential expression of the epidermal growth factors receptor and its ligands in primary non-small cell lung cancers and adjacent benign lung. Cancer Res 1993; 53:2379–2385.

28. Libermann TA, Razon N, Bartal AD, Yarden Y, Schlessinger J, Soreq H. Expression of epidermal growth factor receptors in human head and neck tumors. Cancer Res 1984; 44:753–760.
29. Sherwin S, Minna JD, Gazdar AF, Todaro G. Expression of epidermal and nerve growth factor receptors and soft agar growth factor production by human lung cancer cells. Cancer Res 1981; 41:3538–3542.
30. Cerny T, Barnes D, Hasleton P, et al. Expression of epidermal growth factor receptor (EGF-R) in human lung tumours. Br J Cancer 1986; 54:265–269.
31. Haeder M, Rotsch MM, Bepler G, et al. Epidermal growth factor receptor expression in human lung cancer cell lines. Cancer Res 1988; 48:1132–1136.
32. Damstrup L, Rorth M, Poulsen HS. Growth factors and growth factors receptors in human malignancies, with special reference to human lung cancer. Lung Cancer 1989; 5:49–68.
33. Berger MS, Gullick WJ, Greenfield C, Evans S, Addis BJ, Waterfield MD. Epidermal growth factor receptors in lung tumors. J Pathol 1987; 152:297–307.
34. Tateishi M, Ishida T, Mitsudomi T, Kaneko S, Sugimachi K. Immunohistochemical evidence of autocrine growth factors in adenocarcinoma of the human lung. Cancer Res 1990; 50:7077–7080.
35. Hwang DL, Yay Y-C, Lin SS, Lev-ran A. Expression of epidermal growth factor receptors in human lung tumors. Cancer 1986; 48:2260–2263.
36. Sato JD, Kawamoto T, Le AD, Mendelsohn J. Biological effect in vitro of monoclonal antibodies to human EGF receptors. Molecular Biol Med 1983; 1:511–529.
37. Kawamoto T, Sato JD, Le A, Polikoff J, Sato GH, Mendelsohn J. Growth stimulation of A431 cells by EGF: identification of high affinity receptors for epidermal growth factor by an anti-receptor monoclonal antibody. Proc Natl Acad Sci USA 1983; 80:1337–1341.
38. Gill GN, Kawamoto T, Cochet C, et al. Monoiclonal anti-EGF receptor antibodies which are inhibitors of growth factor binding and antagonists of EGF-stimulated tyrosine protein kinase activity. J Biol Chem 1984; 259:7755–7760.
39. Reiss M, Stash EB, Vellucci VF, Zhou Z-I. Activation of the autocrine transforming growth factor alpha pathway in human squamous carcinoma cells. Cancer Res 1992; 51:6254–6262.
40. Fan Z, Masui H, Atlas I, Mendelsohn J. Blockade of EGF receptor functions by bivalent and manovalent fragments of 225 anti-EGF receptor monoclonal antibody. Cancer Res 1993; 53:4322–4328.
41. Fan Z, Lu Y, Wu X, Mendelsohn J. Antibody-induced epidermal growth factor receptor dimerization and down-regulation block autocrine proliferation of A431 squamous carcinoma cells. J Biol Chem 1994; 269.
42. Masui H, Kawamoto T, Sato JD, Wolf B, Sato G, Mendelsohn J. Growth inhibition of human tumor cells in athymic mice by anti-epidermal growth factor receptor monoclonal antibodies. Cancer Res 1984; 44:1002–1007.
43. Imanishi K-i, Yamaguchi K, Kuranami M, Kyo E, Hozumi T, Abe K. Inhibition of growth of human lung adenocarcinoma cell lines by anti-transforming growth factor-α monoclonal antibody. J Natl Cancer Inst 1989; 81:220–223.
44. Goldenberg A, Masui H, Divgi C, Kamrath H, Pentlow K, Mendelsohn J. EGF receptor overexpression and localization of nude mouse xenografts using indium-

111 labelled anti-EGF receptor monoclonal antibody. J Natl Cancer Inst 1989; 81: 1616–1625.
45. Aboud-Pirak E, Hurwitz E, Pirak ME, Bellot F, Schlessinger J, Sela M. Efficacy of antibodies to epidermal growth factor receptor against KB carcinoma in vitro and in nude mice. J Natl Cancer Inst 1988; 80:1605–1611.
46. Baselga J, Norton L, Masui H, et al. Antitumor effects of doxorubicin in combination with anti-epidermal growth factor receptor monoclonal antibodies. J Natl Cancer Inst 1993; 85:16.
47. Fan Z, Baselga J, Masui H, Mendelsohn J. Antitumor effect of anti-epidermal growth factor receptor monoclonal antibodies plus *cis*-diamminedichloroplatinum on well-established A431 cell xenografts. Cancer Res 1993; 53:4637–4642.
48. Divgi CR, Kris M, Real FX, et al. Phase I and imaging trial of indium-111-labeled anti-epidermal growth factor receptor monoclonal antibody 225 in patients with squamous cell lung carcinoma. J Natl Cancer Inst 1991; 83:97–104.
49. Scott AM, Baselga J, Divgi CR, et al. Comparison of Phase I trials of anti-epidermal growth factor receptor (EGFR) monoclonal antibodies (MAbs) 528 and 225 labelled with I-131 and In-111 (abstr). J Nucl Med 1993; 34:213P.
50. Falcey J, Pfister D, Cohen R, et al. A study of anti-epidermal growth factor receptor (EGFr) monoclonal antibody C225 and cisplatin in patients (pts) with head and neck or lung carcinomas (abstr). Proc Am Soc Clin Oncol 1997; 16:383a.
51. Lax I, Bellot F, Howk R, Ullrich A, Givol D, Schlessinger J. Functional analysis of the ligand binding site of EGF-receptor utilizing chimeric chicken/human receptor molecules. EMBO J 1989; 8:421–427.
52. Perez-Soler R, Donato NJ, Shin DM, et al. Tumor epidermal growth factor receptor studies in patients with non-small cell lung cancer or head and neck cancer treated with monoclonal antibody RG 83852. J Clin Oncol 1994; 12:730–739.
53. Christen RD, Hom DK, Porter DC, et al. Epidermal growth factor regulates the in vitro sensitivity of human ovarian carcinoma cells to cisplatin. J Clin Invest 1990; 86:1632–1640.
54. Kwok TT, Sutherland RM. Enhancement of sensitivity of human squamous carcinomas cells to radiation by epidermal growth factor receptor. J Natl Cancer Inst 1989; 81:1020–1024.
55. Kwok TT, Sutherland RM. Differences in EGF related radiosensitization of human squamous carcinoma cells with high and low numbers of EGF receptors. Br J Cancer 1991; 64:251–254.
56. Nishikawa K, Rosenblum MG, Newman RA, Pandita TK, Hittelman WN, Donato NJ. Resistance of human cervical carcinoma cells to tumor necrosis factor correlates with their increased sensitivity to cisplatin: evidence of a role for DNA repair and epidermal growth factor receptor. Cancer Res 1992; 52:4758–4765.
57. Grant SC, Pisters KMW, Divgi C, et al. Phase I trial of RG 83852, an anti-epidermal growth factor (EGF) receptor monoclonal antibody (MAb) in non-small cell lung cancer (NSCLC). Proc Am Assoc Cancer Res 1992; 33.
58. Modjtahedi H, Hickish T, Nicolson M, et al. Phase I trial and tumor localization of the anti-EGFR monoclonla antibody ICR62 in head and neck or lung cancer. Br J Cancer 1996; 73:228–235.
59. Coussens L, Yang-Feng TL, Liao YC, et al. Tyrosine kinase receptor with extensive

homology to EGF receptor shares chromosomal location with *neu* oncogene. Science 1985; 230:1132–1139.
60. Akiyama T, Sudo C, Ogawara H, Toyoshima K, Yamamoto T. The product of the human c-*erb*B2 gene: a 185,000-dalton glycoprotein with tyrosine kinase activity. Science 1986; 232:1644–1646.
61. Stern DF, Hefferman PA, Weinberg RA. p185, a product of the *neu* proto-oncogene, is a receptor-like protein associated with tyrosine kinase activity. Mol Cell Biol 1986; 6:1729–1740.
62. Huziak RM, Schlessinger J, Ullrich A. Increased expression of the putative growth factor receptor p 185 (HER2) causes transformation and tumorigenesis of NIH3T3 cells. Proc Natl Acad Sci USA 1987; 84.
63. Schechter AL, Hung MC, Vaidyanathan L, et al. The *neu* gene: an *erb*B-homologous gene distinct from and unlinked to the gene encoding the EGF receptor. Science 1985; 229:976–978.
64. DiFiore PP, Pierce JH, Kraus MH, Segatto O, King CR, Aaronson SA. *erb*B-2 is a potent oncogene when overexpressed in NIH/3T3 cells. Science 1986; 237:178–182.
65. Muller W, Sinn E, Patengale P, Wallace R, Leder P. Single-step induction of mammary adenocarcinoma in transgenic mice bearing the activated c-*neu* oncogene. Cell 1988; 54.
66. Kern JA, Schwartz DA, Nordberg JE, et al. p185^{neu} expression in human lung adenocarcinomas predicts shortened survival. Cancer Res 1990; 50:5184–5187.
67. Slamon DJ, Clark GM, Wong SG, Levin WJ, Ullrich A, McGuire WL. Human breast cancer correlation of relapse and survival with amplification of the HER-2/*neu* oncogene. Science 1987; 1987:177–182.
68. Slamon DJ, Gogolphin W, Jones LA, et al. Studies of the HER-2/*neu* proto-oncogene in human breast and ovarian cancer. Science 1989; 244:707–712.
69. Van de Vijver MJ, Peterse JL, Mooi WJ, et al. *Neu*-protein overexpression in breast cancer: association with comedo-type ductal carcinoma in situ and limited prognostic value in stage II breast cancer. N Engl J Med 1988; 319:1239–1245.
70. Wright C, Angus B, Nicholson S, et al. Expression of c-*Erb*B-2 oncoprotein: a prognostic indicator in human breast cancer. Cancer Res 1989; 49:2087–2090.
71. Paik S, Fisher ER, Fisher B, et al. Pathological findings from national Surgical Adjuvant Breast Project (protocol B-06), prognosis significance of *erb*B-2 protein overexpression in primary breast cancer. J Clin Oncol 1990; 8:103–112.
72. Pastorino U, Sozzi G, Miozzo M, Tagliabue E, Pilotti S, Pierotti MA. Genetic changes in lung cancer. J Cell Biochem 1993; 17F(Suppl): 237–248.
73. Urban JL, Shepard HM, Rothstein JL, Sugarman BJ, Schreiber H. Tumor necrosis factor: A potent effector molecule for tumor cell killing by activated macrophages. Proc Natl Acad Sci USA 1986; 83:5233–5237.
74. Hancock MC, Langton BC, Chan T, et al. A monoclonal antibody against c-*erb*B-2 protein enhances the cytotoxicity of *cis*-diamminedichloroplatinum against human breast and ovarian tumor cells. Cancer Res 1991; 51:4575–4580.
75. Stern DF, Kamps MP. EGF-stimulated tyrosine phosphorylation of p185*neu*: a potential model for receptor interactions. EMBO J 1988; 7:995–1001.
76. Wada T, Quian X, Greene MI. Intermolecular association of the p185*neu* pro-

tein and EGF receptor modulates EGF receptor function. Cell 1990; 61:1339–1347.
77. Hudziak RM, Lewis GD, Winget M, Fendly BM, Shepard HM, Ullrich A. p185^{HER2} monoclonal antibody has antiproliferative effects in vitro and sensitizes human breast tumor cells to tumor necrosis factor. Mol Cell Biol 1989; 9:1165–1172.
78. Kasprzyk PG, Song SU, DiFiore PP, King CR. Therapy of an animal model of human gastric cancer using a combination of anti-*erb*B-2 monoclonal antibodies. Cancer Res 1992; 52:2771–2776.
79. McKenzie SJ, Marks PJ, Lam T, et al. Generation and characterization of monoclonal antibodies specific for the human *neu* oncogene product, p185. Oncogene 1989; 4:543–548.
80. Drebin JA, Link VC, Stern DF, Weinberg RA, Greene MI. Down-modulation of an oncogene protein product and reversion of the transformed phenotype by monoclonal antibodies. Cell 1985; 41:695–706.
81. Fendly BM, Winget M, Hudziak RM, Lipari MT, Napier MA, Ullrich A. Characterization of murine monoclonal antibodies reactive to either the human epidermal growth factor receptor or HER2/*neu* gene product. Cancer Res 1990; 50:1550–1558.
82. Kern J, Torney L, Weiner D, Gazdar A, Shepard M, Fendly B. Inhibition of human lung cancer cell line growth by an anti-p185^{HER2} antibody. Am J Respir Cell Mol Biol 1993; 9:448–454.
83. Harwerth IM, Wels W, Schlegel J, Müller M, Hynes NE. Monoclonal antibodies directed to the *erb*B-2 receptor inhibits in vivo tumor cell growth. Br J Cancer 1993; 68:1140–1145.
84. Carter P, Presta L, Gorman CM, et al. HUmanization of an anti-p185^{HER2} antibody for human cancer therapy. Proc Natl Acad Sci USA 1992; 89:4285–4289.
85. Baselga J, Tripathy D, Mendelsohn J, et al. Phase II study of weekly intravenous recombinant humanized anti-p185^{HER2} monoclonal antibody in patients with HER2/*neu*-overexpressing metastatic breast cancer. J Clin Oncol 1996; 14:737–744.
86. Pegram MD, Pietras RJ, Slamon DJ. Monoclonal antibody to HER-2/*neu* gene product potentiates cytotoxicity of carboplatin and doxorubicin in human breast tumor cells. Proc Am Assoc Cancer Res 1992; 33:442.
87. Pietras RJ, Scates S, Howell SB, Slamon DJ. Monoclonal antibody to HER2/*neu* receptor modulates DNA repair and platinum sensitivity in human breast and ovarian carcinoma cells. Proc Am Assoc Cancer Res 1992; 33:3272.
88. Livingston RB. Small cell lung cancer: from the laboratory to the clinic. Anticancer Res 1994; 14.
89. Carney D. Biology of small cell lung cancer. Lancet 1992; 339:843–846.
90. Woll P. Growth factors and lung cancer. Thorax 1991; 46:924–929.
91. Linnoila RI, Mulshine JL, Steinberg SM, et al. Neuroendocrine differentiation in endocrine and non-endocrine lung carcinomas. Am J Clin Pathol 1988; 90:641–652.
92. Moody TW, Cuttitta F. Growth factor and peptide receptors in small cell lung cancer. Life Sci 1993; 52:1161–1173.
93. Lebacq-Verheyden AM, Trepel JT, Sausville EA. Bombesin and gastrin-releasing peptide: neuropeptides, secretogogues, and growth factors. In: Sporn M, Roberts

A, eds. Peptide Growth Factors and Their Receptors. Handbook of Experimental Pharmacology. Vol. II. Berlin, Heidelberg: Springer-Verlag, 1990:71–124.
94. Cuttitta F, Fedorko J, Gu J, Lebacq-Verheyden AM, Linnoila RI, Battey JF. Gastrin-releasing peptide gene-associated peptides are expressed in normal human fetal lung and small cell lung cancer: a novel peptide family found in man. J Clin Endocrinol Metab 1988; 67:576–583.
95. Carney DN, Bunn PA, Gazdar AF, Pagan JA, Minna JD. Selective growth in serum-free hormone-supplemented medium of tumor cells obtained by biopsy from patients with small cell carcinoma of the lung. Proc Na Acad Sci USA 1981; 78: 3185–3189.
96. Cuttitta F, Carney DN, Mulshine J, et al. Bombesin-like peptides can function as autocrine growth factors in human small-cell lung cancer. Nature 1985; 316:823–826.
97. Mahmoud S, Staley J, Taylor J, et al. [Psi^{13,14}] bombesin analogues inhibit growth of small cell lung cancer in vitro and in vivo. Cancer Res 1991; 51:1798–1802.
98. Carney DN, Cuttitta F, Moody TW, Minna JD. Selective stimulation of small cell lung cancer clonal growth by bombesin and gastrin-releasing peptide. Cancer Res 1987; 47:821–825.
99. Giaccone G, Battey J, Gazdar AF, Oie H, Draoui M, Moody T. Neuromedin B is present in lung cancer cell lines. Cancer Res 1992; 52:2732s–2736s.
100. Cardona C, Rabbits P, Spindel ER, et al. Production of neuromedin B and neuromedin B gene expression in human lung tumor cell lines. Cancer Res 1992; 51: 5205–5211.
101. Gazdar AF. The molecular and cellular basis of human lung cancer. Anticancer Research 1994; 14:1B.
102. Mulshine J, Avis I, Carrasquillo J, et al. Phase I study of anti-gastrin releasing peptide monoclonal antibody in patients with lung cancer (abstr): Proc Am Soc Clin Oncol 1990; 9:230.
103. Kelley MJ, Linnoila I, Avis IL, et al. Antitumor activity of a monoclonal antibody directed against gastrin-releasing peptide in patients with small cell lung cancer. Chest 1997; 112:256–261.
104. Daughaday WH, Rotwein P. Insulin-like growth factors I and II. Peptide, messenger ribonucleic acid and gene structures, serum, and tissue concentrations. Endocr Rev 1989; 10:68091.
105. Shigematsu K, Kataoka Y, Kamio T, Kurihara M, Niwa M, Tsuchiyama H. Partial characterization of insulin-like growth factor I in primary human lung cancers using immunohistochemical and receptor autoradiographic techniques. Cancer Res 1990; 50:2481–2484.
106. Nakanishi Y, Mulshine JL, Kasprzyk PG, et al. Insulin-like growth factor-I can mediate autocrine proliferation of human small cell lung cancer cell lines in vitro. J Clin Invest 1988; 82:354–359.
107. Macaulay VM, Everard MJ, Teale JD, et al. Autocrine function for insulin-like growth factor I in human small cell lung cancer cell lines and fresh tumor cells. Cancer Res 1990; 50:2511–2517.
108. Jacques G, Rotsch M, Wegmann C, Worsch U, Maasberg M, Havemann K. Produc-

tion of immunoreactive insulin-like growth factor 1 and response to exogenous IGF-I in small cell lung cancer cell lines. Exp Cell Res 1988; 176:336–343.
109. Zia F, Jacobs S, Kull Jr. F, Cuttitta F, Mulshine JE, Moody TW. Monoclonal antibody αIR-3 inhibits non-small cell lung cancer growth in vitro and in vivo. J Cell Biochem 1996; 24:269–275.
110. Stahel R, Gilks W, Schenker T. Antigens of lung cancer: results of the Third International Workshop on Lung Tumor and Differentiation Antigens. J Natl Cancer Inst 1994; 86:669–672.
111. Rygaard K, Moller C, Bock E, Spang-Thomsen M. Expression of cadherin and NCAM in human small cell lung cancer cell lines and xenografts. Br J Cancer 1992; 65:573–577.
112. Roy DC, Ouellet S, Le Houillier C, Ariniello PD, Perreault C, Lambert JM. Elimination of neuroblastoma and small-cell lung cancer cells with an anti-neural cell adhesion molecule immunotoxin. J Natl Cancer Inst 1996; 88:1136–1145.
113. Kibbelaar RE, Moolenaar KEC, Michalides RJAM, et al. Neural cell adhesion molecule expression, neuroendocrine differentiation and prognosis in lung carcinoma. Eur J Cancer 1991; 27:431–435.
114. Takahashi T, Ueda R, Song X, et al. Two novel cell surface antigens on small cell lung carcinoma defined by mouse monoclonal antibodies NE-25 and PE-35. Cancer Res 1986; 46:4770–4775.
115. Mechtersheimer G, Staudter M, Moller P. Expression of the natural killer cell associated antigens CD56 and CD57 in human neural and striated muscle cells and in their tumors. Cancer Res 1991; 51:1300–1307.
116. Gordon L, Wharton J, Moore S, et al. Myocardial localization and isoforms of neural cell adhesion molecule (N-CAM) in the developing and transplanted human heart. J Clin Invest 1990; 86:1293–1300.
117. Hosano M, Endo K, Hosano MN, et al. Treatment of small cell lung cancer xenografts with iodine-131-anti-neural cell adhesion molecule monoclonal antibody and evaluation of absorbed dose in tissue. J Nucl Med 1994; 35:296–299.
118. Lynch TJ, Lambert JM, Coral F, et al. Immunotoxin therapy of small-cell lung cancer: a Phase I study of N901-blocked ricin. J Clin Oncol 1997; 15:723–734.
119. Goldenberg DM, Kim EE, DeLand FH, Bennett S, Primus FJ. Radioimmunodetection of cancer with radioactive antibodies to carcinoembryonic antigen. Cancer Res 1980; 40:2984–2992.
120. Said JW, Nash G, Tepper G, Banks-Schlegel S. Keratin proteins and carcinoembryonic antigen in lung carcinoma: an immunoperoxidase study of fifty-four cases, with ultrastructural correlations. Hum Pathol 1983; 14:70–76.
121. Holden J, Churg A. Immunohistochemical staining for keratin and carcinoembryonic antigen in the diagnosis of malignant mesothelioma. Am J Surg Pathol 1984; 8:277–279.
122. Krishnamurthy S, Morris J, Antonovic R, et al. Evaluation of primary lung cancer with indium-111 anti-carcinoembryonic antigen (type ZCE-025) monoclonal antibody scintigraphy. Cancer 1990; 65:458–465.
123. Biggi A, Gianfranco B, Ferrigno D, et al. Detection of suspected primary lung

cancer by scintigraphy with indium-111-anti-carcinoembryonic antigen monoclonal antibodies (type F023C5). J Nucl Med 1991; 32:2064–2068.

124. Vuillez J, Moro D, Brambilla E, et al. Immunoscintigraphy using ^{111}In-labelled F(AB')$_2$ fragments of anti-carcinoembryonic antigen (CEA) monoclonal antibody for staging of non-small cell lung carcinoma. Eur J Cancer 1994; 30A:1089–1092.

125. Riva P. Nuclear medicine in staging of lung cancer: immunoscan in detecting small metastatic deposits. Advances in the Biosciences. Vol. 72. New York: Pergamon Press, 1988:75–86.

126. Dienhart DG, Schmelter RF, Lear JL, et al. Imaging of non-small cell lung cancers with a monoclonal antibody, KC-4G3, which recognizes a human milk fat globule antigen. Cancer Res 1990; 50:7068–7076.

127. Kalofonos H, Sivolapenko G, Courtenay-Luck N, et al. Antibody guided targeting of non-small cell lung cancer using ^{111}In-labeled HMFGI F(ab')$_2$ fragments. Cancer Res 1988; 48:1977–1984.

128. Arklie J, Taylor-Papadimitriou J, Bodmer WF, Egan M, Millis R. Differentiation antigens expressed by epithelial cells in the lactating breast are also detectable in breast cancer. Int J Cancer 1981; 28:23–29.

129. Balaban EP, Walker BS, Cox JV, et al. Detection and staging of small cell lung carcinoma with a technetium-labeled monoclonal antibody. A comparison with standard staging methods. Clin Nucl Med 1992; 17:439–445.

130. Morris JF, Krishnamurthy S, Antonovic R, Duncan C, Turner FE, Krishnamurthy BT. Technetium-99m monoclonal antibody fragment (FAb) scintigraphy in the evaluation of small cell lung cancer: a preliminary report. Nucl Med Biol 1991; 18:613–620.

131. Balaban E, Walker B, Cox J, et al. Radionuclide imaging of bone marrow metastases with a Tc-99m labeled monoclonal antibody to small cell lung carcinoma. Clin Nucl Med 1991; 16:732–736.

132. Rusch V, Macapinlac H, Heelan R, et al. NR-LU-10 monoclonal antibody scanning. A helpful new adjunct to computed tomography in evaluating non-small-cell lung cancer. J Thorac Cardiovasc Surg 1993; 106:200–204.

133. Vansant JP, Johnson DH, O'Donnell DM, et al. Staging lung carcinoma with a Tc-99m labeled monoclonal antibody. Clin Nucl Med 1992; 17:431–438.

134. Stewart, JR, Carey J, Merrill W, et al. Radiolabeled monoclonal antibody imaging in non-small cell lung cancer: initial clinical results and implications. Ann Thorac Surg. In press.

135. Friedman S, Sullivan K, Salk D, et al. Staging non-small cell carcinoma of the lung using technetium-99m labeled monoclonal antibodies. Hematol Oncol Clin North Am 1990; 4:1069–1078.

136. Beaumier PL, Venkatesan P, Vanderheyden J-L, et al. ^{136}Re radioimmunotherapy of small cell lung carcinoma xenografts in nude mice. Cancer Res 1991; 51:676–681.

137. Breitz HB, Fisher DR, Weiden PL, et al. Dosimetry of rhenium-186-labeled monoclonal antibodies: methods, prediction from technetium-99m-labeled antibodies and results of Phase I trials. J Nucl Med 1993; 34:908–917.

138. Breitz HB, Weiden PL, Vanderheyden J-L, et al. Clinical experience with rhenium-

186-labeled monoclonal antibodies for radioimmuotherapy: results of Phase I trials. J Nucl Med 1992; 23:1099–1112.
139. Cheresh DA, Harper JR, Schulz G, Reisfeld RA. Localization of the gangliosides GD2 and GD3 in adhesion plaques and on the surface of human melanoma cells. Proc Natl Acad Sci USA 1984; 81:5767–5771.
140. Grant SC, Kostakoglu L, Pisters KMW, et al. Use of the MAb 3F8 in imaging small cell lung carcinoma. Lung Cancer 1991; 7(suppl):A226.
141. Vangsted AJ, Clausen H, Kjeldsen TB, et al. Immunochemical detection of a small cell lung cancer-associated ganglioside (FucGM1) antigen in serum. Cancer Res 1991; 51:2879–2884.
142. Fuentes R, Allman R, Mason MD. Ganglioside expression in lung cancer cell lines. Lung Cancer 1997; 18:21–33.
143. Hanibuchi M, Yano S, Nishioka Y, Yanagawa H, Sone S. Anti-ganglioside GM2 monoclonal antibody-dependent killing of human lung cancer cells by lymphocytes and monocytes. Jpn J Cancer Res 1996; 87:497–504.
144. Cheresh DA, Pierschbacher MD, Herzig MA, Mujoo K. Disialogangliosides GD2 and GD3 are involved in the attachment of human melanoma and neuroblastoma cells to extracellular matrix proteins. J Cell Biol 1986; 102:688–696.
145. Grant SC, Kostakoglu L, Kris MG, et al. Targeting of small-cell lung cancer using the anti-GD2 ganglioside monoclonal antibody 3f8: a pilot trial. Eur J Nucl Med 1996; 23:145–149.
146. Nasi M, Meyers M, Livingston P, Houghton A, Chapman P. Anti-melanoma effects of R24, a monoclonal antibody against GD3. Melanoma Research 1997; 7(Suppl 2):S155–S162.
147. Chapman PB, Houghton AN. Induction of IgG antibodies against GD3 in rabbits by an anti-idiotypic monoclonal antibody. J Clin Invest 1991; 88:186–192.
148. Grant SC, Kris MG, Miller V, Yao TJ, Houghton AN. Long-term survival in 15 patients with small cell lung cancer (SCLC) immunized with BEC2 plus BCG after initial therapy: an update. Proc Am Soc Clin Oncol 1997; 16:1630.

16
Monoclonal Antibody-Based Immunoconjugate Therapy of Cancer: Studies with BR96-Doxorubicin

Mansoor N. Saleh and Albert F. LoBuglio
University of Alabama at Birmingham, Birmingham, Alabama

Pamela A. Trail
Bristol-Myers Squibb, Princeton, New Jersey

I. INTRODUCTION

Monoclonal antibodies directed at tumor-associated antigens provide an attractive means to deliver cytotoxic agents to the tumor target while potentially sparing normal tissue (1–8). An essential prerequisite for the clinical application of most drug-antibody immunoconjugates is the identification of tumor surface antigens that are internalized rapidly upon ligand binding and that thus provide intracellular delivery of the cytotoxic reagent. Following internalization, the drug reagent should be liberated from the carrier antibody molecule and retain its cytotoxic activity (9,10). In this regard, the Lewis y (Le^y) glycoprotein is an especially attractive target for immunoconjugate therapy since it is expressed highly on a majority of human epithelial tumors (including breast, gastrointestinal tract, non-small-cell lung, cervix, ovary, and some melanomas), and is internalized rapidly upon ligand binding (11,12). The immunoconjugate BR96-DOX is composed of the chimeric Anti-Le^y monoclonal antibody linked to the anthracycline doxorubicin. In vitro and in animal models, binding of BR96-DOX to the Le^y antigen results in rapid internalization of the complex and intracellular release of doxorubicin by acid hydrolysis in the acidic environment of endosomes and lysosomes.

The localization of doxorubicin to the nucleus leads to subsequent DNA intercalation and inhibition of cell division (10,12).

This chapter will review the in vitro activity of BR96-Dox as well as the remarkable preclinical animal data that provided the rationale basis for the design of the first clinical application of this novel reagent. The chapter will also provide the results from the Phase I clinical trial of BR96-DOX, with emphasis on the toxicity, pharmacokinetics, and tumor targeting ability of this immunoconjugate.

II. BACKGROUND: BR96-DOX

The BR96-DOX conjugate utilizes an anticarcinoma MAb, termed BR96, to deliver selectively the anthracycline doxorubicin (DOX) to tumor cells. Doxorubicin was chosen for these first-generation anticarcinoma conjugates because it has a broad spectrum of cytotoxic activity and its toxicity profile as a free drug was well understood. BR96 is a chimeric (mouse–human) MAb of the human IgG_1 isotype, produced from murine BR96 as described previously (13). The BR96 MAb binds to the Lewis y (Le^y)-related tumor-associated antigen, which is expressed abundantly (>200,000 molecules per carcinoma cell) on the surface of the majority of epithelial tumors (11,12). In addition to carcinoma cells, BR96 binds to Le^y expressed at low levels on normal cells of the gastrointestinal tract in humans, primarily to differentiated cells of the esophagus, stomach, and intestine, as well as to acinar cells of the pancreas. A similar pattern of reactivity is found in monkeys, dogs, and rats (12,14).

III. CHEMICAL CHARACTERISTICS OF BR96-DOX

The BR96 MAb is rapidly internalized into the acidic environment of lysosomes following antigen-specific binding (11,15). This characteristic of the MAb was used to develop immunoconjugates that contained an acid-labile hydrazone bond to DOX and a thioether linker to the MAb (12,16). Following binding to antigen-expressing cells, the conjugate is internalized into lysosomes, where exposure to the acidic lysosomal environment (pH 4–5) results in the intracellular liberation of biologically active DOX. The BR96-DOX conjugates have a drug/MAb molar ratio (MR) of approximately 8; that is, eight molecules of DOX are bound per MAb. The thioether link in the MAb was introduced by reducing the interchain disulfides of the antibody with dithiothreitol (DTT). With this thiolation method, conjugate MRs of 8 were obtained without a reduction in the binding affinity of the conjugate relative to unmodified MAb (12,16).

Table 1 In Vitro Activity of BR96-DOX Conjugates

Carcinoma line	DOX IC50 (μM)	BR96 expression	IC50 (μM equivalent DOX)	
			BR96-DOX	IgG-DOX
L2987	0.18 ± 0.08	++	2.82 ± 0.85	15.2 ± 2.01
HCT116	0.15 ± 0.06	−	22.2 ± 3.1	18.3 ± 3.52

IV. IN VITRO BIOLOGY OF BR96-DOX CONJUGATES

Several characteristics of the in vitro biology of BR96-DOX conjugates were evaluated. In vitro potency was evaluated against a variety of human carcinoma lines. Antigen-specific cytotoxicity was defined both by evaluating the activity of BR96-DOX on antigen-expressing cell lines (BR96+) and antigen-negative cell lines (BR96-) and by comparing the IC_{50} of BR96-DOX with that of a non-binding human IgG-DOX conjugate against a BR96+ line. In Table 1, the potency of BR96-DOX is compared for two carcinoma lines that have similar sensitivity to unconjugated DOX but differ in that L2987 expresses the BR96 antigen whereas HCT116 does not. The BR96-DOX conjugate was significantly more potent against the BR96+ L2987 line than against the BR96− HCT116 line. Similarly, the BR96-DOX conjugate was significantly more potent than a nonbinding IgG-DOX conjugate evaluated in parallel against L2987 (BR96+). As expected, there was no difference in potency when both conjugates were evaluated against the BR96− HCT116 line. The in vitro potency of BR96-DOX conjugates also was evaluated against a panel of human carcinoma lines expressing different densities of the BR96-defined antigen. As shown in Table 2, the potency of BR96-DOX was related to the quantity of BR96-defined antigen expressed by the various carcinoma lines. As the level of expression of BR96 increased, the potency of BR96-DOX against a given cell line more closely approached that of unconjugated DOX.

Table 2 In Vitro Potency of BR96-DOX Related to Density of Expression of BR96-Defined Antigen

	HCT 116	RCA	L2987	MCF7
Binding ratio[a]	1	5	8	15
IC50 BR96-DOX	20	3	1	0.2
IC50 DOX	0.1	0.2	0.1	0.2

[a] Binding ratio was determined by FACS analysis; mean channel fluorescence for BR96/IgG.

V. ANTITUMOR ACTIVITY OF BR96-DOX

The antitumor activity of BR96-DOX was evaluated in a variety of in vivo model systems (8,12). BR96-DOX conjugates demonstrated antigen-specific antitumor activity against established human breast, colon, and lung carcinoma xenografts in athymic mice. BR96-DOX, administered at tolerated doses, produced complete regressions and/or cures of established DOX-sensitive lung (L2987) tumors (Figure 1a). When evaluated against a colon (RCA) tumor xenograft the BR96-DOX conjugate produced complete tumor regressions and cures of established tumors, even though the tumors were not sensitive to unconjugated DOX (Figure 1b). In the case of the RCA (DOX-insensitive tumor), the dose of BR96-DOX required to produce regressions of established tumors was approximately twice that required for the L2987 (DOX-sensitive) tumor. In each subcutaneous tumor xenograft evaluated, the antitumor activity of the BR96-DOX conjugate was significantly better than that of equivalent doses of nonbinding (IgG-DOX) conjugates or optimized DOX. The lack of activity of matching doses of IgG-DOX conjugates indicates that the antitumor activity of BR96-DOX is not a result of a change in the pharmacokinetics of DOX delivery; i.e., the conjugate does not function as a depot form of DOX, where drug is slowly released off of the antibody protein. BR96-DOX was both more potent and more active than DOX in each tumor model evaluated. Antitumor activity equivalent to BR96-DOX could not be achieved by treatment with MAb BR96 alone or with mixtures of MAb and unconjugated DOX. BR96 was not active against established tumors, and mixtures of MAb and optimal doses of DOX were no more active than DOX alone (8,12).

The use of MAb-directed delivery is designed to increase the therapeutic index by selectively targeting the therapeutic agent to tumor cells. However, few if any MAbs have been described to date that are truly tumor specific. Rather, the MAbs identify tumor-associated antigens that are expressed on a limited number of cells of normal tissues and/or are expressed at a significantly greater density on malignant versus normal cells. It was, therefore, important to evaluate the antitumor activity of BR96-DOX in an animal species that expressed the BR96-defined antigen in normal tissues.

Immunohistologic evaluation demonstrated that several normal human tissues bind BR96 (11,17). The BR96 MAb binds primarily to differentiated cells of the gastrointestinal tract (stomach, esophagus, and intestine) as well as to acinar cells of the pancreas. Normal tissues from some strains of rats, including the Rowett strain of athymic rats (8,12) and immunocompetent Brown Norway rats (18), bind BR96 in similar tissues as that seen in humans. Athymic rats provided a unique model for assessing the antitumor activity of BR96-DOX thioether conjugates using the same human tumor models as those that had been evaluated previously in mice. The BR96-DOX thioether conjugate was shown to produce cures of established L2987 (DOX-sensitive) human lung tumors

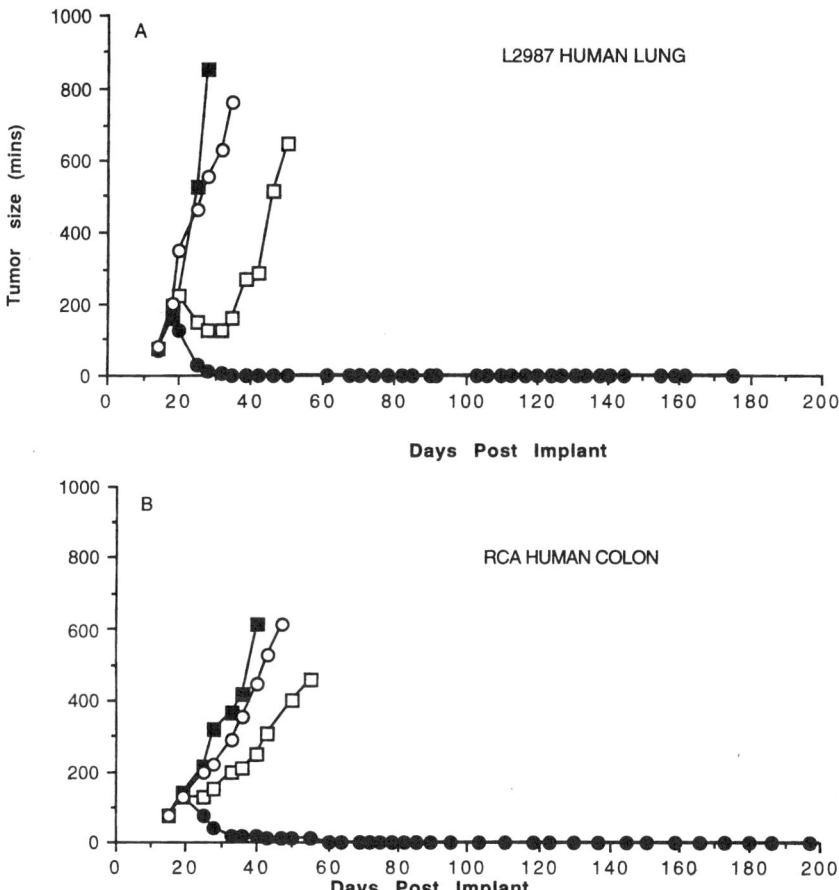

Figure 1 Antitumor activity of BR96-DOX against human tumor after xenografts in athymic mice. All treatments were administered on days 15, 19, and 23 after tumor implant. A: L2987 human lung carcinoma; control mice (■—■), mice treated with BR96-DOX (●—●) or with IgG-DOX (○—○), at a dose of 110 mg/kg conjugate (110 mg/kg antibody, 5 mg/kg equivalent DOX), and mice treated with 8 mg/kg DOX (□—□). B: RCA human colon carcinoma; control mice (■—■), mice treated with BR96-DOX (●—●) or with IgG-DOX (○—○) at a dose of 220 mg/kg conjugate (220 mg/kg antibody, 10 mg/kg equivalent DOX), and mice treated with 8 mg/kg DOX (□—□).

(Figure 2a) when administered at tolerated doses to athymic rats (12). Complete tumor regressions were also seen when athymic rats bearing DOX-insensitive human colon (RCA) tumors (Figure 2b) were treated with BR96-DOX (1,8). Importantly, BR96-DOX conjugates also produced complete regressions and cures of a carcinogen-induced rat colon tumor (BN7005) implanted subcutaneously in immunologically intact rats (18). Taken together, these data demonstrate that it was possible to achieve significant antitumor activity following treatment with tolerated doses of BR96-DOX even when the species used for evaluation expressed the BR96-defined antigen in some normal tissues.

Activity in models of metastatic and/or disseminated disease is an important criterion for evaluating the efficacy of immunoconjugate therapy, even though it is likely that immunoconjugates will be most efficacious when used clinically as adjunctive therapy in the setting of minimal residual disease. The BR96-DOX conjugate produced cures in 70% of mice bearing a large burden of disseminated disease (~0.5 g visible tumor burden) at the initiation of therapy. These mice were treated with a modest dose of conjugate (8 mg equivalent DOX/kg/injection), and cures were defined by histologic evaluation 200 days after tumor implant (12). The median survival time of BR96-DOX–treated mice was significantly increased (>200 days) relative to that of untreated control mice (90 days) or mice treated with the maximum tolerated dose of the unconjugated DOX (94 days).

The preclinical profile of the thioether-linked DOX conjugates was evaluated in a variety of subcutaneous carcinoma models as well as in models of disseminated disease; the antitumor activity of BR96-DOX was superior to that obtained with unconjugated DOX or with nonbinding conjugates in each model evaluated. Administration of BR96-DOX using a multiple-dose regimen consistently produced tumor regressions and cures, and the BR96-DOX conjugate was both more active and more potent than unconjugated DOX. The dose of BR96-DOX required to achieve tumor regressions and cures of the DOX-insensitive

Figure 2 Antitumor activity of BR96-DOX against human tumor xenografts in athymic rats that express the BR96 antigen in normal tissues. All treatments were administered on days 12, 16, and 20 after tumor implant. A: L2987 human lung carcinoma; control rats (■—■), rats treated with BR96-DOX at a dose of 88 mg/kg (●—●) or 44 mg/kg (○—○) conjugate (88 mg/kg BR96, 4mg/kg equivalent DOX and 44 mg/kg BR96, 2 mg/kg equivalent DOX, respectively), and rats treated with 4 mg/kg DOX (□—□). B: RCA human colon carcinoma; control rats (■—■), rats treated with BR96-DOX at a dose of 88 mg/kg (●—●) or 44 mg/kg (○—○) conjugate (88 mg/kg BR96, 4mg/kg equivalent DOX and 44 mg/kg BR96, 2 mg/kg equivalent DOX, respectively), and rats treated with 4 mg/kg DOX (□—□).

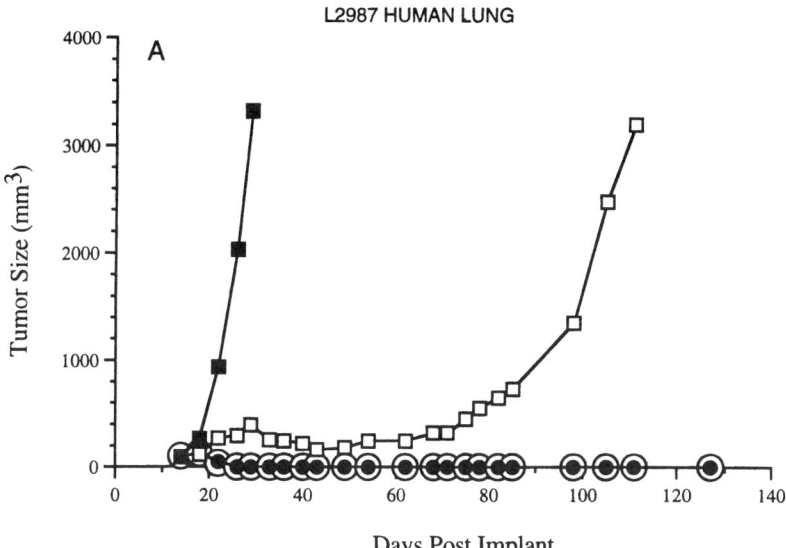
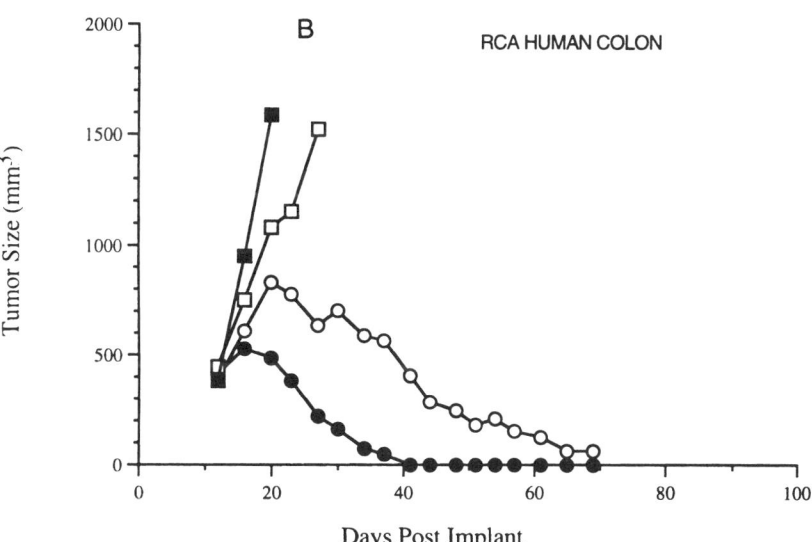

RCA colon tumor xenograft was approximately twice that required for DOX-sensitive L2987 lung carcinoma xenografts. Sensitivity to the parent drug as well as the schedule of administration are critical aspects for defining both the preclinical and the clinical doses of conjugates required to achieve efficacy.

VI. PHASE I CLINICAL TRIALS OF BR96-DOX

The remarkable antitumor activity of BR96-DOX in animal models as demonstrated by Trail et al. (12) provided the impetus for the clinical application of BR96-DOX. Preclinical toxicology studies revealed that dogs, unlike rats and monkeys, were sensitive to the toxic effects of the immunoconjugate and experienced hemorrhagic enteritis as the dose-limiting toxicity. At a single dose of 200 mg/m^2 (doxorubicin equivalent 6 mg/m^2), toxicity was mild and consisted of transient and reversible acute enteritis (toxic dose low, or TDL). Based upon this observation, the Phase I clinical trial in human subjects was initiated at a starting dose of 66 mg/m^2 (one-third the TDL in dogs). The Phase I trials focused primarily on the toxicity and pharmacokinetics of the immunoconjugate as well as on the immunogenicity of the molecule in human subjects (19,20).

The first clinical trial of chimeric BR96-DOX was conducted in patients with pathologically confirmed carcinoma (non-small-cell lung cancer or adenocarcinoma of the breast, GI tract, or ovary) that expressed the Le^y antigen as determined by immunohistochemistry (19). Antigen detection was performed on formalin-fixed primary or metastatic tissue. Eligible patients had to have failed at least one, but not more than two, prior therapeutic regimen. Patients with prior anthracycline exposure were eligible, provided they had not exceeded a cumulative dose of 400 mg/m^2 and had not progressed while on doxorubicin-based therapy. The Phase I study was designed to treat groups of three to six patients per dose level, with dose escalation between patient cohorts. In keeping with the frequency of administration of native doxorubicin, treatment was administered every 3 weeks, and patients were evaluated for evidence of clinical activity every two cycles. The study was initiated at a dose of 66 mg/m^2 of BR96-DOX (2 mg/m^2 doxorubicin equivalent). Dose escalation by 100% was planned until occurrence of grade 1 nonhematologic or grade 2 hematologic toxicity, at which point increases of no more than 50% were permitted. Patients were eligible to receive up to six cycles of treatment unless they experienced dose-limiting toxicity or disease progression.

In this trial a total of 66 patients were entered onto eight dose levels (range 66 mg/m^2 to 875 mg/m^2) (Table 3). The patients received a median of two doses (range one to eight). The immunoconjugate initially was administered as a 2 h infusion. Based upon previous animal data, patients were observed closely for gastrointestinal toxicity, in addition to routine laboratory and clinical toxicity

Table 3 Phase I Dose Escalation of BR96-DOX

Dose level	BR96-DOX (mg/m^2)	DOX equivalent (mg/m^2)	n	Comment
1	66	2	6	No significant toxicity
2	100	3	3	No significant toxicity
3	200	6	6	No significant toxicity
4	300	8	8	Onset of significant GI toxicity
5	400	11	4	—
6	550	15	9	GI toxicity requiring prolonging infusion time from 2 h to 24 h
7	700	17	27	Introduction of antiemetics and gastritis prophylaxis
8	875	25	3	Maximal tolerated dose

monitoring. Patients with metastatic colorectal and breast cancer made up a majority of the study population (50% and 25%, respectively). A majority of the patients (86%) previously had received chemotherapy.

Toxicity at the early dose range (66–300 mg/m^2) consisted primarily of mild to moderate nausea/vomiting, which occurred midway into the infusion and subsided within 24 h. Prophylactic antiemetics consisting of compazine and lorazepam were instituted at the 300 mg/m^2 dose level in patients who experienced >grade 2 nausea/emesis following their first treatment. Emesis requiring interruption of treatment was first observed at the 550 mg/m^2 dose (doxorubicin equivalent 16 mg/m^2). Based upon the suggestion that gastrointestinal toxicity may in part be due to a peak drug-dose effect, the study was amended to allow all subsequent patients to receive the immunoconjugate as a continuous infusion over 24 h. This prolongation of the infusion duration resulted in a modest amelioration of gastrointestinal toxicity and permitted additional dose escalation. Nausea/vomiting was experienced by nearly three-fourths of the patients and was severe (grade 3–4) in nearly half of the patient population. To evaluate the cause of the observed GI toxicity, patients with moderate to severe emesis underwent upper GI endoscopy 24 h following immunoconjugate administration. Endoscopy revealed acute superficial hemorrhagic gastritis, involving principally the gastric body (21). Gastric biopsies revealed focal necrosis, sloughed epithelium, and fibrin pseudomembrane formation (exudative gastritis) (Figure 3a). Immunoperoxidase staining of gastric mucosal tissue obtained at endoscopy revealed deposition of BR96 to the gastric epithelium (Figure 3b). Repeat endoscopy in selected patients on day 14 demonstrated complete resolution of gastritis in all patients. No similar

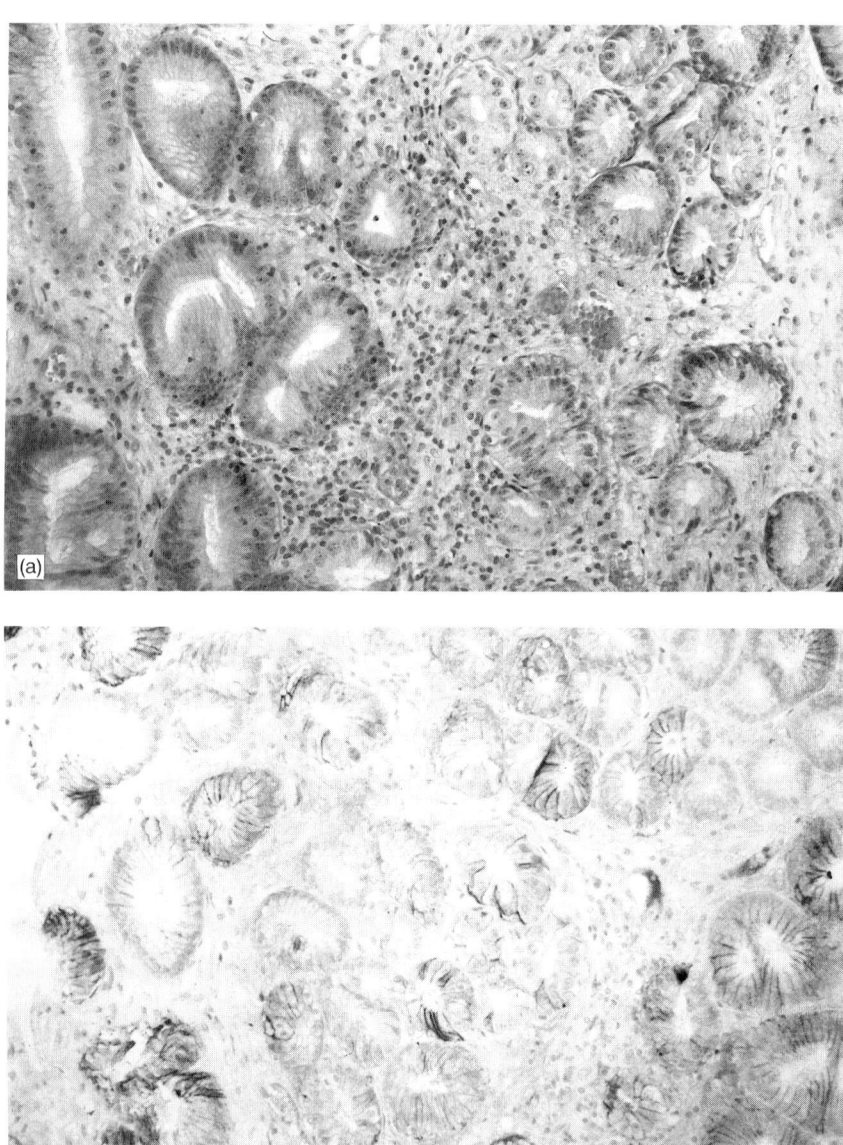

Figure 3 (a) H & E section of gastric mucosal biopsy obtained following BR96-DOX therapy. (b) Immunoperoxidase-based detection of in situ BR96 localization to gastric mucosa following BR96-DOX therapy.

toxicity was observed in the lower GI tract. The restricted location of gastric mucosal damage to areas of acid secretion, as well as the acute and readily reversible nature of the toxicity, suggested the possibility of ameliorating the side effect by prophylactic use of antiacid therapy. An expanded cohort of patients at the 700-mg/m^2 dose thus received various combinations of central as well as peripherally acting antiemetics, GI acid inhibitors, and corticosteroid to ameliorate the gastric toxicity profile. A premedication regime consisting of corticosteroid, Omeprazole (H$^+$/K$^+$ ATPase inhibitor), Kytril (5HT$_3$ antagonist), and lorazepam was noted to provide the most satisfactory amelioration of GI toxicity. Using this combination, the severity of the subjective and endoscopically documented gastritis was reduced, and patients were able to tolerate the administered dose of immunoconjugate with acceptable and transient symptoms (<grade 2).

In preclinical studies, enteritis in the dog model was observed in animals receiving the unconjugated antibody, and it was concluded that toxicity was most likely independent of the doxorubicin component of the immunoconjugate. The critical question of whether the toxicity observed in human subjects was mediated by the BR96 antibody or by the DOX component of the conjugate was studied by administering unconjugated chimeric BR96 antibody to eligible patients. One patient received the unconjugated BR96 antibody at a dose of 550 mg/m^2. The patient experienced bloody diarrhea accompanied by emesis and exudative gastritis. The observation in this patient suggested that the GI toxicity was, as observed in the dog model, most likely due to the biologic activity of the IgG1 chimeric Anti-Le^y antibody. The lack of similar toxicity involving other areas of high Le^y antigen expression in the GI tract, especially the salivary glands, and the lower intestines remains unclear.

Additional toxicity included fever and asthenia, which were observed in approximately half of the patients. Approximately one-third of the patients experienced abdominal pain (Table 4). Laboratory toxicity at higher doses included transient elevation of serum lipase and amylase. The association of abdominal

Table 4 Frequently Observed Adverse Events Associated with BR96-DOX

Toxicity	Any grade (%)	Grade >2 (%)
Nausea	51	30
Vomiting	54	20
Gastritis (endoscopy)	26	17
Fever	39	1
Abdominal pain	23	5
Elevated lipase	31	16
Anemia	30	3

pain and elevation of pancreatic enzymes was felt to be suggestive of antibody-mediated pancreatitis. None of the patients experienced evidence of sustained clinical pancreatitis, and the symptoms as well as laboratory abnormalities resolved over 24–48 h. The 24 h infusion schedule permitted dose escalation up to the 875 mg/m^2 dose, which was determined to be the MTD. Two of the three patients at this dose level experienced grade 4 emesis as well as exudative hemorrhagic gastritis extending into the duodenum, a finding not observed at lower dose levels. The 700 mg/m^2 dose (21 mg/m^2 doxorubicin equivalent) supported by antiemetics and gastritis prophylaxis was thus selected as the Phase II dose (20).

Tumor biopsies were obtained in five patients with accessible lesions. Immunohistochemical studies revealed antibody localized to tumor cells in all cases (22). Antigen saturation was not observed in the tumors specimen studied. Confocal microscopy revealed intranuclear deposition of doxorubicin, thus demonstrating targeted intracellular delivery of the drug conjugate. (Figure 4).

Objective clinical responses were observed in two of sixty-six patients, who received a minimum of two courses of BR96-DOX. A partial response (≥50% reduction in bidimensional tumor measurement) was achieved in one patient with metastatic breast cancer with prior doxorubicin exposure, who received six cycles

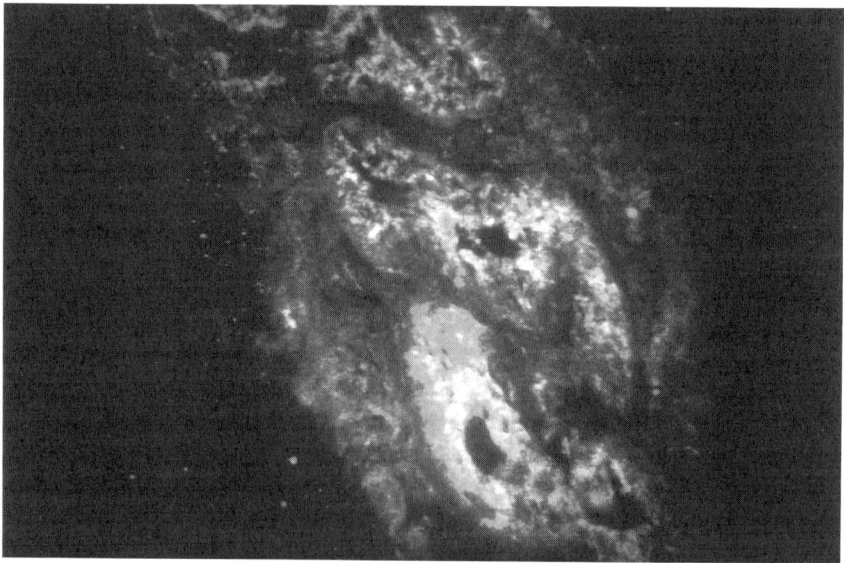

Figure 4 Confocal Microscopy Demonstrating in Situ Localization of BR96 and DOX to Tumor following BR96-DOX Therapy.

of therapy at the 400 mg/m^2 dose level, and in a second patient with advanced, previously untreated gastric cancer, who also received six cycles of therapy. Both patients received BR96-DOX at the 700 mg/m^2 dose level. Twenty-one of sixty-six patients had stable disease following two treatments (17,20).

Pharmacokinetics studies included quantitation of total BR96 by ELISA and total doxorubicin measured by HPLC following acid hydrolysis (22,24). The amount of free doxorubicin in serum as assessed by HPLC was negligible in all patients. Data from the first cycle of treatment revealed a linear relationship for dose and C_{max} as well as dose and AUC (Figure 5). The mean half-life of BR96 at 550 mg/m^2 was calculated to be 300 ± 95 h, with the $t_{1/2}$ for total doxorubicin of 43 ± 4 h (Table 5). The molar ratio of BR96-DOX calculated at the end of the infusion was 6 and maintained over 4 for up to 24 h, indicating a slow and gradual release of doxorubicin from the immunoconjugate in vivo. Minimal levels of anti-BR96 antibodies were detected in 37% of the patients, yet there was no alteration in the clearance kinetics in patients who received repeat therapy in the presence of a low level of anticonjugate antibodies (24). Early animal data with BR96-DOX (12) suggested that the antineoplastic activity was influenced by the schedule of drug administration, with more frequent administration of lower doses being more effective than single large doses administered less frequently (despite equivalent cumulative doses).

Given these data, a second Phase I trial of BR96-DOX administered weekly as a 2 h infusion was initiated (25). Eligibility criteria were similar to those for the every-3-week schedule. Patients were enrolled onto the study at an initial dose level of 100 mg/m^2/week. This was comparable to the dose of 300 mg/m^2 every 3 weeks, which was well tolerated in the previous study. Patients were eligible to receive up to 12 weekly doses. Six dose levels ranging from 100 to 500 mg/m^2/week were studied. A total of 42 patients were enrolled (25). The toxicity profile in this study was similar to that observed with the every 3 week schedule. Patients were able to receive a median of two courses (range one to six). Hematemesis was noted as the dose-limiting toxicity, and the dose of 225 mg/m^2/week was determined as the optimal Phase II dose. The kinetic profile at the weekly dose was comparable to that observed at the every 3 week administration (25). Doxorubicin delivery to tumor tissue was confirmed by confocal microscopic examination of biopsies material. No objective clinical responses were observed in patients treated in the weekly administration study.

VII. SUMMARY

The Phase I study of the immunoconjugate composed of the chimeric Anti-Le^y antibody BR96 linked to doxorubicin demonstrated important clinical features of this novel molecule. The kinetics of doxorubicin administered as the BR96

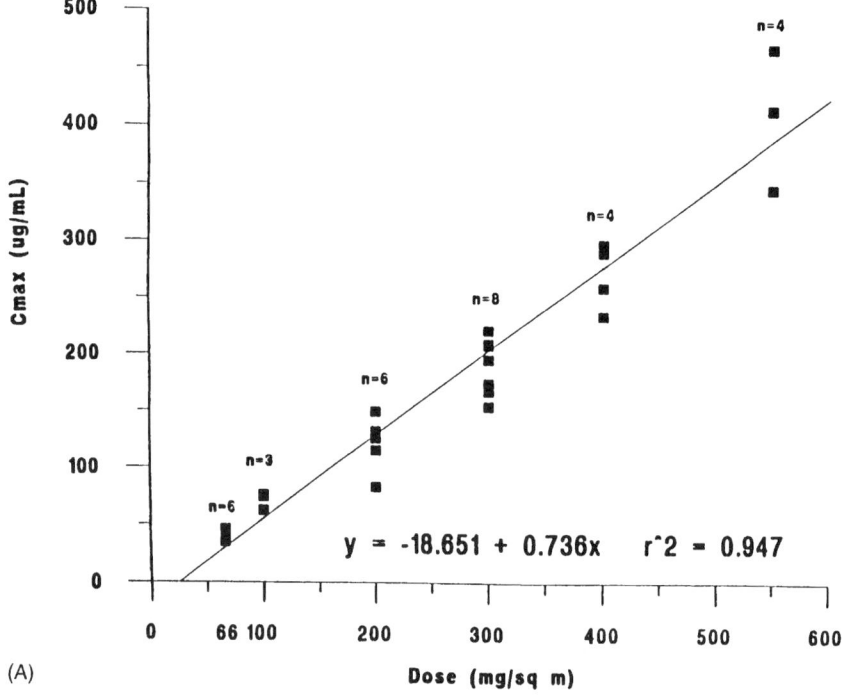

Figure 5 A: Linear relationship between dose and C_{max} for BR96-DOX. B: Linear relationship between AUC and C_{max} for BR96-DOX.

immunoconjugate provided a more prolonged drug exposure than would be expected with native doxorubicin alone (Table 6, Figure 6), and tumor biopsy data confirmed the ability to deliver the drug to the tumor cells via the antibody (22). Interestingly, toxicity of the immunoconjugate appears to be due to the biologic activity of the monoclonal antibody as opposed to doxorubicin. The drug–antibody immunoconjugate was best administered in conjunction with antiemetic and gastritis prophylaxis.

A number of immunoconjugates have been studied over the past decade, and encouraging biologic activity has been observed in hematologic malignancies using antibodies directed at cell-surface CD antigens (2–4,6,7,26–28). Advances in the use of immunoconjugate therapy have been less successful in solid tumors (6,7,29), and this may relate to the inability to deliver adequate levels of toxin to tumor cells within a solid mass as opposed to a highly vascular hematologic malignancy. The objective response observed in a small number of patients in our Phase I study of BR96-DOX is encouraging, especially given that the majority of

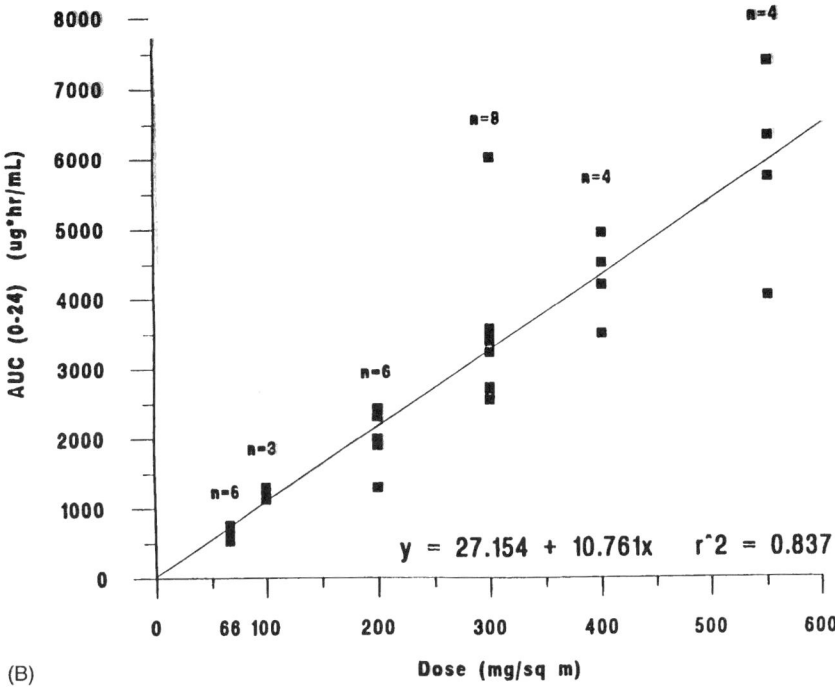

(B)

Table 5 Pharmacokinetic Profile of BR96-DOX

					Dose (mg/m^2)		
					300 ($n = 8$)	400 ($n = 4$)	550 ($n = 4$)
C_{max}(μg/mL)	TBR96	39.5	70.6	122	186	269	409
	TDOX	0.81	1.35	2.62	4.04	5.37	7.59
AUC$_{(0-24)}$ (μg · h/mL)	TBR96	656	1225	2053	3068	4274	5872
	TDOX	11.9	22.1	39.2	60.7	80.8	114.3
$t_{1/2}$(h)	TBR96	205	241	472	285	442	300
	TDOX	26.2	62.8	56.5	52.7	52.3	43.4

Pharmacokinetics: 2-hour infusion.

Table 6 Serum Doxorubicin Kinetics Achieved by BR96-DOX Compared with Native Doxorubicin

	C_{max} (µg/mL)	$AUC_{(0-24)}$ (µg·h/mL)	CLT (mL/min/m^2)	Vss (L/m^2)	$t_{1/2}$ (h)
Total DOX 550 mg/m^2 (14.5 mg/m^2/DOX in 2 h)	7.59	114.3	1.06	4.55	43.4
DOX 14.5 mg/m^2 (simulation: 2 h inf.)	0.358	1.15	~530	~740	~24
DOX 60 mg/m^2 (simulation: 20 min inf.)	2.66	4.58	~530	~740	~24

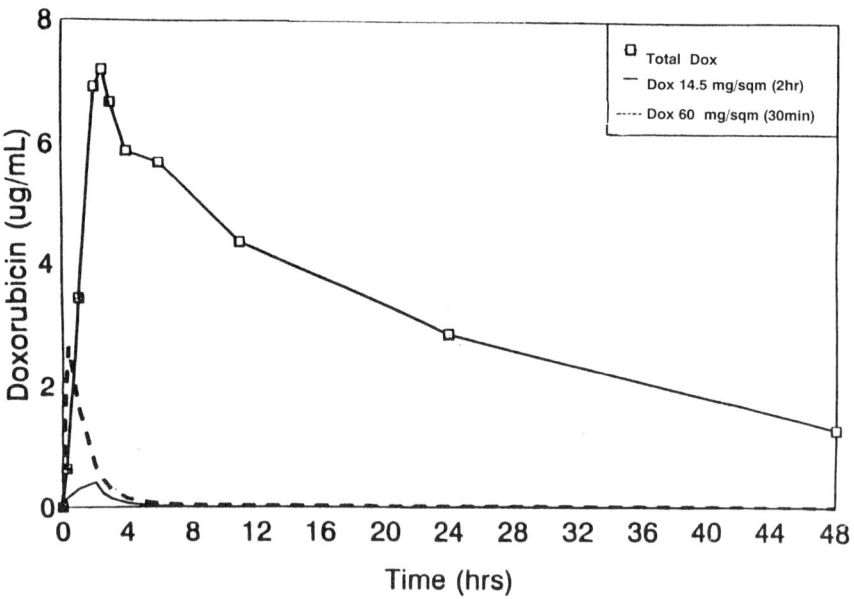

Figure 6 Kinetic profile of serum doxorubicin achieved by BR96-DOX (550 mg/m^2) compared with native doxorubicin. Observed total doxorubicin concentrations for patient at 550 mg/m^2 BR96-DOX.

patients had advanced disease, extensive prior treatment, and tumor types generally felt not to respond to doxorubicin. Targeted delivery of chemotherapy as achieved in this study would, however, need to demonstrate a much higher rate of efficacy in the Phase II setting in order to be clinically acceptable given the associated GI toxicity. As observed with other monoclonal antibody therapies, it is likely that BR96-DOX therapy will be most effective in the settings of minimal residual disease (30,31). The lack of toxicity typically associated with doxorubicin (cardiotoxicity, myelosuppression) was encouraging, especially in view of the substantial prolongation of doxorubicin exposure achieved via the immunoconjugate approach. The broad prevalence of the Le^y antigen, and the wide ranging antitumor activity of doxorubicin, provides the potential for wide clinical utility of BR96-DOX.

VIII. CONCLUSION

Our Phase I study confirms the feasibility of prolonged and tumor-directed delivery of doxorubicin using BR96-DOX. The kinetic and tumor biopsy data demonstrate the feasibility of tumor-directed delivery of doxorubicin via immunoconjugate therapy. Administration of doxorubicin via this route results in a prolonged circulating level of doxorubicin as compared to that achieved with native doxorubicin. The lack of higher response in this Phase I setting is possibly explained by the preponderance of patients with metastatic GI cancer in this study. BR96-DOX was not associated with myelosuppression, cardiac toxicity, or local cutaneous toxicity associated with native doxorubicin. A Phase II study of BR960-DOX as first-line treatment of metastatic breast cancer using the dose 550 mg/m^2 every 3 weeks (doxorubicin equivalent 10 mg/m^2) compared in a randomized fashion with 60 mg/m^2 of single-agent doxorubicin is currently under way. This study will provide important clinical data to determine the further development of this drug and add momentum for the application of this strategy in the treatment of solid tumors.

ACKNOWLEDGMENTS

The authors would like to acknowledge and sincerely thank Diane Healey for assistance and providing relevant clinical data, and review of the manuscript. They also express appreciation to Sandra Shepherd for her help in preparing the manuscript.

REFERENCES

1. Hellström I, Hellström KE, Siegall CB, Trail PA. Immunoconjugates and immunotoxins for therapy of carcinomas. In: August JT, Anders MW, Murad F, Coyle JT, eds. Advances in Pharmacology. San Diego: Academic Press, 1995; 33:349–388.
2. Schlom J. Monoclonal antibodies in cancer therapy. In: DeVita VT Jr, Hellman S, Rosenberg SA, eds. Biologic Therapy of Cancer, 2d ed. Philadelphia: J. B. Lippincott 1995; 20:507–521.
3. Pietersz GA, Krauer K. Antibody-targeted drugs for the therapy of cancer (abstr). J Drug Targeting 1994; 2(3):183–215.
4. Frankel AE, Tagge EP, Willingham MC. Clinical trials of targeted toxins (abstr). Seminars Cancer Biol 1995; 6(5):307–317.
5. Larson S. Radioisotope conjugates. In: DeVita VT Jr, Hellman S, Rosenberg SA, eds. Biologic Therapy of Cancer. 2d ed. Philadelphia: J. B. Lippincott 1995; 20: 534–552.
6. LoBuglio AF, Saleh MN. Monoclonal antibody therapy of cancer. Crit Rev Oncol/ Hematol 1992; 13:271–282.
7. LoBuglio AF, Saleh NM. Monoclonal antibodies. Curr Ther Oncol 1993; 3:41–49.
8. Trail PA, Willner D, Hellström KE. Site-directed delivery of anthracyclines for cancer therapy. Drug Dev Res 1995; 34:196–209.
9. Trail PA, Willner D, Knipe J, Henderson AJ, Lasch SJ, Zoeckler ME, TrailSmith MD, Doyle TW, King HD, et al. Effect of linker variation on the stability, potency, and efficacy of carcinoma reactive BR64-doxorubicin immunoconjugates. Cancer Res 1997; 57:100–105.
10. Trail PA, Willner D, Lasch SJ, Henderson AJ, Greenfield RS, King D, Zoeckler ME, Braslawsky GR. Antigen specific activity of carcinoma reactive BR64-adriamycin conjugates evaluated in vitro and in human tumor xenograft models. Cancer Res 1992; 52:5693–5700.
11. Hellström I, Garrigues HJ, Garrigues U, Hellström KE. Highly tumor-reactive, internalizing, mouse monoclonal antibodies to Le^y-related cell surface antigen. Cancer Res 1990; 50:2183–2190.
12. Trail PA, Willner D, Lasch SJ, Henderson AJ, Hofstead SJ, Casazza AM, Firestone RA, Hellström I, Hellström KE. Cure of xenografted human carcinomas by BR96-doxorubicin immunoconjugates. Science 1993; 261:212–215.
13. Yarnold S, Fell PH. Chimerization of antitumor antibodies via homologous recombination conversion vectors. Cancer Res 1994; 54:506–512.
14. Comereski CR, Peden WM, Davidson TJ, Warner GL, Hirth RS, Frantz JD. BR96-doxorubicin conjugate (BMS-182248) versus doxorubicin: a comparative toxicity assessment in rats. Toxicologic Pathol 1994; 22:473–488.
15. Garrigues J, Garrigues U, Hellström I, Hellström KE. Le^y specific antibody with potent anti-tumor activity is internalized and degraded in lysosomes. Am J Pathol 1993; 142:607–622.
16. Willner D, Trail PA, Hofstead SJ, King HD, Lasch SJ, Braslawsky GR, Greenfield RS, Kaneko T, Firestone RA. (6-Maleimidocaproyl) hydrazone of doxorubicin—a

new derivative for the preparation of immunoconjugates of doxorubicin. Bioconjugate Chem 1993; 4:521–527.
17. Trail PA, Slichenmyer WJ, Birkhofer MJ, Warner G, Knipe J, Willner D, Firestone RA, Sikkema D, Onetto N. BR96-doxorubicin immunoconjugate for treatment of patients with carcinoma. Proc Am Assoc Cancer Res 1996; 37:626.
18. Sjogren HO, Isaksson M, Willner D, Hellström I, Hellström KE, Trail PA. Prerequisites for an immunoconjugate, BR96-DOX, to cure established tumors in preclinical models, including syngeneic colon carcinomas in rats. Cancer Res. In Press.
19. Sugarman S, Murray JL, Saleh MN, Jones D, Daniel C, LeBherz D, Brewer H, Healey D, Kelley S. A Phase I study of BR96-doxorubicin (BR96-DOX) in patients with advanced carcinoma expressing the Lewis antigen (abstr). Proc ASCO 1995; 14:473.
20. Slichenmyer WJ, Bookman MA, Gilewski TA, Murray JL, Saleh MN, Dougan M, Healey D, Onetto N. Phase I clinical trials with the immunoconjugate BR96-doxorubicin (abstr). Am Chemical Soc 1996; 211: Part 1.
21. Saleh MN, LoBuglio AF, Sugarman, Murray J, Onetto N, Warner G, Mezza L, Davidson T, Grizzle WE. Gastrointestinal effects of chimeric BR96-doxorubicin conjugate (abstr). Proc AACR 1995; 36.
22. Trail P, Onetto N, Lasch S, Yelton D, Sikkema D, Sugarman S, Stewart M, Saleh MN, Rosenblum M. Tumor penetration and functional activity of BMS-182248 following administration in a Phase I clinical trial (abstr). Proc AACR 1995; 499.
23. Grasela D, LoBuglio AF, Saleh MN, Murray JL, Raymond R, Birkhofer M, Summerill R, Stewart M. Parametric model for BR96-doxorubicin pharmacokinetics (PK) in cancer patients (abstr). Proc AACR 1995; 36:234.
24. Saleh MN, LoBuglio AF, Sugarman S, Murray J, Khazaeli MB, Rosenblum M, Onetto N, Sikkema D, Warner G. Pharmacokinetics and immunogenicity of chimeric BR96-doxorubicin (BR96-DOX) in patients with Lewis positive metastatic cancer (abstr). Antibody Immunoconjugates Radiopharmaceuticals 1995; 8:61.
25. Giantonio TA, Gilewski TA, Bookman MA, Norton L, Kilpatrick D, Dougan MA, Slichenmyer WJ, Onetto NM, Canetta RM (abstr). A Phase I study of weekly BR96-Doxorubicin (BR96-DOX) in patients (pts) with advanced carcinoma expressing the Lewis^y (Le^y) antigen. Pro ASCO 1996; 443.
26. Grossbard ML, Freedman AS, Ritz J, Coral F, Goldmacher VS, Eliseo L, Spector N, Dear K, Lambert JM. Serotherapy of B cell neoplasm with anti-B4 blocked ricin: a Phase I trial of daily bolus infusion. Blood 1992; 79:576–585.
27. Grossbard ML, Lambert JM, Goldmacher VS, Spector NL, Kinsella, J, Eliseo L, Coral F, Taylor JA, Blattler WA. Anti-B4-blocked ricin: a Phase I trial of 7-day continuous infusion in patients with B-cell neoplasms. J Clin Oncol 1993; 11:726–737.
28. Vitetta ES, Stone M, Amlot P, Fay J, May R, Till M, Newman J, Clark P, Collins R, Cunningham D. Phase I immunotoxin trial in patients with B cell lymphoma. Cancer Res 1991; 51:4052–4058.
29. Pai LH, Wittes R, Setser A, Willingham MC, Pastan I. Treatment of advanced solid tumors with immunotoxin LMB-1: an antibody linked to *Pseudomonas* exotoxin (abstr). Nature Med 1996; 2(3):350–353.

30. Reithmuller G, Schneider-Gadicke E, Schlimok G, Schmiegel W, Raab R, Hoffken K, Gruber R, Pichlmaier H, Hirche H. Randomized trial of monoclonal antibody for adjuvant therapy of resected Dukes' C colorectal carcinoma. Lancet 1994; 343: 1177–1183.
31. Grossbard ML, Gribben JG, Freedman AS, Lambert JM, Kinsella J, Rabinowe SN, Eliseo L, Taylor JA, Blattler WA. Adjuvant immunotoxin therapy with anti-B4-blocked ricin after autologous bone marrow transplantation for patients with B-cell non-Hodgkin's lymphoma. Blood 1993; 81:2263–2271.

17
Immunotoxin Therapy: Past Lessons and Future Directions

Ellen S. Vitetta, Maria-Ana Ghetie, and Victor Ghetie
The University of Texas Southwestern Medical Center at Dallas, Dallas, Texas

I. INTRODUCTION

Immunotoxins (ITs) first were described in the late 1970s by basic scientists who had little appreciation for the issues surrounding clinical development of anticancer drugs. Predictably, the enthusiasm and excitement of the '70s gave way to a more sober view of both translational research and drug development. Looking back over these two decades, we conclude that the expectations concerning these "simple" targeting agents were unrealistic. Nevertheless, within the broader setting of drug development, ITs have proven far from unsuccessful. Indeed, individuals in the IT field continue to predict that ITs and other monoclonal antibody (MAb)-based drugs will find their place alongside chemotherapy and radiotherapy as modalities to treat cancer and other diseases. In this chapter we shall consider the issues relating to both past performance and future prospects.

II. PERFORMANCE OF IMMUNOTOXINS IN RODENTS VERSUS HUMANS

The vast majority of preclinical studies were carried out using rodents. Generally, established cell lines expressing high densities of the targeted antigen were injected into animals shortly before IT therapy was commenced. Animals then were treated with significant doses of the IT (averaging 20–60% of the LD_{50}) and tumor growth was monitored. Such models have been very useful for comparing the potency and stability of different IT constructs. They also have been helpful in evaluating combinatorial approaches using ITs and radiotherapy, chemotherapy, or other agents.

Rodent models have not, however, generally been predictive of the toxicities observed in humans. This has occurred for three reasons.

1. In most cases, mouse MAbs against human tumor cells have been used in mouse xenograft models. Therefore, unpredictable cross-reactions of ITs with normal human tissue have not been observed. In reality, ITs prepared with MAbs against human cells often have spurious cross-reactions with normal humans tissue that can cause life-threatening events in patients (1). These cross-reactions can be subtle and hard to identify even in pre-clinical studies using primates.
2. The toxin portion of the IT can sometimes interact with human tissues or blood proteins in an unpredictable fashion. For example, ricin A-chain reacts with both $\alpha 2$ macroglobulin (2) and fibronectin (3,4) and appears to damage endothelial cells more readily in humans than in mice. Because of these problems, smaller doses of ITs must be used in humans than in animals, leading to narrower therapeutic windows.
3. Phase I trials in humans are carried out in patients with large tumor burdens. Studies in mice usually involve minimal residual diseases (MRD). Because a large tumor sink can reduce blood levels and mask toxicity, information from such trials can lead to an overestimate of the maximum tolerated dose (MTD).

Based on these observations, we recommend that (a) pharmacokinetics play a more prominent future role in evaluating ITs in Phase I trials in humans; (b) efforts be made to determine whether toxicities are related to the active site of the toxin or whether toxins can be genetically or biochemically modified to avoid these side effects and yet retain potency; (c) new biological models be developed to study the toxicity of ITs in human tissue either in SCID mice or in vitro; and (d) Phase I trials (designed to establish safety) be carried out in patients with MRD.

III. THE OPTIMAL SETTING FOR IMMUNOTOXINS IN HUMANS

A. Tumor Burden

It has long been predicted that ITs would have an impact in MRD and, in particular, as adjuvant therapy (5). In addition, it was postulated that solid tumors would not be amenable to IT treatment, except perhaps in the case of early metastatic disease. The predictions have been borne out, largely because the dose-limiting toxicities of ITs have precluded giving amounts large enough to gain access to bulky tumors. In addition, and as predicted, it has become clear that ITs are immunogenic in 30–100% of patients, depending upon their immune status. Because of this, it has not been possible to give chronic or repeated courses of therapy, since in the presence of Anti-IT antibodies, $T_{1/2}$s are too short. This should not be a problem in treating MRD, since one or two courses of IT should suffice to eliminate residual cells. Our own experience has suggested that in patients with more bulky tumors, if antibody titers are allowed to drop to baseline after treatment, another course of IT can be given before new antibodies appear. This is true, however, only in diseases such as lymphoma where the immune system is compromised and the antibody response takes at least 2–3 weeks to develop. It may not be the case in patients with other tumors, where secondary responses can appear within 3–4 days. Such results suggest that (at least in lymphoma patients) careful monitoring of Anti-IT antibody titers should be carried out in individual patients in order to determine when new courses of therapy can be initiated.

B. Dose Schedules

Immunotoxins have been administered to humans both as bolus infusions (BI) (6–10) and continuous infusions (CI) (7,9,11,12). Although, there have been no striking differences between these two approaches, we have noted that in patients who have received prior irradiation, toxicities can be more pronounced using CI regimens. The monitoring of blood levels can be extremely helpful in predicting toxicities, since the administered dose *vs.* the blood levels achieved can be very different from patient to patient. In most trials it has been noted that below the MTD, blood levels of ITs are high enough to be therapeutic (7,11). However, whether this is true in tumor nodules that are less accessible to the bloodstream is unclear. It also should be noted that when tumor cells are present in the circulation, blood levels may be much lower than those in patients with MRD.

Phase I trials frequently are carried out in patients who have had numerous previous therapies and often have compromised organ systems. Hence, ITs could be even more problematic in these patients than in either newly diagnosed patients with MRD or in individuals who have undergone a single course of debulking therapy. In future Phase I trials, efforts should be made to treat patients who will be clinically more similar to those intended for large-scale use of ITs (*i.e.,* postchemotherapy and in MRD). Otherwise, results of Phase I MTDs will be misleading.

C. Side Effects

The dose-limiting side effects of all ITs include liver damage and manifestations of vascular leak syndrome (VLS) (13,14). In some cases, VLS has occurred because the MAb recognizes vascular endothelial cells (VECs). Generally, however, toxins themselves are directly responsible for VLS and hepatotoxicity, even when the MAb is not cross-reactive. Hepatotoxicty is due in some cases to binding of the carbohydrate-containing portions of the toxin by liver cells (15,16). The mechanisms by which toxins induce VLS remain to be elucidated, but, depending on the toxin, they clearly involve damage to VECs (17). Although it is unlikely that modifications in toxin structure will completely solve this problem (18), work along these lines should be encouraged. In addition, new toxins should be evaluated for both VLS-like activity and liver cell binding. In addition, it will be necessary to develop good experimental models of VLS that are relevant to human tissues. Such models would facilitate the testing of agents that decrease this toxicity, keeping in mind, of course, that *mild* VLS may actually improve the delivery and antitumor effect of an IT.

IV. QUESTIONS THAT NEED TO BE ADDRESSED

A. Should IT Therapy Be Carried Out with Single ITs or with Mixtures of ITs?

In our view, IT therapy should be designed to mop up residual tumor cells after debulking therapy in order to achieve a cure. It should, however, be recognized that the residual cells are likely to be heterogeneous. Although it is possible that single ITs may induce significant remissions, it is likely that antigen-negative variants will survive. For this reason, curative therapy probably should include two or more ITs directed against different molecules on the tumor cell surface. In contrast, the use of several different toxins may be less critical, since toxin-insensitive variants are more rare. The use of mixtures of ITs will entail proving that they are safe and that they have an additive effect, at least in some murine tumor models (19–21).

B. What Type and Dose Regimen of Debulking Therapy Should Be Used?

Cells that escape debulking chemotherapy should be sensitive to ITs. The situation, however, may be more complex. For example, chemotherapy and radiotherapy may facilitate the emergence of mutants that are not only resistant to the chemotherapy but that lack certain surface markers as well. Conversely, IT therapy may actually sensitize cells to chemotherapeutic regimens. In our own studies, attempts to combine chemotherapy with IT therapy in mice have shown that chemotherapy given *during* or *after* IT treatment is more effective than chemotherapy given *before* IT treatment (22,23). It is therefore important that the types and temporal order of treatments be evaluated carefully. It also should be noted that debulking therapy involving the use of ^{131}I antibodies (or other MAb-based agents) should be considered and modeled in conjunction with IT therapy.

C. Should Enhancers of IT Activity Be Tested in Humans?

In mice with human and murine tumors, several different IT-enhancing agents, including monensin and chloroquine, improve the potency of ITs (24,25). These agents must now be tested in humans to determine whether they improve the therapeutic index of ITs. If enhancers do not increase toxicity, they should improve the therapeutic index.

D. Are In Vitro Cell Lines in SCID or Nude Mice Predictive of What Will Occur in Humans?

Few studies have been carried out using tumor cells from patients grown in mice, because fresh human tissue is difficult to grow and EBV$^+$ lymphomas often emerge (26,27). Therapy models with fresh tumor tissue should be developed to determine whether, when the density of the targeted antigen is low or heterogeneous, susceptibility to ITs occurs. Although it might not be practical to evaluate the tumors from each individual patient, it might be possible to develop paradigms regarding the relative susceptibilities of different *types* of tumors to ITs.

E. How Much Effort Should Be Spent Improving the Therapeutic Index?

This is the critical area, which must be addressed by using human tissues both in vitro and in SCID mice. The dose-limiting side effects, which thus far have been described for the ITs in clinical trials, have not generally been addressed with regard to mechanisms. Unless we can administer larger doses of the existing ITs, we will be limited to treating *only* MRD, and, at the MTD, idiosyncratic, severe side effects might still occur in humans. Furthermore, not all ITs are potent enough at such low doses. For example, the safe dose chosen for the Phase III trial of B4-blocked ricin showed no efficacy (M. Grossbard, personal communication). Clearly, clinical trials have demonstrated that in cases where multiple courses of ITs can be given, tumors continue to decrease. Although some inroads have been made in understanding VLS and other side effects in humans, a great deal remains to be done.

V. NEW RESEARCH DIRECTIONS

The search for more potent ITs with fewer side effects presently is being conducted in many laboratories, with the aim of improving both the targeting ability of the MAb and the cytotoxicity of the toxin. With regard to MAbs, attempts are being made to target new tumor antigens (28) or other structures supporting tumor growth (29). These are also efforts to decrease IT size and immunogenicity and to increase affinity and tumor penetration without impairing pharmacokinetics.

Toxin improvements aim to increase the cytotoxicity of the presently used toxins (30–32) and to identify or synthesize more potent new toxins with decreased immunogenicity and side effects. Ideally, highly potent human toxins could be developed; research in this key area is ongoing (33).

A. Antibodies Targeting the Vasculature

Monoclonal antibodies can be targeted to antigens present on the activated VECs. The MAb-based ITs can, in some models, prevent tumor angiogenesis (antiangiogenic therapy) or/and exert selective destruction of tumor blood vessels (vascular targeting therapy). In vascular targeting, the ITs destroy or infarct the vasculature of solid tumors and deprive the tumor cells of their blood supply. Furthermore, it is not necessary to destroy all tumor-associated blood vessels, since thousands of tumor cells are dependent upon a small number of capillary endothelial cells. Hence, even incomplete damage to the vasculature should result in extensive tumor destruction. The antibody or IT need not penetrate the tumor mass, since the targets are the endothelial cells lining the blood vessels of the tumor and these are fully accessible to the ligand. Finally, the risk of developing drug-resistant mutants usually generated when tumor is targeted is low, since normal cells, such as endothelial cells, are not prone to generate such mutants.

To test this concept, mice were injected with murine solid tumors (34,35) or with a human breast tumor (36), and the endothelial cells in the tumor vasculature were targeted with specific antibodies conjugated to either dgRTA (34,36) or a truncated form of human recombinant tissue factor (35). Both approaches showed antitumor efficiency (34–36). It should be noted that specificity will be critical in clinical trials, since even minor cross-reactions with normal vasculature will be life threatening (37).

B. Size and Affinity of Antibodies

With regard to improving the therapeutic index, although changes in the size and/or the affinity of ITs are desirable, the issue of making such changes is a complex one. Fragments of antibody with molecular masses of 25 kDa (Fv) or 50 kDa (Fab) will leave the intravascular space and penetrate the surrounding tissues more easily than intact IgG molecules (150 kDa) due to their higher diffusion rates (38). However, decreases in the size of an MAb may also decrease its affinity for its antigen. For example, as a consequence of their reduced affinity, monovalent ITs are less cytotoxic in vitro than their divalent counterparts (39). Fortunately, studies in animals have shown that at least in some cases, the Fab- or Fv-containing ITs are as active as those constructed with intact antibody (40). By removing the Fc portion from the antibody molecule, one also removes the site necessary for persistence of the IT in the circulation (41). Consequently, antibody fragments and ITs constructed with these fragments have a shorter half-life and are rapidly eliminated from the circulation. Since the penetration of the ITs into the tumor tissue is a function of the gradient of concentration between the intra- and extravascular space, the rapid elimination of an IT will decrease this gradient and diminish the advantage of the better diffusion rate conferred by the smaller size of the IT.

Higher affinity does not always lead to better internalization of the IT or to more efficient routing to intracellular targets (42). Successful targeting also depends on the rate of internalization of the ITs bound to the membrane antigen (42,43).Since ITs with Fab or Fv are univalent for their target molecules,they are unable to promote internalization through crosslinking of the adjacent targeted molecules, irrespective of their affinity.Thus, the cytotoxic activity of monovalent ITs will depend primarily on the membrane turnover of the targeted molecule. Importantly, internalization and routing can be more dependent upon the spatial orientation of the molecular epitope recognized by the MAb than on its affinity. For example, in the case of at least two cell-surface molecules, MAbs that recognized epitopes proximal to the plasma membranes made more effective ITs than those directed against epitopes more distal to plasma membrane, irrespective of their affinities for antigen (44).

Decreasing the size of an antibody and/or humanizing an IT can also reduce its immunogenicity. In this regard, ITs containing chimeric antibody already have been constructed (45). However the construction of ITs with lower immunogenicity also will be dependent upon the generation of new, less immunogenic toxins.

Decreasing the size of antibodies to the level of recombinant Fvs with good stability and antigen-binding ability (38) may represent the best option for generating new ITs. It may be possible to make Fv-containing recombinant ITs with high affinity using phage display technology (46). By means of this approach, a specific recombinant IT containing an Fv antibody with a very high affinity was successfully prepared (47). The rapid elimination of the IT-containing Fv fragments might be offset either by continuous administration or by the addition of amino acid structures from the CH2-CH3 interface that control the persistence of IgG molecules in the circulation (48). The rapid dissociation of Fv molecules from tumors might be overcome by engineering multivalent constructs that are retained more effectively (49). The use of Fv fragments will require labile bonds between the Fv and the toxic moiety to allow the intracellular release of the toxin. At present, Fv ITs have been constructed with three toxins, PE, DT, and gelonin (50,51). Highly cytotoxic RTA-containing fusion proteins have been much more difficult to generate (52,53).

C. Toxins

Effectively decreasing the size, immunogenicity, and side effects of the presently used protein toxins will be difficult until we know more about the molecular distribution of the antigenic epitopes and active sites. For example, if the two are the same, it will be difficult to reduce immunogenicity by mutational changes. Even if changes can be made, antigenicity is likely to vary among genetically outbred humans. The search for new toxins presently is directed at identifying protein toxins with smaller molecular masses and/or nonprotein toxic compounds with inherently low immunogenicity.

1. Toxins from Fungi

Mitogillin, α-sarcin, and restrictocin are fungal proteins with small molecular masses (17 kDa) that share high amino acid homology and have ribonuclease activity (54,55). Active ITs have been generated with recombinant restrictocin (56) and mitogillin (57). The recombinant restrictocin produced in *E. coli* was found to be poorly immunogenic, with low nonspecific toxicity in mice (56). Immunotoxins prepared with mitogillin conjugated through an engineered cysteine residue to H65 murine MAb recognizing the human CD5 antigen was at least as potent as H65-RTA in an in vitro cytotoxic assay using CD5$^+$ cells, despite the fact that the mitogillins are only 20–40% as potent as RTA in inhibiting protein synthesis (57). Their toxicity to human VECs has not been tested, but it is possible that ITs constructed with *Aspergillus* toxins will induce less VLS due to their completely different primary structure. In this regard, another toxin, isolated from *Bryonia dioica,* with a molecular mass of 27 kDa and lacking cross-reactivity with RTA, was 5–8-fold less toxic to human endothelial cells than was RTA (58). These new toxins might represent good alternatives to the presently used toxins if they have good activity, lower immunogenicity, and fewer side effects.

2. Toxins of Human Origin

A new class of ITs could be constructed using effector molecules of human origin, such as angiogenin or tumor necrosis factor (TNF), among others (e.g., cytokines) (33,59). These should be less immunogenic (but also less toxic) than the ITs currently available. In this regard, the gene for human angiogenin (a ribonuclease A) was fused to a gene encoding a single-chain Fv antibody against the human transferrin receptor (TR) for the purpose of killing tumor cells selectively. The resulting construct was devoid of immunogenicity and had fewer side effects than bacterial and plant toxins (60). The characteristic RNA-ase activity of angiogenin is responsible for the inhibition of protein synthesis, but only in a cell-free system. The protein by itself is not toxic to cultured human cells (60). The anti-TR fusion ITs were cytotoxic to various TR^+ cells, the most active being a construct with a spacer linking the enzymatic and binding sites (60).

Another IT was constructed using human TNF, a nonglycosylated protein with a low molecular mass (17 kDa) and broad cytotoxic and cytostatic activity. A conjugate of an antimelanoma antibody and TNF had melanoma-selective cytotoxic effects both in vitro (61) and in tumor-bearing nude mice.

3. Cytolytic Toxins

Most ITs have been prepared with toxins that inhibit protein synthesis by inactivating either ribosomes (RIPs) or elongation factor 2 (DT, PE). Both types of toxins must be internalized into the cytosol, and both the degree of internalization and the efficiency of the routing to the intracellular target are variable. Therefore, a promising alternative is to use toxins that damage the plasma membrane. Immunotoxins made with these lytic toxins (*immunolysins*) should be more effective in reaching the core of solid tumors by lysing cells that preclude accessibility of "classical" ITs (62). Given in combination with "classical" ITs, immunolysins may also facilitate the access of the former to the cytosol (62).

A pore-forming toxin, CytA δ-endotoxin from *Bacillus thuringiensis,* was used to construct an IT with an Anti-Thy1 MAb (63). Although this IT did bind specifically to the target cells, it was not cytotoxic. When cells coated with the CytA-antibody IT were treated with dithiothreitol to reduce disulfide bonds linking CytA to the MAb, the Thy-1^+ cells (EL-4) were killed (63). These results suggested that the attachment of CytA to a large molecule(such as the antibody) prevented CytA from penetrating the membrane and/or forming a pore.

Because of this problem, a new class of ITs (called *proimmunolysins*) is being developed (64). These constructs target inactive α-hemolysins (from *S. aureus*) using MAbs that recognize antigenic determinants on the membrane. When brought into contact with the membrane by the MAb, the inactive α-hemolysins are susceptible to activation by cathepsin B, a protease that is secreted by certain metastatic tumor cells. Proteolysis generates active nicked forms of α-hemolysins that can kill the malignant target cells. Mutants of α-hemolysins that are rapidly and preferentially activated/nicked by cathepsin B have been generated using combinatorial library/mutagenesis (64). These mutants are currently being evaluated for their potential antitumor activity when bound to antibody. It should be noted that the activation of ITs by tumor proteases provides a second level of specificity beyond that conferred by the antibody. These two levels of specificity will have limitations, however, since only certain tumor cells express or secrete proteases (65,66). The cytolysins are proteins with molecular masses of 20 kDa and are, therefore, potentially as immunogenic as "classical" toxins.

4. Antineoplastic Drugs

Nonprotein toxic compounds are smaller and less immunogenic. It should be kept in mind, however, that the plant toxins act on the tumor cells in a catalytic manner. The nonprotein toxic compound acts stoichiometrically, so the antibody molecule must deliver a much larger number of molecules to the cell.

Anticancer drugs have been linked to MAbs; recently, completely cleavable linkages between antibody and drugs have been designed (67). New drugs (maytansinoids and calicheamicins), with a toxicity 100–1000 times higher than that of conventional drugs, have been synthesized and are being evaluated (68,69). Maytansinoids and calicheamicins have significant systemic toxicity, which precludes their use at therapeutic doses (68,69). However, when these drugs are bound to antibody, they lose their nonspecific toxicity and demonstrate a significant therapeutic window for treating solid tumors in mice (70). In mice, the toxicity of these drug conjugates was lower than that of ITs containing dgRTA, and the in vitro cytotoxicity against various tumor cells was comparable to that of the most potent ITs (68–70). Immunoconjugates of the maytansinoid drug DM1 linked to various MAbs via disulfide bonds eradicated large tumor xenografts (71) in SCID mice. Calicheamicins (69) as well as doxorubicin (72,73) linked to various MAbs via acid-labile hydrazone bonds have demonstrated significant antitumor activity in nude mice with human breast carcinoma. Doxorubicin/BR96 MAb conjugates directed against multidrug-resistant human breast carcinoma have demonstrated antigen-specific activity both in vitro and in vivo against doxorubicin-resistant cells and xenografts (73).

D. New Ways to Deliver Immunotoxins

Both to increase the efficacy of ITs and to decrease the toxic side effects, cells that preferentially localize in the tumor and secrete ITs have been engineered. Thus, lymphocytes were transfected with the bicistronic vector coding for Fab or Fv antibody fused to PE40 gene (74,75). The transfected lymphocytes remained viable due to the lack of the target antigen on the cell surface or/and possibly to some pecularities in the amino acid sequence at the C-terminal end of PE40 that prevented the retention of the IT in the endoplasmic reticulum (76). To evaluate the potential in vivo application of this strategy, human LAK cells were transfected with Fv Anti-Her2-PE40 chimeric genes, enabling the cells to secrete an IT directed against the Her-2antigen (75). Nude mice were xenografted with a human Her-2^+ tumor and treated with the transfected LAK cells. Tumor growth was efficiently inhibited. Interestingly, if a cell line devoid of tumor tropism (MOLT4) was transfected and administered to tumor-bearing mice, inhibition of tumor growth was also observed, suggesting that the IT was secreted into the blood. Before these IT-secreting cells are used in humans, a way to regulate and/or turn them off must be developed.

VI. CONCLUSIONS

Immunotoxins, as we know them today, represent a distinct class of antitumor agents with remarkable efficacy in the treatment of experimental cancers in animals. Several ITs have been further evaluated in patients with cancer and autoimmune diseases, and the results have clearly indicated that some ITs have activity at safe doses. Ongoing Phase II and III trials will determine whether ITs are effective at treating diseases in humans. In addition to these ongoing clinical studies, basic research is aimed at improving the potency, immunogenicity, and toxicity of ITs in order to increase their therapeutic index in experimental animals. Such studies involve using new antibody and toxin constructs as well as developing ITs to attack other targets, such as the vasculature of solid tumors. Those second- and third-generation molecules that perform well in vitro and in animals will be evaluated further in Phase I trials. Although this process of translational research is tedious and costly, we have learned a great deal over the last two decades and are confidant that some version of these ITs eventually will be used to treat human disease.

ACKNOWLEDGMENTS

We thank Ms. S. Flowers for expert secretarial assistance and the NIH and FDA for supporting aspects of our own work discussed in this review.

REFERENCES

1. Gould BJ, Borowitz MJ, Groves ES, Carter PW, Anthony D, Weiner LM, Frankel AE. Phase I study of an anti-breast cancer immunotoxin by continuous infusion: report of a targeted toxic effect not predicted by animal studies. J Natl Cancer Inst 1989; 81:775–781.
2. Ghetie MA, Uhr JW, Vitetta ES. Covalent binding of human $\alpha 2$-macroglobulin to deglycosylated ricin A chain and its immunotoxins. Cancer Res 1991; 51:1482–1487.
3. Baluna R, Ghetie V, Oppenheimer-Marks N, Vitetta ES. Fibronectin inhibits the

cytotoxic effect of ricin A chain on endothelial cells. Int J Immunopharm 1996; 18: 355–361.
4. Baluna R, Sausville EA, Stone MJ, Stetler-Stevenson MA, Uhr J, Vitetta ES. Decreases in levels of serum fibronectin predict the severity of vascular leak syndrome in patients treated with ricin A-chain-containing immunotoxins. Clin Cancer Res 1996; 2:1705–1712.
5. Byers VS, Baldwin RW. Targeted kill: from umbrellas to monoclonal antibodies. J Clin Immunol 1992; 12:391–405.
6. Grossbard ML, Freedman AS, Ritz J, Coral F, Goldmacher VS, Eliseo L, Spector N, Dear K, Lambert JM, Blattler WA, Taylor JA, Nadler LM. Serotherapy of B-cell neoplasms with anti-B4-blocked ricin: a Phase I trial of daily bolus infusion. Blood 1992; 79:576–585.
7. Stone MJ, Sausville EA, Fay JW, Headlee D, Collins RH, Figg WD, Stetler-Stevenson M, Jain V, Jaffe ES, Solomon D, Lush RM, Senderowicz A, Ghetie V, Schindler J, Uhr JW, Vitetta ES. A Phase I study of bolus versus continuous infusion of the anti-CD19 immunotoxin, IgG-HD37-dgA, in patients with B-cell lymphoma. Blood 1996; 88:1188–1197.
8. Conry RM, Khazaeli MB, Saleh MN, Ghetie V, Vitetta ES, Liu TP, Lobuglio AF. Phase I trial of an anti-CD19 deglycosylated ricin A chain immunotoxin in non-Hodgkin's lymphoma: effect of an intensive schedule of administration. J Immunother 1995; 18:231–241.
9. Kwak LW, Grossbard ML, Urba WJ. Clinical applications of monoclonal antibodies in cancer. In: De Vita VT Jr, Hellman S, Rosenberg SA, eds. Biologic Therapy of Cancer. Philadelphia: Lippincott 1995:553–565.
10. Uckun FM. 1995. B43-pokeweed antiviral protein (B43-PAP) immunotoxin (abstr). Fourth Int Symp Immunotoxins 162.
11. Sausville EA, Headlee D, Stetler-Stevenson M, Jaffe ES, Solomon D, Figg WD, Herdt J, Kopp WC, Rager H, Steinberg SM, Ghetie V, Schindler J, Uhr J, Wittes RE, Vitetta ES. Continuous infusion of the anti-CD22 immunotoxin IgG-RFB4-SMPT-dgA in patients with B-cell lymphoma: a Phase I study. Blood 1995; 85: 3457–3465.
12. Grossbard ML, Lambert JM, Goldmacher VS, Spector NL, Kinsella J, Eliseo L, Coral F, Taylor JA, Blattler WA, Epstein CL, Nadler LM. Anti-B4-blocked ricin: a Phase I trial of 7-day continuous infusion in patients with B-cell neoplasms. J Clin Oncol 1993; 11:726–737.
13. Ghetie MA, Vitetta ES. Recent developments in immunotoxin therapy. Curr Opin Immunol 1994; 6:707–714.
14. Ghetie M, Ghetie V, Vitetta ES. The use of immunoconjugates in cancer therapy. Exp Opin Invest Drugs 1996; 5:309–321.
15. Chaudhary VK, Jinno Y, Gallo G, FitzGerald D, Pastan I. Mutagenesis of *Pseudomonas* exotoxin in identification of sequences responsible for the animal toxicity. J Biol Chem 1990; 265:16,306–16,310.
16. Brinkmann U, Pai LH, FitzGerald DJ, Pastan I. Alteration of a protease-sensitive region of *Pseudomonas* exotoxin prolongs its survival in the circulation of mice. Proc Natl Acad Sci USA 1992; 89:3065–3069.
17. Soler-Rodriguez AM, Ghetie MA, Oppenheimer-Marks N, Uhr JW, Vitetta ES. Ricin

A-chain and ricin A-chain immunotoxins rapidly damage human endothelial cells: implications for vascular leak syndrome. Exp Cell Res 1993; 206:227–234.
18. Kuan C, Pastan I. Deletion analysis of the toxin moiety of the recombinant toxin B3(Fv)PE38 and its therapeutic applications (abstr). Fourth Int Symp Immunotoxins 1997; 54.
19. Ghetie MA, Tucker K, Richardson J, Uhr JW, Vitetta ES. The antitumor activity of an anti-CD22 immunotoxin in SCID mice with disseminated Daudi lymphoma is enhanced by either an anti-CD19 antibody or an anti-CD19 immunotoxin. Blood 1992; 80:2315–2320.
20. Ghetie M-A, Tucker K, Richardson J, Uhr JW, Vitetta ES. Eradication of minimal disease in severe combined immunodeficient mice with disseminated Daudi lymphoma using chemotherapy and an immunotoxin cocktail. Blood 1994; 84:702–707.
21. Flavell D, Noss A, Pulford K, Flavell S. 3BIT, a triple combination cocktail of anti-CD19, -CD22 and -CD38-saporin immunoxtoxins is curative of human B-cell lymphoma in SCID mice. Proc Am Assoc Cancer Res 1997; 38:83.
22. O'Connor R, Liu C, Ferris CA, Guild BC, Teicher BA, Corvi C, Liu Y, Arceci RJ, Goldmacher VS, Lambert JM, Blättler WA. Anti-B4-blocked ricin synergizes with doxorubicin and etoposide on multidrug-resistant and drug-sensitive tumors. Blood 1995; 86:4286–4294.
23. Ghetie MA, Podar EM, Gordon BE, Pantazis P, Uhr JW, Vitetta ES. Combination immunotoxin treatment and chemotherapy in SCID mice with advanced, disseminated Daudi lymphoma. Int J Cancer 1996; 68:93–96.
24. Candiani C, Franceschi A, Chignola R, Pasti M, Anselmi C, Benoni G, Tridente G, Colombatti M. Blocking effect of human serum but not of cerebrospinal fluid on ricin A chain immunotoxin potentiation by monensin or carrier protein-monensin conjugates. Cancer Res 1992; 52:623–630.
25. Ramakrishnan S, Bjorn MJ, Houston LL. Recombinant ricin A chain conjugated to monoclonal antibodies: improved tumor cell inhibition in the presence of lysosomotropic compounds. Cancer Res 1989; 49:613–617.
26. Itoh T, Shiota M, Takanashi M, Hojo I, Satoh H, Matsuzawa A, Moriyama T, Watanabe T, Hirai K, Mori S. Engraftment of human non-Hodgkin lymphomas in mice with severe combined immunodeficiency. Cancer 1993; 72:2686–2694.
27. Meggetto F, Muller C, Henry S, Selves J, Mariamè B, Brousset P, Saati TA, Delsol G. Epstein-Barr virus (EBV)-associated lymphoproliferations in severe combined immunodeficient mice transplanted with Hodgkin's disease lymph nodes: implication of EBV-positive bystander B lymphocytes rather than EBV-infected Reed-Sternberg cells. Blood 1996; 87:2435–2442.
28. Francisco JA, Schreibcr GJ, Comereski CR, Mera LE, Warner GL, Davidson TJ, Ledbetter JA, Siegall CB. In vivo efficacy and toxicities of a single-chain immunotoxin targeted to CD40. Blood 1997; 89:4493–4500.
29. Folkman J. Addressing tumor blood vessels. Nature Biotech 1997; 15:70.
30. Thrush GR, Lark LR, Clinchy BC, Vitetta ES. Immunotoxins: an update. Annu Rev Immunol 1996; 14:49–71.
31. Chignola R, Anselmi C, Serra MD, Franceschi A, Fracasso G, Pasti M, Chiesa E, Lord JM, Tridente G, Colombatti M. Self-potentiation of ligand–toxin conjugates

containing ricin A chain fused with viral structures. J Biol Chem 1996; 270:23,345–351.
32. FitzGerald D, Pastan I. Recombinant immunotoxins for the treatment of cancer. J Controlled Release 1996; 39:261–265.
33. Gadina M, Newton DL, Rybak SM, Wu YN, Youle RS. Humanized immunotoxins. Therap Immunol 1994; 1:59–64.
34. Burrows FJ, Thorpe PE. Eradication of large solid tumors in mice with an immunotoxin directed against tumor vasculature. Proc Natl Acad Sci USA 1993; 90:8996–9000.
35. Huang X, Molema G, King S, Watkins L, Edgington TS, Thorpe PE. Tumor infarction in mice by antibody-directed targeting of tissue factor to tumor vasculature. Science 1997; 275:547–550.
36. Seon BK, Matsuno F, Haruta Y, Kondo M, Barcos M. Long-lasting complete inhibition of growth of human solid tumors in SCID mice by targeting endothelial cells by tumor vasculature with anti-human endoglin immunotoxin. Clin Cancer Res 1997; 3:1031–1044.
37. Burrows FJ, Derbyshire EJ, Tazzari PL, Amlot P, Gazdar AF, King SN, Letarte M, Vitetta ES, Thorpe PE. Up-regulation of endoglin on vascular endothelial cells in human solid tumors: implication for diagnosis and therapy. Clin Cancer Res 1995; 1:1623–1634.
38. Reiter Y, Pastan I. Antibody engineering of recombinant Fv immunotoxins for improved targeting of cancer: disulfide stablized Fv immunotoxins. Clin Cancer Res 1996; 2:245–255.
39. Ghetie V, Vitetta ES. Immunotoxins in the therapy of cancer: from bench to clinic. Pharmacol Ther 1994; 63:209–234.
40. Brinkmann U, Pastan I. Immunotoxins against cancer. Biochim Biophys Acta 1994; 1198:27–45.
41. Ward ES, Ghetie V. The effector functions of immunoglobulins: implications for therapy. Therap Immunol 1995; 2:77–94.
42. Van Horssen PJ, Van Oosterhout YV, De Witte, T, Preijers FN. Cytotoxic potency of CD22-ricin A depends on intracellular routing rather than on the number of internalized molecules. Scand J Immunol 1995; 41:503–509.
43. Yazdi PT, Wenning LA, Murphy RM. Influence of cellular trafficking on protein synthesis inhibition of immunotoxins directed against the transferrin receptors. Cancer Res 1995; 55:3763–3771.
44. May RD, Wheeler HT, Finkelman FD, Uhr JW, Vitetta ES. Intracellular routing rather than cross-linking or rate of internalization determines the potency of immunotoxins directed against different epitopes of sIgD on murine B cells. Cell Immunol 1991; 135:490–500.
45. Hayden MS, Gilliland LK, Ledbetter JA. Antibody engineering. Curr Opin Immunol 1997; 9:201–212.
46. Sollazzo M, Martin F, Venturini S, Esposito G, Traboni C. Engineering and phage-display of antibody fragments and minibody repertoires. In: Zanetti M, Capra JD, eds. The Antibodies. Luxembourg: Harwood Academic, 1995:213–232.
47. Lorimer IAJ, Keppler-Hafkemeyer A, Beers RA, Pegram CN, Bigner DD, Pastan I. Recombinant immunotoxins specific for a mutant epidermal growth factor receptor:

targeting with a single chain antibody variable domain isolated by phage display. Proc Natl Acad Sci USA 1996; 93:14815–14820.
48. Medesan C, Matesoi D, Radu C, Ghetie V, Ward ES. Delineation of the amino acid residues involved in transcytosis and catabolism of mouse IgG. J Immunol 1997; 158:2211–2217.
49. Adams GP, Schier R, Crawford R, McCall AM, Simmons H, Marks JD, Weiner LM. Improved tumor retention and therapeutic potential of single-chain Fv-based diabody molecules. Proc Am Assoc Cancer Res 1997; 38:83.
50. Pai LH, Pastan I. Immunotoxins and recombinant toxins. In: DeVita VT, Hellman S, Rosenberg SA, eds. Biologic Therapy of Cancer. Philadelphia: Lippincott, 1995: 521–533.
51. Better M, Bernhard SL, Fishwild DM, Nolan PA, Bauer RS, Kung AHC, Carroll SF. Gelonin analogs with engineered cysteine residues form antibody immunoconjugates with unique properties. J Biol Chem 1994; 269:9644–9650.
52. O'Hare M, Brown AN, Hussain K, Gebhardt A, Watson G, Roberts LM, Vitetta ES, Thorpe PE, Lord JM. Cytotoxicity of a recombinant ricin-A-chain fusion protein containing a proteolytically cleavable spacer sequence. FEBS Lett 1990; 273:200–204.
53. Spooner RA, Allen RA, Epenetos AA, Lord JM. Expression of immunoglobin heavy chain ricin A chain fusions in mammalian cells. Mol Immunol 1994; 31:117–125.
54. Fernandez-Luna JL, Lopez-Otin C, Soriano F, and Mendez E. Complete amino acid sequence of the Aspergillus cytotoxic mitogillin. Biochemistry 1985; 24:861–867.
55. Bohun E. and Twardowski. T. The α-sarcin domain of large ribosomal RNA is a strategic fragment for plant ribosome function. J Plant Physiol 1994; 143:659–669.
56. Rathore D. and Batra JK. Generation of active immunotoxins containing recombinant restrictocin. Biochem Biophys Res Commun 1996; 222:58–63.
57. Better M, Bernhard SL, Lei SP, Fishwild DM, and Carroll SF. Activity of recombinant mitogillin and mitogillin immunocojugates. J Biol Chem 1992; 267:16712–16718.
58. Siegall CB, Gawlak SL, Chace D, Wolff EA, Mixan B, and Marquardt H. Characterization of ribosome–inactivating proteins isolated from Bryonia dioica and their utility as carcinoma-reactive immunoconjugates. Bioconjug Chem 1994; 5:423–429.
59. Becker JC, Pancook JD, Gillies SD, Mendelson J, and Reisfeld RA. Eradication of human hepatic and pulmonary melanoma metastases in Scid mice by antibody interleukin 2 fusion proteins. Proc Natl Acad Sci USA 1996; 93:2702–2707.
60. Newton DL, Xue Y, Olson KA, Fett JW, Rybak SM. Angiogenin single-chain immunotoxins: influence of peptide linkers and spacers between fusion protein domains. Biochemistry 1996; 35:545–553.
61. Rosenblum MG, Cheung L, Miyoo K, Murray JL. An antimelanoma immunotoxin containing recombinant human tumor necrosis factor: tissue disposition, pharmacokinetic and therapeutic studies in xenograft models. Cancer Immunol Immunother 1995; 40:322–328.
62. Pederzolli C, Belmonte G, Serra MD, Macek P, Menestrina G. Biochemical and cytotoxic properties of conjugates of transferrin with equinatoxin II, a cytolysin from sea anemone. Bioconjug Chem 1995; 6:166–173.
63. Al-Yahyaee SA, Ellar DJ. Cell targeting of a pore-forming toxin, Cyt A δ-endotoxin

from *Bacillus thuringiensis* subspecies *israelensis*, by conjugating CytA with anti-Thy1 monoclonal antibodies and insulin. Bioconjug Chem 1996; 7:451–460.
64. Panchal RG, Cusack E, Cheley S, Bayley H. Tumor protease-activated, pore forming toxins from a combinational library. Nature Biotech 1996; 14:852–856.
65. Sloane BF. Suicidal tumor proteases. Nature Biotech 1996; 14:826–827.
66. Bayley H. Triggers and switches in self-assembling pore-forming proteins. J Cell Biochem 1994; 56:177–182.
67. Greenfield RS, Kaneko T, Daues A, Edson MA, Fitzgerald KA, Olech LJ, Gratt JA, Spitalny GL, Braslawsky GR. Evaluation in vitro of adriamycin immunoconjugates synthesized using an acid-sensitive hydrazone linker. Cancer Res 1990; 50:6600–6607.
68. Chari RVJ, Martell BA, Gross JL, Cook SB, Shah SA, Blattler WA, McKenzie SJ, Goldmacher VS. Immunoconjugates containing novel maytansinoids: promising anticancer drugs. Cancer Res 1992; 52:127–131.
69. Hinman LM, Hamman PR, Wallace R, Menendez AT, Durr FE, Upeslacis J. Preparation and characterization of monoclonal antitumor conjugates of the calicheamicins: a novel and potent family of antitumor antibodies. Cancer Res 1993; 53:3336–3342.
70. Liu C, Tadayoni BM, Bourret LA, Mattocks KM, Derr SM, Widdison WC, Kedersha NL, Arniello PD, Goldmacher VS, Lambert JM, Blattler WA, Chari RV. Eradication of large colon tumor xenografts by targeted delivery of maytansinoids. Proc Natl Acad Sci USA 1996; 93:8618–8623.
71. Liu C, Bourret LA, Derr SM, Widdison WC, Lambert JM, Blattler WA, Chari RVJ. Cure of human small cell lung cancer xenografts in SCID mice by a hN901-maytansinoid immunoconjugates. Proc Am Assoc Cancer Res 1997; 38:29.
72. Trail PA, Willner D, Lasch SJ, Henderson AJ, Hofstead S, Casazza AM, Firestone RA, Hellstrom I, Hellstrom KE. Cure of xenografted human carcinomas by BR96-doxorubicin immunoconjugates. Science 1993; 261:212–215.
73. Lasch SJ, Henderson A, Knipe J, Mosure K, Bianchi A, Fairchild C, Hellstrom I, Hellstrom KE, Trail PA. Activity of carcinoma reactive BR96-DOX immunoconjugate against multidrug resistant human breast carcinoma. Proc Am Assoc Cancer Res 1997; 38:29.
74. Yang AG, Chen SY. A new class of antigen-specific killer cells. Nature Biotech 1997; 15:46–51.
75. Chen S, Yang A, Chen J, Kute T, King CR, Collier J, Cong Y, Yao C, Huang XF. Potent antitumor activity of a new class of tumor-specific killer cells. Nature 1997; 385:78–80.
76. FitzGerald DJP. Antitumor immunotoxin secretion by T cells: absolutely fabulous? Nature Biotech 1997; 15:18–19.

Index

2A11
17-1A
  colorectal cancer, 287, 291, 296, 298
    toxicity, 292, 294
A108
  non-small-cell lung cancer, 372
Abrin, 9
Acute leukemia
  Anti-CD5 immunotoxin, 192
  CD10, 191
  HAMA, 201
  HATA, 201
  immunotoxins, 191, 192, 195, 196, 197
  MAb therapy, 189–203
    barriers, 201–203
    preclinical studies, 191
    target molecules, 193t
    therapeutic use, 192–200
  Thy 1.1, 191
  unconjugated immunotoxins, 201
  unconjugated monoclonal antibodies, 201

Acute lymphoblastic leukemia
  Anti-B4-bR, 195, 245, 248
  Anti-CD7, 245
  Anti-CD22, 196
  Anti-CD38, 197
  Anti-CD22-ricin, 202
  Anti-CD7 saporin, 202
  antigens, 244–245
  Anti-Leu-1, 197
  Anti-TAC antibody, 198
  Anti-TAC-H antibody, 198
  B-lineage, 244
  B43-PAP, 195–196
  BU12-saporin, 196, 202
  CALLA, 194–195
  CD5, 197
  CD10, 194–195
  CD19, 195–196
  CD22, 196
  CD25, 197–198
  CD39, 196–197
  CD52, 199–200
  IL-2 receptor, 197–198
  immunomagnetic bead-mediated purging, 248

[Acute lymphoblastic leukemia]
    immunotoxins, 245–248
    MAb therapy, 189–203
    OKT10-saporin, 197
    progenitor-cell transplantation
            (PCT)
        clinical trials, 248–249
    purging, 245–248
    RFB4-dgA, 196
    T-lineage, 244–245
    Y90 antiTAC-H, 198
Acute myeloid leukemia
    Anti-CD33, 198
    Anti-CD33-calicheamicin, 199
    Anti-My9-bR, 199
    CD33, 198–199
    CD52, 199–200
    iodine-131-M15, 198–199
    M195, 198
    MAb therapy, 189–203
    progenitor-cell transplantation
            (PCT), 236–241
    purging, 236–241
    radioimmunoconjugates, 198–199
    tumor-cell contamination, 231–233
A33-Iodine-131
    colorectal cancer, 297–298
αIR-3
    NSCLC, 375–376
ALL. *see* Acute lymphoblastic leukemia
ALM. *see* Acute myeloid leukemia
Angiogenesis
    tumors, 24
    tumor vasculature, 27–28
    vessels and growth factors, 25
Anti-B4-blocked ricin
    ALL, 195, 245, 248
    animal studies, 95–96
    chronic lymphocytic leukemia,
            107–108

[Anti-B4-blocked ricin]
    clinical trials, 99–108
    combination studies, 97–99
    cytotoxicity, 94
    HIV-related NHL, 106–107
    isobolograms, 14f
    non-Hodgkin's lymphoma, 250–252
    pharmacokinetic studies, 103
    preclinical studies, 95–96
    single-agent studies, 93–97
    in vitro synergy, 97–98
    in vivo cytotoxicity, 97, 98–99
Anti-CALLA monoclonal antibody,
            194–195
Anti-CD3
    GVHD, 219
Anti-CD7
    ALL, 245
Anti-CD19
    Anti-CD22
        NHL combination therapy, 85
Anti-CD22
    ALL, 196
    Anti-CD19
        NHL combination therapy, 85
Anti-CD33
    AML, 198
Anti-CD38
    ALL, 197
Anti-CD52
    clinical trials, 70–71
Anti-CD20 antibody
    clinical trials, 68–70
Anti-CD25 antibody
    lymphoma, 72
Anti-CD33-calicheamicin
    AML, 199
Anti-CD3 immunotoxin
    GVHD, 218
Anti-CD5 immunotoxin
    acute leukemia, 192

Anti-CD10 monoclonal antibody, 194–195
Anti-CD5-ricin
  GVHD, 219, 221, 222
Anti-CD22-ricin
  ALL, 202
Anti-CD5-ricin A-chain immunotoxin
  ALL, 197
Anti-CD7 saporin
  ALL, 202
Anti-CEA(I-1), 287
  toxicity, 294
Anti-CEA-Iodine-131
  thyroid cancer, 301
Anti-erbB2
  breast cancer, 312, 323–324
Antiferritin immunoglobulin, 176
Antiganglioside antibodies
  small-cell lung cancer, 383–384
Antigen modulation, 283, 314
Antigen mutation frequency
  antibody therapy, 56–58
Antigen presentation
  breast cancer, 313
Antiidiotypic antibodies, 54–55, 56, 57, 343
  clinical trials, 64–65
  malignant melanoma, 353–354
  small-cell lung cancer, 384
Anti-IL-6 antibody
  lymphoma, 72
Anti-Leu-1
  ALL, 197
Anti-MY9-bR
  AML, 199
  purging, 240
Antincoplastics, 426
Anti-p185 HER2
  breast cancer, 290
  lung cancer, 373

Anti-Tac antibody
  All, 198
  CD30, 156, 157, 158
  Hodgkin's disease, 155–157
Anti-Tac-H antibody
  ALL, 198
Anti-Tac(sFv)PE38
  Hodgkin's disease, 169
Anti-Tac(sFv)PE40
  Hodgkin's disease, 165
Anti-TAG-72, 316
Anti-thy1.2 ricin
  GVHD, 218
Antitumor mechanisms, 62t

2B1, 288
B3, 325–326
  MAb, 3, 4
B72.3, 325
Bacillus Calmette-Guerin
  breast cancer, 209
BC-2
  gliomas, 287
BC-4, 287
  gliomas, 287, 301
BCG
  breast cancer, 209
BEC2
  small-cell lung cancer, 384, 386
Ber-H2, 157–158
Ber-H2-ricin A-chain
  Hodgkin's disease, 171
Ber-H2-saporin
  Hodgkin's disease, 167–168, 171
Ber-H2-SMPT-dgA
  Hodgkin's disease, 167
Bispecific antibody therapy, 283–284, 288
  breast cancer, 314–315, 322, 324
  clinical data, 161–163
  Hodgkin's disease, 158–163
  preclinical data, 160–161

[Bispecific antibody therapy]
  toxicity, 159–160
Blocked ricin-anti-CEA(I-1)
  colorectal cancer, 298
Bone marrow transplant
  processing and treatment, 229–257
B43-PAP
  ALL, 195–196
  non-Hodgkin's lymphoma, 250
BR55-2
  breast cancer, 300
BR96, 326
  MAb, 3, 4
Brain cancer
  3F8, 346
BR96-DOX, 397–413, 426
  antitumor activity, 400–404
  breast cancer, 404–409
  chemical characteristics, 398
  colorectal cancer, 405–409
  non-small-cell lung cancer, 404–409
  ovarian cancer, 404–409
  pharmacokinetics, 409, 410–413
  phase I clinical trials, 404–409
  toxicity, 405–408
  in vitro biology, 399–400
Breast cancer, 283, 284, 286t, 299–300
  Anti-erbB2, 312, 323–324
  Anti-p185 HER-2, 290
  BCG, 209
  bispecific antibodies, 314–315, 322, 324
  BR55-3, 300
  BR96-DOX, 404–409
  C225, 322
  carcinoembryonic antigen, 324–325
  e23(Fv)PE anti-erbB2, 324

[Breast cancer]
  epidermal growth factor receptors, 317, 323
  ErB2, 323–324
  260F9-ricin A, 283
    toxicity, 294
  260F9-RTA, 299–300
  HER-2/neu, 289–290, 300
  humAB 4D5, 373–374
  immunotherapy, 311–317
    barriers, 312–317
  L6, 300
  levamisole, 209
  MAb therapy, 309–328
  MDX-210, 283, 284, 289, 300
  MDX-447, 322
  MUC-1, 314
  mucin antigens, 325–327
  radioimmunotherapy, 316
  rhu MAbHER2, 315
  T84.66 anti-CEA, 325
Breast cancer-associated antigens, 310–311
BR96(sFv)PE, 326
BU12-saporin
  ALL, 196, 202

C225
  breast cancer, 322
C242
  MAb, 3, 4
CALLA
  ALL, 194–195
CAMPATH-1, 199–200
CAMPATH-1H, 200
  clinical trials, 70–71
  immunosuppression, 56
  lymphoma, 59
Carcinoembryonic antigen
  breast cancer, 324–325
Carcinoembryonic antigen antibodies
  small-cell lung cancer, 378–379

Index

Castlemann's disease, 72
CC49, 286, 325
CC49-Iodine-131
  prostate cancer, 300–301
CD3
  GVHD, 218
  Hodgkin's disease, 154
CD5
  ALL, 197
  cutaneous T-cell lymphomas, 138
  GVHD, 217–218
  lymphoma, 71–72
  mycosis fungoides, 143
CD10
  acute leukemia, 191
  ALL, 194–195
CD19
  ALL, 195–196
  lymphoma antigen, 58
CD20
  antigens, 4
  lymphoma, 58, 63
CD22
  ALL, 196
CD25
  ALL, 197–198
  HD, 85–86
  Hodgkin's disease, 155–157, 164–165, 169–171
  lymphoma, 58, 63
CD30
  Hodgkin's disease, 165–168, 171, 175–176
  lymphoma, 73
CD33
  AML, 198–199
CD34, 230–231
  CLL, 255
  CML, 256
  multiple myeloma, 255
CD39
  ALL, 196–197

CD40, 197
  lymphoma, 73
  lymphoma antigen, 58
CD52
  ALL, 199–200
  AML, 199–200
CD56
  MAb, 3, 4
  small-cell lung cancer, 377–378
CD57
  lung cancer, 367
CD4 antigen
  cutaneous T-cell lymphomas, 139
CD5 antigen
  cutaneous T-cell lymphomas, 139
CD11B
  lung cancer, 367
CD3-CD30
  Hodgkin's disease, 161
CD16-CD30
  Hodgkin's disease, 160, 161, 163
CD28-CD30
  Hodgkin's disease, 161, 163
CDRs. *see* Complementarity-determining regions
CD34 selection
  non-Hodgkin's lymphoma, 253–257
CD2T
  cutaneous T-cell lymphoma, 142–143
C-erb-2, 288, 298
cGVHD. *see* Chronic-graft-versus-host-disease
Ch14.18
  malignant melanoma, 349, 350, 351
ChB72.3-Iodine131
  colorectal cancer, 297
Chemotherapeutic agents. *see* Immunotoxins
Chimeric antibodies, 291

Chronic graft-versus-host disease, 214–215
  clinical manifestations, 216
  therapy, 217
Chronic lymphocytic leukemia
  Anti-B4-blocked ricin, 107–108
Chronic myelogenous leukemia
  CD34, 256
  progenitor-cell transplantation (PCT), 241–243
  purging, 241–243
  tumor-cell contamination, 231–233
Cisplatin
  malignant melanoma, 349–350
Cluster-2 antigen
  lung cancer, 367
Cluster-4 antigen
  lung cancer, 367
  CML. see Chronic myelogenous leukemia
cMT412
  lymphoma antigen, 72
CO17-A
  colorectal cancer, 283, 289
Colorectal cancer, 283, 290–292, 296–298
  17-1A, 287, 289, 291, 296, 298
  A33-Iodine-131, 297–298
  blocked ricin-anti-CEA(I-1), 298
  BR96-DOX, 405–409
  ChB72.3-Iodine131, 297
  CO17-A, 283
  D612, 297
  immunotherapy, 298
  iodine-131-17-Ia, 298
  iodine-131-F19, 290–291
  XomaZyme-791, 298
Complementarity-determining regions, 291

Cutaneous T-cell lymphoma, 137–138
  CD5, 138
  CD4 antigen, 139
  CD2T, 142–143
  conjugated MAb therapy, 140–143
  DAB389IL-2, 143–144
  DAB486IL-2, 143–144
  immunotoxin therapy, 143
  In-111, 141–142
  Leu-1, 138
  ligand fusion toxin therapy, 143–144
  MAb therapy
    limitations, 139–140
    radioimmunoconjugate therapy, 140–143
  T101, 138
  T101-I131, 141–142
  unconjugated MAb therapy, 138–140
    clinical trials, 138–139
  vaccine therapy, 140
  Y90-anti-Tac, 142–143
Cytolytic toxins, 425–426
Cytotoxicity, 94
  immunotoxins, 13t
Cytotoxicity tests
  N901-bR, 12, 13f

4D5
  lung cancer, 373
D612
  colorectal cancer, 297
  gastrointestinal cancer, 289
DAB389IL2
  cutaneous T-cell lymphoma, 143–144
  Hodgkin's disease, 144, 159, 165
  mycosis fungoides, 144
  non-Hodgkin's lymphoma, 144

Index

DAB486IL2
  cutaneous T-cell lymphoma, 143–144
  Hodgkin's disease, 165, 169
  mycosis fungoides, 144
  Sezary syndrome, 144
Deglycosylated ricin A-chain immunotoxins (dgA ITs)
  clinical studies, 81–87
  HD, 86
  VLS, 87
DF3, 326–327
Diphtheria toxin, 5–6, 8, 9
  Hodgkin's disease, 164
DT390-anti-CD3sFv
  GVHD, 219

E23(Fv)PE anti-erbB2
  breast cancer, 324
EGF, 368
Epidermal growth factor, 368
Epidermal growth factor antibodies, 360–372
Epidermal growth factor receptor, 317, 323, 369
Epstein-Barr virus, 152–153
ErB2, 323–324
Extravasation
  blood-borne molecule, 31

1F5
  lymphoma, 69
3F8, 346, 350–351
  brain cancer, 346
  small-cell lung cancer, 383–384
  toxicity, 295
Fab'-RFB4-dgA
  NHL, 82
Ferritin
  Hodgkin's disease, 173–174, 176–178

Fluorescence ratio-imaging microscopy, 28
Fluorescence recovery after photobleaching, 34, 35
260F9-ricin A
  breast cancer, 283, 299–300
  toxicity, 294
Fusion proteins, 191
  GVHD, 219

14G2a, 346
  malignant melanoma, 351
Ganglioside antigens, 343–344
Gangliosides
  lung cancer, 383–386
Gastrin-releasing peptide, 374
GD2, 344, 346
GD3, 343–344, 346
G250-Iodine-131
  renal cell cancer, 300
Gliomas
  BC-2, 287, 301
Graft-versus-host disease
  allogeneic bone marrow transplants, 221
  Anti-CD3, 219
  Anti-CD3 immunotoxins, 218
  Anti-CD5 ricin, 219, 221, 222
  Anti-thy 1.2 ricin, 218
  CD3, 218
  CD5, 217–218
  chronic, 214–215
    clinical manifestations, 216
    therapy, 217
  clinical manifestations, 216
  donor T-cell activation, 212–214
  DT390-anti-CD3sFv, 219
  fusion proteins, 219
  host tissue damage, 212
  H65-RTA, 222–223

[Graft-versus-host disease]
　immune-mediated end organ damage, 214
　immune system, 211–214
　immunotoxin therapy, 217–223
　　animal studies, 218–219
　　human studies, 219–223
　　targets, 217–218
　　toxins, 218
　prophylaxis, 221–222
　T10B9-1A-31, 221
　treatment, 217, 222–223
Growth back-extrapolation assay, 94
Growth factor receptors
　lung cancer, 366–368
Growth factors
　malignant melanoma, 350
　small-cell lung cancer, 374–378
GRP, 374
GVHD. *see* Graft-versus-host-disease

HACA
　lymphoma, 59
HAMA. *see* Human antimouse antibody
HATA, 201
Hematopoietic progenitor-cell graft
　processing and treatment, 229–257
HER-2, 323–324
　non-small-cell lung cancer, 373
HER-2/neu, 300
　breast cancer, 289–290, 300
　non-small-cell lung cancer, 368
High-molecular-weight melanoma-associated antigen, 344
HIV-related NHL
　Anti-B4-blocked ricin, 106–107
HMFG, 379–380
HMFG1, 326–327, 379–380
HMFG2, 326–327

HMFG1-Y90, 287
HMS-MAA, 344
Hodgkin's disease, 81
　Anti-Tac antibody, 155–157
　Anti-Tac(sFv)PE38, 169
　Anti-Tac(sFv)PE40, 165
　Ber-H2-ricin A-chain, 171
　Ber-H2-saporin, 167–168, 171
　Ber-H2-SMPT-dgA, 167
　bispecific antibody therapy, 158–163
　CD3, 154
　CD25, 155–157, 164–165, 169–171
　CD30, 165–168, 171, 175–176
　CD3-CD30, 161
　CD16-CD30, 160, 161, 163
　CD28-CD30, 161, 163
　cell of origin, 150–152
　DAB389IL2, 165, 169
　DAB486IL2, 165, 169
　diphtheria toxin, 164
　EBV, 152–153
　eosinophil peroxidase, 173, 176
　ferritin, 173–174, 176–178
　HRS-3-SMPT-dgA, 167
　immunotoxin therapy, 163–170
　　clinical data, 168–171
　iodine123 HRS1, 175–176
　iodine131 HRS1, 175–176
　Ki-1 antigen, 154
　Leu-Ml, 152, 154
　MAb therapy, 149–180
　markers, 153–154
　passive antibody therapy, 154–158
　radioimmunotherapy, 172–180
　RFT5-SMPT-dg, 165, 169
　RIPs, 163–164
　saporin, 164
　T200, 152
　Tac, 154

Index

[Hodgkin's disease]
  T200 antigen, 153–154
  90Y-antiferritin, 176–179
HRS-3-SMPT-dgA
  Hodgkin's disease, 167
H65-RTA
  GVHD, 222–223
HumAB 4D5
  breast cancer, 373–374
Human and murine immunoglobulin isotypes
  immune effector functions, 63t
Human antimouse antibody, 284, 286, 342–343, 351
  acute leukemia, 201
  development, 315–317
  lymphoma, 59, 60
  mycosis fungoides, 139
Human antimurine antibody response malignant melanoma, 348–349
Human antitoxin antibody, 201
Hydraulic conductivity
  tumors, 32

ICR62
  lung cancer, 372
IDEC-C2B8
  lymphoma, 54, 57, 58, 63, 73
    clinical trials, 68
    radiolabeled antibodies, 56
Idiotype vaccination
  clinical trials, 65, 68
225 IGG, 322
528 IgG2A, 322
IgG-HD37-dgA
  NHL clinical trial, 84–85
  Raynaud's-like syndrome, 86–87
IgG-RFB4-dgA
  NHL, 82, 83, 85
  VLS, 87

Ig-RFT5-dgA
  chemotherapy, 87
  HD, 86
III-In-225
  lung cancer, 370
II-Mel-2
  malignant melanoma, 354
IL-2, 340
  malignant melanoma, 350–351
IL-2 receptor
  ALL, 197–198
Immune effector functions
  human and murine immunoglobulin isotypes, 63t
Immune system
  GVHD, 211–214
Immunoconjugates, 397–413
Immunoglobulin idiotype
  clinical trials, 64–65
Immunolysins, 425
Immunomagnetic bead purging
  ALL, 248
  non-Hodgkin's lymphoma, 250
Immunomagnetic beads, 234
Immunotherapy
  breast cancer, 311–317
  colorectal cancer, 298
  solid tumors, 282–292
Immunotoxin development, 1–20
Immunotoxins
  Anti B4-blocked ricin, 11, 12–15, 17
  blocked ricin, 9, 11–12
  cytoxicity, 13t
  deglycosylated ricin A chain
    clinical studies, 81–87
  drug disposition, 15–17
  efficacy and safety evaluation, 10–19
  genetic engineering, 2–3
  N901-bR, 12
  nonclinical pharmacology, 12–17

[Immunotoxins]
  targeting moiety, 18
  toxicology, 17–19
Immunotoxin therapy, 234, 417–427
  acute leukemia, 191, 192, 195–197, 201
  ALL, 245–248
  AML, 199
  antibody size and affinity, 422–425
  antineoplastics, 426
  cutaneous T-cell lymphoma, 143
  cytolytic toxins, 425–426
  debulking therapy dose regimen, 420–421
  delivery, 426–427
  enhancers
    humans, 421
  future research, 422–427
  GVHD, 217–223, 218
    animal studies, 218–219
    human studies, 219–223
    targets, 217–218
    toxins, 218
  history, 417
  Hodgkin's disease, 163–170
    clinical data, 168–171
  humans, 418–420
    dose schedules, 419
    toxicity, 419–420
    tumor burden, 418–419
  lymphoma
    Anti-B4-blocked ricin, 91–109
  mouse models, 421
  non-Hodgkin's lymphoma, 250
  rodents vs. humans, 417–418
  single therapy vs. mixtures, 420
  small-cell lung cancer, 377–378

[Immunotoxin therapy]
  therapeutic index, 421
  toxicity, 163–164, 294
  vascular leak syndrome, 201, 419, 420
  vascular targeting, 422
In-111
  cutaneous T-cell lymphoma, 141–142
  malignant melanoma, 347
96.5-In-111
  malignant melanoma, 352
225-In-111
  squamous cell lung cancer, 300
In-lll anti CEA ZCE 025
  small-cell lung cancer, 378–379
In-lll-FO23C5
  small-cell lung cancer, 378–379
Insulin-like growth factor
  non-small-cell lung cancer, 375–376
Intact MAb
  vs. MAb fragments, 2–3
Interferon
  96.5, 352
  malignant melanoma, 352
Interstitial pressure
  human tissue, 40t
Intracellular antibodies, 312
Iodine-131-8.2
  malignant melanoma, 347
Iodine-131-96.5
  malignant melanoma, 347
Iodine-131-17-1a
  colorectal cancer, 298
Iodine-131-anti-CD20
  biodistribution, 117
  non-Hodgkin's lymphoma, 121–122
  toxicity, 123
Iodine-131-CC49, 288–289

Iodine-131-F19
  colorectal cancer, 290–291
Iodine-123 HRS1
  Hodgkin's disease, 175–176
Iodine-131-Lym-1
  biodistribution, 118
  dosimetry, 125
Iodine-131-MTS
  AML, 198–199
Isobolograms
  Anti B4-blocked ricin, 14f

KC-4G3
  non-small-cell lung cancer, 380
Ki-1 antigen
  Hodgkin's disease, 154
KM966
  small-cell lung cancer, 383
KS1/4
  lung cancer, 283, 284, 300

L6
  breast cancer, 300
  colorectal cancer, 296
  ovarian cancer, 298
L55-81
  malignant melanoma, 349
L72
  malignant melanoma, 349
L6 antigen, 327
Leu-1
  cutaneous T-cell lymphomas, 138
Leukocyte-endothelial interactions, 37f
Leu-M1
  Hodgkin's disease, 152, 154
Levamisole
  breast cancer, 209
LewisY, 397, 398
LewisY antigen, 325–326, 404, 407

Ligand fusion toxin therapy
  cutaneous T-cell lymphoma, 143–144
Ligands
  lung cancer, 366–368
Liposomes, 316
Lu-171-CC49
  ovarian cancer, 299
Lung cancer, 283, 371, 382
  Anti-p 185HER2, 373
  CD57, 367
  CD11B, 367
  cluster-2 antigen, 367
  cluster-4 antigen, 367
  gangliosides, 383–386
  ICR62, 372
  III-In-225, 370
  KS1/4, 283, 284
  MAb therapy, 365–386
  NCAM, 367
  radioimmunoconjugates, 382–383
  186-Re-NR-LU-10, 382–383
  squamous cell, 300
  surface markers, 365–368
Lymphoma tumor antigens
  characteristics, 55t

M195
  AML, 198
MAb, 225, 369–370
MAb 523, 369
MAb 528, 370
  lung cancer, 371–372
MAbp120, 316
MAb tumor reactivity, 3–4
MAb tumor selectivity, 4–5
MAGE gene family, 340
Magnetic resonance spectroscopy
  tissue-isolated tumors
    tumor metabolism, 28
Malignant melanoma
  96.5, 352

[Malignant melanoma]
   antiidiotypic antibodies, 353–354
   ch14.18, 349, 350, 351
   cisplatin, 349–350
   14.G2a, 351
   growth factors, 350
   human antimurine antibody response, 348–349
   II-Mel-2, 354
   IL-2, 350–351
   III-In-96.5, 352
   indium-111, 347
   interferon, 352
   iodine-131-8.2, 347
   iodine-131-96.5, 347
   L55-81, 349
   L72, 349
   MAb conjugates, 352–353
   MAb therapy, 339–355
      barriers, 342–343
      enhancement, 349–352
   MF11-30, 354
   MK2-23, 354
   p96.5, 347
   R24, 284, 349–350, 351, 354–355
   radioisotope-labeled antibody, 346–348
   225.28S, 347–348
   tumor antigens, 343–344
   tumor immunity, 334–340
   tumor necrosis factor, 351–352
   unconjugated monoclonal antibodies, 344–346
   XOMAZYME-MEL, 353
   ZME-018, 347
Material movement
   interstitial compartment, 24
   microvascular wall, 24
MDX-210, 288
   breast cancer, 283, 284, 289, 300
   ovarian cancer, 298

MDX-447
   breast cancer, 322
ME36.1, 346
Melanocyte lineage proteins, 340
MF11-30
   malignant melanoma, 354
MG22, 351
Microcirculation region, 28
MK2-23
   malignant melanoma, 354
Molecules
   biodistribution schematic, 39f
MUC1 protein, 326–327
   breast cancer, 314
Mucin antigens
   breast cancer, 325–327
MUC1 protein, 326–327
Multiple myeloma, 72
   Anti-B4-blocked ricin, 108
   CD34, 255
Mycosis fungoides, 137–138
   CD-5, 143
   DAB389IL-2, 144
   DAB486IL-2, 144
   HAMA, 139

N901
   human tissue reactivity, 6t–7t
   MAb, 3, 4, 5, 19
   small-cell lung cancer, 287–288
N901-bR
   cytotoxicity tests, 12, 13f
   human tissue reactivity, 6t–7t
   immunotoxins, 12, 19
   small-cell lung cancer, 377–378
NCAM, 367, 376–378
NE 150
   small-cell lung cancer, 377
Necrotic region, 28

Neural cell adhesion antibodies, 367, 376–378
Non-Hodgkin's lymphoma, 53, 60, 91
  Anti-B4-bR, 250–252
  Anti-B4-blocked ricin, 93–108
  Anti-CD20 antibody, 54
  Anti-CD22-dgA, 82–83
  autologous transplantation, 251, 253
  B43-PAP, 250
  blocked ricin, 92–93
  CD19, 115
  CD34 selection, 253–257
  CD45, 115
  DAB389IL-2, 144
  hematopoietic progenitor selection, 253–256
  IDEC-C2B8, 54, 57
  immunomagnetic bead purging, 250
  immunotoxin therapy, 250
    Anti-B4-blocked ricin, 91–109
  immunotoxins, 250
  iodine-131, 115–116
  iodine-131-labeled anti-CD20, 121–122
  progenitor cell transplantation (PCT), 251–252
  purging, 249–257
  radioimmunoconjugate therapy, 113–128
    clinical trials, 118–122
  RIT, 113–114
  unconjugated MAb therapy, 53–73
    antibody administration, 59
    antibody characteristics, 59–61
    antigen characteristics, 55–59
    clinical trials, 64–73
    lymphoid antigens, 54–55
    mechanism, 62–63

[Non-Hodgkin's lymphoma]
    principles, 61–62
    Rituxan, 54, 56–58, 60, 63, 66, 68–70, 73
    tissue distribution, 59
  90Y, 115–116
Non-small-cell lung cancer, 284, 287, 300, 365–366
  αIR-3, 375–376
  A 108, 372
  BR96-DOX, 404–409
  EGF, 368
  epidermal growth factor antibodies, 360–372
  growth factor antibodies, 368–374
  GRP, 374
  HER-2, 373
  HER-2/neu, 368
  HMFG, 379–380
  HMFG1, 379–380
  insulin-like growth factor, 375, 376
  KC-4G3, 380
  KS1/4, 300
  RG83852, 372
  Squamous cell lung cancer, 300
  225-indium-111, 300
NR-LU-10
  lung cancer, 380–383
  small-cell lung cancer, 380–381
NSCLC. see Non-small-cell lung cancer

OKT10-saporin
  ALL, 197
Ovarian cancer, 298–299
  BR96-DOX, 404–409
  L6, 298
  Lu-171-CC49, 299
  MDX-210, 298

[Ovarian cancer]
  OVB3-PE, 299
    toxicity, 294
  radioimmunoconjugates, 287, 299
  90Y-HMFG1, 299
OVB3-PE
  ovarian cancer, 299
    toxicity, 294

P96.5
  malignant melanoma, 347
P97, 343, 344, 346
P240, 343, 346
Passive antibody therapy
  clinical data, 156–158
  Hodgkin's disease, 154–158
  preclinical data, 155–156
  toxicity, 155
PCR, 232, 251, 252
PCT. *see* Progenitor-cell transplantation
PE, 5–6, 8, 9
Pharmacokinetic analysis
  immunotoxin determination, 16–17
Pharmacokinetic parameters
  immunotoxin determination, 16, 17
Phosphorescence quenching microscopy, 28
Polymerase chain reaction, 232, 251, 252
Progenitor-cell transplantation, 229
  ALL
    clinical trials, 248–249
  AML, 236–241
  CML, 241–243
  non-Hodgkin's lymphoma, 251–252
  purging, 233–236
Proimmunolysins, 425
Prostate cancer
  CC49-Iodine-131, 300–301

Pseudomonas exotoxin A, 5–6, 8
Pulmonary infiltrates
  VLS, 86
Purging
  ALL, 245–248
  AML, 236–241
  Anti-MY9-bR, 240
  CML, 241–243
  immunomagnetic bead-mediated ALL, 248
  immunomagnetic beads
    non-Hodgkin's lymphoma, 250
  non-Hodgkin's lymphoma, 249–257

R24, 344–346
  malignant melanoma, 284, 349–350, 351, 354–355
  small-cell lung cancer, 383
  toxicity, 295
Radioimmunoconjugate therapy, 113, 234, 288, 370
  ALL, 198
  AML, 198–199
  biodistribution, 117–118
  biology, 126
  breast cancer, 316, 327
  clinical data, 175–178
  colorectal cancer, 290–291, 297
  cutaneous T-cell lymphoma, 140–143
  dosimetry, 124–125
  effects, 114
  Hodgkin's disease, 172–180
  non-Hodgkin's lymphoma, 113–128
    clinical trials, 118–122
  ovarian cancer, 287, 299
  preclinical data, 173–174
  research, 126–128
  small-cell lung cancer, 378–379

[Radioimmunoconjugate therapy]
  toxicity, 122–124, 172–173
Radioisotope-labeled antibody
  malignant melanoma, 346–348
Radiolabeled antibodies
  IDEC-C2B8, 56
Radiolabeled polyclonal antiferritin, 174
Raynaud's-like syndrome
  IgG-HD37-dgA, 86–87
Reed-Sternberg/Hodgkin cells, 150–152, 173
Renal cell cancer
  G50-Iodine-131, 300
186-Re-NR-LU-10
  lung cancer, 382–383
RFB4-dgA
  ALL, 196
RFT5
  HD, 85–86
RFT5-SMPT-dg
  Hodgkin's disease, 165, 169
RG83852
  non-small-cell lung cancer, 372
RhuMAb HER2, 315
  breast cancer, 315
Ribosome-inactivating proteins, 163–164
Ricin, 9, 92
  capillary leak syndrome, 294–295
RIP, 163–164
RIT. *see* Radioimmunotherapy
Rituxan
  lymphoma, 54, 57, 58, 63
    clinical trials, 68
RS cells, 154

225.28S
  malignant melanoma, 347–348
Saporin
  Hodgkin's disease, 164
SCLC. *see* Small-cell lung cancer

Seminecrotic region, 28
Sezary syndrome, 137–138
  DAB486IL-2, 144
Small-cell lung cancer, 4, 5, 19, 365–366, 375
  2A11, 375
  antiganglioside antibodies, 383–384
  anti-idiotypic IgG2 antibody, 384
  BEC2, 384, 386
  carcinoembryonic antigen antibodies, 378–379
  CD56, 377–378
  3F8, 383–384
  growth factors, 374–378
  immunotoxins, 377–378
  In-111 anti CEA ZCE 025, 378–379
  In-111-FO23C5, 378–379
  KM966, 383
  N901, 287–288
  N901-bR, 377–378
  NE 150, 377
  neural cell adhesion antibodies, 376–378
  NR-LU-10, 380–381
  R24, 383
  radioimmunoconjugates, 378–379
  Tc-99m-NR-LU-10, 381–382
  ZCE 025, 378–379
Solid tumors
  bispecific antibodies, 283–284
  immunotherapy, 282–292
  MAb therapy, 281–301
    toxicities, 292–295
  pathophysiology, 24–26
  radioimmunoconjugates, 287
Stem cell grafts
  quality, 230–233
  tumor-cell contamination, 231–233

T101
    cutaneous T-cell lymphomas, 138
T200
    Hodgkin's disease, 152
Tac
    Hodgkin's disease, 154
T84.66 anti-CEA
    breast cancer, 325
T200 antigen
    Hodgkin's disease, 153–154
T10B9-1A-31
    GVHD, 221
Tc-99m-NR-LU-10
    small-cell lung cancer, 381–382
Therapeutic agents
    categories, 23, 24t
Thy 1.1
    acute leukemia, 191
Thyroid cancer
    Anti-CEA-Iodine-131, 301
T101-I131
    cutaneous T-cell lymphoma, 141–142
Tissue distribution
    antibody therapy, 55–56
Tissue-isolated tumors
    magnetic resonance spectroscopy
    tumor metabolism, 28
Tn antigen, 327
Toxins
    adaptations, 8–10
    selection, 5, 6
Transferrin receptor, 154
Transforming growth factor a, 369
Tumor antigens
    malignant melanoma, 343–344
Tumor-associated glycoprotein, 72, 325
Tumor blood flow
    increase, 41
Tumor cell
    MAb delivery, 23–42

[Tumor cell]
    cell transport, 36–38
    detection and treatment, 40–41
    experimental and theoretical approaches, 24–26
    interstitial space transport, 32–35
    metabolic microenvironment, 28–31
    microvascular wall transport, 31–32
    pharmacokinetic modeling, 38–40
    transvascular transport, 33f
    vascular space distribution, 26–28
Tumor-infiltrating lymphocytes, 340
Tumor metabolism
    magnetic resonance spectroscopy
    tissue-isolated tumors, 28
Tumor necrosis factor, 425
    malignant melanoma, 351–352
Tumor vessels
    leaky, 32

Vaccine therapy
    cutaneous T-cell lymphomas, 140
Vascular leak syndrome (VLS), 83, 86
    dgA ITs, 87
    immunotoxins, 201, 419–420
Vascular permeability
    increase, 41
    tumors, 32
VLS, 83, 86
    dgA ITs, 87
    immunotoxins, 201, 419–420

XomaZyme-791
    colorectal cancer, 298
XOMAZYME-MEL
    malignant melanoma, 353

Y90
  biodistribution, 117
Y90-antiferritin
  Hodgkin's disease, 176–179
Y90-anti-Tac
  cutaneous T-cell lymphoma, 142–143
Y90 anti-Tac-H
  ALL, 198

Y90-2B8
  toxicity, 122–124
Y90-HMFG1
  ovarian cancer, 299

ZCE 025
  small-cell lung cancer, 378–379
ZME-018
  malignant melanoma, 347

About the Editor

MICHAEL L. GROSSBARD is an Assistant Professor of Medicine at Harvard Medical School, Boston, Massachusetts, as well as an Assistant Physician at Massachusetts General Hospital, Boston, Massachusetts. He is the author or coauthor of numerous professional publications reflecting his major research interests in areas such as immunotoxin therapy of lymphoma and leukemia, the development of Phase I agents for cancer therapy, and autologous bone marrow transplantation of lymphomas, among others. A member of the American College of Physicians, the American Society of Hematology, and the American Society of Clinical Oncology, Dr. Grossbard received the M.D. degree (1986) from Yale University School of Medicine, New Haven, Connecticut.

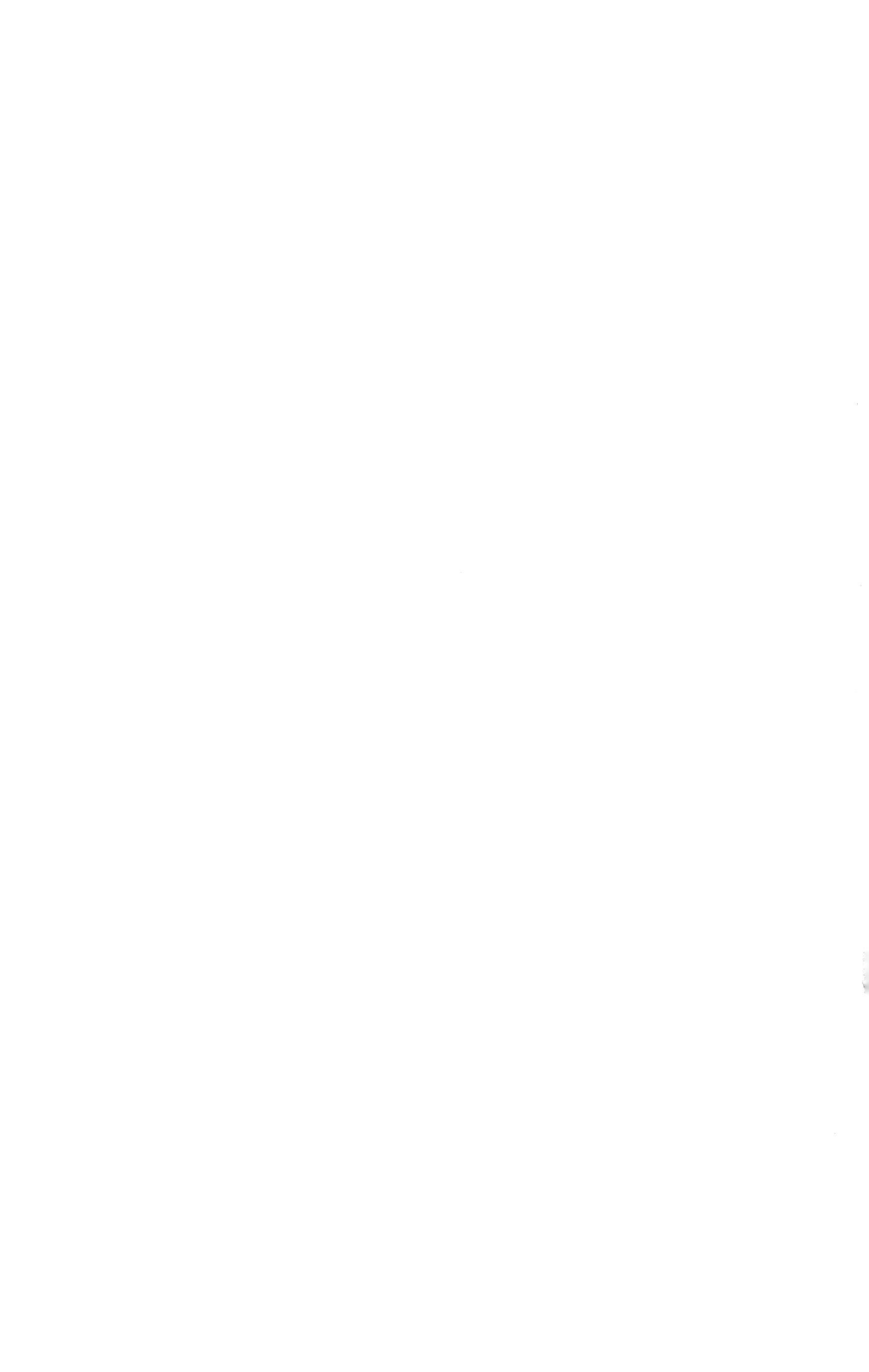